W9-BVN-815

Ivosic

I. voštć

IMMUNOLOGY

A Slide Atlas of Immunology based on the material in this book
is available. Further information may be obtained from:
The C.V. Mosby Company
11830 Westline Industrial Drive, St. Louis, MO63146

IMMUNOLOGY

IVAN M. ROITT
MA DSc(Oxon) FRCPath FRS

Professor and Head of Department
of Immunology
The Middlesex Hospital Medical School
London W1

JONATHAN BROSTOFF
MA DM(Oxon) FRCP FRCPath

Reader in Clinical Immunology
Department of Immunology
The Middlesex Hospital Medical School
London W1

DAVID K. MALE
MA PhD

Research Associate
Department of Immunology
The Middlesex Hospital Medical School
London W1

The C. V. Mosby Company · St Louis · Toronto

Gower Medical Publishing · London · New York · 1985

DISTRIBUTORS

USA and Mexico
The C. V. Mosby Company
11830 Westline Industrial Drive, St. Louis, MO63146

Canada
The C. V. Mosby Company Ltd
120 Melford Drive, Toronto, Ontario M1B 2X5

Japan
Nankodo Company Limited.
42-6, Hongo 3-chome, Bunkyo, Tokyo 113

All other Countries
Churchill Livingstone
Medical Division of Longman Group Limited,
Robert Stevenson House, 1-3 Baxter's Place,
Leith Walk, Edinburgh EH1 3AF

© Copyright 1985 by Gower Medical Publishing Ltd.,
34–42 Cleveland Street, London W1P 5FB, England. All Rights
reserved. No part of this publication may be reproduced, stored in a
retrieval system or transmitted in any form or by any means or
otherwise without the prior permission of the copyright holders.

British Library Cataloguing in Publication Data
Roitt, Ivan M.
  Immunology
  I. Immunology
  I. Title   II. Brostoff, Jonathan
  III. Male, David K.
  574.2'9   QR181

ISBN 0–906923–35–2 (Gower)
        0–443–029121 (Churchill Livingstone)

Library of Congress Cataloging in Publication Data
Roitt, Ivan Maurice
  Immunology
  Bibliography: p.
  Includes index.
  1. Immunology. I Brostoff, Jonathan.
  II. Male, David K., 1954-   . III. Title.
  QR181.R58   1985   616.07'9   85-750

ISBN 0–906923–35–2

Printed in Hong Kong by Mandarin Offset International

Contents

Preface

We believe this to be a remarkably unusual book. We have attempted to present the subject primarily with appealing visual images, many of which are the distillation of much complicated scientific research. These illustrations are complemented specifically by individual captions, and more generally by a concise narrative text which links these images into an evolving conceptual thread. The book covers basic immunology and the fundamental principles relating to clinical immunology. The subject is covered in some depth and much attention is given to the underlying experimental studies. We hope that anyone interested in immunology, be they undergraduate, postgraduate or clinician, will find this an attractive but nonetheless thorough account, which they will find difficult to put down once they have opened it.

We would like to acknowledge the many immunologists and molecular biologists whose research findings have been included to explain particular immunological reactions, and to develop ideas on the function of the immune system. We greatly admire their work, and hope we will be forgiven for not mentioning all these scientists individually. In some cases, we have selected particular items, or simplified experiments to make points more readily understood. Readers who wish to grapple with the fine details of the experiments and hypotheses may locate the original papers by reference to review articles included as further reading at the end of each chapter.

IMR
JB
DKM

Acknowledgements

The editors gratefully acknowledge the following individuals for the major contribution they have made to their respective chapters:

Dr. Ross St.Clair Barnetson, Consultant Physician and Senior Lecturer, Department of Dermatology, The Royal Infirmary, Edinburgh. (*Hypersensitivity – Type IV*)

Dr. David Brown, Consultant Immunologist, Department of Clinical Immunology, Addenbrooke's Hospital, Cambridge. (*Complement*)

Dr. Anne Cooke, Wellcome Senior Lecturer, Department of Immunology, The Middlesex Hospital Medical School, London. (*Genetic Control of Immunity*)

Dr. Michael Crumpton, Deputy Director of Research, Imperial Cancer Research Fund Laboratories, London. (*Major Histocompatibility Complex*)

Dr. Marc Feldman, Senior Research Scientist, Department of Zoology, University College, London. (*The Antibody Response*)

Professor Carlo Grossi, Professor of Pathology, Department of Pathology, University of Alabama in Birmingham, Alabama. (*Cells Involved in the Immune Response; The Lymphoid System; Development of the Immune Response*)

Dr. Tony Hall, Department of Microbiology and Immunology, The Oregon Health Sciences University, Portland, Oregon. (*Hypersensitivity – Type I*)

Dr. Frank Hay, Reader in Immunology, Department of Immunology, Middlesex Hospital Medical School, London. (*Generation of Antibody Diversity; Hypersensitivity – Type III*)

Dr. John Horton, Reader in Immunology, Department of Zoology, University of Durham, Durham. (*Evolution of Immunity*)

Dr. James Howard, Director of Biochemical Research, The Wellcome Research Laboratories, Beckenham. (*Immunological Tolerance*)

Dr. Peter Lydyard, Honorary Senior Lecturer and Research Associate, Department of Immunology, The Middlesex Hospital Medical School, London. (*Cells Involved in the Immune Response; The Lymphoid System; Development of the Immune Response*)

Dr Kenneth McLennan, Lecturer in Histopathology, Bland Sutton Institute of Histopathology, Middlesex Hospital, London. (*The Lymphoid System; Development of the Immune Response*)

Dr. Michael Moore, Head of the Division of Immunology, Paterson Laboratories, Christie Hospital and Holt Radium Institute, Manchester. (*Immunity to Tumours*)

Dr. Michael Owen, Staff Scientist, Imperial Cancer Research Fund, University College, London. (*Major Histocompatibility Complex*)

Dr. Graham Rook, Department of Pathology, The Middlesex Hospital Medical School, London. (*Cell-Mediated Immunity; Immunity to Viruses, Bacteria and Fungi*)

Professor Michael Steward, Professor of Immunology, Department of Medical Microbiology, London School of Hygiene and Tropical Medicine, London (*Antigen-Antibody Reactions; Immunological Tests*)

Dr. Janice Taverne, Research Associate, Department of Immunology, The Middlesex Hospital Medical School, London (*Immunity to Protozoa and Worms*)

Dr. Roger Taylor, Reader in Immunology, Department of Pathology, University of Bristol, Bristol. (*Regulation of the Immune Response*)

Professor John Turk, Professor of Pathology, Department of Pathology, The Royal College of Surgeons, London. (*Hypersensitivity – Type IV*)

Dr. Malcolm Turner, Reader in Immunology, Department of Immunology, Institute of Child Health, London. (*Antibody Structure and Function*)

Dr. Kenneth Welsh, Head of Tissue Typing (South Eastern and South Western Regions), Tissue Typing Laboratory, Guy's Hospital, London. (*Transplantation and Rejection*)

Project Editor   David Bennett
Designer   Celia Welcomme
Assistant designer   Mary Ross

Line Artist (diagrams)   Karen Cochrane
Line Artist (line drawings)   Jeremy Cort
Index   Janine Ross

1 Adaptive and Innate Immunity

Our environment contains a large variety of infectious microbial agents – viruses, bacteria, fungi and parasites. Any of these can cause pathological damage and if they multiply unchecked will eventually kill their host. It is evident that the great majority of infections in normal individuals are of limited duration and leave very little permanent damage. This is due to the individual's immune system which combats infectious agents.

The immune system is divided into two functional divisions, namely the innate immune system and the adaptive immune system. Innate immunity acts as a first line of defence against infectious agents and most potential pathogens are checked before they establish an overt infection. If these first defences are breached the adaptive immune system is called upon. The adaptive system produces a specific reaction to each infectious agent which normally eradicates that agent. Furthermore, the adaptive immune system remembers that particular infectious agent and can prevent it causing disease later (Fig. 1.1). For example, diseases such as measles and diphtheria produce a life-long immunity following an infection.

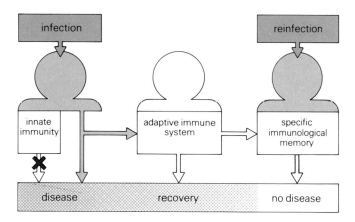

Fig. 1.1 Adaptive and innate immunity. When an infectious agent enters the body it first encounters elements of the innate immune system. These may be sufficient to prevent disease but if not, a disease will result and the adaptive immune system is activated. The adaptive immune system produces recovery from the disease and a specific immunological memory is established so that following reinfection with the same agent no disease results; the individual has acquired immunity to the infectious agent.

The innate and adaptive immune systems consist of a variety of molecules and cells distributed throughout the body whose functions are described below (Fig. 1.2). The most important cells are the leucocytes or white blood cells which are described fully in 'Cells Involved in the Immune Response'. The leucocytes fall into two broad categories: 1) phagocytes, including neutrophil polymorphs, monocytes and macrophages, which form part of the innate immune system; 2) lymphocytes, which mediate adaptive immunity. Cells of the immune system (lymphoid cells) are organized into organs as described in 'The Lymphoid System'.

	Innate Immune System	Adaptive Immune System
	resistance not improved by repeated infection	resistance improved by repeated infection
soluble factors	lysozyme, complement, acute phase proteins eg CRP, interferon	antibody
cells	phagocytes natural killer (NK) cells	T lymphocytes

Fig. 1.2 The major elements of the innate and adaptive immune systems. There is considerable interaction between the two systems. Immunity due to soluble factors is sometimes referred to as humoral immunity.

THE INNATE IMMUNE SYSTEM

The exterior of the body presents an effective barrier to most organisms; in particular, most infectious agents cannot penetrate intact skin (Fig. 1.3).

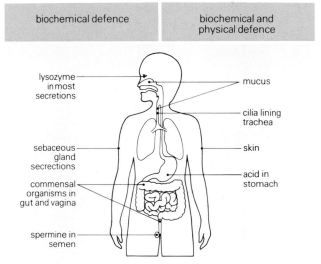

Fig. 1.3 Exterior defenses. Most of the infectious agents which an individual encounters do no penetrate the body's surfaces, but are prevented from entering by a variety of biochemical and physical barriers. The body tolerates a number of commensal organisms which compete effectively with many potential pathogens.

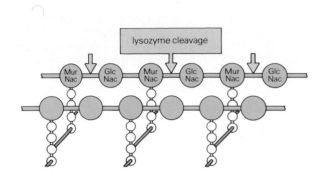

Fig. 1.4 Action of lysozyme on the cell wall of *S. aureus*.
In the structure of *S. aureus* cell wall proteoglycan the
backbone of N-acetylglucosamine (GlcNac) alternates with
N-acetylmuramic acid (MurNac) crosslinked by amino acid
side chains (yellow) and bridges of 5-glycine residues (orange).
Lysozyme splits the molecule at the places indicated.

The importance of this barrier is made abundantly clear
when an individual suffers serious burns. In this case
prevention of infection via the damaged skin is a major
concern. Most infections enter the body via the epithelial surface of the nasopharynx, gut, lungs and
genito-urinary tract. A variety of physical and biochemical defences protect these areas from most infections. For
example, lysozyme is an enzyme distributed widely in
different secretions which is capable of splitting a bond
found in the cell walls of many bacteria (Fig. 1.4).

Phagocytes

If an organism penetrates an epithelial surface it encounters phagocytic cells of the reticuloendothelial system.
These cells are of several different types but they are all

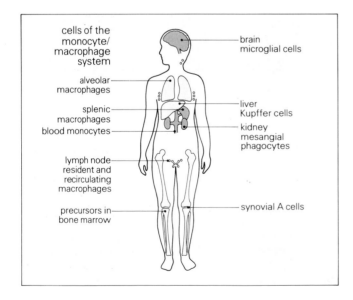

Fig. 1.5 Phagocytes of the reticuloendothelial system.
Many organs contain phagocytic cells. Cells of the monocyte/
macrophage series (listed left) are derived from blood
monocytes which are manufactured in the bone marrow.
Monocytes pass out of the blood vessel and become
macrophages in the tissues. The other phagocytes listed are
also derived from bone marrow stem cells.

derived from bone marrow stem cells. Their function is to
engulf particles, including infectious agents, internalize
them and destroy them. For this purpose they are strategi-
cally placed where they will encounter such particles; for
example, the Kupffer cells of the liver line the sinusoids
along which blood flows while the synovial A cells line
the synovial cavity (Fig. 1.5). The blood phagocytes include the neutrophil polymorph and the blood monocyte
(Fig. 1.6). Both of these cells can migrate out of the blood
vessels into the tissues in response to a suitable stimulus
but they differ in that the polymorph is a short-lived cell
while the monocyte develops into a tissue macrophage.

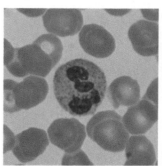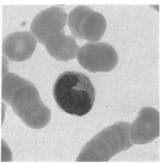

Fig. 1.6 Phagocytes. Apart from the fixed cells of the
reticuloendothelial system there are polymorphonuclear
neutrophils (left) and blood monocytes (right), both derived
from bone marrow stem cells. Courtesy of Dr. P. M. Lydyard.

NK Cells and Soluble Factors

Natural killer (NK) cells are leucocytes capable of recognizing cell surface changes on virally-infected cells. The
NK cells bind to these target cells and can kill them. The
NK cells are activated by interferons which are themselves components of the innate immune system (Fig.
1.7). Interferons are produced by virally-infected cells
and sometimes also by lymphocytes. Apart from their
action on NK cells, interferons induce a state of viral
resistance in uninfected tissue cells. Interferons are produced very early in infection and are the first line of resistance against many viruses.

The serum concentration of a number of proteins increases rapidly during infection. These are referred to as
acute phase proteins. The concentrations of these acute
phase proteins can increase from 2 to 100-fold by comparison with their normal levels and they remain elevated
throughout the infection. An example of this is C-reactive
protein, so-called because of its ability to bind the C
protein of pneumococci. C-reactive protein bound to
bacteria promotes the binding of complement which
facilitates their uptake by phagocytes; this process of
protein coating to enhance phagocytosis is known as
opsonization (Fig. 1.8). Complement is a group of about
twenty serum proteins, rather like the blood clotting system, which interact with each other and with other components of the innate and adaptive immune systems. The
complement system is spontaneously activated by the
surface of a number of microorganisms by the so-called
alternative complement pathway. Following activation
some complement components can cause opsonization
of the microorganisms for phagocytes while others attract
phagocytes to the site of infection.

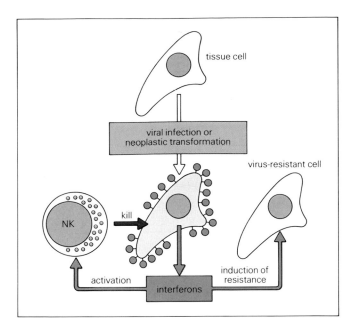

Fig. 1.7 Interferon and NK cells. When a cell becomes infected by virus, or transforms into a cancerous cell its surface molecules are altered. These alterations can sometimes be recognized by natural killer (NK) cells which engage the cell and kill it. Virally-infected cells produce interferons which can signal to neighbouring tissue cells and put them into a state capable of resisting viral replication, so preventing virus spread. Additionally, interferons can activate NK cells and enhance their cytotoxic action.

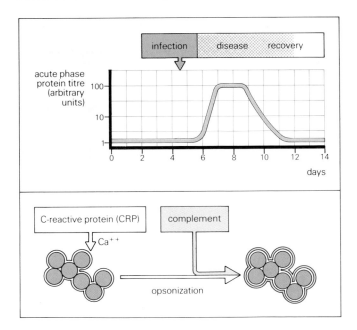

Fig. 1.8 Acute phase proteins. Acute phase proteins (here exemplified by C-reactive protein) are serum proteins which increase rapidly in concentration (up to 100 fold) following infection (graph). They are important in the innate immunity to infection. C-reactive protein (CRP) recognizes and binds, in a Ca^{++} dependent fashion, to molecular groups found on a wide variety of bacteria and fungi. In particular it binds the phosphorylcholine moiety of pneumococci. The CRP acts as an opsonin and also activates complement with all the associated sequelae.

A further group of complement components causes direct lysis of the cell membranes of bacteria by the 'lytic pathway' (Fig. 1.9). Although the various molecules of the innate immune system have been described separately, *in vivo* they act in concert. For example, the destruction of bacterial cell walls by lysozyme facilitates an attack on the cell membrane by the lytic pathway complement components. As will become evident later the complement system performs a number of functions in addition to its action in opsonization and lysis of microorganisms. These can be summarized as the control of inflammation.

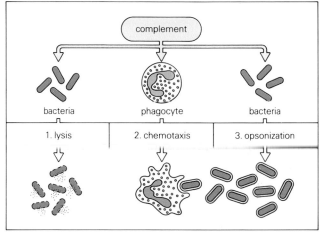

Fig. 1.9 Complement functions. The complement system has an intrinsic ability to lyse the cell membranes of many bacterial species (1). Complement products released in this reaction attract phagocytes to the site of the reaction –. chemotaxis (2). Once they arrive at the site of reaction other complement components coating the bacterial surface allow the phagocyte to recognize the bacteria and facilitate bacterial phagocytosis — opsonization (3). These are all functions of the innate immune system, although the reactions can also be triggered by the adaptive immune system.

INFLAMMATION

Inflammation is the body's reaction to an injury such as an invasion by an infectious agent. In just the same way as it is necessary to increase the blood supply to active muscles during exercise to provide glucose and oxygen so it is also necessary to direct elements of the immune system into sites of infection. Three major things occur during this response namely:
1. An increased blood supply to the infected area,
2. Increased capillary permeability caused by retraction of the endothelial cells. This permits larger molecules to traverse the endothelium than would ordinarily be capable of doing so and thus allows the soluble mediators of immunity to reach the site of infection,
3. Leucocytes, particularly neutrophil polymorphs and to a lesser extent macrophages, migrate out of the capillaries and into the surrounding tissue. Once in the tissue they migrate towards the site of infection by a process known as chemotaxis. These three events manifest themselves as inflammation.

Chemotaxis

Chemotaxis is the process by which phagocytes are attracted to sites of inflammation (Fig. 1.10). It can be demonstrated *in vitro* that phagocytes will actively migrate up a concentration gradient of certain (chemotactic) molecules. Particularly active is C5a, a fragment of one of the complement components. When purified C5a is applied to the base of an ulcer *in vivo* neutrophil polymorphs can be seen sticking to the endothelium of the nearby capillaries shortly afterwards. Initially this occurs on the side of the capillary nearest the point of application but as the C5a diffuses further the neutrophils stick to all

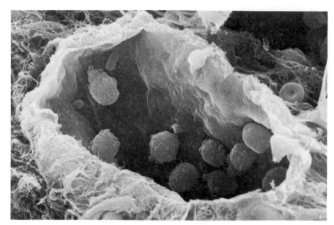

Fig. 1.12 Scanning electron micrograph showing leucocytes adhering to the wall of a venule in inflamed tissue. ×16,000. Courtesy of Professor M. J. Karnovsky.

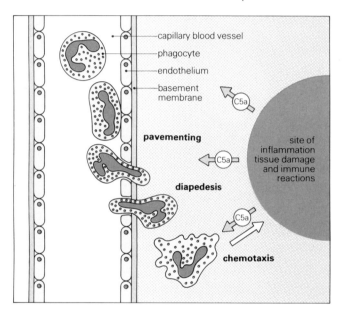

Fig. 1.10 Chemotaxis. At a site of inflammation tissue damage and complement activation by the infectious agent cause the release of chemotactic peptides (eg. C5a, a fragment of one of the complement components, which is one of the most important chemotactic peptides). These peptides diffuse to the adjoining capillaries causing passing phagocytes to adhere to the endothelium (pavementing). The phagocytes insert pseudopods between the endothelial cells and dissolve the basement membrane (diapedesis). They then pass out of the blood vessel and move up the concentration gradient of the chemotactic peptides towards the site of inflammation.

sides of the endothelium before traversing the endothelium, crossing the basement membrane and migrating up the gradient of the chemotactic molecule. Adherence and diapedesis of leucocytes is illustrated in figures 1.11 and 1.12. Both neutrophil polymorphs and macrophages are attracted by C5a but neutrophils are the predominant cell in sites of acute inflammation reflecting their numerical preponderance in the blood.

Phagocytosis

Once they have arrived at a site of inflammation the phagocytes have to recognize the infectious agent. They have receptors on their surface which allow them to attach non-specifically to a variety of microorganisms, but the attachment is greatly enhanced if the microorganism has been opsonized by the C3b component of complement. Complement activation at the site of infection causes C3b to be deposited on the infectious agent and since both neutrophils and macrophages have receptors which specifically bind to C3b this allows the phagocytes to recognize their targets (Fig. 1.13). The importance of complement opsonization can be seen in those very rare patients who are genetically deficient in complement component C3. These patients suffer from recurrent bacterial infections and septicaemia.

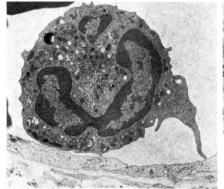
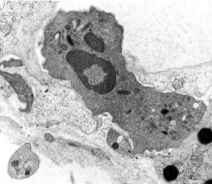
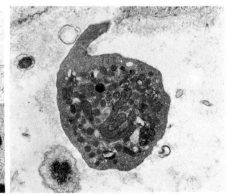

Fig. 1.11 Electron micrographs showing the three phases of diapedesis. The first micrograph shows a leucocyte adhering to the capillary endothelium (left) before it penetrates the endothelium (middle). The third micrograph illustrates a leucocyte which has traversed the endothelium (right). X 4000. Courtesy of Dr. I. Jovis.

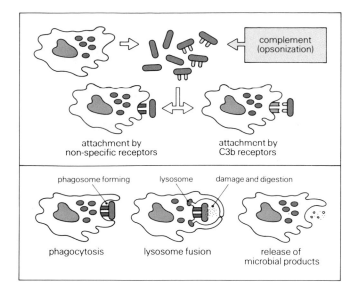

After attachment the phagocytes proceed to engulf the microorganism by extending pseudopods around it. These fuse and the microorganism is internalized in a phagosome (Fig. 1.14). Lysosomes fuse with the phagosome and destroy the trapped microorganism. The mechanisms involved are described more fully in 'Immunity to Viruses, Bacteria and Fungi' and 'Immunity to Protozoa and Worms'.

ANTIBODY — A FLEXIBLE ADAPTOR

Problems arise when the phagocytes are unable to recognize the infectious agent either because they lack a suitable receptor for it or because the microorganism does not activate complement and so cannot become attached to the phagocyte via the C3b receptor. Ideally, what is needed is a flexible adaptor that can attach at one end to the microorganism and at the other to the phagocyte. In answer to this requirement molecules known as antibodies have evolved and these are fully described in 'Antibody Structure and Function'. Antibodies are a class of molecules produced by B lymphocytes of the adaptive immune system which act as flexible adaptors between the infectious agents and phagocytes (Fig. 1.15).

Fig. 1.13 Phagocytosis. Phagocytes arrive at a site of inflammation by chemotaxis. They may then attach to microorganisms via their non-specific cell surface receptors, or if the organism is opsonized with a fragment of the third complement component (C3b) through activation of the complement system, attachment will be through the cell surface receptors for C3b. If the membrane now becomes activated by the attached infectious agent, it is taken into a phagosome by pseudopods which extend around it. Once inside, lysosomes fuse with the phagosome forming a phagolysosome and the infectious agent is killed by a battery of microbicidal mechanisms. Undigested microbial products may be released to the outside.

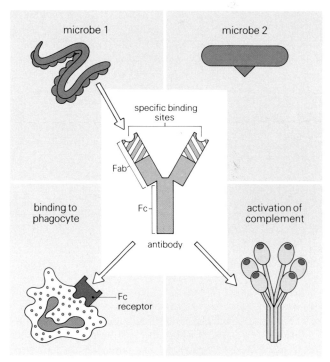

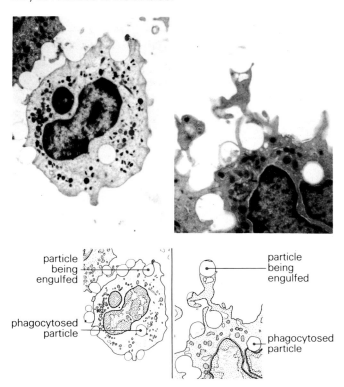

Fig. 1.14 Electron micrographic study of phagocytosis. These two micrographs show human phagocytes engulfing latex particles. ×3000 (left), ×4500 (right). Courtesy of Professor C. H. W. Horne.

Fig. 1.15 Antibody — a flexible adaptor. When a microorganism lacks the inherent ability to activate complement or phagocytes, the body provides a class of flexible adaptor molecules with a series of different shapes which can attach to the surface of different microbes. These flexible adaptor molecules are, of course, antibodies and the body can make several million different antibodies able to recognize a wide variety of infectious agents. Thus the antibody illustrated binds microbe 1, but not microbe 2, by its 'antigen binding portion' (Fab) while the 'Fc portion' (which may activate complement) binds to Fc receptors on host tissue cells, particularly phagocytes.

phagocyte	opsonin	binding
1 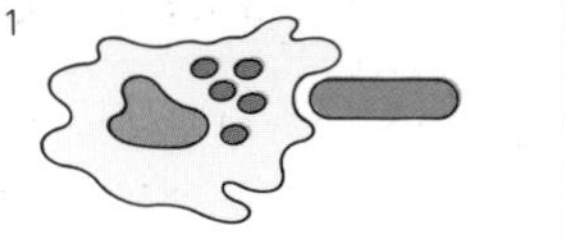	–	±
2 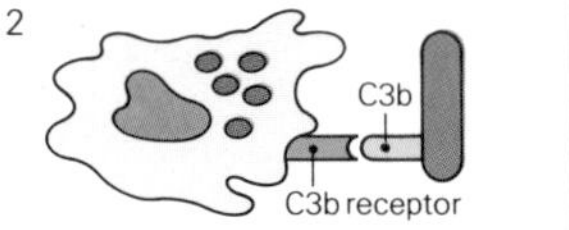 (C3b / C3b receptor)	complement C3b	+ +
3 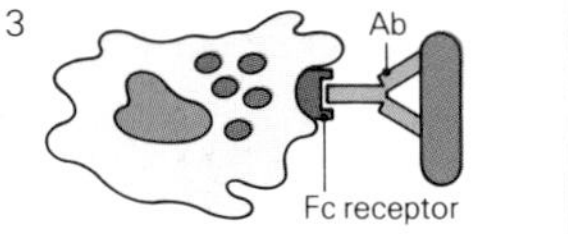 (Ab / Fc receptor)	antibody	+
4 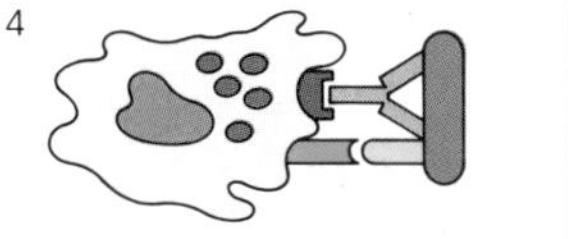	antibody and complement C3b	+ + + +

Fig. 1.16 Opsonization. Phagocytes have some intrinsic ability to bind directly to bacteria and other microorganisms (1), but this is much enhanced if the bacteria have activated complement (C3b) so that they can bind the bacteria via their C3b receptor (2). Opsonization of organisms which do not activate complement well, if at all, is performed by antibody (Ab) which acts as a bridge to attach the microbe to the Fc receptor on the phagocyte (3). If both antibody *and* C3b opsonize, binding is greatly enhanced (4).

Any particular antibody molecule can only bind to one type of infectious agent, the other end of the molecule binds to the phagocyte via a receptor, the Fc receptor. Macrophages, neutrophils and all other cells of the reticuloendothelial system have Fc receptors. Since antibodies also cause the activation of complement by the so-called 'classical pathway' infectious agents will often have both antibody and C3b bound to their surface. In this case the phagocyte will recognize the agent via both its Fc receptors and its C3b receptors so that attachment and phagocytosis are greatly enhanced (Fig. 1.16).

It should be evident that antibodies are effectively bifunctional molecules. One part, which is extremely variable between different antibodies, is responsible for binding to the many different infectious agents the body may encounter while the second, constant portion binds to the Fc receptors of cells and also activates complement. In fact, antibodies act as adaptors not just for phagocytes but also for other cells and different antibodies can act as adaptors for different cell types.

ANTIGEN

Antibody molecules do not bind to the whole of an infectious agent. Each antibody molecule binds to one of many molecules on the microorganism's surface. Molecules to which antibodies bind are called antigens (*antibody generators*). Different antibodies will bind to different antigens since each antibody is specific for a

particular antigen. Indeed, a particular antigen specifically induces the production of the antibodies which can bind to it. The way in which a sufficient diversity of antibody molecules are generated able to recognize different antigens, is explained in the 'Generation of Antibody Diversity'. Each antibody binds to a particular part of the antigen called an antigenic determinant or epitope. Note that the terms antigenic determinant and epitope are synonymous. A particular antigen can have several different epitopes or may have several identical epitopes (Fig. 1.17). In reality, the antibodies are specific for the epitopes rather than for the whole antigen molecule but since each antigen has its own particular set of epitopes which are not usually shared with other antigens the collection of antibodies in an antiserum are effectively specific for the antigen. The characteristics of antigenantibody combination are discussed in 'AntigenAntibody Reactions'.

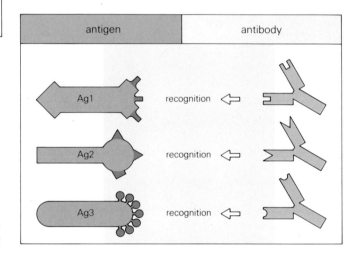

Fig. 1.17 Antigens. Foreign molecules which generate antibodies are called antigens. Antigen molecules each have a set of antigenic determinants also called epitopes. The epitopes on one antigen (Ag1) are usually different from those on another (Ag2). Some antigens (Ag3) have repeated epitopes. Epitopes are molecular shapes recognized by the antibodies and cells of the adaptive immune system. Each cell recognizes one epitope rather than the whole antigen. Even simple microorganisms have many different antigens.

ADAPTIVE IMMUNITY AND CLONAL SELECTION

The specificity of the adaptive immune system is based on the specificity of the antibodies and lymphocytes. It is found that each lymphocyte is only capable of recognizing one particular antigen. Since the immune system as a whole can specifically recognize many thousands of antigens this means that the lymphocytes recognizing any particular antigen are a very small proportion of the total. How then is an adequate response to an infectious agent generated? The answer is by clonal selection. Antigen binds to the small number of cells which can recognize it and induces them to proliferate so that they now constitute sufficient cells to mount an adequate immune response, that is the antigen selects the specific clones of antigen-binding cells (Fig. 1.18).

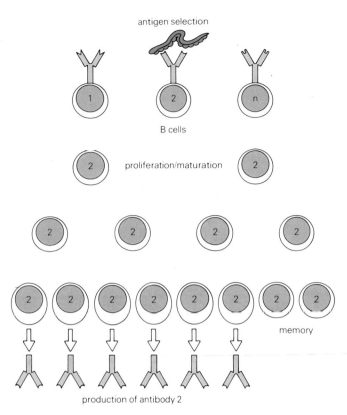

antigen selection

B cells

proliferation/maturation

memory

production of antibody 2

Fig. 1.18 Clonal selection. Each antibody-producing cell (B cell) is programmed to make just one antibody, which is placed on its surface as an antigen receptor. Each B cell has a different antigen binding specificity (1-n). Antigen binds to only those B cells with the appropriate surface receptor. These cells are stimulated to proliferate and mature into antibody-producing cells and the longer-lived, memory cells, all with the same antigen binding specificity (2).

This process occurs both for the B lymphocytes, which proliferate and mature into antibody-producing cells and for the T lymphocytes, which are involved in the recognition and destruction of virally-infected cells.

This raises the question of exactly what the immune system is capable of recognizing. Broadly speaking, the immune system regards all molecules not belonging to the individual as 'non-self' and reacts against them, and it recognizes many of the individual's own molecules as 'self' but does not react against them. The failure to react to a potentially antigenic molecule is referred to as tolerance (see 'Immunological Tolerance'). The critical importance of self/non-self discrimination is outlined in figure 1.19 in the context of the adaptive and non-adaptive immune response. The body must both tolerate its own tissues and react effectively against all infective agents if disease is to be avoided.

INTEGRATED DEFENCE MECHANISMS

It will be appreciated that the innate and adaptive immune systems do not act in isolation. Antibodies produced by lymphocytes help phagocytes to recognize their targets. Following clonal activation by antigen, T lymphocytes produce lymphokines which stimulate phagocytes to destroy infectious agents more effectively. The macrophages in turn help the lymphocytes by transporting antigen from the periphery to lymph nodes and other lymphoid organs where it is presented to lymphocytes in a form they can recognize (Fig. 1.20).

The immune system is not the only system which protects the body from injury; the clotting, fibrinolytic and kinin systems are also involved in mediating inflammation and in the resolution of tissue damage. These systems interact to maintain the integrity of the vascular system and to limit the spread of tissue damage whether it is caused by physical damage or infectious agents.

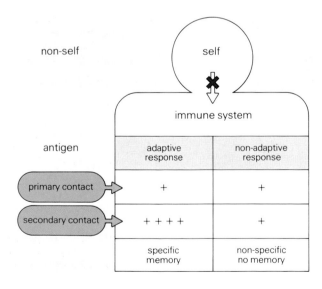

Fig. 1.19 Summary of self/non-self discrimination. The immune system discriminates self from non-self, and reacts against non-self molecules (antigens). Following a primary contact with antigen, there are weak adaptive, and non-adaptive responses, but if the same antigen persists or is encountered a second time there is a much enhanced specific response to that antigen. The characteristics of an adaptive immune response are specificity and memory.

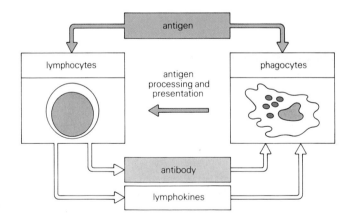

Fig. 1.20 Interaction between lymphocytes and phagocytes. The adaptive and non-adaptive areas of the immune system interact at all levels. Lymphocytes are responsible for specific recognition: they produce antibody and lymphokines, soluble molecules which help the phagocytes combat the infection. Antigen processed by phagocytes and other cells which cannot themselves specifically recognize antigen, present the antigen to lymphocytes which can recognize it.

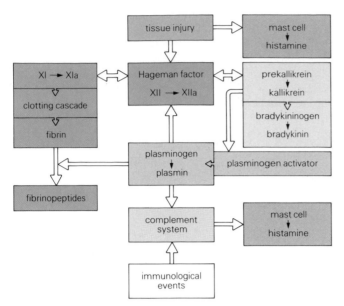

Fig. 1.21 The plasma enzyme systems in inflammation.
This diagram summarizes the four plasma enzyme systems which interact in the control of inflammation. These are the clotting system (turquoise), the kinin system (light blue), the fibrinolytic system (pink) and the complement system (green). When tissue injury occurs enzymes are released and surfaces are exposed which activate Hageman factor XII and trigger mast cells to release histamine. Activated Hageman factor (XIIa) activates, and is reciprocally activated by, factor XIa and kallikrein. The kinin system produces bradykinin which induces pain, increased vascular permeability and vasodilation. Kallikrein activates the fibrinolytic system to produce plasmin which can activate Hageman factor and complement components and splits fibrin to produce chemotactic fibrinopeptides. Immunological events (for example, the combination of antibody with antigen) interact with these systems and modulate inflammation via the complement system. Different components (for example, C3a and C5a) trigger mast cells to release histamine producing vasodilation, increased capillary permeability and chemokinesis. (Other factors act as spasmogens, cause endothelial cell retraction, and are chemotactic for phagocytes.)

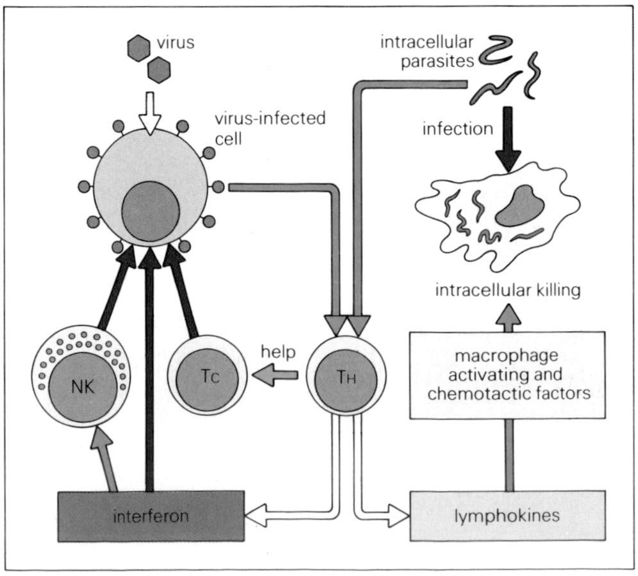

Immunological events can interact with this integrated system of damage control via the complement system (Fig. 1.21). Complement components released from sites of inflammation act directly on the local vasculature and the fragments C3a and C5a can also activate mast cells. These cells are widely distributed throughout the body and contain mediators which cause vasodilation and increased vascular permeability. The immune system can

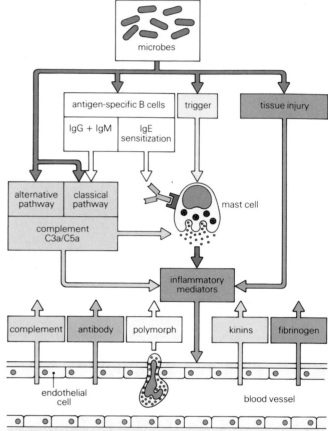

Fig. 1.22 Immune system in acute inflammation. The adaptive immune system modulates inflammatory processes via the complement system. Antigen from microbes stimulates antigen-specific B cells to produce antibody; some (IgE) binds to mast cells while others (IgG and IgM) activate complement. Complement can also be activated directly by microbes via an alternative pathway. When triggered by microbial antigens the sensitized mast cell releases mediators. In association with complement (which also activates mast cells via C3a and C5a) the mediators induce local inflammation facilitating the arrival of phagocytes and more plasma enzyme system molecules.

Fig. 1.23 Innate and acquired mechanisms of killing intracellular organisms. Viruses and intracellular parasites stimulate T cells of the adaptive immune system (yellow). T-helper cells (TH) cooperate in the maturation of T-cytotoxic cells (Tc) and release lymphokines, including interferon. Tc cells and NK cells can kill virally-infected cells. Interferons (also produced by the infected cell) stimulate NK cells and inhibit viral replication directly. Other lymphokines attract macrophages to the site of infection and enable them to kill intracellular organisms which would otherwise persist.

also interact directly with mast cells via a type of antibody (IgE) which binds to Fc receptors on the mast cell (Fig. 1.22). The inflammatory reaction effects the arrival of molecules and cells to the site of infection where they activate the macrophages to destroy their intracellular parasites (Fig. 1.23).

VACCINATION

Specificity and memory, two of the key elements of the adaptive immune response are exploited in vaccination since the adaptive immune system mounts a much stronger response on second encounter with antigen. The principle is to alter a microorganism or its toxins in such a way that they become innocuous without losing antigenicity. Take for example, vaccination against diphtheria. The diphtheria bacterium produces a toxin which is cytotoxic for muscle cells. The toxin can be chemically modified by formalin treatment so that it retains its antigenic epitopes but loses its toxicity; the resulting toxoid is used as a vaccine (Fig. 1.24). Other infectious agents such as polio can be attenuated so that they retain their antigens but lose their pathogenicity.

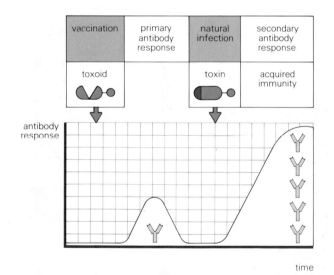

Fig. 1.24 **Principle of vaccination.** The principle of vaccination is illustrated by immunization with diphtheria toxoid. Diphtheria toxoid retains some of the epitopes of the diphtheria bacillus toxin so that a primary antibody response to these epitopes is produced following vaccination with toxoid. In a natural infection the toxin restimulates B memory cells which produce the faster and more intense secondary antibody response to the epitope so neutralizing the toxin.

IMMUNOPATHOLOGY

Up to this point the immune system has been presented as an unimpeachable asset. It is certainly true that deficiencies in any part of the immune system leave the individual exposed to a greater risk of infection, although other parts

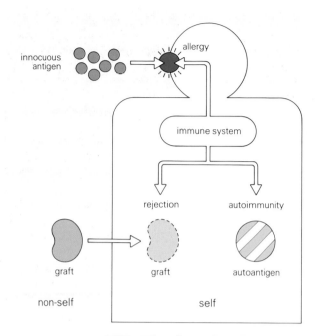

Fig. 1.25 **Undesirable consequences of immunity.** Tissue damage may occur through the operation of immune mechanisms, either because the immune response is excessive or the antigen is persistent. Thus, in allergic patients, some innocuous antigen, such as pollen provokes an immune reaction out of proportion to any damage it might do; we speak of hypersensitivity reactions. The immune system recognizes foreign tissue grafts like any other antigen and rejects them. Sometimes the self/non-self recognition system breaks down and the body's own components are recognized as non-self (autoantigens) in which case autoimmune diseases can ensue.

of the system often partly compensate for such deficiencies. Clearly strong evolutionary pressures from infectious agents have led to the development of the system in its present form.

Nevertheless, there are occasions when the immune system is itself a cause of disease or other undesirable consequences (Fig. 1.25).

It has been stated that the immune system is established on a principle of self/non-self recognition. In some cases tolerance of self antigens breaks down and autoimmune disease may develop (see 'Autoimmunity and Autoimmune Disease'). In other cases innocuous antigens such as pollen are recognized and the immune system mounts an inappropriate response to them giving rise to symptoms of allergy. This is referred to as hypersensitivity and is discussed in 'Hypersensitivity Types 1, 2, 3, and 4'. Hypersensitivity reactions can also occur during infections. In some infections the amount of tissue damage produced by the immune reactions to a resistant microorganism may be comparable to that produced by the infection itself. It is often not possible to say where an advantageous reaction to an infection ends and hypersensitivity begins, particularly since the fundamental mechanisms underlying both are the same. In spite of these drawbacks it must always be remembered that overwhelming selective pressures have led to the development of the immune system as we see it today.

FURTHER READING

Golub E. S. (1981) *The Cellular Basis of the Immune Response*. Sinauer Associates, Massachusetts.

McConnell I., Munro A. & Waldmann H. (1981) *The Immune System: a Course on the Molecular and Cellular Basis of Immunity,* 2nd edn. Blackwell Scientific Publications, Oxford.

Nisonoff A. (1982) *Introduction to Molecular Immunology*. Sinauer Associates, Massachusetts.

Roitt I. M. R. (1984) *Essential Immunology,* 5th edn. Blackwell Scientific Publications, Oxford.

Sites D. P., Stubo J. D., Fudenberg H. H. & Wells J. V. (1984) *Basic and Clinical Immunology,* 5th edn. Lange Medical Publications, Los Altos, California.

2 Cells Involved in the Immune Response

The immune system of vertebrates consists of a number of organs and several different cell types which have evolved to accurately and specifically recognize non-self antigens on microorganisms and to eliminate those organisms. By contrast, lower animals have more primitive defence mechanisms to protect themselves. These include proteins (with low specificity) which can recognize and agglutinate a wide variety of microorganisms, and cells which are capable of engulfing and digesting the microbes – phagocytes.

Phagocytes are an important defence in all animals, including the vertebrates. The key development which has occurred in vertebrate immune systems is the evolution of lymphoid cells and lymphoid organs. The lymphoid cells function to produce the high degree of specificity involved in the recognition of non-self antigens by vertebrate immune systems.

All the cells of the immune system arise from pluripotent stem cells through two main lines of differentiation (Fig. 2.1):
1. the lymphoid lineage – producing lymphocytes
2. the myeloid lineage – producing phagocytes and other cells.
There are two different kinds of lymphocytes which subserve different functions – T cells and B cells. T cells differentiate initially in the thymus whilst B cells differentiate in foetal liver, spleen, and in mammals in the adult bone marrow. In birds B cells differentiate in an organ found only in birds, the bursa of Fabricius.

There is also a population of 'null cells' (also called non T, non B cells or third population cells) which do not have characteristics corresponding to either T or B cells and their differentiation sequence is uncertain. All three cell types can be distinguished functionally but T and B cells are morphologically identical. The majority of lymphoid 'null cells' can be distinguished from T and B cells by their intracytoplasmic granules (see below).

The phagocytes are also of two basic kinds, monocytes and polymorphonuclear granulocytes. The latter are more usually referred to as polymorphs and they may be neutrophil, basophil, or eosinophil depending on the histological staining of their granules. In addition, there are a number of auxiliary cells derived from the myeloid lineage, these include:
1. platelets which are involved in blood clotting and inflammation
2. mast cells which have structural and functional similarities to basophil polymorphs.
The important features of these cell types will now be described in greater detail.

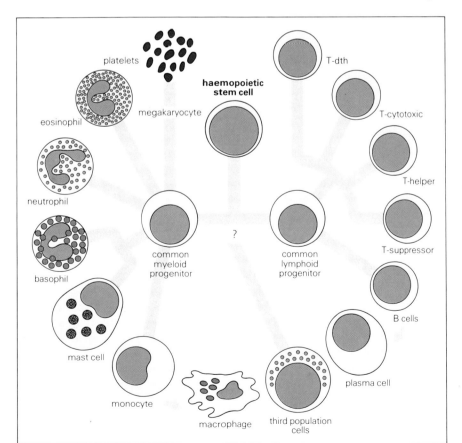

Fig. 2.1 Origin of cells involved in the immune response. All the cells are derived from pluripotent stem cells. These give rise to two distinct progenitors, one for lymphoid cells and the other for myeloid cells. The common lymphoid progenitor has the potential to differentiate into either T or B cells depending on the microenvironment to which it 'homes', that is, thymus or foetal liver/bone marrow. The origin of lymphoid cells which are not obviously T or B cells – the 'third population' – is still uncertain. They might have a lymphoid or myeloid origin but might also represent a distinct cell lineage. The myeloid cells differentiate into the 'committed' cells shown here.

LYMPHOID CELLS

Lymphocytes are produced in the primary lymphoid organs (thymus and adult bone marrow) and at a high rate (10^9/day). Some of these cells migrate via the circulation into the secondary lymphoid tissues namely, the spleen, lymph nodes and unencapsulated lymphoid tissue. The average human adult has about 10^{12} lymphoid cells and the lymphoid tissue as a whole represents about 2% of total body weight. Lymphoid cells represent about 20% of the total white blood cells (leucocytes) present in the adult circulation – the majority of white cells being polymorphonuclear (PMN). Many mature lymphoid cells are long-lived and may persist as memory cells for several years.

Morphological Heterogeneity of Lymphocytes
Lymphocytes in a conventional blood smear are heterogeneous in both size (6-10 μm in diameter) and morphology. Differences are seen in the nuclear (N) to cytoplasmic (C) ratio, in the degree of cytoplasmic staining with histological dyes and the presence or abesence of azurophilic granules.

Two distinct types of resting lymphoid cells can be distinguished in the cirulation by light microscopy using a haematological stain such as Giemsa. The typical small lymphocyte is agranular and possesses a high nuclear to cytoplasmic ratio. Others, with a lower nuclear to cytoplasmic ratio and containing intracytoplasmic azurophilic granules are currently referred to as large granular lymphocytes (LGL), not to be confused with polymorphonuclear granulocytes (Fig. 2.2).

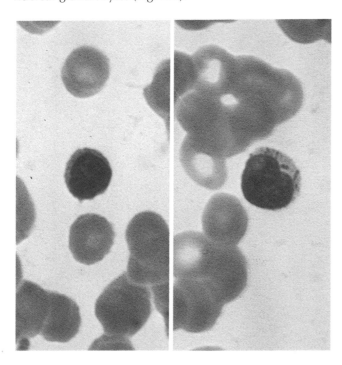

Fig. 2.2 Morphological heterogeneity of lymphocytes. The small lymphocyte (left) is agranular with a high N/C ratio. The large granular lymphocyte (right) has a low N/C ratio and azurophilic granules in the cytoplasm. Condensed chromatin produces dark nuclear staining. Giemsa stain, ×6,000.

T cells
The small lymphocyte population comprises both B cells and T cells. Although they appear similar, T cells and B cells can be distinguished from one another since they carry different cell surface proteins which act as 'markers'. For example, human T cells, but not B cells, carry a marker which binds to sheep erythrocytes (Fig. 2.3).

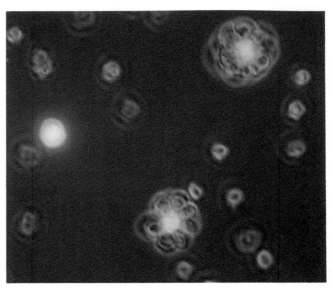

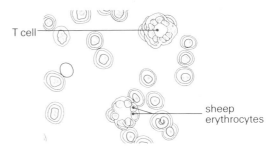

Fig. 2.3 Typical marker of human T cells. Human T cells from blood and tissues have the fortuitous property of binding to sheep erythrocytes (SE). Following their centrifugation together, T cells are distinguishable by their ability to form 'rosettes' with SE. The nucleated cells are distinguished from the SE by green fluorescent staining of the nuclei and cytoplasm with acridine orange. The formation of 'rosettes' with SE by T cells also provides a means for the physical separation of T from non-T cells.

Markers are also demonstrable using fluorescent antibodies as probes. In this case the surface marker proteins act as antigens (Fig. 2.4). The antibody probes may be raised in a different member of the same species (alloantibodies) or a different species (heteroantibodies). Hybridoma technology for making these antibody probes, together with flow cytometry techniques, which allows the separation of cells on the basis of size and fluorescence intensity, has revolutionized studies on the functional activities of lymphoid cell populations.

Markers have been used to define mouse and human T cell subpopulations and they are summarized in figure 2.5. Thy 1 (or θ, MW = 19-35 KD) is a glycoprotein found on (or expressed by) all mouse peripheral T cells. Most human T cells express three surface glycoproteins

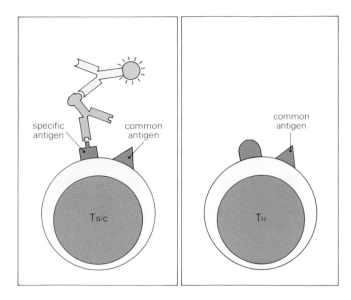

Fig. 2.4. Immunofluorescent method for the demonstration of T cell markers. Mouse antibodies directed towards T cell subset-specific antigen on a suppressor or cytotoxic T cell (Ts/c) will bind to this antigen but not to the T cell-specific antigen common to the T helper subset. The bound antibody is detected using antibodies to mouse immunoglobulin coupled to a fluorescent molecule.

detected by the monoclonal antibodies T11, T1 and T3. (T is the prefix indicating that the antibodies were prepared by Ortho and those with the prefix Leu by Becton Dickinson). T11 (MW = 55 KD) reacts with the receptor for sheep erythrocytes (SE), whilst T3 (MW = 20 KD) recognizes a glycoprotein involved in T cell triggering. The function of the molecule recognized by the T1 anti body (MW = 67 KD) is unknown. It also occurs on a subpopulation of B cells.

Some markers occur on some cell subpopulations only. Mouse helper T cells express Ly1 antigens (MW = 67 KD, which are probably equivalent to that detected by T1 in man). Most helper T cells (~ 60%) also express Qa1 antigens (MW = 64 KD) which are thought to be involved in the regulation of the immune response and are present

	mouse T cell			human T cell		
all T cells		Thy1			(T1), T3, T11	
T$_H$, T-dth	Ly1	Qa1	L3T4	T4/Leu 3a		T1
Ts, Tc		Ly2,3			T8/Leu 2a	
all activated.T cells		Ia		HLA-DR		TAC

Fig. 2.5 Summary of the surface markers on mouse and human peripheral T cells. These markers have been identified using specific antibodies. Some (eg. Thy 1) are found on all T cell subpopulations whereas others occur on only some of these subpopulations. T1 molecules appear on the majority of T cells but are probably restricted to the T$_H$/ T-dth subset. Equivalent molecules on mouse and human cells are in the same shade of brown.

only on T cells. Mouse T cells also express an antigen, L3T4 (MW = 55KD) which is equivalent to the molecule recognized by the T4 and Leu 3a monoclonal antibody (MW=55KD). These surface molecules appear to be involved in the recognition of antigen by T cells in association with class 2 MHC products. The mouse Ly2,3 antigens (MW=35K), equivalent to the glycoproteins on most human helper T cells recognized by T8/Leu 2a (MW=32KD), appears to help these T cells to recognize antigen in association with class 1 MHC products.

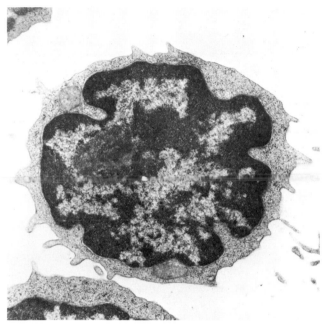

Fig. 2.6 Electron micrograph showing the T cell ultrastructure. The majority of circulating resting T lymphocytes have a thin rim of cytoplasm containing few mitochondria and polysomes, and little organized rough endoplasmic reticulum. ×20,000.

Mouse Ia antigens and human HLA-DR antigens consist of two polypeptide chains (MW = 28KD and 33 KD) and are expressed on B cells but only on T cells when they are activated by antigens/mitogens. In addition, the interleukin 2 receptor (TAC, MW = 50 KD) is detected (by a monoclonal antibody) on human T cells following activation. Unlike B cells, which have immunoglobulin for their antigen receptors, T cells carry a surface glycoprotein made up of two chains (52KD and 42KD), which can be identified by monoclonal antibody YT35.

Other surface antigens, such as receptors for the Fc region of antibody, are found on both T and B cells; they probably play a role in the regulation of lymphocyte responses.

Monoclonal antibodies directed to surface markers on human functional T cell subsets have also been extremely valuable in defining different stages of differentiation of early T cells in the thymus.

The majority of normal human blood T cells (about 65-80% in the adult circulation) have an ultrastructure characteristic of small lymphocytes, possessing a high nuclear to cytoplasmic ratio and few intra-cytoplasmic organelles (Fig. 2.6).

Mouse and human T cells contain a number of lysosomal acid hydrolases which appear in a distinct pattern when demonstrated by cytochemical staining. Detection of the acid hydrolases, β glucuronidase, acid phosphatase and alpha naphthyl acid esterase (ANAE) by cytochemical procedures shows that in the majority of T cells the enzyme is localized in one or a few 'dot-like' regions of the cytoplasm corresponding to the gall bodies. Figure 2.7 shows T cells stained for ANAE.

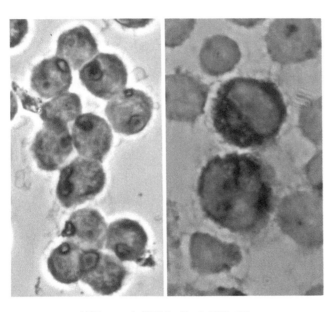

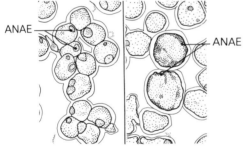

Fig. 2.7 T cells stained in suspension for the lysosomal enzyme ANAE. ANAE is localized in discrete 'dots' in the cytoplasm, corresponding to the gall body (left). (This pattern is also seen on tissue sections.) Most B cells do not stain for ANAE whereas monocytes have a distinctive diffuse staining pattern (right).

B cells
B lymphocytes represent about 5-15% of the circulating lymphoid pool and are classically defined by the presence of endogenously produced immunoglobulins (antibody). These molecules are inserted into the surface membrane where they act as specific antigen receptors. They are detected on the surface of mature cells by staining cell suspensions with fluorescent labelled, specific antibodies to the appropriate immunoglobulin of the species under investigation. Staining of cells in the cold results in the detection of the fluorescence in the 'ring-like' (or patchy) appearance over the cell (Fig. 2.8).

The majority of human peripheral blood B lymphocytes express both surface IgM and IgD antibodies. Very few

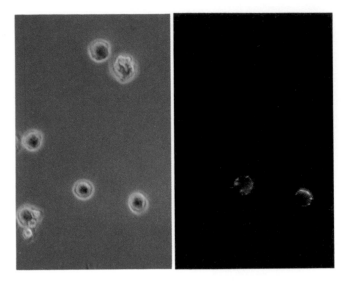

Fig. 2.8 B cells stained for surface immunoglobulin. Human blood B cells stained in the cold with fluoresceinated anti-human immunoglobulin show a patchy surface fluorescence viewed under ultraviolet light. Under phase contrast light microscopy (right) it can be seen that only 2 out of the 6 cells in this field are B lymphocytes. The lower cell shows 'capping' of the fluorescent antibody (see below).

cells express surface IgG, IgA or IgE in the circulation although these are present in larger numbers in specific locations in the body, for example, IgA-bearing cells in the gut. Since other cells, in addition to B cells also carry surface receptors which non-specifically bind to antibodies, care should be taken in evaluating the number of B cells. Antibodies bound to these receptors (Fc receptors) can also stain with fluoresceinated anti-human immunoglobulin (Fig. 2.9).

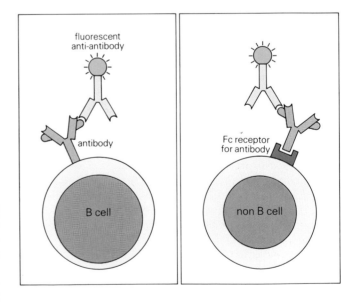

Fig. 2.9 Visualization of antibody bound to B cells and non-B cells by immunofluorescence. The surface antibody on the B cell is detected using a fluorescein/anti-antibody conjugate (left). This conjugate will also 'detect' non-B cells carrying receptors for the Fc part of the antibody and which have antibody on their surface (right).

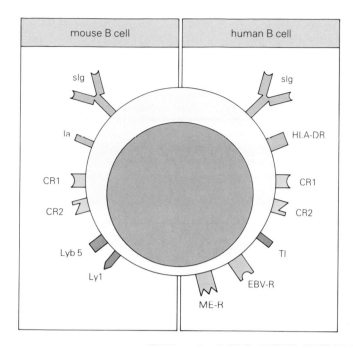

Fig. 2.10 Summary of the surface markers on mouse and human peripheral B cells. Equivalent molecules are in the same colour.

Divalent antibodies will cross-link antigens on surface membrane glycoproteins and be seen as 'patches' of cross-linked antigen-antibody complexes on the cell surface. Most of these complexes are actively swept along the cell surface and are seen as a 'cap' over one pole of the cell (see Fig. 2.8, right). This phenomenon is not peculiar to immunoglobulin on B cells but may also be seen with surface glycoproteins on other cell types when multivalent antibodies are attached to them.

A number of other markers are carried by both mouse and human B cells but not resting T cells (Fig. 2.10). B cells are defined as those cells carrying endogenously produced immunoglobulins. The majority of B cells also carry class 2 MHC products — Ia (mouse) or HLA-DR (human). These products are functionally important in the regulation of the immune response. Complement receptors for C3b (CR1) and C3d (CR2) are found on more mature B cells. Lyb5 (a mouse alloantigen) also appears on B cells later in their differentiation. Ly1 is primarily a mouse T cell marker but, like the human T1 marker of T cells, it is also present on a distinct subpopulation of B cells. Human B cells carry a surface receptor (EBV-R) for the Epstein-Barr virus — a herpes virus. A subpopulation of human B cells also carry a receptor for mouse erythrocytes (ME-R). This marker (together with T1) is probably a marker of immature B cells and has been useful in the diagnosis of human lymphoproliferative disorders.

Lymphocyte Proliferation and Maturation

During their development, both T and B lymphocytes acquire specific receptors for antigen which commit them to a single antigenic specificity for the rest of their life-span. The cells are activated when they bind their specific antigen in the presence of accessory cells; the resting 'virgin' lymphocytes then proliferate and mature into effector cells. This clonal selection through antigen recognition results in expansion of specific clones which either terminally differentiate into effectors or give rise to memory cells (Fig. 2.11). The 'resting' lymphocytes (in particular memory cells) recirculate through the body tissues and lymphoid organs via the blood and the thoracic duct thus allowing surveillance of the body tissues for invading microorganisms.

Antigen-induced lymphocyte proliferation normally occurs outside the blood and thoracic duct and can be visualized *in vitro* by cultivating lymphoid cells with specific antigens. Using the same experimental system, it can be demonstrated that mitogenic lectins (a lectin is a protein which binds and cross-links specific cell surface carbohydrate determinants), will polyclonally stimulate lymphoid cells. These mitogenic lectins (mitogens) are derived from various plants and bacteria. Lymphocyte activation by either antigens or mitogens results in intracellular changes and the subsequent development into a lymphoblast. Mitogen stimulation of lymphocytes *in vitro* is believed to mimic the series of events which occur *in vivo* following their stimulation by specific antigens. T and B cells are activated by different mitogens. Phytohaemagglutinin (PHA) and Concanavalin A (Con A) stimulate human and mouse T cells.

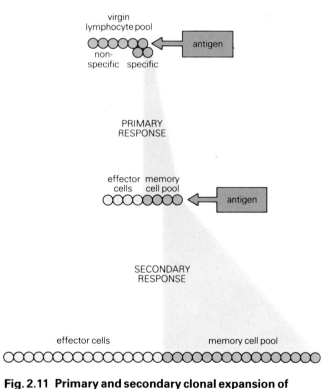

Fig. 2.11 Primary and secondary clonal expansion of lymphocytes in response to specific antigenic stimulation. T and B lymphocytes carrying specific antigen receptors are produced in the primary lymphoid organs and form the 'virgin' lymphoid pool. Following stimulation by specific antigen these cells proliferate and differentiate as clones into either: (1) effector cells (eg. T cells with cytotoxic or other functions, or antibody-secreting plasma cells from mature B cells), or (2) memory cells constituting the memory cell pool. This cellular proliferation is the primary response. When the memory cells are again stimulated by antigen they also proliferate (the secondary response) and some cells of the clone mature into effector cells whilst other cells remain as memory cells.

2.5

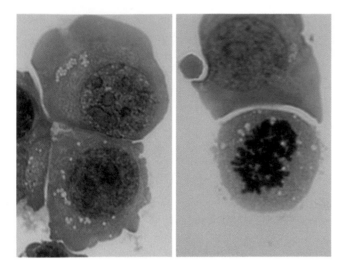

Fig. 2.12 Mitogen/antigen-induced lymphocyte blastogenesis. The human T and B cells shown here have been stimulated by pokeweed mitogen (PWM). There is increased basophilia in the cytoplasm and an increase in cell volume (left). The chromosomes condense and can be clearly seen during metaphase (right). Giemsa stain, ×4000.

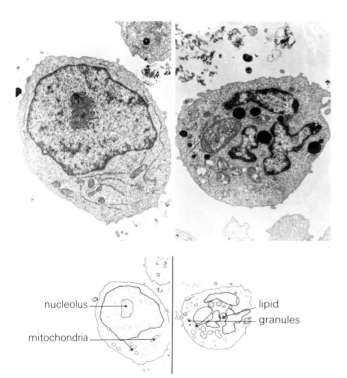

nucleolus

mitochondria

lipid granules

Fig. 2.13 Electron micrographs showing the ultrastructure of T cell blasts. T cell blasts developing after antigen or mitogen stimulation are large cells with extended cytoplasm containing a variety of organelles, including mitochondria and free polyribosomes. The blasts may be 'agranular' (left) or granular (right) depending on the presence or absence of electron-dense granules. Note also the lipid droplets in the granular blast. Studies on T cell clones (ie. populations derived from a single cell) have shown that in humans all the cytotoxic and suppressor clones are granular. Studies on the mouse have shown that both cytotoxic and suppressor clones are granular, whilst those clones without these functions are agranular. ×3200.

Lipopolysaccharide (LPS) stimulates mouse B cells. Pokeweed mitogen (PWM) stimulates both human T and B cells (Fig. 2.12).

Following T and B cell activation by mitogen or antigen, distinctive differentiation features are observed at the ultrastructural level (Figs. 2.13 and 2.14).

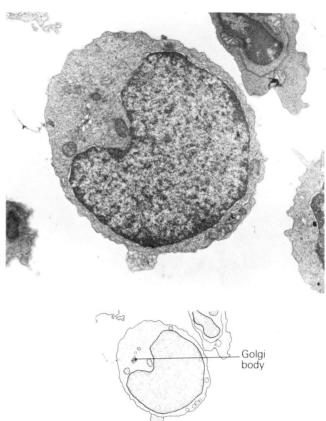

Golgi body

Fig. 2.14 Electron micrograph showing the ultrastructure of B cell blasts. The main feature of activated B cells is the development of the machinery for immunoglobulin synthesis. This includes smooth and rough endoplasmic reticulum, free polyribosomes and the Golgi apparatus, which is involved in glycosylation of the immunoglobulins. ×7500.

Ultimately, many B cell blasts mature into terminally differentiated plasma cells. Some B blasts do not develop membrane-bound polyribosomes. These cells are found in germinal centres and named follicle centre cells or centroblasts – they are the putative B memory cells (Fig. 2.15). Under light microscopy, the cytoplasm of the plasma cell is basophilic due to the large amount of RNA being utilized for antibody synthesis in the rough endoplasmic reticulum (RER) (Fig. 2.16). At the ultrastructural level, the RER is often seen in parallel arrays (Fig. 2.17). This is the 'production line' of the antibody-producing factory. Plasma cells are seldom seen in the circulation (less than 0.1% of lymphocytes) and are normally restricted to the secondary lymphoid organs and tissues. Antibodies produced by a single plasma cell are of one specificity and immunoglobulin class. Immunoglobulins are visualized in the plasma cell cytoplasm by staining with fluorescent-labelled specific antibodies (Fig. 2.18).

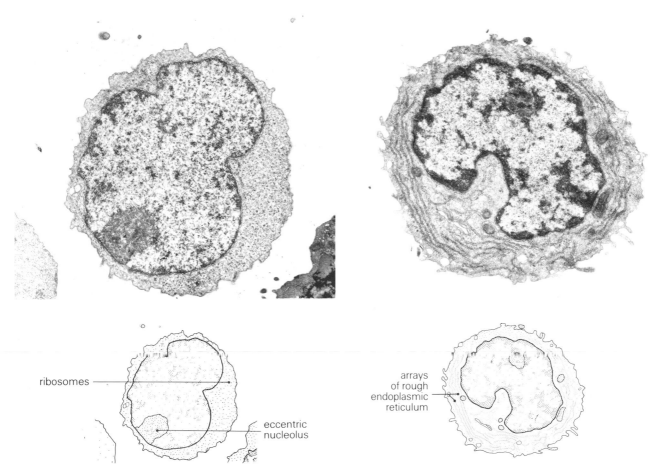

Fig. 2.15 Electron micrograph showing the follicle centre cell. This shows extended cytoplasm with polyribosomes and a few strands of RER. The large eccentric nucleolus is of note. This cell is frequently seen as a tumour cell in lymphoproliferative disorders. ×8500.

Fig. 2.17 Electron micrograph showing the ultrastructure of the plasma cell. The plasma cell is characterized by parallel arrays of RER. In mature cells these cisternae become dilated with immunoglobulins. ×6000. Courtesy of Professor A. Zicca.

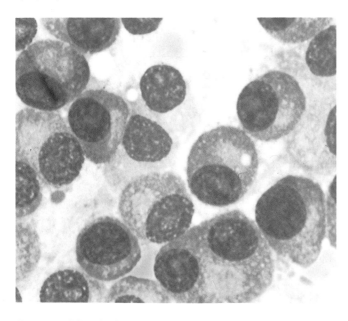

Fig. 2.16 Morphology of the plasma cell. The mature plasma cell has an eccentric nucleus with a large amount of basophilic cytoplasm, due presumably to the abundant RNA required for protein synthesis. May-Grünewald-Giemsa stain, ×4000.

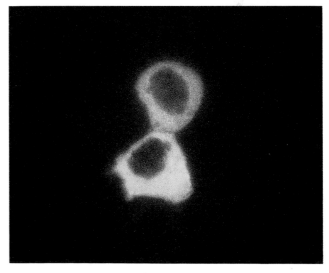

Fig. 2.18 Immunofluorescent staining of intracytoplasmic immunoglobulin in plasma cells. Fixed human plasma cells treated with fluoresceinated anti-human IgM (green) and rhodaminated anti-IgG (red) show extensive intracytoplasmic staining. The distinct staining (red or green) of the two plasma cells indicates that plasma cells normally only manufacture one class of antibody. ×3000.

'NULL' OR 'THIRD POPULATION' CELLS

There is a population of lymphoid cells which does not consistently carry markers of either T or B cells. In the circulation the majority of these null cells are lymphocyte-like and since they are not obviously either T or B cells they have been called 'third population' cells. They are characterized by the possession of Fc receptors for IgG and although probably of bone marrow origin their exact lineage is uncertain. They have been shown to share some characteristics with monocytes and even display some T cell markers. The ultrastructure of a third population cell is typical of a large granular lymphocyte (Fig. 2.19).

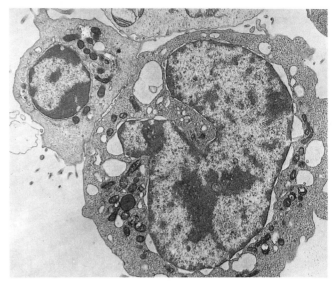

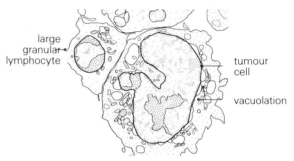

Fig. 2.20 Electron micrograph of a large granular lymphocyte (LGL) killing a tumour cell. LGLs bind to and kill IgG antibody-coated, and even non-coated, tumour cells. It is essential for the membranes of the two cells to be closely apposed in order for the LGL to deliver the 'kiss of death'. Note the vacuolation of the tumour cell cytoplasm, characteristic of a dying cell. ×4500.

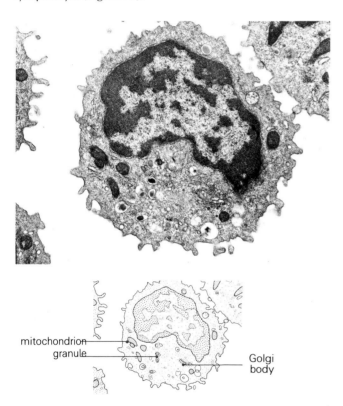

Fig. 2.19 Electron micrograph showing the ultrastructure of a large granular lymphocyte. These cells characteristically have electron-dense (peroxidase-negative) granules close to the well-developed Golgi apparatus and also scattered in the cytoplasm. They have an expanded cytoplasm which contains a variety of vesicles (apart from the granules) and mitochondria. ×6000.

It is currently believed that this population of cells contains the majority of natural killer and antibody dependent cellular cytotoxic effectors. Natural killer (NK) cells non-specifically kill tumour cells and virally-infected cells and play a role in regulating the immune response. Antibody dependent cellular cytotoxic cells (ADCC) also kill non-specifically but this occurs via antibodies bound to their target cells. Figure 2.20 shows an ADCC effector cell delivering the 'kiss of death' to a tumour cell. A minority of circulatory null cells are myeloid stem cells and immature T or B cells.

MONONUCLEAR PHAGOCYTIC SYSTEM (MONOCYTES)

Bone marrow derived myeloid progenitors give rise to the cells of the mononuclear phagocyte system which has two main functions, performed by two different types of cells.
1. the 'professional' phagocytic macrophages whose predominant role is to remove particulate antigens and,
2. antigen-presenting cells (APC) whose role is to present antigen to specific antigen-sensitive lymphocytes.

The Reticuloendothelial System
The phagocytic tissue macrophages form a network – the reticuloendothelial system (RES) which is found in many organs (Fig. 2.21). Intravenously injected carbon particles become localized in these tissues (Fig. 2.22).

Promonocytes in the bone marrow give rise to the blood monocytes and these represent a circulating pool which migrate into the various organs and tissue systems and become macrophages. Since the blood monocyte is the most easily obtainable phagocytic cell of this class it has been studied in greatest detail.

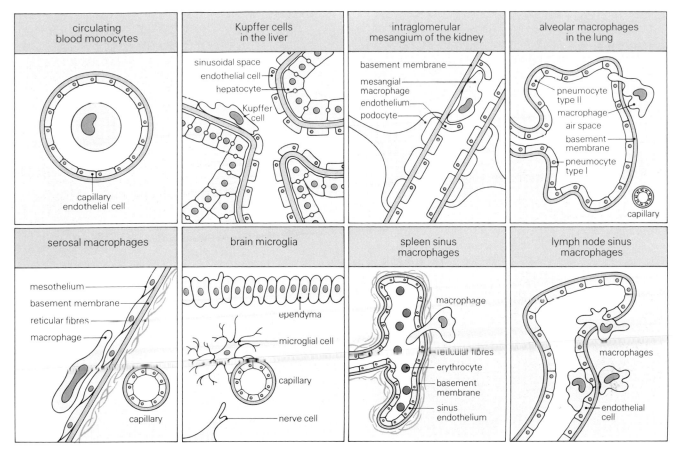

Fig. 2.21 The reticuloendothelial system. The cells of this system include circulating blood monocytes and dispersed phagocytes in connective tissue (eg. in the liver known as Kupffer cells) or fixed to the endothelial layer of the blood capillaries. Endothelium-fixed phagocytes include intraglomerular mesangial cells in the kidney. Alveolar and serosal macrophages, and microglial cells of the brain are examples of 'wandering' macrophages.

The human blood monocyte is a large cell (10–18 μm diameter) relative to the lymphocyte which usually has a horseshoe-shaped nucleus and often contains faint azurophilic granules (Fig. 2.23).

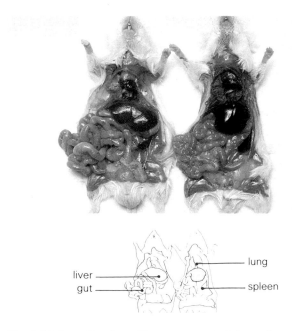

Fig. 2.22 Localization of intravenously injected particles in the RES. A mouse was injected intravenously with fine carbon particles and killed five minutes later. Carbon accumulates in organs rich in mononuclear phagocytes – lungs, liver, spleen and areas of the gut wall. The normal organ colour is shown in the control mouse on the left.

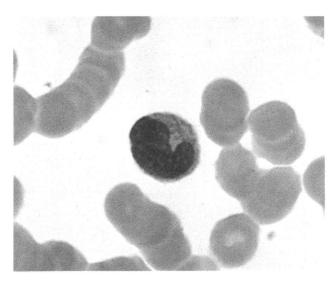

Fig. 2.23 Morphology of the monocyte. Blood monocytes have a characteristic horseshoe-shaped nucleus and are larger than most circulating lymphocytes. Giemsa stain, ×2500.

At the ultrastructural level, the monocyte possesses prominent microvilli and undulating membranes, a well-developed Golgi complex and many intracytoplasmic lysosomes (Fig. 2.24). These lysosomes contain several acid hydrolases and peroxidase which is important in the intracellular killing of microorganisms. Monocytes/macrophages adhere strongly to glass and plastic surfaces and will actively phagocytose organisms or even tumour cells *in vitro*.Ingestion and adherence by monocytes is promoted when the cells bind the microorganisms through specialized receptors for IgG (Fc$^\gamma$ receptors) and complement (eg. C3b) with which the microorganism is coated. Monocytes carry other surface markers, including small amounts of HLA-DR (Ia) (Fig. 2.25). In general, the markers are not lineage specific, except perhaps for the glycoprotein F4/80 (MW=160KD) on mouse macrophages. In the mouse, Fc receptors are of two kinds – those binding IgG1 and IgG2b (MW=47-60KD), and those binding IgG2a. Some human cells also possess receptors for IgE (Fc$^\varepsilon$R). Ia and HLA-DR molecules are present on only a small number of monocytes and (possibly activated) macrophages. The complement receptors for C3b (CR1, MW=250KD) and inactivated C3b (CR3, MW=260KD) have been found. (CR3 is probably equivalent to the MAC-1 antigen recognized by a monoclonal antibody.) Thus, together with Fc receptors, complement receptors are important in the adherence and phagocytosis of microorganisms.

In addition to all of these molecules, monocytes and macrophages must also have receptors for lymphokines such as γ-interferon and migration inhibition factor. These receptors have not yet been clearly characterized.

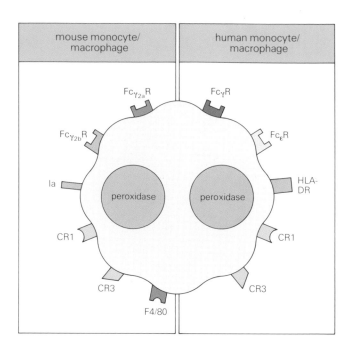

Fig. 2.25 Summary of the surface markers on mouse and human monocytes/macrophages. Equivalent molecules are shown in the same colour.

Like neutrophils, monocytes and macrophages contain peroxidase, which inactivates peroxide ions generated during killing of ingested microorganisms.

The functions of monocytes and macrophages can be enhanced by factors released from T cells. In addition, monocyte/macrophages produce complement components, prostaglandins, interferons and monokines such as interleukin I (see Fig. 11.14).

Antigen-Presenting Cells

Antigen-presenting cells (APC) are found primarily in the skin, lymph nodes, spleen and thymus. Their main role is to present antigens to antigen-sensitive lymphoid cells (Fig. 2.26). The archetypal APC is the Langerhan's cell in the skin. These cells with characteristic 'tennis-racket' granules termed Birbeck granules (see Fig. 22.5) migrate via the afferent lymphatics as 'veiled cells' into the paracortex of the draining lymph nodes. Within the paracortex the cells 'interdigitate' with many T cells (Fig. 2.27). This provides an efficient mechanism to present antigen, carried from the skin, to T cells in the draining lymph nodes. These APCs are rich in class 2 MHC antigens which are important for presenting antigen to the T cells. Other specialized APCs, the follicular dentritic cells, are found in the secondary follicles of the B cell areas of the lymph nodes and spleen.

Recently APCs have been found in the thymus. These interdigitating follicular cells which are specially abundant in the thymus medulla are rich in self-antigens (including class 2 MHC antigens). The thymus is of crucial importance in the development and maturation of T cells. It appears that the immature T cells learn to discriminate self antigens from non-self antigens during this maturation step. The interdigitating cells carry self antigen and therefore are thought to play a role in selecting out T cells that react against self antigen.

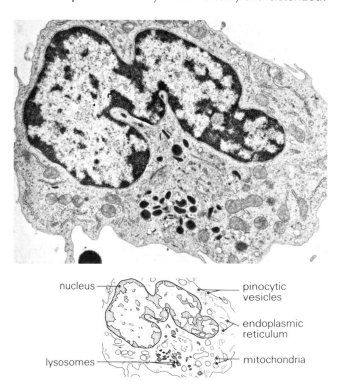

Fig. 2.24 Electron micrograph showing the ultrastructure of the monocyte. This shows the 'horseshoe' nucleus, pinocytic vesicles, lysosomal granules, mitochondria and isolated RER. ×8000. From *Journal of Cell Biology*, 1971, Vol. 50, article by Nichols *et al.*

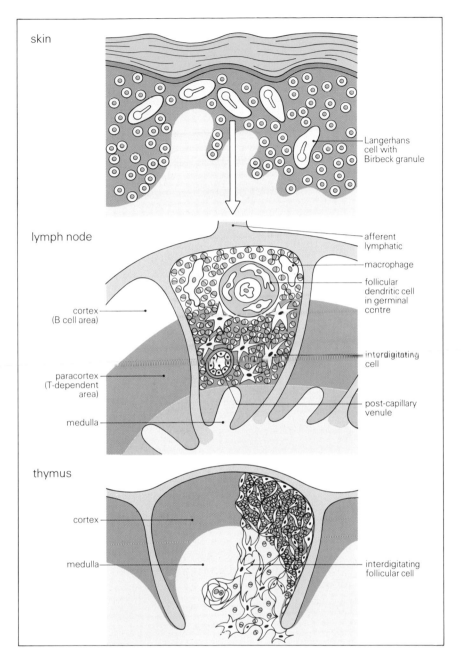

skin

Langerhans cell with Birbeck granule

lymph node

afferent lymphatic

macrophage

follicular dendritic cell in germinal centre

cortex (B cell area)

interdigitating cell

paracortex (T-dependent area)

post-capillary venule

medulla

thymus

cortex

medulla

interdigitating follicular cell

Fig. 2.26 Antigen-presenting cells.
Bone-marrow derived antigen-presenting cells are found especially in lymphoid tissues and in the skin. APCs are represented in the skin by Langerhan's cells, present in the epidermis and characterized by specialized granules (the tennis racket-shaped Birbeck granules). These cells, rich in Ia (mouse) or HLA-DR (human) determinants, are believed to carry antigens and migrate via the afferent lymphatics (where they appear as 'veiled' cells) into the paracortex of the draining lymph nodes where they interdigitate with T cells. These 'interdigitating cells' localized in the T cell dependent areas of the lymph node present antigen to the antigen-sensitive lymphocytes. Follicular dendritic cells are found in the B cell areas of the lymph nodes and in particular in the germinal centres. Some macrophages located in the outer cortex and marginal sinus may also act as antigen-presenting cells. In the thymus, APCs occur as interdigitating follicular cells.

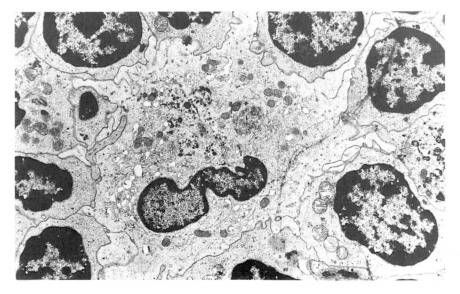

Fig. 2.27 Electron micrograph showing the ultrastructure of an interdigitating cell (IDC) in the T cell area of the rat lymph node. Intimate contacts are made with the membranes of the surrounding T cells. The cytoplasm contains relatively few organelles and does not show the Birbeck granules characteristic of the skin Langerhans cell, but these appear after antigenic stimulation. ×2000. Courtesy of Dr. B. H. Balfour.

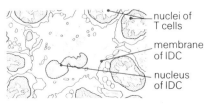

nuclei of T cells

membrane of IDC

nucleus of IDC

THE POLYMORPHONUCLEAR GRANULOCYTES (POLYMORPHS)

Granulocytes are produced in the bone marrow at a rate of eighty million per minute and are short-lived (2-3 days) relative to monocyte/macrophages which may live for months or years. Granulocytes represent about 60 to 70% of the total normal blood leucocytes but are also found in extravascular sites. Polymorphs are able to adhere to and penetrate the endothelial cells lining the blood vessels. As the name suggests, the mature forms usually contain a multi-lobed nucleus and many granules. They are classified into neutrophils, eosinophils and basophils on the basis of the staining reaction of their granules by histological dyes.

Although these cells do not show any specificity for antigens they play an important role in acute inflammation and, together with antibodies and complement, in protection against microorganisms. The predominant role of polymorphs is phagocytosis and their importance in protection is emphasized by the great increase in susceptibility to infections found in individuals with low numbers of circulating polymorphs.

Neutrophils

Neutrophils represent over 90% of the circulating granulocytes and are 10-20µ in diameter (Fig. 2.28). They possess two main types of granules. The primary (azurophilic) granules (lysosomes) contain acid hydrolases, myeloperoxidase and muraminidase (lysozyme) whilst the secondary or specific granules contain lactoferrin in addition to lysozyme. These granules can be seen at the ultrastructural level (Fig. 2.29). Ingested organisms are contained within vacuoles termed phagosomes which fuse with the enzyme-containing granules to form the phagolysosomes (Fig. 2.30).

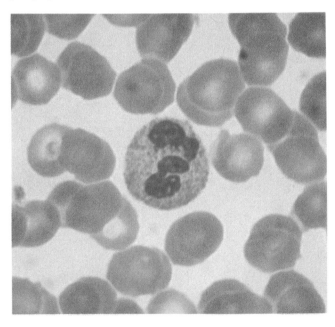

Fig. 2.28 Morphology of the neutrophil. This blood smear shows a neutrophil with its characteristic polymorphonuclear shape and neutrophilic cytoplasm. Giemsa stain, ×4500.

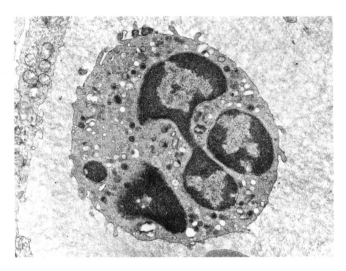

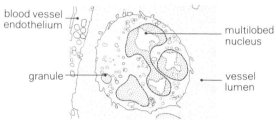

Fig. 2.29 Electron micrograph showing the ultrastructure of the neutrophil. This mouse neutrophil lies within a skin blood vessel. The neutrophil cytoplasm contains primary and secondary granules of different electron opacity. ×10,000. Courtesy of Dr. D. McLaren.

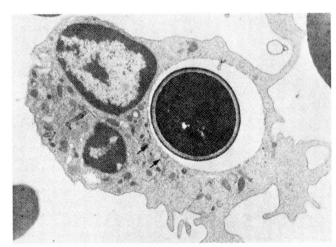

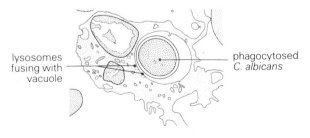

Fig. 2.30 Electron micrograph showing a neutrophil containing phagocytosed *Candida albicans*. Two lysosomal granules may be seen fusing with the vacuole containing the organism. ×7000. Courtesy of Dr. H. Valdimarsson.

Eosinophils

Eosinophils comprise 2-5% of blood leucocytes in healthy, non-allergic individuals (Fig. 2.31). Like neutrophils they do appear to be capable of phagocytosing and killing ingested microorganisms, although it is not their primary function. The granules in mature eosinophils are membrane-bound organelles with a 'crystalloid' or 'core' differing in electron opacity from the surrounding matrix (Fig. 2.32). Human blood eosinophils usually have only a bilobed nucleus and many cytoplasmic vesicles. They possess many ribosomes, mitochondria, and microtubules, suggesting that they are metabolically active.

Eosinophils (as well as basophils and mast cells described below) can be triggered to degranulate by appropriate stimuli. Degranulation involves fusion of the intracellular granules with the plasma membrane. The contents are released to the outside of the cell. This type of reaction is the only way that these cells can use their 'granule armament' against large targets which cannot be phagocytosed. Eosinophils are thought to play a specialized role in the immunity to helminth infections using this mechanism (see 'Immunity to Protozoa and Worms').

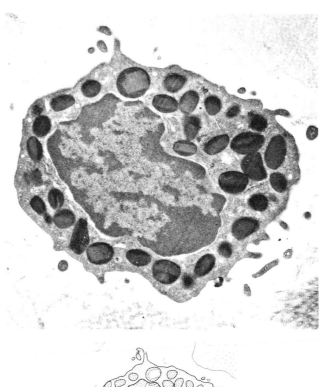

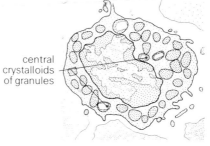

central
crystalloids
of granules

Fig. 2.32 Electron micrograph showing the ultrastructure of a guinea pig eosinophil. The mature eosinophil contains granules with central crystalloids. ×11,500. Courtesy of Dr. D. McLaren.

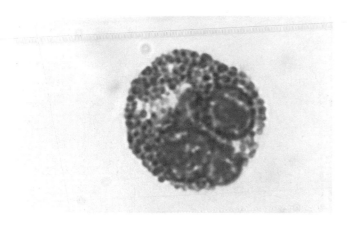

Fig. 2.31 Morphology of the eosinophil. This blood smear enriched for granulocytes shows an eosinophil with its multilobed nucleus and heavily-stained cytoplasmic granules. Leishman stain, ×5000.

Eosinophils are attracted by products released from T cells, mast cells and basophils (Eosinophil Chemotactic Factor of Anaphylaxis, ECF-A). They bind schistosomulae coated with IgG antibody, degranulate, and release a toxic protein ('major basic protein'). Eosinophils release histaminase and aryl sulphatase, which inactivate the mast cell products histamine and Slow Reactive Substance of Anaphylaxis (SRS-A) respectively. The net effect of these factors is to dampen down the inflammatory response and reduce granulocyte migration into the site of invasion.

Basophils and Mast Cells

Basophils are found in very small numbers in the circulation (less than 0.2% of the leucocytes) and are characterized by deep violet blue granules (Fig. 2.33). The mast cell is often indistinguishable from the basophil in a number of its properties and although they are both of bone marrow origin its relationship to the basophil is not completely clear.

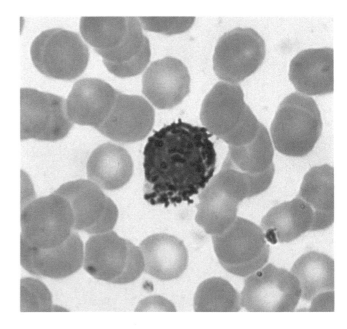

Fig. 2.33 Morphology of the basophil. This blood smear shows a typical basophil with its deep violet-blue granules. Wright's stain, ×4500.

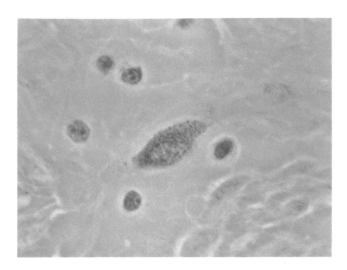

Fig. 2.34 Histological appearance of human (gut) connective tissue mast cells. This micrograph shows the dark blue cytoplasm with brownish granules. Alcian blue and Safranin, ×2500.

Mast cells are found associated with mucosal epithelial cells where they appear to be dependent on T cells for their proliferation. In addition, they are commonly found in the connective tissue where they are T cell independent. Under light microscopy, they can be visualized with Alcian blue (Fig. 2.34).

Mature blood basophils have randomly distributed granules surrounded by, and containing membranes (Fig. 2.35). These granules in both basophils and mast cells

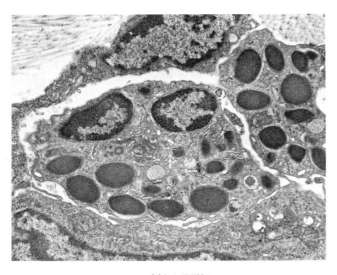

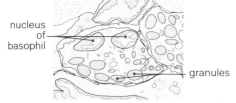

Fig. 2.35 Electron micrographs showing the ultrastructure of the basophil. Basophils in guinea pig skin showing the characteristic randomly distributed granules. ×10,000. Courtesy of Dr. D. McLaren.

contain heparin, SRS-A and ECF-A and these are released on degranulation initiated by the appropriate stimulus. This is usually an allergen which cross-links specific IgE molecules bound to the surface of the mast cell or basophil via Fc receptors for IgE (Fig. 2.36). Pharmacological mediators released following degranulation cause the adverse symptoms of allergy but, on the positive side, they may also play a role in immunity against parasites. Granulocyte markers are summarized in figure 2.37.

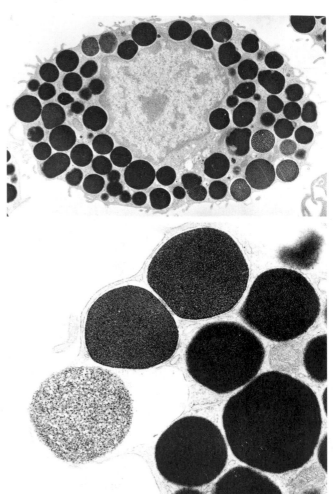

Fig. 2.36 Electron micrographs of rat peritoneal mast cells. These show the undegranulated cell with its electron-dense granules (upper, ×6000) and a granule in the process of exocytosis (lower, ×30,000). Courtesy of Dr. T. S. C. Orr.

Platelets

The final myeloid cell to be considered here is the blood platelet. In addition to their role in blood clotting, platelets are also involved in the immune response, especially in inflammation. They possess class 1 MHC products and receptors for both IgG and IgE. Platelets are derived from large megakaryocytes in the bone marrow and are seen to contain granules at the ultrastructural level (Fig. 2.38). Following endothelial injury, platelets adhere to and aggregate at the endothelial surface releasing permeability-increasing substances and factors responsible for activating complement components to attract leucocytes.

	FcεR	FcγR	C3aR	C5aR	CR1	CR3	peroxidase	acid phosphatase	alkaline phosphatase
neutrophil	−	+	+	+	+	+	+	+	+
eosinophil	+	+	+?	+	+	+	+	+	
basophil	+	+	+	+	+	+	+		
mast cell	+	+	+	+	+	+		+	+

Fig. 2.37 Summary of the surface markers on mature human granulocytes. All cells possess Fc receptors for IgG (FcγR). Only basophils and mast cells have high affinity receptors for IgE (FcεR); eosinophils have low affinity receptors. All cells carry receptors for complement components: receptors for C3a and C5a are important for chemotaxis; and CR1 and CR3 are involved in adherence and phagocytosis. The granules in different cell types vary qualitatively in their enzyme content.

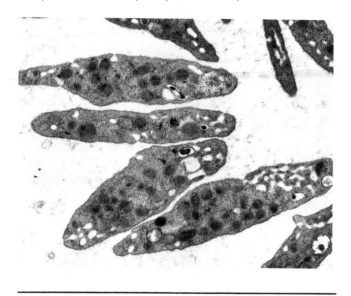

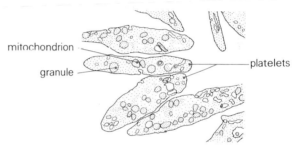

mitochondrion

granule

platelets

Fig. 2.38 Electron micrograph showing the platelet ultrastructure. The cytoplasmic organelles, including granules and mitochondria, are randomly dispersed. ×20,000. Courtesy of Dr. J. G. White.

SUMMARY

There are several types of cells involved in the immune response. Some cells possess the basic primitive function of phagocytosis and intracellular killing. This can be augmented by antibodies and complement components. Other cells, which are not phagocytic, present antigen to the more advanced lymphocytes. T and B lymphocytes with specialized functions are able to respond, specifically through complex cellular interactions, to defined antigenic determinants. Unlike the primitive immune system of lower animals, the vertebrate immune system exhibits memory. That is to say that a secondary antigenic challenge usually produces a greater and more effective response than the primary challenge. The function of memory, as well as specificity, is dependent on the lymphocytes.

FURTHER READING

Ezekowitz R.A.B., Hill M. & Gordon S. (1983) Macrophage plasma membrane and activation. *Transactions of the Royal Society of Tropical Medicine and Hygiene* **77,** 604.

Feaison D.T. (1984) Cellular receptors for fragments of the third component of complement. *Imunology Today* **5,** 105

Friedman P.S. (1981) The Immunobiology of the Langerhans Cells. *Immunology Today* **2,** 124.

Jarrett E.E.E. & Haig D.M. (1984) Mucosal mast cells *in vivo* and *in vitro*. *Immunology Today* **5,** 115.

Lydyard P.M., Banga P., Guamotta G., Walker P., Mackenzie L. & Mackanday S. (1985) Human lymphocyte antigens – a mini review. *Transactions of the Biochemical Society* (in press).

Playfair J.H.L. (1984) *Immunology at a Glance,* 2nd edition. Blackwell Scientific Publications, Oxford.

Roitt I.M. (1984) *Essential Immunology,* 5th edition. Blackwell Scientific Publications, Oxford.

Zucker-Franklin D., Greaves M.F., Grossi C.E. & Marmont A.M. (1980). Atlas of Blood Cells: Function and Pathology. Edi. Ermes, Milan and Lea & Febiger, Philadelphia.

3 The Lymphoid System

The cells involved in the immune response are organized into tissues and organs in order to perform their functions most effectively. These structures are collectively referred to as the lymphoid system and are illustrated and described below.

Primary and Secondary Lymphoid Tissue

The lymphoid system is comprised of lymphocytes, epithelial and stromal cells and is arranged either into discretely capsulated organs or accumulations of diffuse lymphoid tissue. Lymphoid organs contain lymphocytes at various stages of development and are classified into either primary/central lymphoepithelial organs or secondary/peripheral lymphoid organs (Fig. 3.1). The primary lymphoid organs are the major sites of lymphopoiesis. Here, lymphocytes differentiate from lymphoid stem cells, proliferate and mature into functional effector cells. In mammals, including man, T lymphocytes are produced in the thymus and B lymphocytes in the foetal liver and bone marrow. In avian species there is a specialized site of B cell generation, the bursa of Fabricius. In the primary lymphoid organs the lymphocytes acquire their repertoire of specific antigen receptors in order to cope with the antigenic challenges the individual receives during its life. They also learn to discriminate between self antigens, which are tolerated, and non-self antigens which, generally are not.

Secondary lymphoid organs include lymph nodes, spleen and mucosal associated tissue including the tonsils and Peyer's patches of the gut. The secondary lymphoid tissue creates the environment in which lymphocytes can interact with each other and with antigens and disseminates the immune response once generated. These functions are performed by phagocytic macrophages, antigen-presenting cells, and mature T and B lymphocytes in the secondary lymphoid organs.

PRIMARY LYMPHOID ORGANS

The Thymus

The thymus in mammals is bilobed, located in the thorax and overlies the heart and major blood vessels. Each lobe is organized into lobules or follicles separated from each other by connective tissue trabeculae (Fig. 3.2).

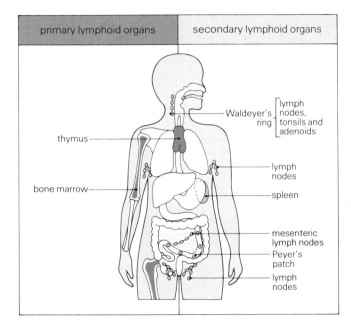

primary lymphoid organs	secondary lymphoid organs

Waldeyer's ring — lymph nodes, tonsils and adenoids

thymus

lymph nodes

bone marrow

spleen

mesenteric lymph nodes

Peyer's patch

lymph nodes

Fig. 3.1 Major lymphoid organs and tissues. The thymus produces T cells and the bone marrow, B cells. The secondary lymphoid organs and tissues contain mature T and B cells and accessory cells. In the mammalian foetus the B cells are initially generated in the liver. In man the adult bone marrow is also a secondary lymphoid organ. Lymph nodes are present throughout the body (only a few are depicted here) and are usually found at the junctions of lymphatic vessels. The group of lymph nodes including the tonsillar and adenoidal lymphoid tissue in the area of the neck and throat is called the Waldeyer's ring of lymphoid tissue. Lymph nodes drain the tissue spaces and the lymphocytes at these sites generally respond well to lymph-borne antigens whilst lymphoid cells in the spleen respond well to blood-borne antigens. Peyer's patches are unencapsulated masses of lymphoid tissue in the small intestine.

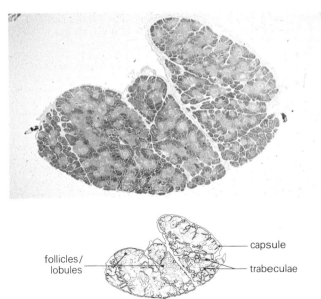

follicles/lobules

capsule

trabeculae

Fig. 3.2 Thymus section showing the lobular structure. This low power cross-section shows a collagenous capsule with the thymocytes (young T lymphocytes) organized into follicles/lobules separated from each other by connective tissue trabeculae. Haematoxylin and Eosin stain, × 3.5.

3.1

Within each lobule the lymphoid cells (thymocytes) are arranged into an outer cortex and an inner medulla (Fig. 3.3). The tightly packed cortex contains the majority of relatively immature proliferating cells whilst the medulla contains more mature cells. There is a network of epithelial cells throughout the lobules which probably play a role in the differentiation process from stem cells to T lymphocyutes. In addition, interdigitating cells (derived from bone marrow) are superimposed on the epithelial network especially in the medulla. These cells, which are rich in the major histocompatibility class 2 antigens, are thought to be important in the process of learning to recognize self antigens in the thymus: (major histocompatibility complex – MHC – class 2 antigens are important in regulating interactions between cells of the immune system and in determining how antigen is recognized by helper T cells).

Hassall's corpuscles are found in the thymus medulla. Their function is unknown but they appear to contain degenerating epithelial cells.

The Bursa of Fabricius and its Mammalian Equivalent

In birds, B cells differentiate in the bursa of Fabricius, hence the name 'B' cells. The bursa is like a modified piece of intestine with plicae directed towards a central lumen (Fig. 3.4). The bursal follicles are organized into cortex and medulla and lie along the margins of the plicae. Mammals have no bursa, instead, islands of haemopoietic cells in the foetal liver and in the foetal and adult bone marrow give rise directly to B lymphocytes. As well as being a site of B cell generation the adult bone marrow contains many mature T cells and antibody producing, plasma cells: that is to say, in man it is also an important secondary lymphoid organ.

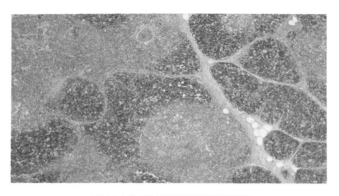

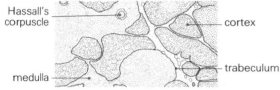

Fig. 3.3 Thymus section showing the lobular organization. This high power section shows the lobules to consist of two main areas – an outer cortex of rapidly dividing immature cells and an inner medulla of more mature cells. Structures of unknown function known as Hassal's corpuscles are found in the medulla. H & E stain, × 25.

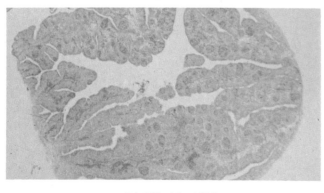

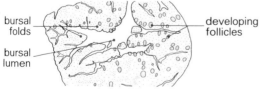

Fig. 3.4 Bursa section showing the follicular structure. The avian bursa of Fabricius is a lympho-epithelial organ (like the thymus) and is found dorsal to the hindgut. The lumen of the bursa opens into the cloaca. The bursa is composed of folds or plicae penetrating the central lumen and the follicles are arranged along their surfaces in close contact with the epithelial lining cells. Like the thymic follicles, bursal follicles are arranged into an outer cortex and inner medulla. The bursa, like the thymus, atrophies with age. H & E stain, × 10.

SECONDARY LYMPHOID ORGANS

The generation of lymphocytes in primary lymphoid organs is followed by their migration into the secondary peripheral organs; this flow is part of the 'lymphocyte traffic' which occurs between organs. The secondary lymphoid organs include the well organized encapsulated spleen and lymph nodes and non-encapsulated accumulations of lymphoid tissue throughout the body.

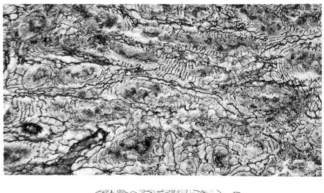

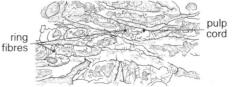

Fig. 3.5 Spleen section showing the connective tissue framework. This high power section is stained for reticulin and shows the architecture of the red pulp cords and the ring fibres which support phagocytic macrophages. × 125.

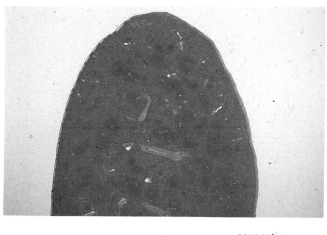

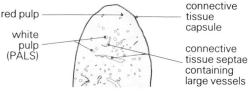

red pulp — connective tissue capsule

white pulp (PALS) — connective tissue septae containing large vessels

Fig. 3.6 Spleen section showing the cellular organization. This low power cross-section of the spleen shows the lymphoid tissue localized in the white pulp around arterioles. This lymphoid tissue in the periarteriolar lymphoid sheath – PALS – is easy to distinguish from the red pulp of the spleen. The red pulp is mainly involved in destruction of effete erythrocytes, but also contains some lymphocytes and plasma cells. H & E stain, × 7.

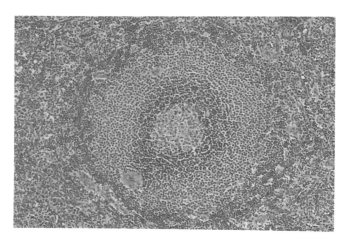

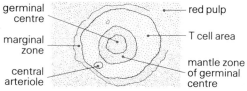

germinal centre — red pulp

marginal zone — T cell area

central arteriole — mantle zone of germinal centre

Fig. 3.7 Spleen section showing the periarteriolar lymphoid sheath (PALS). This high power view shows the lymphoid tissue arranged around an arteriole. The T cells are found close to the central arteriole and the B cell area has a germinal centre. In the 'unstimulated' state the B cell area consists of a primary follicle. The lymphoid tissue is separated from the red pulp by the marginal zone. This contains blood vessels and is the site of entry of blood-borne lymphocytes into the splenic lymphoid areas. H & E stain, × 125.

Much of this lymphoid tissue is associated with mucosal surfaces and is referred to as MALT (mucosa associated lymphoid tissue) of the gut, respiratory tract and the urinogenital tract. It has commonly been called GALT or gut associated lymphoid tissue when associated with the alimentary tract.

The Spleen

The spleen lies at the upper left of the abdomen behind the stomach and close to the diaphragm. It is surrounded by a collagenous capsule containing smooth muscle fibres, which penetrate into the parenchyma of the organ. These trabeculae, together with the reticular framework support the variety of cells found within the organ (Fig. 3.5). There are two main types of tissue: the red pulp, which is mainly concerned with the destruction of effete erythrocytes, and the white pulp, which contains the lymphoid tissue (Fig. 3.6). The bulk of the lymphoid tissue is arranged around a central arteriole – the periarteriolar lymphoid sheath (PALS). The PALS is composed of T and B cell areas, the T cells being found around the central arteriole while the B cells are found beyond this zone. The B cells may be present as either primary, 'unstimulated' follicles, or secondary 'stimulated' follicles possessing a germinal centre (Fig. 3.7). Figure 3.8 shows a schematic diagram of the spleen indicating the structures of the PALS in relation to the blood supply.

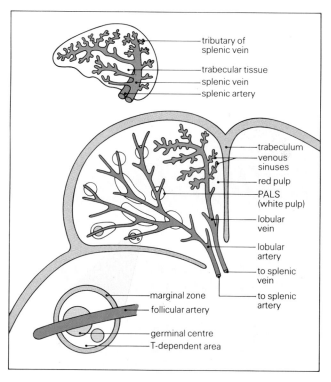

tributary of splenic vein
trabecular tissue
splenic vein
splenic artery

trabeculum
venous sinuses
red pulp
PALS (white pulp)
lobular vein
lobular artery
to splenic vein
to splenic artery

marginal zone
follicular artery
germinal centre
T-dependent area

Fig. 3.8 The structure of a spleen lobule. The red pulp contains a reticular network, splenic cords lined by macrophages, and venous sinuses which drain into the lobular vein. The lymphoid tissue of the white pulp forms a sheath around the arterioles and contains both T and B cells together with macrophages and specialized antigen-presenting cells. The periarteriolar lymphoid sheaths contain germinal centres. The lymphoid tissue is surrounded by the marginal zone which contains specialized antigen-presenting cells, macrophages and slowly recirculating B cells.

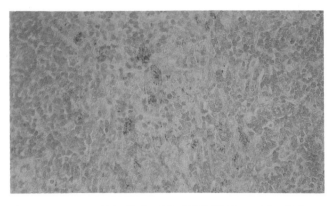

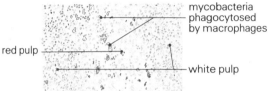

mycobacteria
phagocytosed
by macrophages

red pulp

white pulp

Fig. 3.9 Spleen section showing the red pulp macrophages. Microorganisms in the blood become trapped in the red pulp macrophages of the spleen, which are part of the reticulo-endothelial system. This high power view shows intravenously injected mycobacteria phagocytosed by the red pulp macrophages. Modified Ziehl-Neelsen stain, × 125. Courtesy of Dr. I. Brown

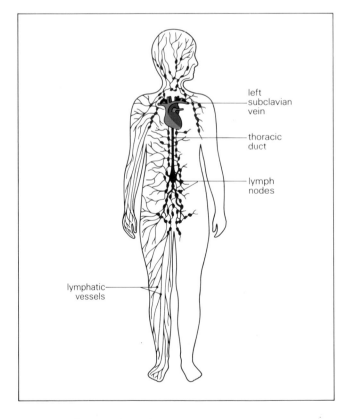

left
subclavian
vein

thoracic
duct

lymph
nodes

lymphatic
vessels

Fig. 3.10 The lymph node network. Lymph nodes are found at junctions of lymphatic vessels and form a complete network draining and filtering extravasated lymph from the tissue spaces. They are either superficial or visceral, draining the internal organs of the body. The lymph eventually collects in the thoracic duct which drains into the left subclavian vein and thus into the circulation.

Dendritic reticular cells and phagocytic macrophages are also found in germinal centres. Specialized macrophages are found in the marginal zone – the area surrounding the PALS. These, together with the dendritic follicular cells of the primary follicles, are the cells which present antigen to B cells. Lymphocytes are free to leave and enter the PALS via capillary branches of the central arterioles in the marginal zone and both T and B cells are found in this area. Some lymphocytes, especially maturing plasma-blasts, can pass across the marginal zone via bridges into the red pulp. The red pulp consists of sinuses lined by phagocytic macrophages, lymphocytes and in particular plasma cells (Fig. 3.9).

Lymph Nodes and the Lymphatic System

Lymph nodes form part of a body network which filters antigen from the tissue fluid or lymph during its passage from the periphery to thoracic duct (Fig. 3.10). Human lymph nodes are 1 to 25mm in diameter, round or kidney shaped and have an indentation, the hilus, where blood vessels enter and leave the node. Lymph nodes frequently occur at branches of the lymphatic vessels. Figure 3.11 shows a section across a typical lymph node which, like the spleen, is surrounded by a collagenous capsule which penetrates the organ.

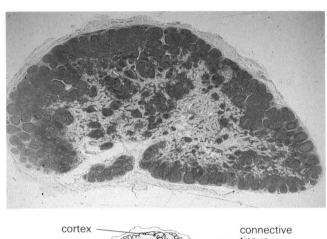

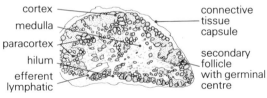

cortex

medulla

paracortex

hilum

efferent
lymphatic

connective
tissue
capsule

secondary
follicle
with germinal
centre

Fig. 3.11 Lymph node section. The lymph node is surrounded by a connective tissue capsule and organized into three main areas – the cortex (B cell area), the paracortex (T cell area) and the medulla, which contains cords of lymphoid tissue (T and B cell area). H & E stain, × 5. Courtesy of Mr. C. Symes.

The radial trabeculae together with reticulin fibres support the various cellular components within the lymph node. The lymph node is composed of a B cell area (cortex), a T cell area (paracortex) and central medulla which is also shown schematically in figure 13.12. The paracortex contains many antigen-presenting cells (interdigitating cells) which have large quantities of MHC class 2 antigens on their surface. The bulk of the lymphoid tissue is

Fig. 3.12 The structure of a lymph node. Beneath the collagenous capsule is the subcapsular sinus which is lined by phagocytic cells. Lymphocytes and antigens (if present) pass into the sinus via the afferent lymphatics from surrounding tissue spaces or adjacent nodes (see section below on lymphocyte traffic). The cortex contains aggregates of B cells (primary follicles) most of which (secondary follicles) have a focus of active proliferation (germinal centres). The paracortex mainly contains T cells, many of which are found in close apposition to the interdigitating cells (antigen-presenting cells). Each node has its own arterial and venous supply. Lymphocytes enter the node from the circulation through the specialized high endothelial vessels in the paracortex (high endothelial venule – HEV). The medulla contains both T and B cells and most of the lymph node

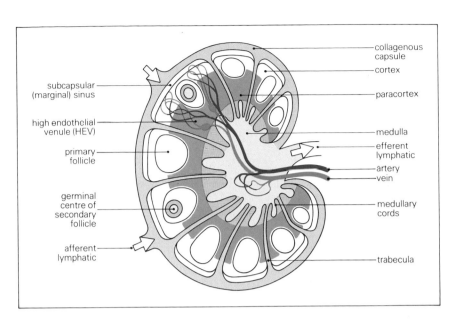

plasma cells organized into cords of lymphoid tissue. Lymphocytes can only leave the node through the efferent lymphatics.

found in the cortex and paracortex. Some lymphoid tissue extends into the medulla where it is found along strands of connective tissue fibres. These medullary cords are separated by large sinuses and contain the majority of plasma cells in the lymph node (Fig. 3.13). In addition, scavenger phagocytic cells are arranged along these fibres especially in the medulla. During passage of the lymph across the node from the afferent to the efferent lymphatics particulate antigens are removed by these phagocytic cells (Fig. 3.14).

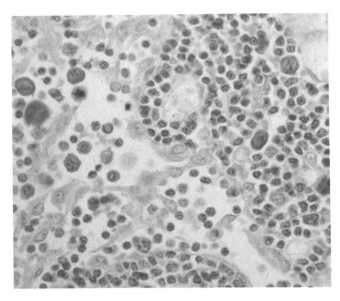

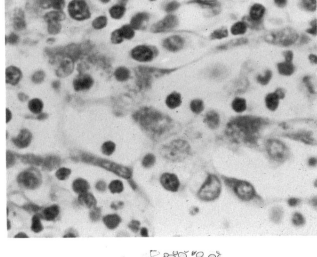

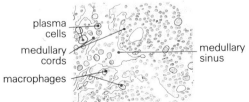

Fig. 3.13 Section of lymph node medulla showing plasma cells and phagocytic macrophages. This high power view shows typical plasma cells in the medullary cords and sinuses. Recirculating macrophages are also seen in this region. Methyl green pyronin stain, × 200.

Fig. 3.14 Section of lymph node medulla showing phagocytic macrophages. The macrophages which line the medullary cords can be seen following their uptake of the red dye, lithium carmine (counterstained with haematoxylin). × 330.

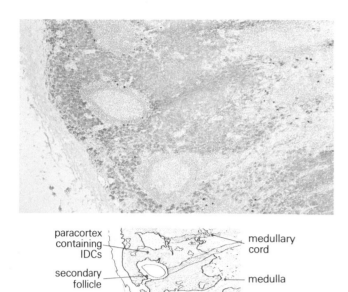

paracortex containing IDCs

secondary follicle

capsule

medullary cord

medulla

Fig. 3.15 Lymph node section showing paracortical proliferation. This micrograph shows a lymph node draining the skin area of a patient with chronic eczema. Antigens penetrating the skin are carried to draining lymph nodes by antigen-presenting cells which are normally present in the dermis – Langerhans cells. These cells are seen as 'veiled' cells in the afferent lymphatics and they settle in the paracortex as interdigitating reticulum cells (IDC), here stained with enzyme linked monoclonal antibody. T cell proliferation in response to specific antigen results in paracortical expansion. Haematoxylin counterstain, × 40.

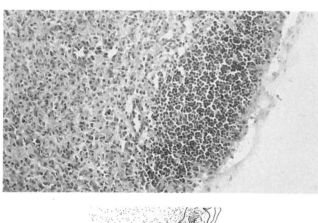

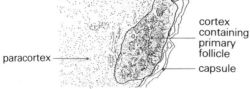

paracortex

cortex containing primary follicle

capsule

Fig. 3.16 Lymph node section from a congenitally athymic ('nude') mouse showing paracortical depletion. This high power view of the lymph node from a 'T-less' mouse shows few cells in the T-dependent paracortex. There are, however, large numbers of interdigitating reticulum cells within the paracortex in this node. The cortex is also poorly developed since T cells are required for the organization of the follicles. H & E stain, × 125. Courtesy of Dr. H. Dockrell.

The cortex contains aggregates of B cells (primary or secondary follicles) whilst T cells are localized primarily in the paracortex. If an area of skin is challenged by a T-dependent antigen, examination of the lymph nodes draining that area of skin shows active T cell proliferation in the paracortex (Fig. 3.15). On the other hand, patients with congenic thymic aplasia (DiGeorge syndrome) and neonatally thymectomized, or cogenitally athymic ('nude') mice or rats have fewer cells in the paracortex than normals (Fig. 3.16).

Germinal centres or secondary follicles are seen in antigen-stimulated lymph nodes. These are similar to the germinal centres seen in the B cell areas of the splenic PALS. The proliferative activity within the germinal centres is dependent on the age of the centre: young centres contain many centroblasts (follicle centre cells) whilst few are seen in old centres. The areas of active proliferation are surrounded by a mantle of lymphocytes (Fig. 3.17). The B lymphocytes in this area are rich in surface antibody of the IgD class, as detected by immunohistochemical staining (Fig. 3.18).

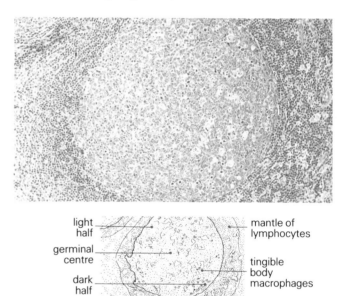

light half

germinal centre

dark half

mantle of lymphocytes

tingible body macrophages

Fig. 3.17 Secondary lymphoid follicle section showing a germinal centre. This human lymph node germinal centre contains actively proliferating B cells. Zoning of this centre may be seen as a light part and a more actively proliferating dark part, which contains the tingible body macrophages. There is a well developed mantle or corona of small resting lymphocytes. Giemsa stain, × 40.

In some secondary follicles this thickened mantle or corona is orientated towards the capsule of the node. Secondary follicles contain dendritic antigen-presenting cells and some macrophages in addition to a few T cells and natural killer cells (Fig. 3.19). These, together with specialized marginal sinus macrophages, appear to play a role in development of B cell responses and in particular B cell memory, which is probably the primary function of the germinal centres. Proliferating B cells within the germinal centres have a clearly defined nuclear shape which has been useful in defining malignant lymphoid proliferation (see 'Cells Involved in the Immune Response').

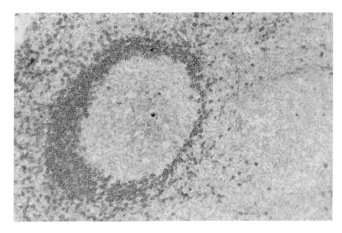

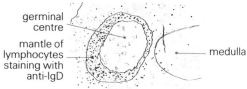

germinal centre

mantle of lymphocytes staining with anti-IgD

medulla

Fig. 3.18 Secondary lymphoid follicle section showing the mantle of lymphocytes around the germinal centre. High power magnification of a human lymph node germinal centre stained by anti-human IgD antibody labelled with horse radish peroxidase. Note that there are few IgD-positive cells in the centre itself. (Both areas, however, contain IgM-positive cells.) × 40.

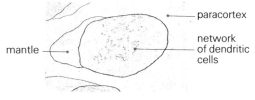

paracortex

network of dendritic cells

mantle

Fig. 3.19 Secondary lymphoid follicle section showing the reticular cell network. This lymph node germinal centre is stained with peroxidase-labelled monoclonal antibody to dendritic cells and macrophages. Note the extension of the network of reticulum cells into the mantle. Haematoxylin counterstain, × 40.

Mucosal Associated Lymphoid Tissue (MALT)
Dispersed aggregates of non-encapsulated lymphoid tissue are frequently found in a variety of organs, especially in the submucosal areas of the gastrointestinal,

respiratory and urinogenital tracts. These systems normally provide the main portal of entry into the body for foreign microorganisms. The lymphoid cells are present either as diffuse aggregates or organized into nodules containing germinal centres. Figure 3.20 illustrates diffuse accumulations of lymphoid tissue in the lamina propria of the intestinal wall. The Peyer's patches of the lower ileum are particularly prominent in young animals and frequently contain secondary follicles (Fig. 3.21).

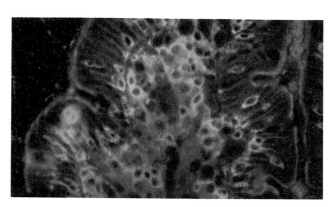

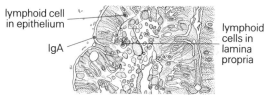

lymphoid cell in epithelium

IgA

lymphoid cells in lamina propria

Fig. 3.20 Section of human jejunum showing MALT. This shows lymphoid cells in the epithelium and lamina propria fluorescing green (using an anti-leucocyte monoclonal antibody, 2D1). Red cytoplasmic staining is obtained with anti-IgA antibody, which detects plasma cells in the lamina propria and IgA in the mucus. Courtesy of Professor G. Janossy.

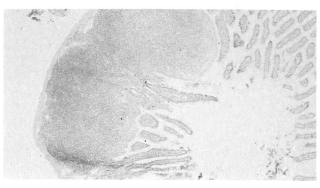

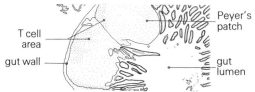

T cell area

gut wall

Peyer's patch

gut lumen

Fig. 3.21 Section of mouse ileum showing Peyer's patches in the MALT. The section shows the lymphoid tissue in the intestinal wall organized into Peyer's patches. Note the T cell areas, which are stained with peroxide labelled monoclonal antibody to the Thy–1 antigen on the T cell. Haematoxylin counterstain, × 40. Courtesy of Dr. E. Andrew.

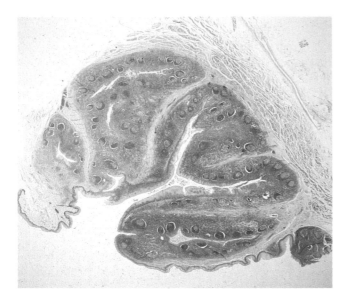

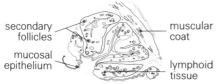

secondary follicles — muscular coat
mucosal epithelium — lymphoid tissue

Fig. 3.22 Section of human tonsil showing MALT. This low power view shows the large number of germinal centres frequently found in the tonsilar lymphoid tissue. H & E stain, × 4. Courtesy of Mr. C. Symes.

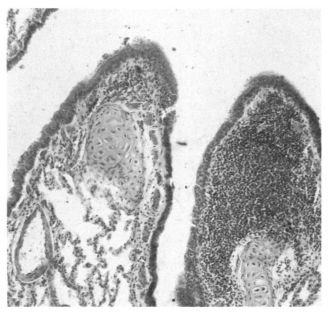

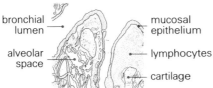

bronchial lumen — mucosal epithelium
alveolar space — lymphocytes
— cartilage

Fig. 3.23 Section of lung showing the MALT. This section shows a diffuse accumulation of lymphocytes in the bronchial wall. H & E stain, × 40.

The gut epithelium overlying the Peyer's patches is specialized to allow transport of antigens into, and possibly secretory IgA out of, the lymphoid tissue. Secretory IgA is an antibody which can traverse mucosal membranes and acts to protect them against infection. In man, the tonsils contain a considerable amount of lymphoid tissue which usually contains many germinal centres (Fig. 3.22). Similar accumulations of lymphoid tissue are seen lining the bronchi (Fig. 3.23) and along the urinogenital tract. Mucosal associated lymphoid tissue is important in the local immune response at mucosal surfaces.

LYMPHOCYTE RECIRCULATION

The migration of lymphocytes from the primary to secondary lymphoid tissues has already been described. Once in the secondary tissues the lymphocytes do not simply remain there but many move from one lymphoid organ to another through the blood and lymphatics. The recirculation routes are shown in figure 3.24.

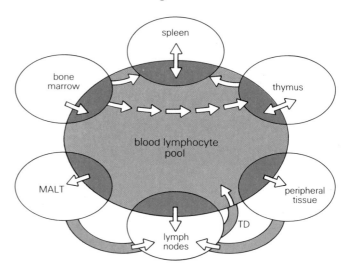

Fig. 3.24 Lymphocyte traffic. The lymphocytes in a mature animal move through the circulation (red) and the lymphatic ducts (orange) between various organs. The lymphocytes can traverse the endothelium (arrows) in particular organs and may become temporarily parked in the various organs which contain accumulations of lymphoid tissue. Newly formed T and B lymphocytes migrate into peripheral tissues and become functionally mature. Lymphocytes leave the vasculature via the high endothelial venule of the MALT and at other peripheral sites. They eventually return to the blood stream via the afferent lymphatics, lymph nodes, efferent lymphatics and ultimately through the thoracic duct (TD) into the venous circulation.

Although some lymphocytes can leave the blood circulation through non-specialized venules, the main exit route is through a specialized section of the post-capillary venules known as the high endothelial venule (HEV) (Fig. 3.25). In the lymph nodes these are mainly in the paracortex; recirculating lymphocytes interact with the columnar-shaped high endothelial cells of the HEV and pass between them (Fig. 3.26). In the lymph nodes all the lymphocytes return to the circulation via the efferent lymphatics which pass via the thoracic duct into the left subclavian vein. Some lymphocytes, primarily T cells, arrive from the drainage area of the node by way of the afferent lymphatics; this is the main route by which antigen enters the nodes.

Under normal conditions there is a continuous active flow of lymphocyte traffic through the nodes, but when antigen enters the lymph node of an animal already sensitized to the antigen there is a temporary shutdown in the traffic which lasts for approximately 24 hours. Thus, antigen-specific lymphocytes are preferentially retained in the lymph nodes draining the source of antigen, in particular blast cells do not recirculate but appear to remain in one particular site.

Lymphocytes also enter non-encapsulated lymphoid tissues such as tonsils and Peyer's patches via the HEV and pass into the afferent lymphatics of the draining lymph nodes. The main route of lymphocyte traffic into the spleen from the circulation is via the group of capillaries forming the marginal zone of the PALS. They leave through the marginal zone bridging channels into the splenic veins.

Each hour about 1 to 2% of the total recirculating lymphocyte pool migrates in this way. The overall effect of this process allows a large number of antigen-specific lymphocytes to 'home to' and come into contact with their appropriate antigen in the micro-environment of the peripheral lymphoid organs. This is particularly important since lymphoid cells are monospecific and there is only a finite number of lymphocytes capable of recognizing any particular antigenic shape. In addition to antigen-specific lymphocyte homing there is now evidence for a non-random migration of lymphocytes to particular lymphoid compartments. For example, lymphocytes which home to the gut are selectively transported across gut specific HEV. Other lymphocytes would home to lung tissue, and so on.

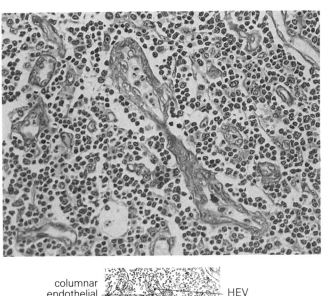

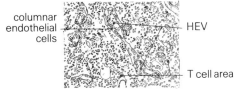

Fig. 3.25 Section of lymph node showing the high endothelial venule. This high power section of lymph node paracortex shows the specialized columnar-shaped high endothelial cells lining the HEV through which lymphocytes leave the circulation and enter the node. Giemsa stain (resin section), × 180.

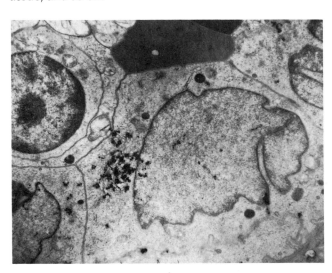

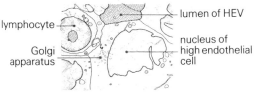

Fig. 3.26 Electron micrograph showing a high endothelial venule in the thymus dependent area of a lymph node. A lymphocyte can be seen in transit through the specialized capillary wall. The high endothelial cell is labelled with ^{35}S and grains occur over the Golgi apparatus. × 5000. Courtesy of Professor W. L. Ford.

FURTHER READING

McConnell I., Munro A. & Waldmann H. (1981) *The Immune System,* 2nd edition. Blackwell Scientific Publications, Oxford.

Osmond D.G. & Lala P.K. (1984) The Immune System. *Am.J.Anatomy,* **3.**

Stein H., Gerders J. & Mason D.Y. (1982) The normal and malignant germinal centre. In *Clinics in Haematology.* Janossy, G (ed.). W.B. Saunders, London.

Weiss L. (1972) The cells and tissues of the immune system: structure function interactions. Prentice-Hall, New Jersey.

4 Major Histocompatibility Complex

It has long been recognized that successful blood transfusion is dependent on matching the blood groups of donor and recipient red cells. In his Nobel lecture of 1931, Landsteiner suggested that similar 'blood groups' would be involved in the acceptance or rejection of other transplanted tissues. This idea led Gorer to the identification of a group of antigens in mice which, when matched between donor and recipient animals, markedly improved the ability of a graft to survive. The name histocompatibility antigens was coined for these antigens involved in graft rejection. It was also noted that the products of one particular region of the genome were of predominant importance in the rejection process. This region is the Major Histocompatibility Complex (MHC), referred to as H-2 in the mouse and located on chromosome 17. Analogous major histocompatibility systems have been found in all mammalian species studied so far. In man the major histocompatibility complex is the HLA gene cluster on chromosome 6. Recombination between extreme ends of the gene complex occurs at about 1% in human family studies, from which it can be calculated that HLA occupies about 1/3000th of the total genome. This means that there is room for several hundred individual genes. Although the MHC was originally identified by its role in transplant rejection, it is now recognized that proteins encoded in this region are involved in many aspects of immunological recognition, including interaction between different lymphoid cells, as well as between lymphocytes and antigen-presenting cells.

INHERITANCE OF MHC GENES

An individual inherits one maternal and one paternal chromosome 6, that is to say, one HLA haploid genotype (haplotype) is derived from each parent. Since there are a large number of gene loci in the MHC and much polymorphism within the loci, a normal population will have a very large number of different haplotypes. Many of the genetic studies on the MHC have been performed with inbred strains of mice.

Inbred Mouse Strains
In a normal outbred population the chromosome derived from the mother will differ from the same numbered chromosome derived from the father. To simplify the genetic analysis of complicated systems such as the MHC it is highly desirable to have animals with identical chromosomes from each parent (inbred animals), since progeny from these animals will have identical sets of autosomes (non-sex chromosomes) in all their gametes and therefore their offspring will have a predictable genotype.

It is possible to produce an inbred mouse strain by repeatedly inbreeding a strain with brother X sister

matings in successive generations. On average 50% of the chromosomes in two siblings derived from crossing outbred animals will be identical. If those two F_1 siblings were crossed there is a 25% chance (50% x 50%) that any particular pair of chromosomes in their F_2 progeny would be identical. All the descendants from crossing two such F_2 mice will now have identical pairs of that particular chromosome (Fig.4.1). Using this method of repeated inbreeding all the chromosome pairs will eventually become identical.

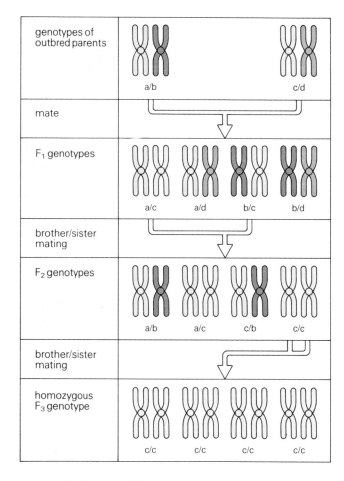

Fig.4.1 Production of inbred mice from two outbred parents. The parents in the normal outbred population differ at the same chromosome locus, that is, they have different haplotypes (a/b and c/d). An F_1 individual inherits one haplotype from each parent so that four possible genotypes may occur in the F_1 generation. Mating two F_1 individuals (eg. a/c and b/c) will give rise to F_2 offspring, some of which possess identical haplotypes (c/c). They are used as parents to produce a population of inbred individuals (F_3), all having identical sets of autosomes – c/c. Note that in this simplified scheme only one chromosome has become homozygous – about 20 generations will be required to produce animals identical with respect to all their autosomes.

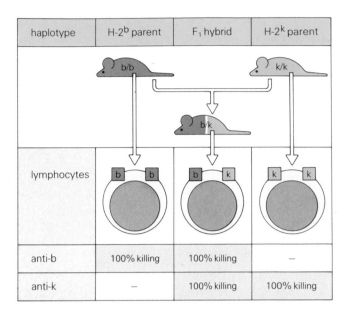

haplotype	H-2^b parent	F$_1$ hybrid	H-2^k parent
lymphocytes	b b	b k	k k
anti-b	100% killing	100% killing	—
anti-k	—	100% killing	100% killing

Fig. 4.2 Codominant expression of MHC antigens. Mice of two different genotypes, b/b (strain of haplotype H–2^b) and k/k (strain of haplotype H–2^k) are crossed. (In this diagram MHC antigens displayed on the lymphocyte surface are represented by squares.) Antiserum raised to lymphocytes of either parent (anti–b, anti–k) is found to kill lymphocytes of the F$_1$ hybrid. It is concluded that the F$_1$ hybrid is of genotype b/k and that its cells express the histocompatibility antigens of both parents.

Fig.4.3 The mouse MHC – a genetic map of the region of chromosome 17 in the mouse showing the H–2 and TLA gene complexes. The complexes are subdivided into regions, which produce the polypeptides indicated. Regions shaded emerald produce class 1 proteins, turquoise, class 2 proteins and light green, class 3 proteins (that is complement components). Earlier functional and serological studies subdivided the I region. The I–A region apparently corresponds to the section encoding Aβ, Aα and Eβ. The I–J region does not appear to encode a polypeptide directly and is therefore the subject of controversy. The I–E region (also called I–E/C) contains the Fα gene.

Fig.4.4 The human MHC – a genetic map of the region of chromosome 6 in the human showing the HLA gene complex. Regions B, C and A encode class 1 molecules, region D encodes α and β chains of the class 2 proteins, SB, DC and DR (carrying specificities DP, DQ and DR respectively – see Fig.4.11). The region between D and B encodes class 3 (complement) proteins including the tandem alleles of C4 and the genes for C2 and factor B (Bf). Polypeptides are bracketed if the precise gene order is uncertain.

Inbred individuals have identical haplotypes at the H-2 gene loci of both chromosomes. F$_1$ hybrids between two such inbred strains express (carry) histocompatibility antigens of both parental strains – expression of the MHC antigens is codominant (Fig.4.2).

ARRANGEMENT OF MHC GENES

As previously stated the MHC gene complex contains a large number of individual genes, and although the complex as a whole performs similar functions in different species, the detailed arrangement of genes within the MHC differs between species. For example, in mice the H-2 complex is divided into four regions, K, I, S and D.

Originally the different gene loci of the MHC were identified by functional and serological analysis but more recently complete genetic maps have been made of the mouse MHC. This has clarified which loci encode particular polypeptides, but there is still incomplete understanding of the way in which the polypeptides and proteins determine all the functions which have been mapped to the MHC. Since many of the MHC– encoded proteins were first identified by serological analysis they are frequently called MHC *antigens*.

The MHC proteins are of three different generic types as determined by their structures and functions. Class I proteins consist of two polypeptides. The larger peptide is encoded by the MHC, and this is non-covalently associated

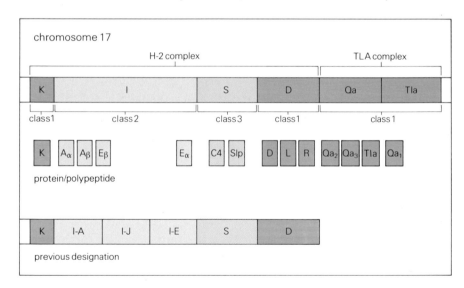

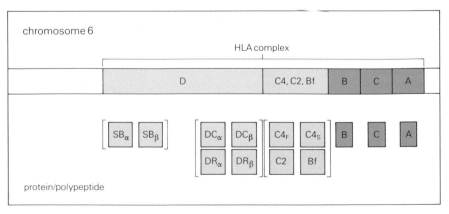

with the polypeptide β_2-microglobulin which is encoded outside the MHC. Class 2 proteins consist of two non-covalently associated peptides referred to as α chains and β chains both of which are encoded by the MHC. Class 3 proteins are those complement components which are coded by the MHC. There are additional gene loci outside the H-2 complex (the TLA complex) which also encode class 1 proteins and since these appear to have immunological functions they are also included on the genetic map of the region set out in figure 4.3.

In man the main regions are D, B, C and A (Fig.4.4). It appears that the A and B regions in man perform analogous functions to K and D in the mouse, that is they act as cell surface recognition molecules which can be identified by cytotoxic T cells. The D region of man is apparently analogous to the mouse I-region and contains genes for class 2 proteins which are involved in cooperation and interaction between cells of the immune system. Products of the mouse I region are termed Ia antigens, which is also the generic term of antigens encoded by the human D region. It is found that the strength of an immune response in mice is partly determined by immune response genes (Ir-genes) which map to the H-2I region. There is an enormous degree of structural polymorphism in the MHC of all the animals in which it has been studied as discussed in 'The Genetic Control of Immunity'.

CELLULAR DISTRIBUTION OF MHC ANTIGENS

In man essentially all nucleated cells carry the antigens of the A, B and C regions in varying amounts, but the antigens coded by the D region have a restricted distribution as do the analogous mouse I region antigens. I region antigens occur only on B lymphocytes, macrophages, monocytes and possibly epithelial cells; some I region antigens occur on suppressor T cells while some activated human T cells also have class 2 antigens (Fig.4.5).

MHC subregion		tissue distribution of antigen
H-2	HLA	
K, D, L	A, B, C	all nucleated cells and platelets, erythrocytes (mouse)
I-A I-E	D	B lymphocytes macrophages monocytes epithelial cells (?) melanoma cells activated T cells (human)
I-J		suppressor T lymphocytes

Fig. 4.5 The tissue distribution of the MHC antigens.
Emerald and turquoise colours are used here as in the previous figures to indicate the analogous functions performed by H–2 and HLA antigens. It should be noted that whereas mouse erythrocytes carry H–2K, D and L antigens, human erythrocytes do not carry the analogous HLA–A, B and C antigens. The genes of the mouse I–A and I–E regions encode the class 2 Ia antigens. A product for the I–J region has not been found but the region has been implicated in suppressor T cell function.

RECOMBINATION BETWEEN INBRED STRAINS

On rare occasions crossing over occurs within the H-2 region of F_1 mice of two parental inbred strains of different haplotype. These variants contain chromosomes with H-2 regions matching each parental strain in some of the regions only. The strains derived from these variants have been particularly valuable in determining the region of H-2 involved in each MHC function, since it is possible, for example, to transplant cells into a recipient that differs from the donor at only a small subregion of H-2. Examples of strains resulting from recombination between two inbred parental strains are given in figure 4.6.

strain	haplotype	K	I-A	I-E	S	D
B10	H-2^b	b	b	b	b	b
				X		
DBA/2	H-2^d	d	d	d	d	d
			⇩			
B10.GD, D2.GD	H-2^{g2}	d	d	b	b	b
other examples						
B10.A(4R)	H-2^{h4}	k	k	b	b	b
B10.A(2R)	H-2^{h2}	k	k	d	d	b
A.TH	H-2^{t2}	s	s	s	s	d

Fig.4.6 H–2 regions of some recombinant mouse strains.
The haplotype of an inbred strain is designated by a superscript, for example H–2^b and H–2^d, and the polypeptides produced by the MHC regions of a particular strain are designated by the same superscript. Mating F_1 individuals from two inbred strains (H–2^b and H–2^d) may sometimes result in a crossover in the I region, giving rise to a recombinant strain, for example of haplotype H–2^{g2}. Further crossovers involving other inbred strains produce the other examples of recombinant strains shown here.

STRUCTURAL VARIATION IN MHC ANTIGENS – PUBLIC AND PRIVATE SPECIFICITIES

If the antigens of a particular MHC region from different strains are examined they are found to have similar basic structures, but the fine structure of each antigen differs with each haplotype. These fine differences may be assessed by employing allo-antisera against the antigens. The antigens produced by an inbred strain will induce antibodies in strains lacking that haplotype and the reaction between the two will be characteristic. A standard panel of antisera has been established covering a wide range of inbred strains. Thus, particular MHC antigens may now be compared and defined with reference to the standard panel of antisera.

Using antisera it is possible to recognize antigenic determinants common to several different class 1 molecules or haplotypes, termed 'public' specificities, and also antigenic determinants unique to a particular molecule and haplotype termed 'private' specificities. The term specificity is derived from the 'specificity' of the 'tissue typing' antisera which are used to determine and define the antigenic determinants present on cells. An illustration of the difference between public and private specificities is given in figure 4.7.

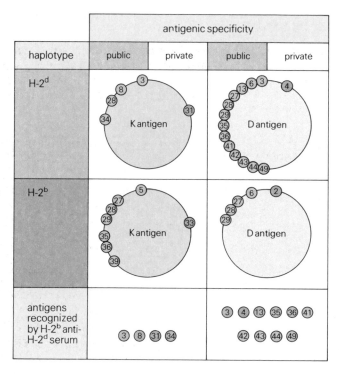

Fig.4.7 H–2 public and private specificities. In this figure large circles represent K and D antigens and the antigenic specificities carried by these antigens are indicated by circled numbers. Some specificities are shared between antigens and haplotypes, for example specificity 28 is carried on the K and D antigens of both the H–2^d and H–2^b strains. These are known as *public* specificities, shown here all on the left for convenience. A smaller number of specificities are unique to a particular antigen and haplotype and are known as *private* specificities. If an antiserum were raised in the H–2^b strain against antigens of the H–2^d strain it will recognize the private determinants (eg. 31 on the K antigen) and also the public determinants absent from its own cells (eg. 3, 8 and 34 on the K antigen) but not public determinants which it shares with the other strain (eg. 28).

Tissue Typing

The technique of using standardized antisera to investigate structural variation between MHC antigens has been mentioned. When such antisera are used in tissue typing (cf. blood typing) the tissue is said to have been typed serologically. This method of tissue typing is performed by applying antisera of defined specificity to the cells to be tested (usually lymphocytes) together with complement and then observing whether the test cells are killed (Fig.4.8). Other techniques of visualizing antibody binding by cells are also used occasionally.

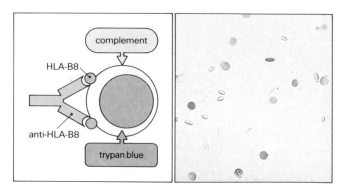

Fig.4.8 Tissue typing – serological. Tissue typing is performed serologically by adding typing antisera of defined specificity (eg. anti–HLA–B8), complement and trypan blue stain to test cells on a microassay plate. Cell death, as assessed by trypan blue staining, confirms that the test cell carried the antigen in question (HLA–B8). Dead, trypan blue-stained cells (dark staining) are shown on the right.

A second method of tissue typing exploits the fact that T lymphocytes are stimulated to grow in the presence of cells carrying foreign histocompatibility class 2 antigens, hence the name of the test, the Mixed Lymphocyte Reaction (MLR). In particular, the two types of cell must differ within the I region (mouse) or the HLA-D region (human) for this stimulation to occur. The test lymphocytes are mixed with homozygous typing cells (B lymphocytes with two identical haplotypes at the MHC) of defined specificity. In culture, test cells lacking the specificity of the typing cell recognize it as foreign and so are stimulated to undergo transformation and proliferation (Fig. 4.9).

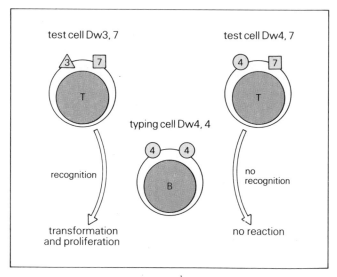

Fig.4.9 Tissue typing – Mixed Lymphocyte Reaction. In this example the homozygous typing cell is HLA–Dw 4,4 and antigenic specificities are represented by differently numbered shapes. Two different test lymphocytes are shown, Dw 3,7 and Dw 4,7. Dw 4,7 carries the typing cell's specificity (4), does not recognize Dw 4,4 as foreign, and does not react to the typing cell. Dw 3,7 recognizes the typing cell as foreign. This is revealed by the test cell transforming and proliferating. (Typing cells are treated to stop them dividing in response to the test cells.)

Proliferation may be detected by the uptake of ^{3}H-thymidine into DNA and transformed lymphocytes may be distinguished by their characteristic appearance (Fig. 4.10). HLA antigens determined by this technique are D specificities. It has recently proved possible to detect HLA–D region antigens serologically and these are called DR specificities. When the two typing procedures are apparently detecting identical antigens, identical numbers are given to both D and DR specificities but it is questionable whether the two techniques identify exactly the same part of the molecule. If a particular specificity has not been sufficiently well defined the letter w (for workshop) is added to the designation.

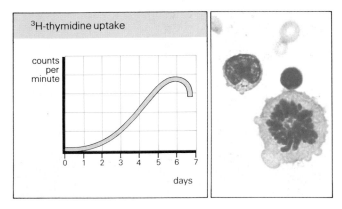

Fig.4.10 Lymphocyte proliferation and transformation in the MLR typing test. Proliferation of the test lymphocytes may be assessed by the uptake of radioactive thymidine (^{3}H thymidine) into DNA over a period of days (left). The appearance of transformed lymphocytes is shown on the right, with one cell in the process of division.

CURRENTLY RECOGNIZED HLA SPECIFICITIES AND LINKAGE DISEQUILIBRIUM

Many different specificities can be detected at each gene locus in the human population (Fig.4.11). Since virtually any A region antigen may be linked with any of the B, C or D antigens the number of haplotypes present in the human population is very large and, with two non-identical chromosomes, the total number of possible genotypes is correspondingly enormous. Under ideal conditions (a random breeding population at equilibrium) the frequency with which two specificities occur together in a population is given by the product of the individual gene frequencies. For example, if 16% of the population have a particular HLA-A antigen (A1) and 10% of the population have a particular HLA-B antigen (B8) the chance of finding A1 genetically linked to B8 on the same chromosome is given by the product of their gene frequencies (16% × 10% = 1.6%). In practice this does not always occur. Certain combinations of A and B specificities occur more frequently together than would be expected if their association were random. For example, the combination of A1 and B8 is found at a frequency of 8.8% in human populations, compared to an expected frequency of 1.6%. Such paired specificities are said to be in linkage disequilibrium (Fig.4.12). Two mechanisms may account for linkage disequilibrium:

DR		DQ (DC)	DP (SB)	B		C	A
DR1	Dw1	DQw1	DPw1	Bw4	Bw47	Cw1	A1
DR2	Dw2	DQw2	DPw2	B5	B48	Cw2	A2
DR3	Dw3	DQw3	DPw3	Bw6	B49	Cw3	A3
DR4	Dw4		DPw4	B7	Bw50	Cw4	A9
DR5			DPw5	B8	B51	Cw5	A10
DRw6			DPw6	B12	Bw52	Cw6	A11
DR7	Dw7			B13	Bw53	Cw7	Aw19
DRw8	Dw8			B14	Bw54	Cw8	A23
DRw9				B15	Bw55		A24
DRw10				B16	Bw56		A25
DRw11	Dw5			B17	Bw57		A26
DRw12				B18	Bw58		A28
DRw13	Dw6			B21	Bw59		A29
DRw14	Dw9			Bw22	Bw60		A30
DRw52				B27	Bw61		A31
DRw53				B35	Bw62		A32
				B37	Bw63		Aw33
				B38	Bw64		Aw34
				B39	Bw65		Aw36
				B40	Bw67		Aw43
				Bw41	Bw70		Aw66
				Bw42	Bw71		Aw68
				B44	Bw72		Aw69
				B45	Bw73		
				Bw46			

Fig.4.11 Currently recognized HLA specificities. This table lists the distinct antigenic specificities detected at each HLA subregion. HLA–A, –B, –C and DR (D-related) antigens are detected serologically. HLA–D specificities are also detected in the MLR. Specificities not yet sufficiently defined are designated by the subscript 'w'.

a) the origin of a specificity has occurred relatively recently and there has been insufficient time to allow the recombination events which distribute new specificities at random among the chromosomes in the population, or
b) some mechanism, evolutionary or otherwise, favours the association of that pair of genes (although any such mechanism remains obscure).

The phenomenon is not uncommon. For example, of the 300 possible combinations of known A and B locus alleles, 8 pairs show significant association. Linkage disequilibria are very common between B locus alleles and the closely genetically linked C locus alleles.

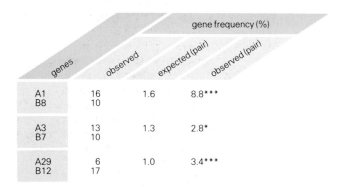

genes	observed	gene frequency (%)	
		expected (pair)	observed (pair)
A1 B8	16 10	1.6	8.8***
A3 B7	13 10	1.3	2.8*
A29 B12	6 17	1.0	3.4***

Fig.4.12 Examples of linkage disequilibrium. This table gives the frequencies of particular genes observed in European caucasoid populations, the frequency at which pairs of genes would be expected to occur on the same chromosome, and the frequency at which the pairs are actually observed together. The three pairs of genes shown here are more frequently associated than would be expected by chance. χ^2 analysis may be applied to the observed linkages (*=p<5%, ***=p<0.01%).

STRUCTURE OF THE MHC ANTIGENS

Recent work on the isolated MHC antigens has led to the elucidation of their structure. As might be anticipated for molecules involved in cell/cell recognition, the majority of the cellular MHC antigens are found in the plasma membrane. They are transmembrane glycoproteins and to perform structural analysis on them they must first be dissociated from the membrane. This may be achieved in two ways:

a) by releasing the intact proteins from the plasma membrane fraction with detergent, or
b) using the enzyme papain to clip off the section of the MHC molecule exposed at the cell surface.

When the molecules are dissociated enzymatically they are found to differ from the native MHC antigens, since they lack the part of the antigen which traverses the plasma membrane. Purification of the solubilized antigens may be performed by conventional biochemical techniques, including affinity chromatography, using lectins or antisera to the antigens under investigation (Figs. 4.13 & 4.14).

fraction	isolation	relative purity	
		HLA-A2	HLA-la
cells	lysis / sucrose density gradient	1	1
plasma membrane		45	45
detergent-soluble proteins	detergent	41	51
gel filtration fractions	gel filtration	136	158
purified fraction	lentil lectin columns (la, A2)	1240	1390

Fig. 4.13 Biochemical purification of the HLA–A2 (emerald) and la (turquoise) antigens from human lymphoblastoid cells. This illustration charts the isolation of the MHC products from cells and gives the relative purity of the antigens at each stage of purification, expressed as specific MHC protein/total protein. The purity increases as MHC antigens are separated from non-MHC proteins (blue), in successive steps. In the first stage the cells are lysed and the subcellular components separated by ultracentrifugation in a sucrose density gradient. The fraction containing the plasma membrane (rich in MHC and other proteins) is treated with detergent (sodium deoxycholate) in order to release the proteins, which are then subjected to gel filtration (on AcA34). The fractions containing HLA–A2 and la antigens are further purified on lentil lectin columns which specifically bind the HLA antigens. The antigens are eluted by adding sugar which competitively binds to the lectin.

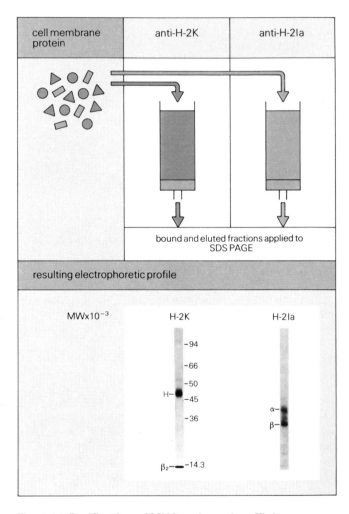

Fig. 4.14 Purification of MHC antigens by affinity chromatography. This technique employs columns carrying antibodies directed against specific MHC antigens. Protein, isolated from cell membrane is introduced into columns containing antibody against specific MHC proteins. The columns are washed thoroughly to remove unbound membrane proteins, then specific antigens are eluted from the columns in conditions which dissociate the antigen/ antibody interaction. They are then subjected to electrophoresis in reducing conditions (sodium dodecyl sulphate polyacrylamide gel electrophoresis—SDS PAGE). SDS PAGE separates the constituent polypeptides on the basis of molecular weight. The electrophoretic profile reveals that the H–2K and la proteins each consist of two subcomponents of different molecular weight (H and β_2, α and β respectively). Affinity chromatography makes it possible to isolate individual antigens in a single step.

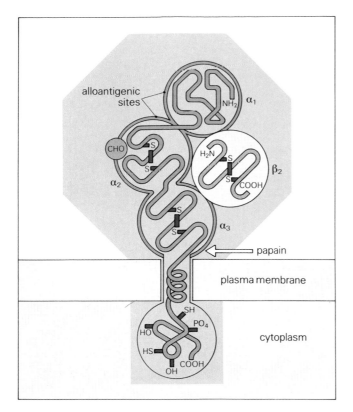

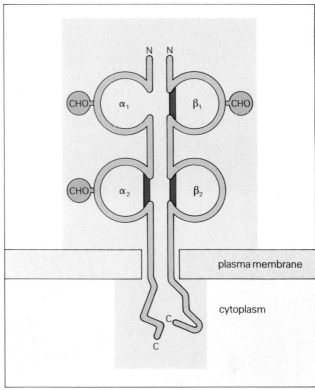

Fig.4.15 Structure of an intact class 1 antigen (HLA–A, –B) in plasma membrane. The MHC-encoded chain has three globular domains (termed α1, α2 and α3 shown in green). The α3 domain is closely associated with the non-MHC-encoded peptide, β₂–microglobulin (grey). β₂–microglobulin is a small globular peptide of molecular weight 12,000 which is stabilized by an intrachain disulphide bond (red) and has a similar tertiary structure to an immunoglobulin domain. A short hydrophilic section of the MHC–encoded component at the –COOH terminus lies within the cytoplasm. A hydrophobic section traverses the membrane and the majority of the polypeptide, comprising the three globular domains, protrudes from the cell surface. Alloantigenic sites (carrying determinants specific to each individual) occur on the α1 and α2 domains and there is a carbohydrate unit attached to the α2 domain (CHO). Papain cleaves the molelcule at the point indicated, close to the outer margin of the plasma membrane.

Fig.4.16 Schematic representation of a class 2 antigen (HLA–DR). The HLA–DR antigens consist of two non-identical peptides (α and β) non-covalently bound together which traverse the plasma membrane towards the C terminus. Both chains have two globular domains. These are structurally related to immunoglobulin domains and all except the α1 domain are stabilized by intrachain disulphide bonds (red). Both chains have carbohydrate units attached. The shorter, β chain (mol. wt. 28,000) contains the alloantigenic sites although there is also some structural polymorphism in the α chain of some class 2 molecules.

Purification of MHC antigens by affinity chromatography on monoclonal antibody columns possesses several advantages over biochemical purification techniques. In particular, the 'one-step' nature of the approach results in rapidity, high yield and minimal degradation. Contamination is, however, often a problem due to non-specific adherence of other membrane proteins, in particular actin. This can be overcome by using a combination of the two approaches, for example, applying a glycoprotein fraction, isolated using lentil lectin chromatography, to a monoclonal antibody column.

The structure of the class 1 antigens differs from that of the class 2 antigens. Each class 1 antigen consists of one glycosylated polypeptide chain of molecular weight about 45,000 non-covalently associated with a non-glycosylated peptide (β₂–microglobulin) (about

12,000D) (Fig.4.15). β₂–microglobulin also occurs free in serum or urine as a small globular peptide which has a similar tertiary structure to an immunoglobulin constant region domain. It is bound non-covalently to the α₃ domain of the class 1 heavy chain on the outer side of the plasma membrane. Although β₂–microglobulin does not form part of the antigenic site of the HLA molecule, it is necessary for processing and expression of the class 1 molecules and thus if a cell congenitally lacks β₂–microglobulin the class 1 antigenic determinants are not expressed. The gene for β₂–microglobulin lies on a separate chromosome to that containing the MHC gene loci. Comparison of the amino acid sequences from different haplotypes of the human HLA–A and –B antigens and the mouse H–2K and H–2D antigens implies that the alloantigenic sites occur on the α₁ and α₂ domains (see 'The Genetic Control of Immunity').

The structure of the class 2 antigens is less well established: they consist of two distinct polypeptide chains (α and β) held together by non-covalent forces, both chains traversing the plasma membrane. The shorter chain contains the alloantigenic sites, and both chains carry carbohydrate units (Fig.4.16).

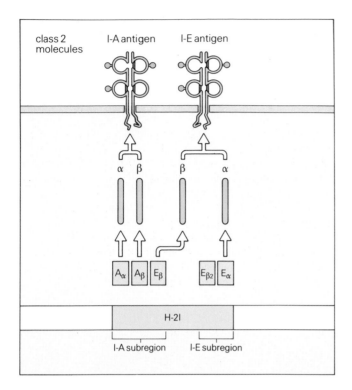

Fig. 4.17 Genetic organization of the mouse H–2I region.
The H–2I region codes for antigens consisting of α and β
chains. The two types of antigen identified (I–A and I–E) are of
similar size but differ in detailed structure. The genes for the
Aα and Aβ chains are in the I–A subregion, which also
probably includes the gene for Eβ. Another Eβ gene (Eβ₂) and
the Eα gene are in the I–E subregion.

The genetic organization of the mouse H–2I region is
better understood than the human HLA–D region, and
genetic analysis of crossovers within this region has
allowed subdivision of the H–2I region. Although structurally similar molecules are produced by all H–2I region
genes so far studied, different subcomponents of the same
H–2I molecule are encoded within different sub-
regions (Fig. 4.17).

Examination of the isolated α and β peptides of I–E antigens from mice of different haplotypes indicates that the
majority of allotypic variation occurs in the β chain (as is
the case with the HLA–D antigen). There is also some
evidence that limited allotypic variation may also occur
in the α chain of the H–2I antigens. A demonstration of β
chain variability is described in figure 4.18.

FUNCTIONS OF THE MHC ANTIGENS

The MHC antigens are essential for reactions of immune
recognition. Different MHC antigens are recognized by
different T cell types as summarized in figure 4.19. Cytotoxic T cells involved in recognition and rejection of virally infected cells and foreign tissue grafts recognize H–2K
and H–2D molecules (HLA–A and –B in human) on the
foreign cells, and in cooperation with T–helper cells they
will cause destruction of the foreign cells. Evidently the
rejection of foreign tissue grafts has no normal physiological function, but the processes involved in recognition
of foreign antigenic determinants on cell surfaces are
similar to those necessary for recognition of viral antigens
displayed on the membranes of infected cells.

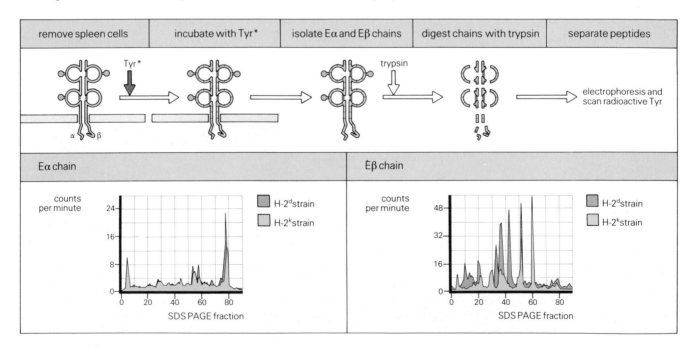

**Fig. 4.18 An experimental demonstration of β chain
variability in I–E antigens.** Spleen cells of two different mice
strains (H–2ᵏ and H–2ᵈ haplotypes) were removed and
incubated with ³H–labelled tyrosine (Tyr). When Tyr had
become incorporated into the I–E antigen the Eα and Eβ
chains were isolated, digested with trypsin and the resulting
peptides analysed electrophoretically. The two graphs

(referred to as tryptic peptide maps) display the radioactivity
(³H–tyrosine) in each fraction. The radioactivity of each
fraction of Eα chain is similar for the two haplotypes,
indicating that the peptides produced are similar. By contrast,
the profiles of the Eβ chains are totally dissimilar for the two
haplotypes, indicating that allotypic variation is primarily
confined to the β chains in these antigens.

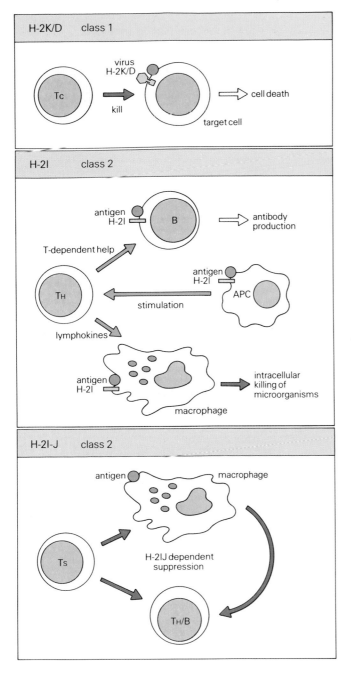

Most virally-infected cells display viral antigens on the surface of their plasma membranes–these antigens are recognized by T–cytotoxic cells. Furthermore it may be demonstrated that T–cytotoxic cells recognize the viral antigens in association with their recognition of the H–2K and –D antigens present on the surface of the infected cells. In this way T–cytotoxic cells of a particular H–2 haplotype from an animal infected with a virus are primed to kill cells infected with that virus. However, it is found that they will not kill cells of a different haplotype infected by the same virus. This phenomenon is referred to as haplotype restricted killing. Since the T–cytotoxic cells have been primed by a combined recognition of H–2 and viral antigens they can only subsequently kill cells carrying both antigen types. In effect the H–2 molecules on the surface of the virally-infected cell act as a code, guiding the T–cytotoxic cell to its target, and allowing it to differentiate the target cell from other tissues carrying the viral antigens (Fig. 4.20).

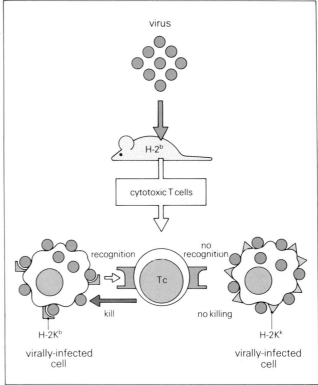

Fig.4.20 Killing of virally-infected target cells and haplotype restricted killing. A mouse of the H–2^b haplotype is primed with virus, and the cytotoxic T cells thus generated are then isolated. These T cells are then tested for their ability to kill cells of the H–2^b and H–2^k haplotypes infected with the same virus. The Tc cells kill H–2^b infected cells but not infected cells of a different haplotype, H–2^k. It is concluded that the T cell is recognizing a specific structure resulting from the association between the H–2K (or H–2D) product and viral antigen (eg. a virus/H–2K complex). The association between antigen and MHC protein may be at the molecular level or at the cellular level as shown in the next figure. (As a control measure, both groups are treated with anti-viral antibody, which does not exhibit haplotype restriction: infected cells of both haplotypes are killed by anti-viral antibody and complement.)

Fig.4.19 A summary of the biological functions of the MHC in the mouse.
H-2K/D. Cytotoxic T cells (Tc) recognize foreign antigen (eg. virus) when associated with either H–2K or H–2D products and kill the target cell.
H-2I. Helper T cells (Tн) recognize foreign antigen in association with H–2I gene products on antigen-presenting cells (APC). Tн cells can cooperate with B cells to induce antibody production and they can also release lymphokines, which help macrophages to kill intracellular microorganisms.
H-2IJ. Suppressor T cells (Ts) specifically suppress the action of macrophages, B cells and T–helper cells which are induced by particular foreign antigens. The action of Ts cells is apparently related to their I–J region haplotype and the interaction between Ts and their targets is most efficient when Ts and target share the same I–J haplotype. Products of the I–J region have not been found and the basis for this observation is still under investigation.

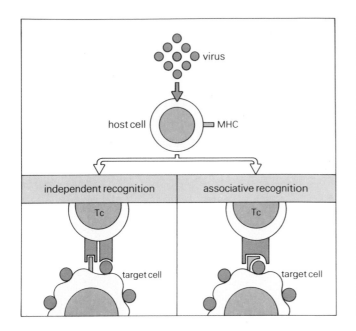

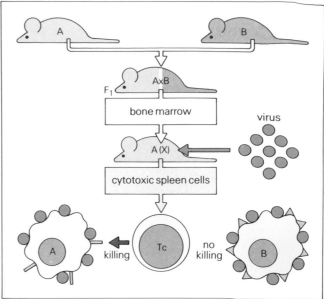

Fig.4.21 Two hypotheses for the recognition by Tc cells of viral and MHC antigens on infected target cells. Once a cell becomes infected by a virus and carries the viral antigens on its surface, it becomes a target for the host's Tc cells. The Tc cells may either recognize the viral and MHC antigens independently, or a combination of viral and MHC antigen. In associative recognition the T cell may recognize either antigen and MHC together or altered MHC (as shown here).

It is still not certain how the T– cytotoxic cell recognizes the dual specificity of viral and MHC antigen expressed on the target cell, either:
1. the T–cytotoxic cell recognizes both the viral antigen and the MHC antigen independently, or
2. a combination of the viral antigen and the MHC antigen in association on the cell surface produces an altered conformation of the MHC molecule. This condition may be recognized as altered self.
These two hypotheses are illustrated in figure 4.21. The principle of haplotype restricted killing described above,

Fig.4.22 Host education of cytotoxic T cells. Two inbred mice (A,B) are crossed. Bone marrow cells are transferred from the F_1 (A×B) into a mouse of parental strain A, whose own immune system has been destroyed by X–irradiation (X). This strain A mouse is then primed with virus. Cytotoxic cells are isolated from the spleen and it is found that these F_1 cells will kill virally-infected cells of strain A but not strain B. This haplotype restricted cytotoxicity to strain A virus-infected target cells indicates that the F_1 (A×B) Tc cells recognize virus in association with host (A) MHC antigens since they have been educated in a strain A environment. Other experiments show that the thymus is the important organ in producing this MHC specificity.

suggests that during priming, an individual's T cells recognize both the foreign antigen and MHC determinants. Immature T cells initially learn to discriminate between self and non-self determinants in the thymus, a process termed thymic education. Normally this thymic environment is the individual's own thymus, consequently

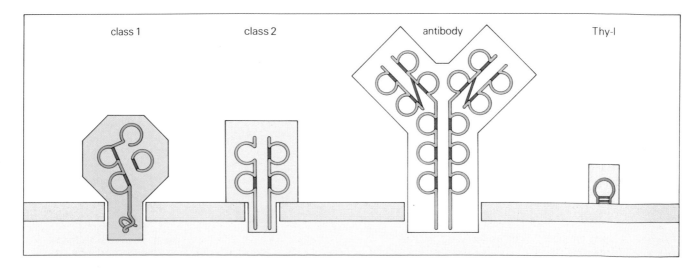

Fig.4.23 Molecules of the immune system. The MHC class 1 and 2 antigens, the immunoglobulins and the T cell surface marker Thy–1 all have related domain structures and are probably evolutionarily related.

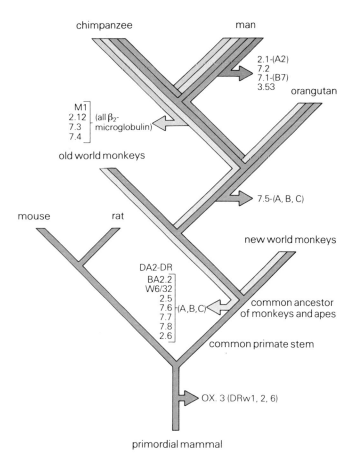

Fig.4.24 **Development of MHC specificities.** This evolutionary tree traces the appearance of new MHC determinants. It should be emphasized that the shape of the tree is not derived from the MHC determinants but is based on other considerations. The older specificities shown are named after the monoclonal antibodies employed to detect them. Thus OX.3 is a monoclonal antibody recognizing rat Ia antigens and also a cross-reacting determinant on HLA.DR1, 2.6. W6/32 is a monoclonal antibody which recognizes a determinant common to the HLA—A, —B, —C antigens and transplantation antigens of old world monkeys. The colours show the representation of the various determinants in different species. The molecules recognized are bracketed.

T cells are educated to recognize foreign antigen and self MHC. However, experimental situations may be created in which an individual's T cells are developed in a thymic environment of a different haplotype (Fig. 4.22).

Similar principles of haplotype restriction apply to T—helper cells which recognize antigen on macrophages and B cells in association with H—2I region antigens. In this case the I region antigens act as recognition signals between antigen-presenting cells and the lymphocyte.

One rationalization for the evolution of a joint recognition system for MHC antigen plus viral antigen is that by recognizing viral antigen in association with MHC antigen, receptors on cytotoxic T cells do not become saturated with free virus: saturation would inhibit the cytotoxic T cells from killing virally—infected cells.

Many of the functions of the MHC will be discussed more fully in connection with other aspects of the immune system since the MHC is involved in most

disease	antigen	frequency of antigen		
		control	patients	relative risk
Ankylosing spondylitis	B27	8	90	87.8
Reiter's disease	B27	9	80	35.9
Rheumatoid arthritis	DRw4	31	64	4.0
Multiple sclerosis	A3	21	33	1.8
	B7	18	35	2.0
	Bw2	21	74	1.9
	DRw2	22	42	3.8
Myasthenia gravis	B8	16	39	3.4
	DRw3	17	40	3.0
Psoriasis	A1	26	39	2.1
	B13	6	21	8.7
	Bw37	2	4	8.1
	Cw6	23	70	4.3
Addison's disease	Dw3	21	70	8.8
Grave's disease	B8	18	44	2.5
	Bw35	20	57	5
	Dw3	53	18	5.5
Coeliac disease	B8	20	67	8.6
	Dw3	27	96	73.0
Hemochromatosis	A3	20	71	9.0
Active chronic hepatitis	B8	16	36	9.2
	DRw3	7	79	4.6

Fig.4.25 **Disease associations of HLA antigens in European caucasoids.** This table lists some diseases which are associated with particular HLA antigens. The extent to which an individual carrying the antigen is more likely to contract the disease, relative to an individual without the determinant, is given in the relative risk column. (The Bw 35 association is based on a study in Japan.)

reactions of immune recognition. Indeed recent evidence suggests that the MHC and other molecules involved in immune recognition share sequence homologies and may therefore be related evolutionarily to a basic primordial recognition molecule as discussed in 'The Genetic Control of Immunity' (Fig.4.23).

It is pertinent to speculate at this point on the enormous amount of allotypic variation observed in the MHC region antigens. The development of new MHC specificities can be seen in different but related species (Fig.4.24). The reason for the great variation is not known, but it has been suggested that by carrying a large number of different MHC molecules there is less likelihood that a microbe could evade the body's immune system by imitating one of the recognition molecules of the system. Moreover when seen at a population level the self/non-self recognition systems of different individuals are all different, though working on the same principle. Since the immune system of each individual is different the 'perfect pathogen' cannot evolve to spread through a population. Despite this, it is known that the possession of particular MHC antigens renders that individual more susceptible to particular diseases, some examples of which are given in figure 4.25.

FURTHER READING

Kaufman J.F., Auffray C., Korman A.J., Shackelford D.A. & Strominger J.L. (1984) The Class II Molecules of the Human Murine Major Histocompatibility Complex. *Cell* **36,** 1.

Owen M.J. & Crumpton M.J. (1980) Biochemistry of major human histocompatibility antigens. *Immunol. Today* **1,** 117.

Ploegh H.L., Orr H.T. & Strominger J.L. (1981) Major Histocompatibility Antigens: The Human (HLA-A, -B, -C) and Murine (H-2K, H-2D) Class I Molecules. *Cell* **24,** 287.

Strominger J.L. et al (1980) In *The Role of the Major Histocompatibility Complex in Immunobiology.* Benacerraf B. & Dorf M. (eds.) Garland Publishing Inc., New York.

Zinkernagel R.M. & Doherty P.C. (1979) MHC-Restricted Cytotoxic T Cells: Studies on the Biological Role of Polymorphic Major Transplantation Antigens Determining T-Cell Restriction – Specificity, Function, and Responsiveness. *Adv. Immunol.* **27,** 51.

5 Antibody Structure and Function

The immunoglobulins, or antibodies are a group of glyco-proteins present in the serum and tissue fluids of all mammals. Their production is induced when the host's lymphoid system comes into contact with immunogenic foreign molecules (antigens) and they bind specifically to the antigen which induced their formation. They are therefore an element of the adaptive immune system.

present nomenclature	shorthand	previous nomenclature
immunoglobulin G	IgG	γ G globulin 7S γ-globulin
immunoglobulin A	IgA	γ A globulin β₂ A-globulin
immunoglobulin M	IgM	γ M globulin 19S γ-globulin γ -IM γ -macroglobulin
immunoglobulin D	IgD	γ -SJ
immunoglobulin E	IgE	Reagin, IgND

Fig. 5.1 Nomenclature of the five classes of immunoglobulin molecule. These are the five classes recognized in most higher mammals.

THE FIVE IMMUNOGLOBULIN CLASSES

Five distinct classes of immunoglobulin molecule are recognized in most higher mammals, namely IgG, IgA, IgM, IgD and IgE (Fig. 5.1). These differ from each other in size, charge, amino acid composition and carbohydrate content. In addition to the differences between classes the immunoglobulins within each class are also very heterogeneous. Electrophoretically the immunoglobulins show a unique range of heterogeneity which extends from the γ to the α fractions of normal serum. In general it is the IgG class which exhibits most charge heterogeneity, the other classes having a more restricted mobility in the slow β and fast γ regions (Fig. 5.2). The basic four chain polypeptide structure of the immunoglobulin molecule is represented in figure 5.3.

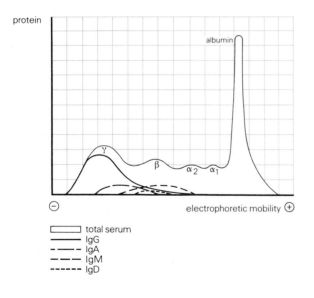

Fig. 5.2 Immunoelectrophoresis of human serum showing the distribution of the four major immunoglobulin classes. Serum proteins are separated according to their charge in an electric field, and classified as α₁, α₂, β, and γ, depending on their mobility. (The IgE class has a similar mobility to IgD but cannot be represented quantitatively because of its low level in serum.) IgG exhibits most charge heterogeneity, the other classes having a more restricted mobility in the slow β and fast γ regions. These fractions suffer marked depletion following absorption with antigen suggesting a role for them in the immune response.

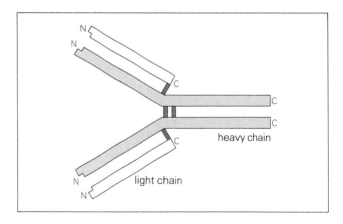

Fig. 5.3 The basic immunoglobulin structure. The unit consists of two identical light polypeptide chains and two identical heavy polypeptide chains linked together by disulphide bonds (red). Note the position of the amino (N) and carboxy (C) terminal ends of the peptide chains.

ANTIBODY FUNCTION

Essentially each immunoglobulin molecule is bi-functional; one region of the molecule is concerned with binding to antigen while a different region mediates binding of the immunoglobulin to host tissues, including various cells of the immune system, some phagocytic cells, and the first component (C1q) of the classical complement system.

IMMUNOGLOBULIN CLASSES AND SUBCLASSES

The basic structure of all immunoglobulin molecules is a unit consisting of two identical light polypeptide chains and two identical heavy polypeptide chains linked together by disulphide bonds. The class and subclass of an immunoglobulin molecule is determined by its heavy chain type. Thus the four human IgG subclasses (IgG1, IgG2, IgG3 and IgG4) have heavy chains called $\gamma1$, $\gamma2$, $\gamma3$, and $\gamma4$ which differ only slightly although all are recognizably γ heavy chains. The differences between the various subclasses within an immunoglobulin class are less than the differences between the different classes; thus IgG1 is more closely related to IgG2, 3, or 4 than to IgA, IgM, IgD or IgE.

The four subclasses of human IgG occur in the approximate proportions of 66, 23, 7 and 4 per cent respectively. There are also known to be subclasses of human IgA (IgA1 and IgA2) but none have been unambiguously described for the other classes. Immunoglobulin subclasses appear to have arisen after speciation and the human subclasses cannot be compared with, for example, the four known subclasses of IgG which have been identified in the mouse.

THE OCCURRENCE AND PHYSICOCHEMICAL PROPERTIES OF IMMUNOGLOBULINS

IgG is the major immunoglobulin in normal human serum accounting for 70-75% of the total immunoglobulin pool. IgG is a monomeric protein with a sedimentation coefficient of 7S and a molecular weight of 146,000. However, studies of IgG subclasses have indicated that IgG3 proteins are slightly larger than the other subclasses and this increase is due to the slightly heavier $\gamma3$ chain. The IgG class is distributed evenly between the intra- and extravascular pools, is the major antibody of secondary immune responses and the exclusive anti-toxin class.

IgM accounts for about 10% of the immunoglobulin pool. The molecule has a pentameric structure in which individual heavy chains have a molecular weight of approximately 65,000 and the whole molecule has a molecular weight of 970,000. This protein is largely confined to the intravascular pool and is the predominant 'early' antibody frequently directed against antigenically complex infectious organisms.

IgA represents 15-20% of the human serum immunoglobulin pool. In man more than 80% of IgA occurs as the basic four chain monomer but in most mammals the IgA in serum is mainly polymeric, occurring mostly as a dimer. IgA is the predominant immunoglobulin in seromucous secretions such as saliva, tracheobronchial secretions, colostrum, milk and genito-urinary secretions. Secretory IgA (sIgA) which may be of either subclass, exists mainly in the 11S, dimeric form and has a molecular weight of 385,000. sIgA is abundant in seromucous secretions and is protected from proteolysis by combination with another protein – the secretory component.

IgD accounts for less than 1% of the total plasma immunoglobulin but it is known to be present in large quantities on the membrane of many circulating B lymphocytes. The precise biological function of this class is not known but it may play a role in antigen-triggered lymphocyte differentiation.

IgE though a trace serum protein, is found on the surface membrane of basophils and mast cells in all individuals. This class may play a role in active immunity to helminthic parasites but in Western countries is more commonly associated with immediate hypersensitivity diseases such as asthma and hayfever.

All immunoglobulins appear to be glycoproteins but the carbohydrate content ranges from 2-3% for IgG to 12-14% for IgM, IgD and IgE. The physicochemical properties of the immunoglobulins are summarized in figure 5.4. The diversity of structure of the different classes suggests that they perform different functions, in addition to their primary function of antigen binding. In spite of this diversity all antibodies have a common basic structure.

Immunoglobulin	IgG1	IgG2	IgG3	IgG4	IgM	IgA1	IgA2	sIgA	IgD	IgE
heavy chain	γ_1	γ_2	γ_3	γ_4	μ	α_1	α_2	$\alpha_1 or \alpha_2$	δ	ϵ
mean serum concentration (mg/ml)	9	3	1	0.5	1.5	3.0	0.5	0.05	0.03	0.00005
sedimentation constant	7S	7S	7S	7S	19S	7S	7S	11S	7S	8S
molecular weight	146,000	146,000	170,000	146,000	970,000	160,000	160,000	385,000	184,000	188,000
molecular weight of heavy chain	51,000	51,000	60,000	51,000	65,000	56,000	52,000	52-56,000	69,700	72,500
number of heavy chain domains	4	4	4	4	5	4	4	4	4	5
carbohydrate (%)	2-3	2-3	2-3	2-3	12	7-11	7-11	7-11	9-14	12

Fig. 5.4 Physicochemical properties of human immunoglobulin classes. Each class possesses a characteristic type of heavy chain. Thus IgG possesses γ chains; IgM, μ chains; IgA, α chains, IgD, δ chains and IgE, ϵ chains. Variation in heavy chain structure within a class gives rise to immunoglobulin subclasses. For example the human IgG pool consists of four subclasses reflecting four distinct types of γ heavy chain. The physicochemical properties of the immunoglobulins vary between the different classes. Note that IgA occurs in a dimeric form (sIgA) in association with a protein chain termed the secretory piece.

ANTIBODY STRUCTURE

In 1962 Rodney Porter proposed a basic four chain model for immunoglobulin molecules (as shown in Fig. 5.3) which is based on two distinct types of polypeptide chain. The smaller (light) polypeptide chain has a molecular weight of 25,000 and is common to all classes of immunoglobulin whereas the larger (heavy) chain has a molecular weight of 50,000-77,000 and is structurally distinct for each class or subclass. The polypeptide chains of immunoglobulins are linked together by covalent and non-covalent forces to give a four chain structure based on pairs of identical heavy and light chains. IgG, IgD and IgE occur only as monomers of the four chain unit, IgA occurs in both monomeric and polymeric forms and IgM occurs as a pentamer with five four-chain subunits linked together.

The light chains of most vertebrates have been shown to exist in two distinct forms called kappa (κ-type) and lambda (λ-type). They may be distinguished by their behaviour as antigens – antisera may be raised to one type which do not react with the other. Either of the light chain types may combine with any of the heavy chain types, but in any one molecule both light chains are of the same type and hybrid molecules do not occur naturally.

The work of Hilschmann, Craig and others in 1965 established that when light chains of the same type are sequenced they are found to consist of two distinct regions. The carboxyterminal half of the chain (approximately 107 amino acid residues) is constant except for certain allotypic and isotypic variations (see below) and is called the C_L (Constant:Light chain) region, whereas the amino terminal half of the chain shows much sequence variability and is known as the V_L (Variable: Light chain) region.

The IgG molecule may be considered as a typical example of the basic antibody structure. As shown in figure 5.5 IgG has two intrachain disulphide bonds in the light chain – one in the variable and one in the constant region. Similarly, there are four such bonds in the heavy (γ) chain, which is twice the length of a light chain. Each disulphide bond encloses a peptide loop of 60-70 amino acid residues and if the amino acid sequences of these loops are compared a striking degree of homology is revealed. Essentially this means that each immunoglobulin peptide chain is composed of a series of globular regions with a very similar secondary and tertiary structure (folding). The peptide loops enclosed by the disulphide bonds represent the central portion of a 'domain' of about 110 amino acid residues. In the light chain these domains correspond with V_L and C_L for the variable and constant regions respectively. In the heavy chain, the N-terminal region is called the V_L domain and in γ, α and δ chains there are three in the constant part of the chain called C_H1, C_H2 and C_H3. In μ and ε chains there is an additional domain which is referred to as C_H4 (in fact the additional domain is situated after C_H1 and so the final domain in the chain, referred to as $C\mu4$ for convenience, is homologous to $C\gamma3$).

A specific nomenclature may be used to describe the domains of different classes; for example $C\gamma1$, $C\gamma2$ and $C\gamma3$ for IgG and $C\mu1$, $C\mu2$, $C\mu3$ and $C\mu4$ for IgM.

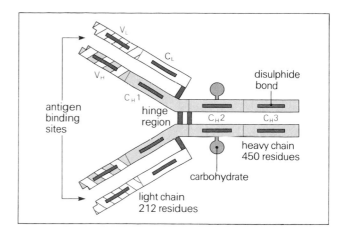

Fig. 5.5 The basic structure of IgG. The amino terminal end is characterized by sequence variability (V) in both the heavy (H) and light (L) chains which are referred to as the V_H and V_L regions respectively. The rest of the molecule has a relatively constant (C) structure. The constant portion of the light chain is termed the C_L region. The constant portion of the heavy chain is further divided into three structurally discrete regions: C_H1, C_H2 and C_H3. These globular regions, which are stabilized by intrachain disulphide bonds, are referred to as 'domains'. The sites at which the antibody binds antigen are located in the variable domains. The hinge region is a vaguely defined segment of heavy chain between the C_H1 and C_H2 domains. Flexibility in this area permits variation in the distance between the two antigen binding sites, allowing them to operate independently. Carbohydrate moieties are attached to the C_H2 domains.

IgG Although the four chain structure of human IgG1 shown in figure 5.5 is a useful model for all immunoglobulins there exist differences of detail in every class. Even with human IgG, no two subclasses are identical in the number and distribution of interchain disulphide bonds. Indeed, the light-heavy chain bonds in IgG2, 3 and 4 are linked to the junction between the variable and constant regions of the heavy chains and this pattern is the one most frequently observed. Similarly the number of inter-heavy chain bonds may be two (IgG1 and IgG4), four (IgG2) or fifteen (IgG3) (Fig. 5.6).

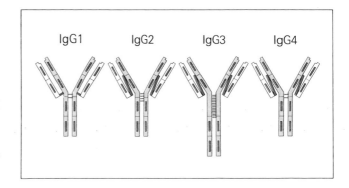

Fig. 5.6 Polypeptide chain structure of the four human IgG subclasses. The subclasses have different numbers and arrangements of the interchain disulphide bonds. In IgG1 the bond linking the light and heavy chains goes to the hinge region, whereas in the IgG2, IgG3 and IgG4 subclasses it goes to the junction between the variable and constant regions.

This type of heterogeneity is also seen within the IgG subclasses of other species (Fig. 5.7).

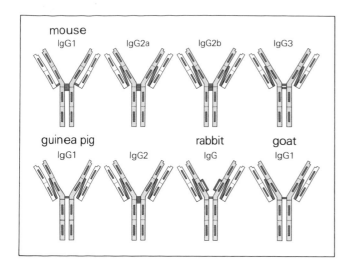

Fig. 5.7 Polypeptide chain structure of IgG subclasses in mouse, guinea pig, rabbit and goat. The different IgG molecules in these species vary in their molecular structures and the number of isotypes they carry in their genomes (see below). Note that the Cγ1 domain in the rabbit has two intrachain disulphide bonds.

IgM The four chain basic structure consisting of two heavy and two light chains is common to all the immunoglobulin classes, but for some classes the whole molecule may be a polymer of this basic unit. IgM is a pentamer of the basic unit which in this case consists of two μ heavy chains and two light chains (Fig. 5.8). The μ chains not only differ from γ chains in amino acid sequence but also

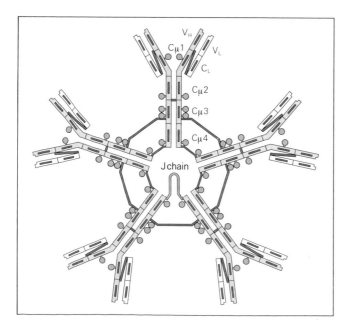

Fig. 5.8 Pentameric polypeptide chain structure of human IgM. IgM heavy chains have five domains with disulphide bonds cross-linking adjacent Cμ3 and Cμ4 domains of different units. Also shown are the carbohydrate side chains and possible location of the J chain.

in the number of constant region domains. The subunits are held together by disulphide bonds between the Cμ3 domains and the complete molecule consists of a densely packed central region with radiating arms. This structure is clearly seen in many of the electron micrographs of IgM molecules. Photographs of IgM antibodies binding to bacterial flagella have shown molecules cross-linking two flagella as well as molecules adopting a 'staple' configuration (Fig. 5.9). The latter suggests that flexion readily occurs between the Cμ2 and Cμ3 domains although this region is not structurally homologous to the IgG hinge. Two other features characterize the IgM molecule. There is an abundance of oligosaccharide units associated with the μ chain and there is an additional peptide chain called the J (joining) chain which is thought to assist the process of polymerization prior to secretion by the antibody-producing cell.

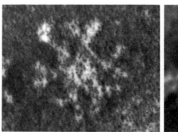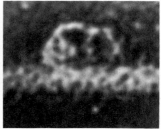

Fig. 5.9 Electron micrographs of IgM molecules: in free solution adopting the characteristic star-shaped configuration (left, ×5.2 × 10⁶, courtesy of Dr. R. Dourmashkin), and a crab-like configuration due to cross-linkage with a single flagellum (right, ×5.2 × 10⁶, courtesy of Dr. A. Feinstein).

IgA Polymeric serum IgA and all secretory IgA molecules also contain the J chain (but this peptide is not associated with IgG, IgD or IgE). The primary structure of a human IgA1 molecule has been determined; the 472 amino acid residues of the α chain are arranged in four domains (V_H, Cα1, Cα2 and Cα3) (Fig. 5.10). A feature shared with IgM is the presence of an additional C-terminal octapeptide with a penultimate cysteine residue, which is able to bind covalently to the J chain in polymeric molecules. The Cα1 and Cα2 domains possess an additional intrachain disulphide bond and in each Cα2 domain there are two cysteine residues of unknown function. Electron micrographs of IgA dimers show double Y-shaped structures which suggest that the monomeric subunits are linked end to end through the C-terminal Cα3 regions (Fig. 5.11). Secretory IgA (sIgA) exists mainly in the form of a molecule sedimenting at 11S and having a molecular weight of 380,000. The complete molecule is made up of two four chain units of IgA, one secretory component (molecular weight 70,000) and one J chain (molecular weight 15,000) (Fig. 5.12). It is not clear how the various peptide chains are linked together. In contrast to the J chain, the secretory component is not synthesized by the plasma cells but by epithelial cells. IgA held in the dimer configuration by a J chain and secreted by submucosal plasma cells actively binds secretory component (SC) as it traverses epithelial cell layers. Bound SC may both facilitate transport of secretory IgA into secretions as well as protect the immunoglobulin from proteolytic attack.

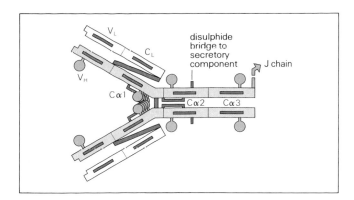

Fig. 5.10 Polypeptide chain structure of human IgA1. This diagram shows intra- and interchain disulphide bonds and the possible location of carbohydrate units. An additional disulphide bond stabilizes the Cα2 domain, and a further disulphide bond cross-links to the J chain in polymeric IgA.

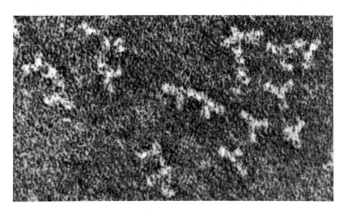

Fig. 5.11 Electron micrograph of a human dimeric IgA myeloma protein. The double Y-shaped appearance suggests that the monomeric subunits are linked end to end through the C-terminal Cα3 domain. × 1.6 × 10⁶. Courtesy of Dr. R. Dourmashkin.

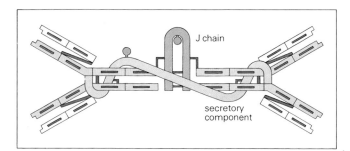

Fig. 5.12 Structure of human secretory IgA1 (sIgA1). The secretory component is probably wound around the sIgA dimer as shown and attached by disulphide bonds to the Cα2 domain of each IgA monomer. The J chain is required for the joining of the two subunits. For simplicity the domains are not labelled and the additional disulphide bond extending from the Cα2 domain to the hinge region has been omitted.

IgD IgD is a trace immunoglobulin in serum (less than 1% of the total). The protein is more susceptible to proteolysis than IgG1, IgG2, IgA or IgM and has a tendency to undergo spontaneous proteolysis. IgD has a structure similar to that shown in figure 5.13. There appears to be a single disulphide bond between the δ chains and a high content of carbohydrate distributed in multiple oligosaccharide units. One of these units is rich in N-acetylgalactosamine, a sugar which occurs also in IgA1, but in no other known immunoglobulin.

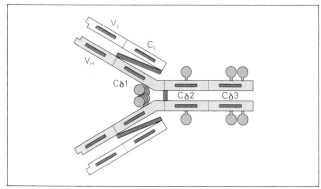

Fig. 5.13 Polypeptide chain structure of human IgD. This diagram shows the intra- and interchain disulphide bonds, and the possible location of oligosaccharide units.

IgE Despite the low serum concentration of IgE the complete amino acid sequence of the human molecule is available following work on an IgE myeloma protein. The higher molecular weight of the ε chain (72,500) suggests that there are approximately 550 amino acid residues in this heavy chain distributed amongst four constant region domains (Cε1, Cε2, Cε3 and Cε4). When IgE is cleaved by the proteolytic enzyme, papain, a 5S fragment of molecular weight 98,000 is released. This fragment (Fc), which contains many of the IgE specific determinants of the whole molecule and binds to the mast cell surface also shares some antigenic determinants with the F(ab')₂ fragment produced when the molecule is cleaved by another proteolytic enzyme, pepsin. A fragment corresponding to the region of overlap (Fc'') of these two fragments has also been isolated but does not retain mast cell binding activity (Fig. 5.14).

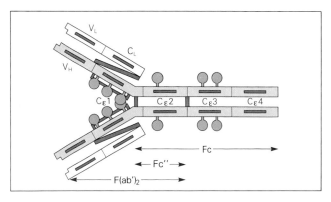

Fig. 5.14 Polypeptide chain structure of human IgE. The four constant region domains, the intra- and interchain disulphide bonds and the location of oligosaccharide units are shown. IgE can be cleaved by enzymes to give the fragments F(ab')₂ (Fab = Fragment antigen binding), Fc (Fc = Fragment crystalline) and Fc''.

THE GENETIC BASIS OF ANTIBODY HETEROGENEITY

Recent work has shown that the mRNA for an immunoglobulin polypeptide is made by splicing together sections of mRNA coding for different parts of the polypeptide. For example, the production of light chain mRNA involves the splicing together of 2 mRNA segments – for the V domain and the C domain. The segment of DNA coding for the V genes is, in turn, produced by recombination of two germ line genes. (This subject is dealt with fully in a later chapter). Since a single polypeptide is produced from several genes this creates problems in analysing the genetic variability of a single polypeptide. Nevertheless the variability of antibodies can be divided into three types.

Isotypic variation The genes for isotypic variants are present in *all* healthy members of a species. For example, the genes for $\gamma 1, \gamma 2, \gamma 3, \gamma 4, \mu, \alpha 1, \alpha 2, \delta, \varepsilon, \kappa$ and λ chains are all present in the human genome and these are therefore isotypes.

Allotypic variation This refers to genetic variation within a species involving different alleles at a given locus. *Not all* healthy members of a species have a particular allotype (cf. allelic forms in blood groups). For example, the variant of IgG3 called G3m (b0) (an allotype characterized by having phenylalanine at position 436 of its heavy chain) is not found in all people, and is therefore an allotype. Allotypes occur mostly as variants of heavy chain constant regions.

Idiotypic variation Variation in the variable domain (particularly in the highly variable segments known as hypervariable regions) produces idiotypes. Idiotypes are usually specific for the individual antibody clone (private idiotypes) but are sometimes shared between different antibody clones (public, cross-reacting or recurrent idiotypes). The exact genetic basis of idiotypic variability is only partially understood. These forms of genetic variability are summarized in figure 5.15.

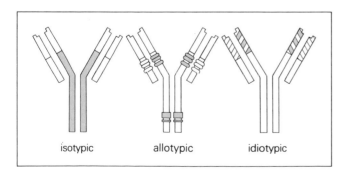

Fig. 5.15 Antibody variants. Isotypic variation refers to the different heavy and light chain classes and subclasses: the variants produced are present in *all* healthy members of a species. Allotypic variation occurs mostly in the constant region: *not all* variants are present in all healthy individuals. Idiotypic variation occurs in the variable region only and idiotypes are specific to each antibody molecule.

ANTIBODY EFFECTOR FUNCTIONS

As previously stated the primary function of an antibody is to bind the antigen but, aside from those cases where this has a direct neutralizing effect (eg. on bacterial toxin or viral penetration of cells) such interactions would generally be without significance if secondary 'effector' functions did not then become manifest.

The activation of the complement system is one of the most important effector mechanisms of IgG1 and IgG3 molecules. The complement system is a complex group of serum proteins which mediate inflammatory reactions. Having bound to antigen, IgM, IgG1 and IgG3 may activate the complement enzyme cascade. IgG2 appears to be less effective in activating complement, while IgG4, IgA, IgD and IgE are ineffective in this respect.

In man IgG molecules of all subclasses cross the placenta and confer a high degree of passive immunity to the newborn. In other species in which maternal immunoglobulin reaches the offspring postnatally (eg. the pig) it is again IgG derived from the maternal milk which selectively crosses the gastro-intestinal tract (Fig. 5.16).

properties of human immunoglobulins								
immunoglobulin	IgG1	IgG2	IgG3	IgG4	IgM	IgA	IgD	IgE
complement fixation	++	+	+++	−	+++	−	−	−
placental transfer	+	±	+	+	−	−	−	−
reactivity with staphylococcal protein A	+	+	−	+	−	−	−	−

Fig. 5.16 Major properties of human antibody classes and subclasses. Classes and subclasses differ in the ability to fix complement, cross the placenta and react with staphylococcal protein A. (Staphylococcal protein A is a cell wall protein of staphylococci which binds to the Fc region of certain immunoglobulins and as such is a natural receptor for antibody.) These properties are determined by the Fc region.

cell binding functions of human immunoglobulins								
immunoglobulin	IgG1	IgG2	IgG3	IgG4	IgM	IgA	IgD	IgE
mononuclear cells	+	−	+	−	−	−	−	?
neutrophils	+	−	+	+	−	+	−	−
mast cells and basophils	−	−	−	?	−	−	−	+++
T and B lymphocytes	+	+	+	+	+°	+°	−	+°
platelets	+	+	+	+	−	−	−	?

Fig. 5.17 Cell binding functions of human immunoglobulins. The binding ability varies between the different classes and subclasses. In some cases binding by lymphocytes is restricted to a subpopulation of these cells (+°).

The immunoglobulins also display a complex pattern of interactions with various cell types and some of these are tabulated in figure 5.17. Some of this data is still controversial, particularly that relating to the interactions with lymphocytes, and further clarification may follow from improved definition of cell subpopulations.

STRUCTURE IN RELATION TO FUNCTION

The plant proteinase papain cleaves the IgG molecule in the hinge region between the $C\gamma1$ and $C\gamma2$ domains to give two identical Fab fragments and one Fc fragment. The fragments generated by papain have been of enormous value in structure/function studies on the antibody molecule. It was noted that the Fab region is concerned with binding to antigen while the Fc region mediates effector functions such as complement fixation, monocyte binding and placental transmission.

Another useful enzyme for such studies is pepsin which generates two major fragments: the $F(ab')_2$ fragment which broadly encompasses the two Fab regions linked by the hinge region, and the pFc' fragment, which corresponds to the $C\gamma3$ domain of the molecule. Papain also generates, after prolonged digestion periods, a degraded fragment of the $C\gamma3$ region which is called the Fc' fragment. Some of these major points of enzymic cleavage are shown in figure 5.18. Many other enzymes are known to cleave the immunoglobulin molecule. Brief trypsin digestion of acid-treated Fc fragment yields the $C\gamma2$ domain, and isolation of this fragment has permitted extensive structural and functional comparisons with other subfragments such as pFc'.

The recognition of immunoglobulin domains as functional subunits led Edelman in 1970 to suggest that each had evolved to subserve a specific function. There was already clear evidence that the V_H and V_L domains interact to form the antigen binding surfaces of the antibody molecule, and subsequent crystallographic work (see later) has amply confirmed this prediction. Edelman suggested that the other domains would be shown to mediate the other (effector) functions of immunoglobulin. Precise structural location of these other sites has still to be achieved but there is good evidence that the C1q component of complement interacts with the $C\gamma2$ domain (in the case of IgG) and that a site controlling the rate of catabolism of the whole molecule is in the same domain.

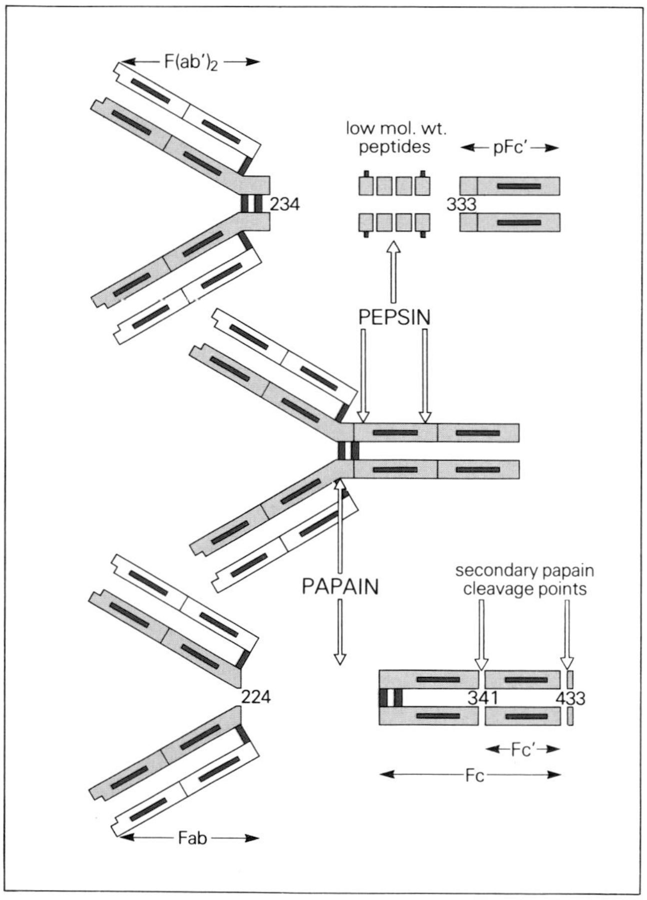

Fig. 5.18 Enzymic cleavage of human IgG1. Pepsin cleaves the heavy chain at the amino acid residues, 234 and 333, to yield the $F(ab')_2$ and pFc' fragments. Further action reduces the central fragment to low molecular weight peptides. Papain splits the molecule in the hinge region (at residue 224) yielding two Fab fragments and the Fc fragment. Secondary action on the Fc fragment at residues 341 and 433 gives rise to Fc'.

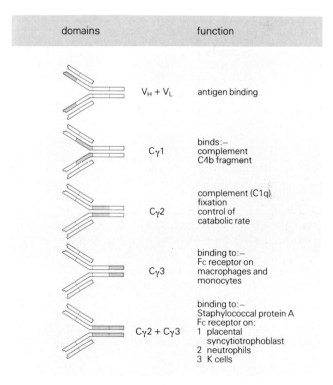

domains	function
$V_H + V_L$	antigen binding
$C\gamma1$	binds:— complement C4b fragment
$C\gamma2$	complement (C1q) fixation control of catabolic rate
$C\gamma3$	binding to:— Fc receptor on macrophages and monocytes
$C\gamma2 + C\gamma3$	binding to:— Staphylococcal protein A Fc receptor on: 1 placental syncytiotrophoblast 2 neutrophils 3 K cells

Fig. 5.19 Functions of IgG domains. The relevant domains are shown shaded, together with the functions they perform.

There is much data to suggest that interactions with macrophages and monocytes occurs through a site in the $C\gamma3$ domain but an adjunctive function for the $C\gamma2$ domain in such reactions appears likely. Similarly there is evidence that interaction with other cell structures either occurs through sites spanning the two Fc domains ($C\gamma2 + C\gamma3$) or requires some synergistic activity between these two domains. The functions performed by domains of the IgG antibody are summarized in figure 5.19.

STRUCTURE IN RELATION TO ANTIGEN BINDING

When the primary amino acid structure of a large number of light and heavy polypeptide chains is examined it is found that the variability between their V domains is not distributed evenly throughout the length of these regions. Some short polypeptide segments show exceptional variability and these segments are termed hypervariable regions. In both κ and λ light chains such hypervariable regions are located near positions 30, 50 and 95 (Fig. 5.20). It is now generally accepted that such hypervariable regions are involved directly in the formation of the antigen binding site. Hypervariable regions are sometimes referred to as Complementarity Determining Regions (CDR) and the intervening peptide segments as Framework Regions (FR). In both light and heavy chain V regions there are three CDRs (CDR1-CDR3) and four FRs (FR1-FR4).

variability
150
100
50
0
0
25
50
75
100
position
FR1 CDR1 FR2 CDR2 FR3 CDR3 FR4

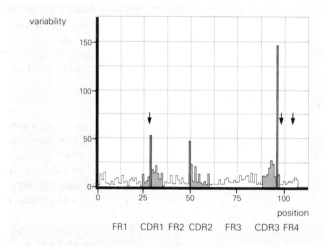

Fig. 5.20 Amino acid variability in the variable region of immunoglobulin light chains. Variability is calculated by comparing the sequences of many individual chains and, for any position, is equal to the ratio of the number of different amino acids (found at that position) to the frequency of the most common amino acid. The areas of greatest variability, of which there are three in the V_L domain, are the hypervariable regions. In some sequences studied, extra amino acids are found but these have been excluded here to enhance comparison and their positions are indicated by arrows. The areas shaded orange denote regions of hypervariability (CDR), and the most hypervariable positions are shaded red. The four framework regions (FR) are shown in yellow. Courtesy of Professor E. A. Kabat.

When sequences are examined for evidence of homology the variable regions of κ, λ and heavy chains may each be divided into subgroups depending on their framework amino acid sequences. The numbers of such recognizable subgroups differ from species to species: in man there are four major κ-chain subgroups, six λ-chain subgroups and three heavy chain subgroups. The prototype sequences of the light chain subgroups are shown in figure 5.21.

κ chains
VκI D I T S P S S V G R V T I C
VκII V T S P L L V G A C
VκIII I V T S P T L S S P G L S C
VκIV D V Q S P L A V S G A T C
λ chains
VλI Z S L T P P S S P G C
VλII Z S L Q P S S S P G T S C
VλIII Y L P P S S V P G I T C
VλIV S L Q V G I C
VλV Z S A L T Q P P S A S G S G Q S V T I S C
VλVI L P S S S P G S C

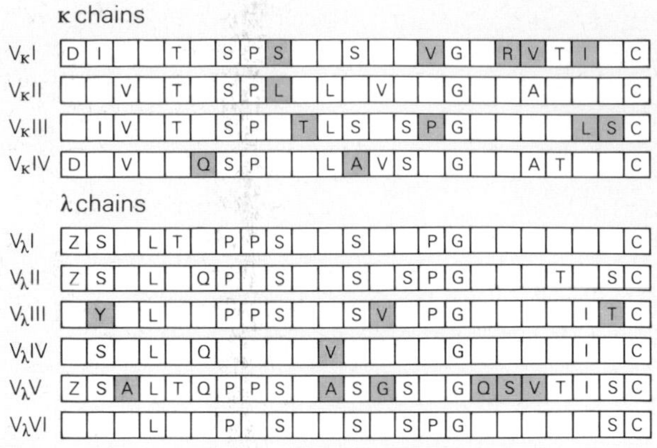

Fig. 5.21 Prototype sequences in the FR1 region of different human κ and λ V region subgroups. The first 23 amino acid residues (N-terminal) of the FR1 framework sequences of the four κ and six λ chain subgroups are shown. Amino acid residues not occurring at the same position in any other subgroup of that chain are coloured red. Empty boxes could represent any amino acid residue. (Amino acids are indicated by the single letter code given in Fig. 13.22.)

Within the past decade the three-dimensional structure of immunoglobulins has been investigated by X-ray diffraction techniques. Such studies have shown that the immunoglobulin domains share a basic folding pattern with several straight segments of polypeptide chain lying parallel to the long axis of the domain. These parallel sections are arranged in two layers running in opposite directions with many hydrophobic amino acid side chains between the layers. One of the layers is composed of four segments, the other has three segments and both are linked by a single disulphide bridge (Fig. 5.22).

N-terminus
96
26
53
C-terminus
V_L
C_L

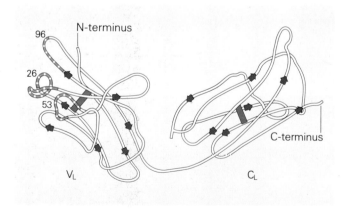

Fig. 5.22 The basic folding pattern of the variable and constant domains of the light chain. The domains are essentially comprised of two layers of polypeptide chain; one is composed of four segments (arrowed red) and the other of three segments (arrowed black). The segments of these layers, which are joined by disulphide bonds (red), run in opposite directions. Folding of the V_L domains causes the hypervariable regions to become exposed in three separate but closely disposed loops. One numbered residue from each hypervariable region is identified.

Homologous domains of the light and heavy chains are paired in the Fab regions as are the C_H3 domains of the γ-heavy chains; $C\gamma2$ domains tend to be separated by carbohydrate moieties. Despite the structural similarities between domains there are striking differences at the level of domain interaction. For example, the variable domains associate through their three segment layers, whereas the constant domains associate through the four segment layers. A further difference between the constant and variable domains is the presence of an additional loop of peptide in the variable regions. The variable regions of the light and heavy chains are folded in such a way that the regions of hypervariability are brought together to create the surface structures which bind antigen. As shown in figure 5.22 these regions are, in the main, associated with bends in the peptide chain. X-ray crystallography is now yielding structural data on complete IgG molecules and it is possible to construct both a provisional α-carbon skeleton and computer generated atomic models for this class (Figs. 5.23 and 5.24). These show the general Y-shaped structure with three limbs which has also been visualized by electron micrography. An appropriate analogy of the antigen-antibody interaction is illustrated in figure 5.25.

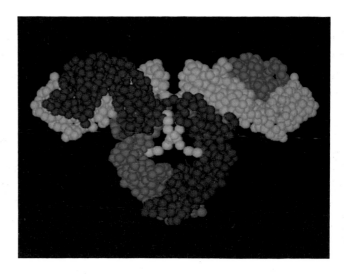

Fig. 5.24 Computer generated model of IgG. One heavy chain is shown in blue and one in red with two light chains being depicted in green. Carbohydrate bound to the Fc portion of the molecule is shown in turquoise. The structure of immunoglobulin was determined by David R. Davies et al (*Proc. Nat. Acad. Sci.* USA, 1977; *74*). The figure was generated by computer graphics using the system developed by Richard J. Feldmann at the National Institutes of Health.

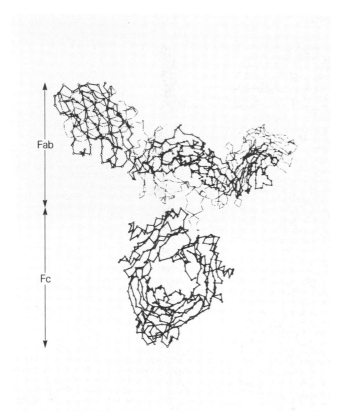

Fab

Fc

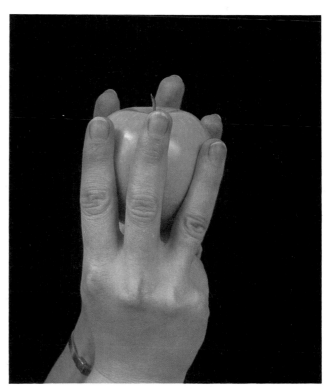

Fig. 5.23 Provisional model of the α-carbon backbone of human IgG1. This model is based on X-ray crystallography studies which reveal that the polypeptide is folded into globular domains forming a Y-shaped structure. The antigen binding surfaces formed between the variable regions of the light and heavy chains are located at the tips of the arms. The model clearly shows the hinge region between the Fab and Fc regions, as well as suggesting weak interaction between the $C\gamma2$ domains and strong interaction between the $C\gamma3$ domains. Courtesy of Professor R. Huber.

Fig. 5.25 Analogy for antigen-antibody binding. Binding of antigen to antibody is represented by an apple (antigen) being held by the fingers of two hands (heavy and light chains) representing hypervariable loops formed into a cleft (the antigen binding site). If the apple were still attached to the tree it might also serve to illustrate the point that there are usually many such antigenic determinants displayed on the surface of even simple microorganisms.

FURTHER READING

Capra D. & Edmundson A.B. (1977) The antibody combining site. *Scientific* American **236,** 50.

Hahn G.S. (1982) Antibody structure, function and active sites. In *Physiology of Immunoglobulins: Diagnostic and Clinical Aspects.* S.E. Ritzmann (ed.) Alan Liss Inc., New York.

Nisonoff A. (1982) *Introduction to molecular immunology.* Sinauer Associates. Blackwell Scientific Publications, Oxford.

Turner M.W. (1977) Structure and function of immunoglobulins. In *Immunochemistry: An Advanced Textbook.* L. E. Glynn & M. W. Steward (eds.) John Wiley & Sons, Chichester.

Turner M.W. (1983) Immunoglobulins. In *Immunology in Medicine. A comprehensive Guide to Clinical Immunology.* 2nd Edition. E.J. Holborow & W.G. Reeves (eds.) Grune & Stratton, London.

6 Antigen-Antibody Reactions

The basic Y-shaped immunoglobulin molecule is a bifunctional structure: the V domains are primarily concerned with antigen binding, while the remaining constant (C) domains are concerned with the ability of the different immunoglobulins to interact with host tissue. Although the C domains do not form the antigen binding sites, the arrangement of the C domains and hinge region confer segmental flexibility on the molecule which allows it to combine with separated antigenic determinants.

ANTIGEN-ANTIBODY BINDING

Certain segments of the V domains have particularly heterogeneous primary amino acid sequences and it has been shown by X-ray crystallography that particular amino acids in these hypervariable regions make contact with the antigen (Fig. 6.1). Although the remaining 'framework' residues of the V region do not come into direct contact with the antigen, they are essential in producing the folding of the V domains and maintaining the integrity of the binding site.

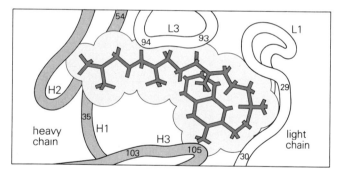

Fig. 6.1 The antibody combining site. The antigen molecule nestles in a cleft formed by the antibody combining site. The example shown is based on X-ray crystallography studies of human IgG (the myeloma protein NEW) binding γ-hydroxyl vitamin K. The antigen makes contact with 10-12 amino acids in the hypervariable regions of both heavy and light chains. The numerals refer to amino acids identified as actually making contact with the antigen.

The binding of antigen to the antibody takes place by the formation of multiple non-covalent bonds between the antigen and amino acids of the binding site. Although the attractive forces (namely, hydrogen bonds, electrostatic, Van der Waals and hydrophobic) involved in these bonds are individually weak by comparison with covalent bonds, the multiplicity of the bonds leads to a considerable binding energy. The non-covalent bonds are critically dependent on the distance (d) between the interacting groups. The force is proportional to $1/d^2$ for electrostatic forces and to $1/d^7$ for Van der Waals forces; thus the interacting groups must be close in molecular terms before these forces become significant (Fig. 6.2). The consequence of this is that an antigenic determinant and the antigen combining site must have complementary structures to be able to combine, meaning:
1. there must be suitable atomic groupings on opposing parts of the antigen and antibody
2. the shape of the combining site must fit the antigen, so that several non-covalent bonds can form simultaneously.
If the antigen and the combining site are complementary in this way, there will be sufficient binding energy to resist thermodynamic disruption of the bond. However, if electron clouds of the antigen and antibody happen to overlap steric repulsive forces come into play which are inversely proportional to the twelfth power of the distance between the clouds ($F \propto 1/d^{12}$). These forces are very likely to play a vital role in determining the specificity of the antibody molecule for a particular antigen and its ability to discriminate between antigens since any variation from the ideal complementary shape will cause a fall in the total binding energy through increased repulsive forces and decreased attractive forces.

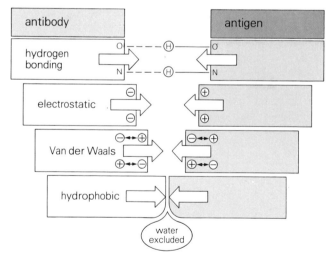

Fig. 6.2 The intermolecular attractive forces binding antigen to antibody. These forces require the close approach of the interacting groups. *Hydrogen bonding* results from the formation of hydrogen bridges between appropriate atoms; *electrostatic forces* are due to the attraction of oppositely charged groups located on two protein side chains. *Van der Waals bonds* are generated by the interaction between electron clouds (here represented as induced oscillating dipoles) and *hydrophobic bonds* (which may contribute up to half the total strength of the antigen-antibody bond) rely upon the association of non-polar, hydrophobic groups so that contact with water molecules is minimized. The distance of separation between the interacting groups which produces optimum binding varies for the different types of bond.

Examples of a good fit and poor fit between antigen and antibody are illustrated in figure 6.3.

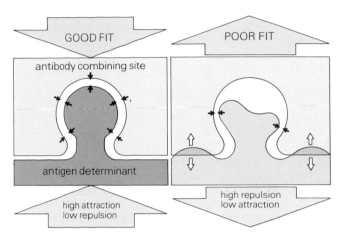

Fig. 6.3 Good fit and poor fit between antigen and antibody. A good fit between the antigenic determinant and the binding site of the antibody will create ample opportunities for intermolecular attractive forces to be created and few opportunities for repulsive forces to operate. Conversely, when there is a poor fit the reverse is true, that is, high repulsive forces are generated when electron clouds overlap, which dominate any small forces of attraction.

ANTIBODY AFFINITY

The strength of a single antigen-antibody bond is termed the antibody affinity and it is produced by summation of the attractive and repulsive forces described above (Fig. 6.4). The interaction of the antibody combining site with an antigen can be investigated thermodynamically.

To measure the affinity of a single combining site it is necessary to use a monovalent antigen or even a single isolated antigenic determinant – a hapten. Since the non-

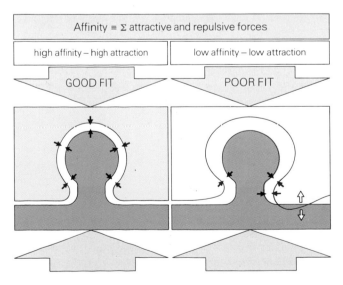

Fig. 6.4 Antibody affinity. The affinity with which antibody binds antigen results from a balance between the attractive and repulsive forces. A high affinity antibody implies a good fit and conversely, a low affinity antibody implies a poor fit.

covalent bonds between antibody and hapten are dissociable the overall combination of an antigen and antibody must also be reversible; thus the Law of Mass Action can be applied to the reaction and the equilibrium constant, K determined. This is the affinity constant (Fig. 6.5).

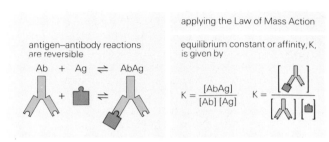

Fig. 6.5 Reversibility of the antigen-antibody bond and the calculation of antibody affinity. All antigen-antibody reactions are reversible and the Law of Mass Action has been applied, from which antibody affinity (given by the equilibrium constant, K) can be calculated at equilibrium. (Square brackets refer to the concentration of reactants.)

AFFINITY AND AVIDITY

Since each 4 polypeptide chain antibody unit has two antigen binding sites, antibodies are potentially multivalent in their reaction with antigen. In addition, antigen can also be monovalent or multivalent. A hapten has only one antigenic determinant and so can only react with one antigen combining site – it is therefore monovalent.

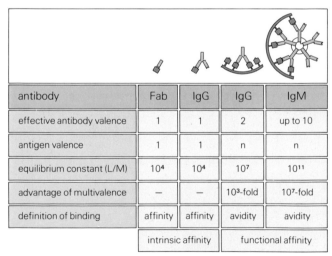

antibody	Fab	IgG	IgG	IgM
effective antibody valence	1	1	2	up to 10
antigen valence	1	1	n	n
equilibrium constant (L/M)	10^4	10^4	10^7	10^{11}
advantage of multivalence	–	–	10^3-fold	10^7-fold
definition of binding	affinity	affinity	avidity	avidity
	intrinsic affinity		functional affinity	

Fig. 6.6 Affinity and avidity. Multivalent binding between antibody and antigen (avidity or functional affinity) results in a considerable increase in stability as measured by the equilibrium constant, compared to simple monovalent binding (affinity or intrinsic affinity, here arbitrarily assigned a value of 10^4 L/M). This is sometimes referred to as the 'bonus effect' of multivalency. Thus there may be a 10^3-fold increase in binding energy of IgG when both valencies (combining sites) are utilized, and 10^7-fold increase when IgM binds antigen in a multivalent manner. Monovalent antigen combines with multivalent antibody with no greater affinity than it does with monovalent antibody (eg. an Fab fragment).

Many molecules however, have more than one antigenic determinant. Microorganisms have a very large number of antigenic determinants exposed on their surfaces, hence all these are multivalent. When a multivalent antigen combines with more than one of an antibody's combining sites, the binding energy between the two is considerably greater than the sum of the binding energies of the individual sites involved since all the antigen-antibody bonds must be broken simultaneously before the antigen and antibody will dissociate.

The strength with which a multivalent antibody binds a multivalent antigen is termed *avidity* to differentiate it from the *affinity* of the bond between a single antigenic determinant and an individual combining site. Thus the avidity of an antibody for its antigen is dependent on the affinities of the individual combining sites for the determinants on the antigen, but is greater than the sum of these affinities if both antigen and antibody are multivalent (Fig. 6.6). In normal physiological situations avidity is likely to be more relevant since naturally occurring antigens are multivalent; however, the precise measurement of hapten-antibody reactions is more likely to give an insight into the immunochemical nature of the antigen-antibody reaction.

ANTIBODY SPECIFICITY

Antigen-antibody reactions can show a high level of specificity, that is, the binding sites of antibodies directed against determinants on one antigen are not complementary to determinants of another antigen. For example, antibodies to a virus like measles will bind to the measles virus and confer immunity to this disease, but will not combine with, or protect against, an unrelated virus such as polio. The specificity of an antiserum is the result of the summation of actions of the various antibodies in the total population each reacting with a different part of the antigen molecule and even different parts of the same determinant (Fig. 6.7). However, when some of the determinants of an antigen, A, are shared by another antigen, B, then a proportion of the antibodies directed to A will also react with B. This is termed *cross-reactivity*. The specificity and cross-reactivity expressed by an antiserum are properties which result from the antibody molecules within the serum.

Radical (R)	sulphonate	arsonate	carboxylate
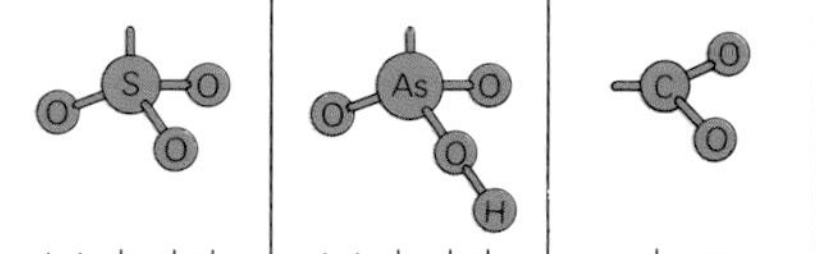	tetrahedral	tetrahedral	planar
ortho	+ +	−	−
meta	+ + +	+	±
para	±	−	−

Fig. 6.8 An example of specificity and cross-reactivity: recognition by antibody of overall antigenic structure rather than chemical composition. An antiserum is raised to the meta isomer of amino benzene sulphonate (the immunizing antigen). This antiserum is then reacted with the ortho and para isomers of amino benzene sulphonate and also with the three isomers (ortho, meta, para) of two different but related antigens: aminobenzene arsonate and amino benzene carboxylate. The antiserum reacts specifically with the sulphonate group (which has a tetrahedral structure) in the meta position but will give a cross-reaction (though weaker) with sulphonate in the ortho position. Further, but weaker, cross-reactions are possible when this antiserum is reacted with either the tetrahedral arsonate group or the planar carboxylate group in the meta, but not in the ortho or para position. The arsonate group is larger than sulphonate and has an extra H atom, while the carboxylate is smaller and planar. These results suggest that the overall configuration of the antigen is as important as individual chemical groupings.

There is evidence that the antibody recognizes the overall configuration of the antigen rather than its chemical composition and it is envisaged that antibodies are directed against particular three-dimensional electron cloud shapes rather than specific chemical structures (Fig. 6.8). In addition, there is frequently an inverse relationship between the charge of an antigen and the antibodies it induces (Fig. 6.9).

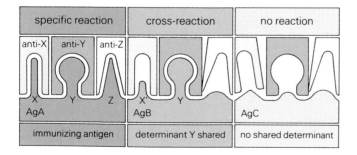

Fig. 6.7 Specificity, cross-reactivity and non-reactivity. Antiserum specificity results from the action of a population of individual antibody molecules (anti-X, anti-Y, and anti-Z) directed against different determinants (XYZ) on the antigen molecule (AgA). Antigen A (AgA) and antigen B (AgB) share determinant Y in common. Antiserum raised against AgA (anti-XYZ) not only reacts *specifically* with AgA but *cross-reacts* with AgB (through recognition of shared determinant Y and weak recognition of determinant X'). The antiserum gives *no reaction* with AgC (no shared determinants).

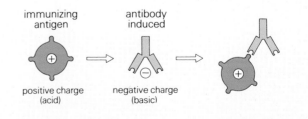

Fig. 6.9 Charge specificity. Antigen induces formation of, and complexes with, antibody of a charge opposite to its own.

Antibodies are capable of expressing remarkable specificity and are able to distinguish between small differences in the primary structure of the antigen, and differences in charge, optical configuration and steric comformation. Further examples of antibody specificity are illustrated in figures 6.10-6.12.

antiserum	antigen	
	α-helical	non-helical
	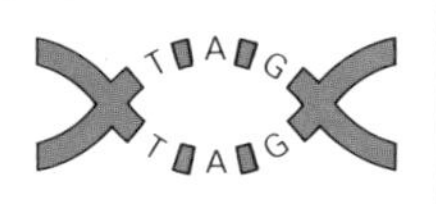 T A G / T A G	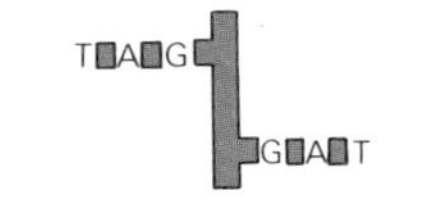 T A G / G A T
anti α-helical	+ + +	−
anti-non-helical	−	+ + +

Fig. 6.10 Configurational specificity I. Antibody is able to discriminate between an α-helical tripeptide and the same tripeptide in a non-helical form.

antiserum	antigen		
	p aminophenol α glucoside 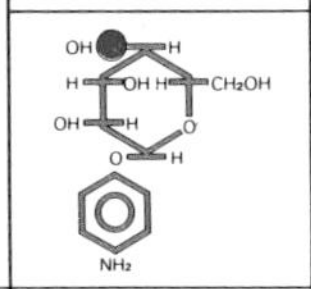	p aminophenol β glucoside 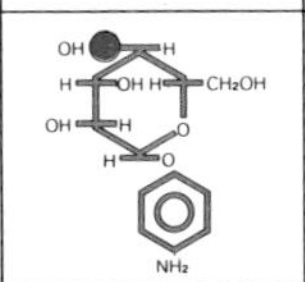	p aminophenol β galactoside 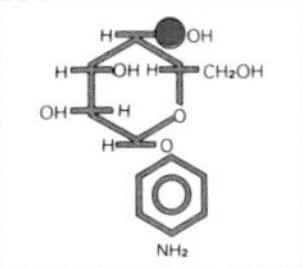
anti-α glucoside	+ + +	+ +	−
anti-β glucoside	+ +	+ + +	−
anti-β galactoside	−	−	+ + +

Fig. 6.11 Configurational specificity II. Antibody was raised to each of three different, but very similar antigens: p aminophenol α glucoside, p aminophenol β glucoside and p aminophenol β galactoside and the ability of each antibody to cross-react with the other two antigens was assessed.

antiserum	antigen		
	lysozyme 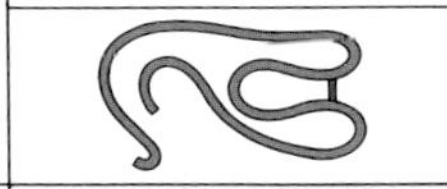	isolated 'loop' peptide 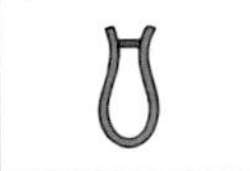	reduced 'loop' 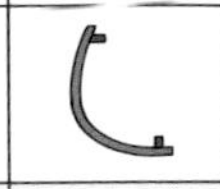
anti-lysozyme	+ +	+	−
anti-'loop'peptide	+	+ +	−

Fig. 6.12 Configurational specificity III. The lysozyme molecule possesses an intrachain bond (red) which produces a loop in the peptide chain. Antisera may be raised against either whole lysozyme (anti-lysozyme) or the isolated loop (anti-'loop' peptide) and are found to distinguish between the two. Neither antiserum reacts with the isolated loop in its linear, reduced form. This demonstrates the importance of tertiary structure in determining antibody specificity.

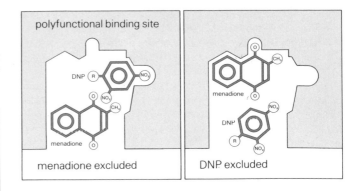

Fig. 6.13 Competitive binding. The antibody combining site may bind more than one antigen determinant. For example, antibody 460 has two different sites in the binding cleft which are 1.2-1.4 nm apart. The antibody binds the haptens menadione and DNP competitively, that is, the binding of one excludes binding of the other. Binding sites which are capable of specifically binding more than one antigenic determinant are termed polyfunctional binding sites.

Over the past few years research has suggested that an antibody molecule may be complementary to several dissimilar antigens. The binding of these antigens is competitive, and it appears that there are spatially separated positions within the combining site (Fig. 6.13).

On this basis the specificity of a population of antibodies would not necessarily arise because *all* the antibodies have the same exlusive specificity, but if a large number of different polyfunctional antibodies all had a site which could combine with a particular antigen A, the net reactivity of those antibodies would be high to A but low to all other antigens. Thus specificity would be a population phenomenon, an average characteristic of all the antibodies in an antiserum (Fig. 6.14).

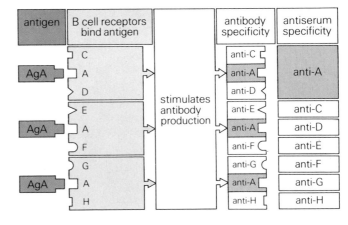

Fig. 6.14 Polyfunctional binding sites – specificity as a population phenomenon. A single antigen (AgA) may bind to the antigen receptors (essentially, antibody molecules) of different B cells which are specific not only for A but also other antigens C, D, E, F etc. – ie. the receptors possess polyfunctional binding sites. Each B cell stimulated by AgA produces antibody specific not only to AgA but also the other antigens. Since all the B cells stimulated are AgA specific, but not all specific to the other antigens, the concentration of antibody to AgA would be high but low to the other antigens.

THE PHYSIOLOGICAL SIGNIFICANCE OF HIGH AND LOW AFFINITY ANTIBODIES

The determination of antibody affinity and avidity has provided considerable information on the nature of the antigen-antibody bond, and it has become clear that binding affinity is not merely a matter of theoretical interest, since affinity and avidity affect the physiological and pathological properties of the antibodies. High affinity antibody is superior to low affinity antibody in a number of biological reactions (Fig. 6.15). Also, antibody affinity may have immunopathological significance since in experimental animals antigen-antibody complexes containing low affinity antibody persist in the circulation, localize on the glomerular basement membrane of the kidney and induce impaired renal function. High affinity complexes are more rapidly removed from the circulation, localize in the mesangium of the kidney, and have little effect on renal function.

haemagglutination
haemolysis
complement fixation
passive cutaneous anaphylaxis
immune elimination of antigen
membrane damage
virus neutralization
protective capacity against bacteria
enzyme inactivation

Fig. 6.15 Biological reactions in which high affinity antibody is superior to low affinity antibody.

DETERMINATION OF AFFINITY AND AVIDITY

Since the affinity of an antibody can affect its action, it is frequently necessary for research purposes to determine this parameter. A number of methods are available for the determination of affinity and avidity. In each procedure a system is set up in which antigen and antibody are allowed to come to equilibrium: $Ab + Ag \rightleftharpoons AbAg$ The quantities of free antigen and complexed antigen are then measured without disturbing the equilibrium. There are several ways of doing this, including separation of free antigen from bound antigen by physical methods such as dialysis, gel filtration, centrifugation and selective precipitation or by utilization of changes in the fluorescence properties of the complexed antigen or antibody. Data from these systems can be analysed by application of the Law of Mass Action to give the affinity constant, K since:
$$K = \frac{[AbAg]}{[Ab][Ag]}$$
where [AbAg] is the concentration of complexed antigen, [Ag] is the concentration of free antigen and [Ab] is the concentration of free binding sites at equilibrium. When half the binding sites are occupied by antigen, [Ab]=[AbAg] and it follows that K=1/[Ag]. In other words a high affinity antibody only requires a low antigen concentration to achieve binding of antigen to half its combining sites.

ANTIBODY AFFINITY HETEROGENEITY

When enzymes interact with their substrate the equilibrium constant (K value) for the reaction at different substrate concentrations is invariant. The reaction between an antigen and an antiserum differs from this: K varies with antibody concentration reflecting the heterogeneity of a normal antibody population. For many years it was assumed that in any particular population of antibodies, the affinities would have a Gaussian (normal) distribution (Fig. 6.16). Average affinity (K_o) is defined as the reciprocal of the free antigen concentration at equilibrium when half of the total antigen binding sites are occupied:
$$K_o \equiv \frac{1}{[Ag_{free}]}$$
When the equilibrium constant for the reaction between an antiserum and antigen is analysed however, (using different antigen concentrations), a non-Gaussian range of K values (affinities) is obtained (Fig. 6.17).

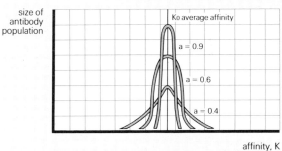

Fig. 6.16 Gaussian distribution of affinities. The heterogeneity of affinity has been assumed to be described by a normal, Gaussian, distribution (that is, equal distribution of affinities around the average affinity, Ko). The peak of the curve represents the average affinity, Ko. With an assumed Gaussian distribution of affinities, the heterogeneity index (a) represents the distribution of affinities around Ko. Thus a perfectly homogeneous antiserum would have a heterogeneity index of 1, as may be seen with monoclonal antibodies.

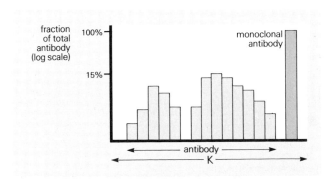

Fig. 6.17 Affinity heterogeneity. This histogram shows a typical distribution of antibody affinities (K) in an antiserum to an antigenic determinant, compared to the single affinity with which a monoclonal antibody binds its antigenic determinant. Note that the distribution of antibody affinities does not have a normal distribution.

This distribution creates problems in determining the average affinity of an antiserum. This finding should not cause surprise, given that even with a simple hapten, antibodies may be raised against different parts of the hapten's structure. The binding affinities of these antibodies will depend upon the number and type of secondary bonds formed between antigen and antibody, discussed previously. The number of possible antibodies that may be produced to an antigen is high because antigens, which are three-dimensional structures, present many different configurations to the antibody-producing cells.

While the affinity of an antibody is very important in relation to its primary function of antigen binding, it should be remembered that the other biological properties of an antibody are largely determined by its class and subclass, which returns us to the central concept of antibody as a bifunctional molecule.

FURTHER READING

Day E.D. (1972) *Advanced Immunochemistry.* Williams & Wilkins, Baltimore.

Karush F. (1962) Immunologic specificity and molecular structure. *Advanc. Immunol.* **2,** 1.

Steward M.W. (1977) In *Immunochemistry. An Advanced Textbook.* L.E. Glynn & M.W. Steward (eds.) Wiley, Chichester.

Steward M.W. (1983) *Antibodies: their structure and function.* Chapman and Hall, London.

Steward M.W. & Steensgaard J. (1983) *Antibody affinity: Thermodynamic aspects and biological significance.* C. R. C. Press, Boca Raton, Florida.

Weir D.M. (ed.) (1978) *Handbook of Experimental Immunology,* 3rd edition. Blackwell Scientific Publications, Oxford.

7 Complement

Antibody was discovered between 1880 and 1890, but it was revealed soon after that the ability of antibody to inactivate foreign material depended upon the collaboration of another factor, complement. Complement consists of a complex series of proteins many of which are proteinases. This system of enzymes non-specifically complements the immunologically specific effects of antibody by the opsonization and lysis of red cells (in experimental systems) and bacteria. However, this minimal definition requires some expansion in the light of more recent knowledge about the biological activities of complement. In particular, low molecular weight peptides released during firing of the complement cascade (the sequential activation of complement enzymes) have powerful effects on inflammatory cells. This effect can be defined by the general term 'cell activation'. The complement system performs three vital functions (Fig. 7.1):

1. cell activation
2. cytolysis
3. opsonization: rendering cells vulnerable to phagocytosis by the adherence of opsonins, for example, complement components.

The proteins of the complement system form two inter-related enzyme cascades, termed the classical and alternative pathways (see Fig. 7.6), providing two routes to the cleavage of C3, the central event in the complement system: a third set of plasma proteins become assembled into the structures (membrane attack complexes) responsible for the lytic lesions in the lipid bilayers of foreign membranes, lethal to the invading microorganism.

The enzyme cascades are generated by the activation of enzyme precursors which are fixed in turn to biological membranes. Each enzyme precursor is activated by the previous complement component or complex, which is a highly specialized proteinase. This converts the enzyme precursor to its catalytically active form by limited proteolysis, during which a small peptide fragment is cleaved, a nascent membrane binding site is exposed, and the major fragment binds, so forming the next active complement enzyme of the sequence (Fig. 7.2). Because each enzyme can activate many enzyme precursor molecules, each step is amplified, the whole system forming an amplifying cascade resembling the reactions seen in blood clotting and fibrinolysis. The main difference is that the complement system is predominantly a membrane or immune complex associating one and acts locally in its normal role.

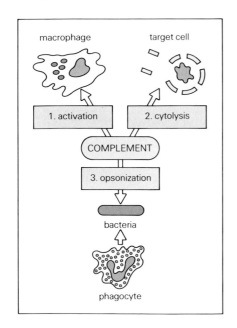

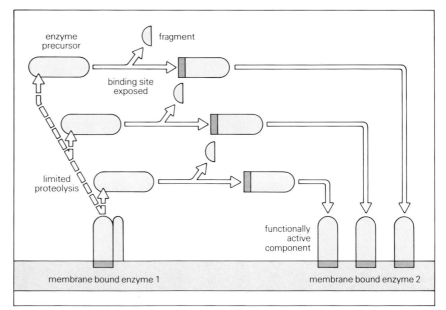

Fig. 7.1 The three major biological activities of the complement system. (1) Activation of the immune system eg. macrophages, (2) cytolysis of target cells, and (3) opsonization, where complement facilitates the phagocytosis of antigen eg. bacteria.

Fig. 7.2 Enzyme cascades of the complement system. Inactive enzyme precursor molecules are activated, through limited proteolysis, by membrane-bound enzymes, (membrane bound enzyme 1). A small fragment is lost from the enzyme precursor and a nascent membrane binding site revealed. The major fragment then binds to the membrane as the next functionally active enzyme of the sequence (membrane-bound enzyme 2). Since each enzyme is able to activate many enzyme precursors the system forms an amplifying cascade. In this and subsequent figures, broken arrows are used to indicate activation processes.

THE COMPLEMENT PROTEINS

Proteins of the Classical Pathway

Before discussing the complement pathways in detail, the principal components which are involved will be described. The classical pathway components are numbered C1-C9, though the scientifically correct sequence of activation of the components (C1, 4, 2, 3, 5, 6, 7, 8, 9) is slightly at odds with the original discovery and numbering of the components. This system is still adhered to. Most components are β globulins with molecular weights of around 2000K (K=1000) and consist mainly of one peptide chain or two peptide chains joined by disulphide bonds. The main exceptions are C4 with three peptide chains and C1q with its unique structure. There is one proteinase inhibitor in the classical pathway which is a specific inhibitor of the serine proteinases C1s and C1r. This inhibitor is discussed later in connection with angioedema. (C3b inactivator is considered separately as part of the feedback loop.)

The complement proteins are collectively a major fraction of the β_1 and β_2 globulins. C3 is present in plasma in the largest quantities (600-1800 mg/L) and fixation of C3 is the major reaction of the complement sequence in molar terms (Fig. 7.3). It is analogous to the conversion of fibrinogen to fibrin in the clotting sequence. Almost all the complement components can be made by monocytes or macrophages in culture, though whether these cells are the major synthetic source of complement *in vivo* is still debatable. It seems likely that these cells make complement for their own use in their immediate environment and that the bulk of the plasma complement components are made in hepatic parenchymal cells. C1 is an exception and for reasons that are not fully explained its principal site of synthesis is the epithelium of the gastrointestinal and urogenital tracts.

Proteins of the Alternative Pathway

The proteins of the alternative pathway (also known as the complement feedback loop) form an alternative reaction pathway to the classical one for the conversion of C3 to C3b. Strictly speaking C3b is both a product and a reactant of the feedback loop, though it is not listed as an alternative pathway component. The proteins are β globulins of high molecular weight (100K-200K) with the exception of factor D. The two inhibitory proteins (β_1H and C3 INH) are an integral part of this pathway and play a key role in C3 breakdown (fig. 7.4)

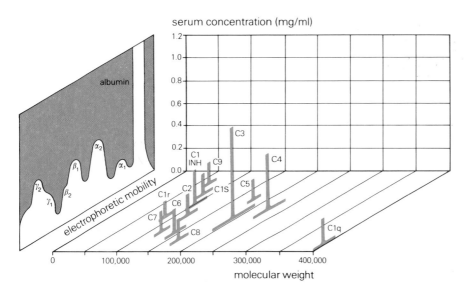

Fig. 7.3 Proteins of the classical complement pathway. They are represented here by vertical bars in a three-dimensional plot to illustrate (x) molecular weight, (y) serum concentration and (z) electrophoretic mobility compared to serum globulins (gamma, beta, alpha and albumin).

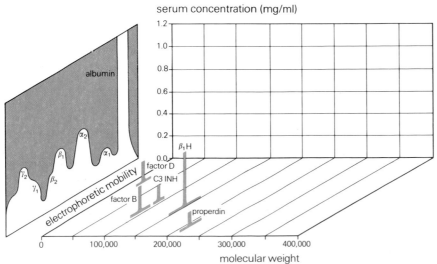

Fig. 7.4 Proteins of the alternative complement pathway. The proteins are represented in the same way as are those in the previous figure. (C3 inhibitor, C3 INH, is also referred to as C3 inactivator, C3 INA or factor I: β_1H is also called factor H.)

A PRIMITIVE COMPLEMENT SYSTEM

Looking back in evolutionary terms, a simple non-adaptive complement effector system causing opsonization of pathogenic microorganisms can be envisaged as arising by any simple mechanism which might bring about limited proteolysis of C3 to C3b (Fig. 7.5).

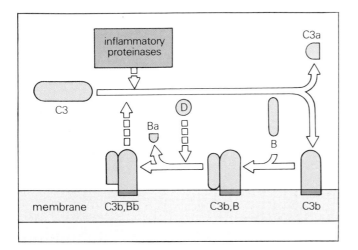

Fig. 7.5 A primitive complement system. Proteinases released during inflammation catalyse the tranformation of C3 into C3b with the release of C3a (anaphylatoxin). Factor B then combines with C3b, to form C3b,B, on the bacterial cell membrane. C3b,B possesses only a weak C3-splitting activity. A non-inhibitable proteinase, factor D (or other proteinases), proteolytically splits the C3, B complex releasing Ba; the resulting C3b,Bb has powerful C3-splitting activity and will amplify the reaction by positive feedback. (The convention of using a horizontal bar above a complement component to designate its activation will be adopted here.) A mechanism to control C3 conversion operates, principally by limiting the functional activity of the C3b molecule and its ability to combine with factor B.

The C3b formed would coat the target particle which would then become susceptible to immuneadherence (or cytoadherence) by phagocytic cells bearing receptors for C3b on their surface. Such a mechanism could arise during acute inflammation since it is known that the common serine-histidine proteinases – trypsin, plasmin, thrombin and elastase – cause limited proteolysis of C3 in a manner which is similar to the action of the natural complement C3 convertases. Only one other protein is required in this primitive scheme and that is factor B. This stabilizes and amplifies the reaction by combining with C3b to form C3b,B with weak C3-splitting activity. Complexed factor B is itself split by serine-histidine proteinases and a 33K fragment, Ba, is lost. The resultant C3b,Bb has powerful C3-splitting activity and will amplify the reaction by positive feedback and so increase the C3b coating of microorganisms at inflammatory loci. In practice a non-inhibitable proteinase specific for factor B seems to have evolved (factor D). Some control mechanism is required to prevent the reaction going to exhaustion, and this principally operates by limiting the

functional activity of the C3b molecule (control site) and its capacity to combine with factor B. It seems likely that C3 and factor B evolved before the proteins of the early part of the classical pathway. It appears that C2 evolved by gene duplication from factor B and that C4 and C5 evolved from C3.

COMPARISON OF THE CLASSICAL AND ALTERNATIVE PATHWAYS

Figure 7.6 compares the classical and alternative complement pathways. The alternative pathway provides non-specific 'innate' immunity, whereas the classical pathway represents a more recently evolved mechanism, which confers specific 'adaptive immunity', associated with 'memory'.

The first stage leading to C3 fixation by the classical sequence is the complexing of antigen to its specific antibody (either IgG or IgM). C3 fixation by the alternative pathway does not require complexed antibody, the sugar component of the microorganism's cell membrane often initiates the reaction sequence. The alternative pathway may provide a mechanism for C3 fixation whenever sufficient quantities of specific antibody are unavailable,

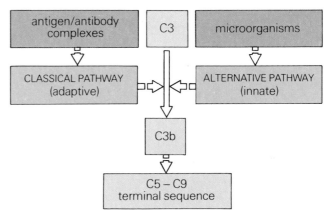

Fig. 7.6 Comparison of the classical and alternative complement pathways. Both generate a C3 convertase, which converts C3 to C3b, the central event of the complement pathway. C3b in turn activates the terminal lytic complement sequence, C5-C9. The first stage leading to C3 fixation by the classical sequence is the complexing of an antigen with its specific antibody. C3 fixation by the alternative pathway does not require complexed antibody since it can be promoted by the sugar component of the microorganism's cell membrane. The alternative pathway provides non-specific 'innate' immunity, whereas the classical pathway probably represents a more recently evolved adaptive mechanism.

for example, early after primary infection. Although it is possible to analyse the effects of classical and alternative pathways separately *in vitro*, it is probable, under normal physiological conditions, that the firing of one pathway also leads to the activation of the other. These two reaction pathways will now be discussed, starting with the classical complement pathway.

THE CLASSICAL COMPLEMENT PATHWAY

The sequence of events comprising this pathway will be considered in three stages: recognition, enzymatic activation, and membrane attack leading to cell death. The recognition unit of the complement system is the C1 complex.

Fixation of C1 by Immunoglobulin

The C1 complement protein complex is a unique feature of the classical complement cascade leading to C3 conversion. C1 fixation occurs when the C1q subcomponent binds directly to immunoglobulin. The other two sub-components, C1r and C1s, do not bind to the immunoglobulin but are involved in the subsequent classical pathway activation. Whether or not C1 fixation occurs depends on a number of constraints. Firstly, only certain subclasses of immunoglobulin can fix C1 even under optimal conditions. For example, these are IgG1, IgG3 and IgM in man, IgG2a and IgM in mice, IgG2 in guinea pigs and IgG1 in ruminants. Secondly, there are spacial or configurational constraints which are still only partially understood. If the amount of C1 fixed is plotted against the concentration of antibody bound to red cells (in model systems) then it can be shown that for IgM the amount of C1 fixed increases in direct proportion to the antibody concentration (slope=1.0), whereas for IgG the amount of C1 fixed increases as the square of the antibody

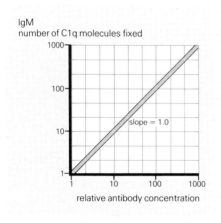

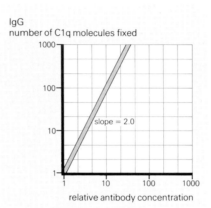

Fig. 7.7 C1q fixation versus bound antibody concentration. The amount of C1q fixed by IgM increases in direct proportion to the antibody concentration, slope = 1, whereas for IgG the amount of C1q fixed increases as the square of the antibody concentration, slope = 2. Therefore, whereas a single IgM molecule is capable of fixing C1q, at least a pair of IgG molecules are required to achieve this result. (The relative antibody concentration refers to antibody bound to red cells.)

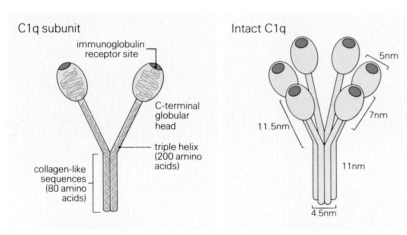

Fig. 7.8 The structure of C1q. 18 peptide chains are formed into three subunits of six chains each. Each subunit consists of a Y-shaped pair of tripe helices joined at the stem and ending in a globular head. The receptors for the attachment to complexed immunoglobulin are situated in the globular heads.

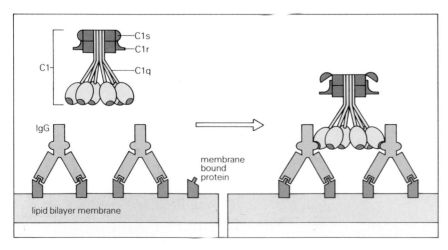

Fig. 7.9 C1qrs fixation. A pair of IgG molecules are bound to a repeating protein antigen (membrane bound protein). C1 fixes to the C_H2 domain of IgG. The activation of C1r and C1s is by internal cleavage represented diagrammatically by the alteration in their orientation on the C1q component.

concentration; slope=2.0 (Fig. 7.7). It can be concluded from this evidence that whereas a single IgM molecule is potentially able to fix C1 at least a pair of IgG molecules are required for this purpose.

The C1q molecule is potentially multivalent for attachment to the complement fixation sites of immunoglobulin. The sites are on the C_H2 domain of IgG and probably on the C_H4 domain of IgM. The appropriate peptide sequence of the complement fixing site may become exposed following complexing of the immunoglobulin or the sites may always be available but require multiple attachment by C1q with critical geometry to achieve the necessary avidity. C1q is a 400K protein formed from 18 peptide chains in three subunits of six. Each 6 peptide subunit consists of a Y-shaped pair of triple peptide helices joined at the stem and ending in a globular non-helical head. The 80 amino acid helical components of each triple peptide contain many Gly-X-Y sequences, where X and Y are proline, isoleucine or hydroxylysine; they therefore strongly resemble collagen fibrils. Electron microscopy views of C1q molecules are compatible with the shape and dimensions given in figure 7.8. It is assumed that the globular ends are the sites for multivalent attachment to the complement fixing sites in immune complexed immunoglobulin.

C1 fixation is demonstrable by binding IgG to a repeating protein antigen inserted into a lipid bilayer for example, a red cell (Fig. 7.9). C1 fixes to the C_H2 domain of IgG and its subunits are held together as they are in plasma by a Ca^{++} ion acting as a ligand. The ultrastructure of C1r and C1s is now known. They are chemically similar, 83K proteins, though a distinctive difference between them is that C1r dimerises whereas C1s binds monovalently to C1r. They form a tetrameric complex which binds to C1q in the presence of a Ca^{++} ion. How C1q activates C1r is a mystery, since C1q itself has no known enzymic activity. It is known, however, that C1r and C1s activate in sequence still attached to C1q and that both proteins become typical DFP-inhibitable (diisopropylflurophosphate) serine-histidine esterases on activation. There are also marked amino acid sequence and functional homologies between the two proteins and they almost certainly arose by gene duplication. The active catalytic site is a 27K peptide resembling the corresponding peptide in trypsin and plasmin, which are also serine-histidine esterases. However, C1r and C1s differ in enzymic specificity. C1s is the only substrate for C1r,

while C1s, but not C1r, will activate C4 and C2, the following components in the classical complement sequence. C1q, C1r and C1s are best envisaged as an interlocking enzyme system.

Fixation and Activation of C4 and C2 by the C1qrs Complex

C1s splits a 6K peptide (C4a) from the N-terminal part of the α chain of C4 leaving a large fragment called C4b. This occurs in the 'fluid phase' of the plasma around the C̄1s catalytic site and a nascent, but labile, reactive internal thioester bond is revealed on C4b. The reaction is efficient, but the stable binding of C4b molecules to membranes is inefficient (less than 10%). These bind in close proximity to their site of activation, either to the C̄1qrs complex, or to the adjacent red cell membrane. C4b molecules which fail to bind decay in the medium, through loss of the active site.

C̄1s is weakly proteolytic for free intact C2 but highly active against C2 which has complexed with C4b molecules in the presence of Mg^{++} ions. This reaction will only occur if the C4b, C2 complexes form close to the C̄1s. A smaller, C2a fragment (30K) is lost to the surrounding medium and the larger, C2b fragment (70K) joins with C4b to form the C̄4b2b enzyme whose catalytic site is probably in the C2b peptide. Overall, the fixation and activation of C2 is inefficient. The C̄4b2b enzyme is unstable and decays with a half life of 5 minutes at 37°C due to release and decay of C2b (Fig. 7.10).

There are two major constraints on the action of C̄1s on C4 and C2, and on the stable formation of the C̄4b2b complex. The first is the action of the proteinase inhibitor, C1 esterase inhibitor or α2-neuraminoglycoprotein, which stoichiometrically binds to C̄1s and C̄1r. This reaction may not be important in restraining the action of C̄1s at a local membrane site, but is extremely important in preventing the excessive action of free C1 on C4 and C2 in the fluid phase, a point discussed later with regard to hereditary angioedema. Membrane-bound C4b is susceptible to decay by C3b-inactivator, which destroys the acceptor site for C2 in the same way that it acts on C3b to prevent formation of the C3b,B complex.

There has recently been a change in the nomenclature of this part of the complement system. Previously, the larger fragment of C2 was C2a and the smaller fragment, C2b. The names of the fragments were reversed to accord with the system used for other parts of the pathway.

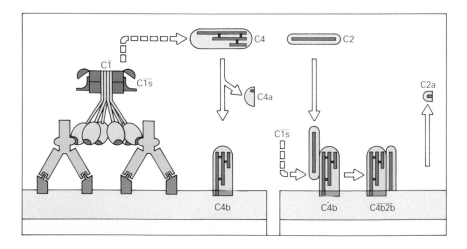

Fig. 7.10 Generation of C̄4b2b – the classical pathway C3 convertase. C̄1s splits C4 releasing the fragment C4a. The resulting C4b binds to the adjacent membrane through reaction with its nascent thioester bond. C2 from the serum binds to C4b in a magnesium-dependent complex and is then split by C̄1s, releasing C2a, resulting in the formation of C̄4b2b, the classical pathway C3 convertase. In this diagram dark green bars represent peptide chains of the molecules cross-linked by disulphide bonds (red).

Action of the C$\overline{\text{4b2b}}$ Complex on C3 to Form C4b2b3b

The C$\overline{\text{4b2b}}$ complex, which is often termed 'classical pathway C3 convertase' activates C3 molecules by splitting a 9K peptide, the C3 anaphylatoxin, from the N-terminal end of the peptide of C3 revealing a nascent thioester reactive binding site on the larger fragment, C3b. Clusters of C3b molecules are thus activated and bound near the C$\overline{\text{4b2b}}$ complex (Fig. 7.11). The overall efficiency of the reaction is low (less than 10%), but because C3 is present in such a high concentration, each

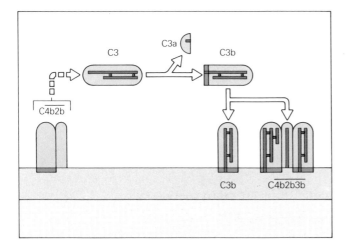

Fig. 7.11 Action of the C$\overline{\text{4b2b}}$ complex on C3 – formation of the C$\overline{\text{4b2b3b}}$ complex and uncomplexed C3b. The C$\overline{\text{4b2b}}$ complex splits C3 molecules by cleaving the C3a anaphylatoxin from the N-terminal end of the α peptide of C3. (Anaphylatoxins are small peptides released during complement activation which cause histamine release from mast cells, and smooth muscle contraction and in this sense mimic anaphylactic reactions. They also show chemotactic activity for neutrophil polymorphs but C3a is relatively weak in this respect.) An internal thioester bond is exposed on the C3b which causes C3b molecules to bind near the C$\overline{\text{4b2b}}$ complex. One of these molecules will bind to C$\overline{\text{4b2b}}$ to form C$\overline{\text{4b2b3b}}$, the classical pathway C5 convertase.

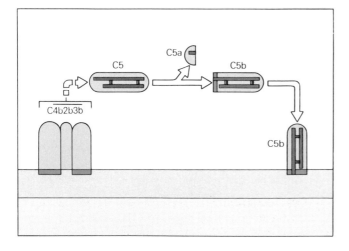

Fig. 7.12 C5 fixation. C$\overline{\text{4b2b3b}}$ cleaves C5a (a 15K peptide) from the α chain of C5. C5b fixation initiates the events leading to the formation of the membrane attack complex described later. A membrane binding site is thus revealed on the major fragment, C5b.

catalytic site can bind several hundred C3b molecules. Only one favourably sited C3b molecule combines with C$\overline{\text{4b2b}}$ to form the final proteolytic complex of the complement sequence.

Action of C3b on C5

C3b splits a 15K peptide, C5a, from the α chain of C5, to initiate C5b fixation and the beginning of the membrane attack complex (Fig. 7.12).

No further proteinases are generated in the classical complement sequence. Other bound C3b molecules not involved in the C$\overline{\text{4b2b3b}}$ complex form an opsonic macromolecular coat on the red cell or other target particle rendering it susceptible to immuneadherence by C3b receptors on phagocytic cells. The classical complement pathway is summarized in figure 7.13.

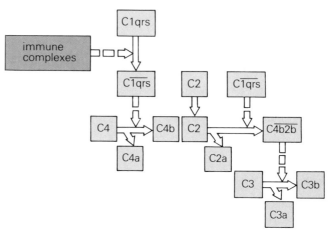

Fig. 7.13 Summary of the classical complement pathway. Immune complexes activate C1qrs, which cleaves C4 releasing C4a. The major fragment, C4b, binds C2, which is in turn cleaved by C$\overline{\text{1}}$, releasing the minor fragment, C2a. The major fragment, C2b, remains bound to C4b to constitute the C3 convertase, C$\overline{\text{4b2b}}$, which cleaves C3 into C3a and C3b, the most abundant reaction of the classical complement pathway.

C3b (C4b) COATINGS AND IMMUNEADHERENCE

There seems little doubt that the generation of a C3b macromolecular coating on target particles is the major biological function of complement and it is the culminating step for the classical pathway enzyme cascade and the feedback loop. C3b receptors are present on neutrophils, eosinophils, monocytes and macrophages, including Kupffer cells and alveolar macrophages. They are also present on primate red cells (the receptor cell in the original immuneadherence reaction), on the platelets of many non-primate species, excluding ruminants, and on B lymphocytes, where they may also act as receptors for the EB virus.

C3b-coated particles of all descriptions adhere avidly to the phagocytic cells mentioned above. While this ability of C3b to promote immuneadherence is not in question, there is controversy about the role of the C3b coating in the induction of phagocytosis. That C3b alone can induce phagocytosis does seem to be the case for many bacteria of low virulence, particularly those lacking the complete O-somatic polysaccharide side chains to their endotoxins (ie. rough forms) or lacking other anti-phagocytic devices, such as capsules. It may not be true that C3b alone can induce phagocytosis of red cells by

neutrophils and monocytes, and this suggests that the bacteria of low virulence are providing some accessory signal. Activated macrophages, which have more C3b receptors than monocytes per unit surface area, have a greater activity for immuneadherence and phagocytosis and on present evidence, it seems that they can ingest cells coated with C3b alone.

Another broad generalization can be made about the role of C3b in effector cell reactions. C3b coatings on target cells almost always augment the cytotoxic activity of an effector cell directed against an IgG-coated target cell. The effect of C3b coatings are summarized in figure 7.14. Figure 7.15 shows the appearance of C3b coatings on bacterial flagelli under electron microscopy.

Since most effector cells lack receptors for IgM, C3b fixation to target particles is probably a critical opsonizing event during the early IgM phase of a primary immune response. Later, when high avidity IgG antibody appears, the augmenting opsonizing effects of C3b, though present, may no longer be so necessary since multivalent binding of IgG to Fc receptors itself can induce phago-cytosis. C4b coatings act similarly to C3b coatings but are less effective.

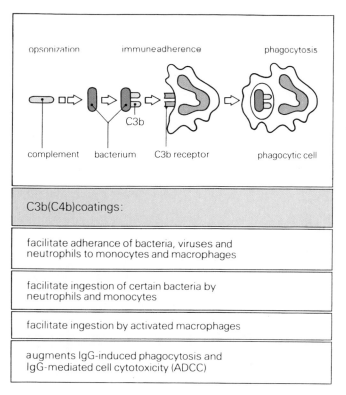

<table>
<tr><td>C3b(C4b)coatings:</td></tr>
<tr><td>facilitate adherance of bacteria, viruses and neutrophils to monocytes and macrophages</td></tr>
<tr><td>facilitate ingestion of certain bacteria by neutrophils and monocytes</td></tr>
<tr><td>facilitate ingestion by activated macrophages</td></tr>
<tr><td>augments IgG-induced phagocytosis and IgG-mediated cell cytotoxicity (ADCC)</td></tr>
</table>

Fig. 7.14 C3b coatings and immuneadherence.
This diagram represents the processes of opsonization, immuneadherence and phagocytosis. The main functions of C3b coatings are listed underneath.

ANAPHYLATOXIN FORMATION

C3a and C5a are split from the N-terminal ends of the α-chain of C3 and C5 respectively by their convertase enzymes. In the case of C3, a 77 amino acid sequence is cleaved at a point where a carboxyterminal arginine is revealed: in the case of C5 a 74 amino acid peptide is cleaved, again exposing a carboxyterminal arginine (Fig. 7.16). Both C3a and C5a have 'spasmogenic' properties which are critically dependent on the possession of the carboxyterminal arginine.

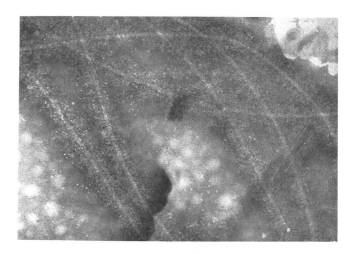

Fig. 7.15 EM appearance of C3-coated *Salmonella* flagellae. The flagellae have been incubated with anti-flagella antibody and complement. The electron-dense material extending 30nm on either side of each flagellum is believed to be C3b. The interpretation of this is that complement fixation by antibody results in a heavy macromolecular coating of C3b on biological membranes to which complement has been fixed. ×900,000. Courtesy of Drs. A. Feinstein and E. Munn.

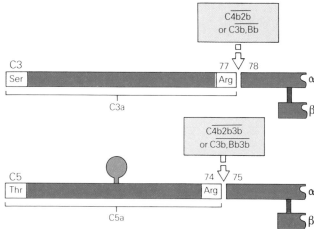

Fig. 7.16 Anaphylatoxin formation. The N-terminal ends of C3 and C5 alpha chains are shown. A 77 amino acid peptide, C3a, is split from the C3 molecule, revealing a carboxyterminal arginine, by the C3 convertase C4b2b (classical pathway) or C3b,Bb (alternative pathway). In the case of C5, a 74 amino acid peptide, C5a, is split from C5 also revealing a carboxyterminal arginine, by the C5 convertase, C4b2b3b (classical pathway) or C3b,Bb3b (alternative pathway). C5a contains a carbohydrate moiety indicated by a blue circle.

BIOLOGICAL EFFECTS OF C3a

C3a causes smooth muscle contraction in a wide variety of animal tissues, for example, guinea pig ileum and rat uterus, and given intravenously or intradermally causes endothelial cell contraction in post-capillary venules. The effect on skin is an almost immediate erythema and oedema at concentrations as low as 10-100mol. At least some of the vascular effects are indirect and are due to the release of histamine from mast cells. C3a is inactivated shortly after its formation in serum and body fluids by carboxypeptidase B, an enzyme which rapidly removes the arginine group. Loss of the arginine destroys all the biological functions of C3a. The whole C3a peptide sequence is known and all the biological activities appear to reside in the carboxyterminal octapeptide which includes the arginine.

BIOLOGICAL EFFECTS OF C5a

C5a is ten to twenty times more active than C3a on a molar basis, though its net effectiveness may be less since fewer C5a molecules are generated in the complement cascade. C5a also has a wider biological activity than C3a. The important features of C5a are:
1. it is the major chemotactic factor for neutrophils liberated during complement activation and causes their margination in vessels leading to blood neutropenia
2. it appears to activate neutrophils by triggering the bactericidal oxidative burst, and increased procoagulant activity and glucose uptake
3. it switches on neutrophil production of leukotrienes, particularly B4, which prolongs the increased permeability phase induced by C5a
4. it increases vascular permeability
5. it causes mast cell degranulation, especially if the C5a is located on a solid surface.
6. it causes smooth muscle contraction.
A further important point about C5a is that its cell activating properties are maintained, albeit in a weaker form, in the desarginine (desArg) peptide, though like C3a, the spasmogenic activities are lost (Fig. 7.17).

ASSEMBLY OF THE C5-9 MEMBRANE ATTACK COMPLEX

The fixation of C5b to biological membranes is followed by the sequential addition of four more proteins C6, C7, C8 and C9 (Fig. 7.18). Fully assembled in the correct molar ratios they form the membrane attack complex. The C5b-C6 complex is hydrophilic, but the addition of C7 in some way results in the exposure of apolar groups in the C567 complex which have detergent and phospholipid binding properties. In free solution, nascent C567 has a half life of about 0.1 second and is 'contagious' in the sense that it can attach to any lipid bilayer within its effective diffusion radius producing the phenomenon of 'reactive lysis' on innocent bystander cells. Once membrane bound, C567 is relatively stable and can interact with C8 and C9.

Another characteristic of C567 is its strongly amphiphilic nature due to the exposed apolar groups. This occurrence of both hydrophobic and hydrophilic groups within the same complex may account for its tendency to polymerize and form small protein micelles. C5-8 polymerizes C9 to form a tubule, known as the membrane attack complex, traversing the membrane. This is a highly amphiphilic, 33S, 1700K hollow cylinder, 15 nm long and 10 nm in diameter. It is inserted end on into the lipid bilayer, and projects from it.

The micellar arrangement of the membrane insertion region is conjectural. A structure of this form can be assumed to perturb the lipid bilayer sufficiently to allow the free exchange of electrolytes and water across the membrane. The consequence of this for a living cell will be the net influx of Na^+ and H_2O due to high internal colloid osmotic pressure, which will eventually lead to lysis. Additionally, it appears that the formation of complement micelles can lead to the piecemeal disassembly of viral envelope membranes, where osmosis is unlikely to be an important factor in the lytic event. The membrane attack complex is seen under electron microscopy in figure 7.19.

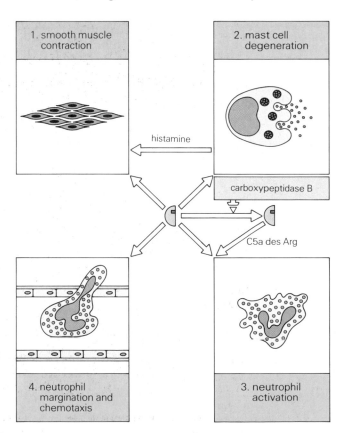

Fig. 7.17 Biological effects of C5a and C5a des Arg. C5a causes (1) smooth muscle contraction, (2) mast cell degranulation, (3) neutrophil activation and (4) margination and chemotaxis of neutrophils. Smooth muscle is further affected by histamine released following mast cell degranulation. Loss of the C-terminal arginine residue, following cleavage by carboxypeptidase B, produces C5a des Arg, which possesses weak cell-activating properties.

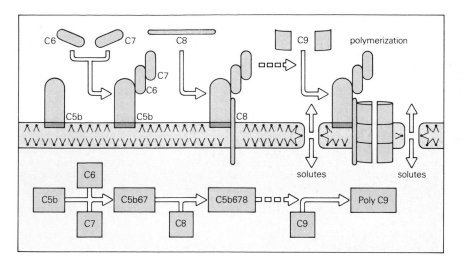

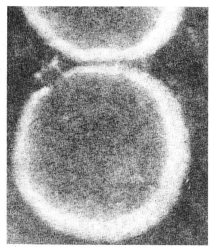

Fig. 7.18 Assembly of the C5-9 membrane attack complex. Once C5b is membrane bound, C6 and C7 attach themselves to form the stable complex, C5b67, which interacts with C8 to yield C5b678. This unit has some effect in disrupting the membrane, and it also causes the polymerization of C9 to form tubules traversing the membrane. The tube may remain associated with the C5b678 and is referred to as a membrane attack complex (MAC). Disruption of the membrane by this structure permits the free exchange of solutes, which is primarily responsible for cell lysis.

Fig. 7.19 Electron micrograph of the membrane attack complex. The funnel-shaped lesion is due to a human C(5b-9) complex that has been reincorporated into lecithin liposomal membranes. ×234,000. Courtesy of Professor J. Tranum-Jensen and Dr. S. Bhakdi.

THE ALTERNATIVE PATHWAY

The components of the alternative pathway collaborate to cause various immunological responses, such as phagocytosis and inflammation, through the activation of C3. Activated alternative pathway enzymes assemble themselves on the target membrane – usually without antibody involvement – and cleave a C3b fragment from C3, the initial step of the membrane attack sequence. A simple C3b feedback loop, the primitive complement system, was described above and it was suggested that the complement system may have started here, with the classical pathway evolving later. The central controlling element of such a pathway is a mechanism which prevents the association between C3b and factor B, since such a mechanism will block the formation of C3b,Bb, the catalytically active C3 convertase of the feedback loop. This is achieved by factor H (previously β_1H), which competes with factor B for its combining site on C3b, eventually leading to C3 inactivation (Fig. 7.20).

Factors H and B appear to occupy a common site on C3b and which factor is preferentially bound to C3b depends on the nature of the surface to which C3b is attached. Certain surfaces, usually polysaccharides, are also called 'activator' surfaces and for reasons which are still not really understood, favour the uptake of factor B onto the chain of C3b, with the corresponding displacement of factor H. In this environment, binding of factor H is inhibited and consequently factor B will replace H at the common binding site. In the condition known as paroxysmal nocturnal haemoglobinuria (PNH), the patient's red blood cells act as an activator surface, leading to complement fixation by the alternative pathway, and lysis by the terminal complement components. When factor H is excluded, C3b, thought to be formed

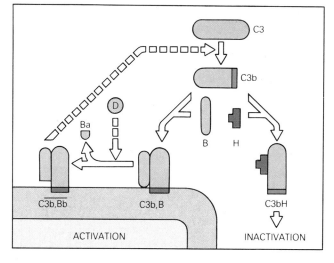

Fig. 7.20 The Alternative pathway. C3b and factor B combine to form C3b,B, which is converted into an active C3 convertase, C3b,Bb by the loss of a small fragment, Ba, through the action of the enzyme, factor D. C3b,Bb then converts more C3 to C3b, which binds more factor B and so the feedback cycle continues. The uptake of factor B onto C3b occurs when C3b is bound to an activator surface. However, C3b in the fluid phase or attached to a non-activator surface will preferentially bind factor H and so prevent C3b,B formation.

continuously in small amounts by a 'tickover mechanism' possibly involving proteolytic enzymes in body fluids, is able to combine with factor B to form the complex C3b,B which is susceptible to enzymatic cleavage by factor D. The smaller, 33K Ba fragment, is lost and the C3b,Bb enzyme is formed. C3b,Bb is a C3 convertase which fixes more C3b to the activator surface so that more B binding sites are exposed, and the feedback cycle continues.

In theory, there is no restraint on this system, when it excludes the influence of factor H, and in practice, incubation of zymosan or inulin (both activator polysaccharides) with serum or injection of inulin intravenously in experimental animals results in the conversion of large amounts of C3 to C3b. Another controlling point in the amplification loop depends on the stability of the C3b,Bb convertase. Ordinarily this decays by the loss of Bb with a half life of approximately 5 minutes. However, if properdin (P) binds to C3b,Bb, forming C3b,BbP, the half life is extended to 30 minutes, thus potentiating the action of the alternative pathway C3 convertase. The alternative pathway was originally called the properdin pathway because purified properdin apparently caused complement activation by this mechanism. Properdin levels are elevated in some diseases. The analogous action of the classical and alternative pathways is illustrated in figure 7.21.

BREAKDOWN OF C3b

C3b formed in the fluid phase in the reaction above or C3b fixed to a non-activator surface, for example, a sheep red cell, is susceptible to factor H binding. This alters the α chain of C3b in some way that allows it to be cleaved by the enzyme C3b inactivator, originally called KAF, then C3bINA and now factor I. The α chain is 117K in length and is split into a 68K and a 43K portion with the loss of a 3K fragment. At this stage C3b loses its haemolytic and immuneadherence activity. Further action of an uncharacterized trypsin-like enzyme in plasma, breaks the α chain, to leave a 29K fragment, C3d, on the red cell. The inactive main fragment, C3c, is removed by the reticuloendothelial system (Fig.7.22).

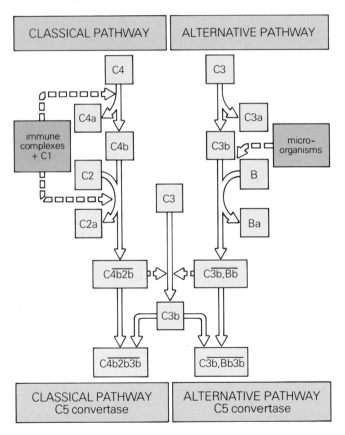

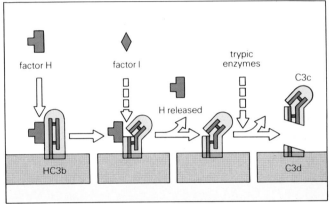

Fig. 7.22 C3b inactivation. The C3b fixed to a non-activator surface may bind factor H which allows an inactivator enzyme, factor I to cleave the α chain of C3b. Factor H is released and C3b is left susceptible to the action of tryptic enzymes which break the α chain releasing an inactive main fragment, C3c, and leaving a smaller fragment, C3d bound to the surface.

Fig. 7.21 Analogous action of the classical and alternative pathways. Both pathways generate a C3 convertase: C4b2b (classical pathway) and C3b,Bb (alternative pathway). In the classical sequence, C1 activated by complexed antibody splits C4 and C2 with the loss of the small fragments C4a and C2a: the major components form C4b2b. In the alternative route, pre-existing C3b binds factor B, which is split releasing a small fragment, Ba. The major fragment, Bb, remains bound to form C3b,Bb. This converts more C3 so continuing the feedback cycle. Activator surfaces, on microorganisms for example, facilitate the combination of factor B and C3b, and promote alternative pathway activation. The C3 convertases of both pathways may bind further C3b to yield the enzymes which activate the next component of the complement system, C5: classical pathway C5 convertase, C4b2b3b, and alternative pathway C5 convertase C3b,Bb3b.

COBRA VENOM FACTOR (CVF) AND C3 NEPHRITIC FACTOR (C3 Nef)

The C3b,Bb complex can be stabilized 'non-physiologically' by several mechanisms, with predictable results on C3 conversion. The simplest way of doing this (at least in principle) is to remove factor H, the competitor of factor B, or to remove factor I, which breaks down C3b. Both inhibitors can be removed from serum in vitro by precipitation with the appropriate F(ab')₂ antibody and in both cases, fluid phase stabilized C3b,Bb is formed in the presence of properdin, and excessive C3 to C3b conversion occurs. This phenomenon also occurs in vivo in a group of very rare patients with an inherited deficiency of factor I, which presents clinically as severe C3 hypocomplementaemia and pyogenic infections.

Non-physiological stabilization of C3b,Bb occurs in two other pathological states. Cobra venom contains, among its many toxins and enzymes, cobra C3b. This appears to be resistant to the action of human factor H and I and the C3b(cobra), Bb(human) complex formed when cobra C3b (cobra venom factor) is added to human serum is a highly stable enzyme. The complex is also formed if purified CVF is injected into animals. Here, the stable convertase has a half life of 37 hours and causes massive conversion of C3 to C3b, by discharging the feedback loop to exhaustion and by forming the alternative pathway C5 convertase, causing C5-9 consumption. It remains the most effective way of producing experimental complement depletion *in vitro*.

A rather similar effect is produced clinically by nephritic factor (NEF). Nephritic factor(s) is an unusual IgG3 subclass autoantibody against the C3b,Bb enzyme complex. Possibly it stabilizes the complex by preventing the displacement of factor B by factor H. The clinical consequences of this stabilization are marked C3 hypocomplementaemia without infection. Nephritic factors of this classical type are found in the plasma of patients with Type II mesangiocapillary glomerulonephritis.

the IgM phase of a primary immune response, the localization of antigen on dendritic cells in germinal centres is blocked by prior decomplementation with CVF and is, therefore, dependent on C3-9 fixation. Failure of antigen localization can interfere quantitively but not absolutely with the development of a B cell memory to thymus dependent antigens and to late IgG responses. One awkward fact which still needs to be explained fully is the virtually normal IgG antibody responses in patients who are homozygously deficient in C3. Once possible explanation is that the initial cycle of antigen localization and memory is dependent on IgM and C3 for its optimal performance, but that once small amounts of IgG antibody appear this dependence is circumvented and with time, normal IgG responses build up (Fig. 7.23). Thus, a role for C3-9 is postulated in the generation and function of memory cells after primary intravenous immunization with thymus-dependent antigen.

EFFECT OF C3-9 DEPLETION ON THE ADAPTIVE IMMUNE RESPONSE

For several years there was controversy surrounding the role of complement in the immune response and some conflict between observations made *in vivo* and *in vitro*. It was concluded that in some way, C3-9 depletion could interfere with the IgG, but not the IgM, response to thymus dependent antigens *in vivo*. Some of the controversy has been resolved since it has been recognized that during

INHERITED COMPLEMENT DEFICIENCIES AND THEIR EFFECTS IN MAN

The great majority of deficiencies have an autosomal recessive mode of inheritance and there is usually a total absence of the complement protein implying the absence of a functional structural gene (ie. a null structural gene). Main points of note are:
1. the high association between complement deficiency and immune complex-like or lupus-like disorders.

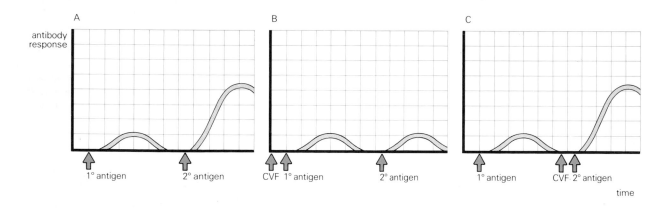

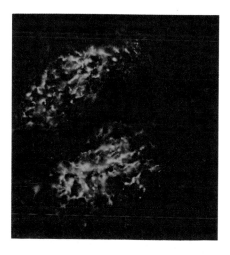

Fig. 7.23 Effect of complement depletion on the IgG response.
Injection of priming (1°) and boosting (2°) doses of antigen produces a classical primary and secondary immune response (A). If the animal is complement-depleted by the addition of cobra venom factor (CVF) prior to the primary response, immunological memory fails to develop, and on subsequent antigen challenge the animal produces another primary response (B). The effect of CVF is only produced if complement is depleted prior to the primary response – depletion subsequent to the primary response does not hinder a normal secondary response (c). The effect of depletion is thought to be related to poor localization of antigen-antibody complexes in the germinal centres of complement-depleted animals. The immunofluorescence picture shows antigen localized in the germinal centres of mouse spleen (24 hours after injection of 1mg of aggregated human IgG, here acting as an antigen) and bound predominantly to the dendritic cells. This localization does not occur in complement-depleted mice. Courtesy of Professor John Holborow.

This association is possibly due to failure of complement-dependent mechanisms for the elimination of immune complexes.

2. the relatively large number of patients (and pedigrees) with C2 deficiency. The C2 deficiency gene is in marked disequilibrium with the HLA haplotype A10,BW18,Bfs,Dw2.

3. the total absence of C3 (in homozygous C3 deficiency) and the virtual absence of C3 (in C3bINA deficiency) are associated with severe life threatening infections, particularly with pneumococcal or meningococcal septicaemia, meningitis and peritonitis.

4. the high association of C5, C6, C7 and C8 deficiency with disseminated meningococcal and gonococcal infections. The obvious implication of this association is that complement lysis of *Neisseria* is a major mechanism for controlling the dissemination of the organisms from local sites such as the nasopharynx, urethra and vagina. There is no association between neutropenic states and disseminated neisserial infections, suggesting that neutrophil phagocytosis is not a critical factor. In mixtures of *Neisseria* with complement and neutrophils *in vitro*, the bactericidal effect on the *Neisseria* resides entirely in the capacity of complement to generate the C5-9 step and not on the presence of the neutrophils.

Figure 7.24 lists the rare inherited complement deficiencies in man.

component	disease associations
classical C1-C4	lupus like syndromes including glomerulonephritis, arthralgia, vasculitis
C3	disseminated infections particularly with pyogenic bacteria
lytic pathway C5-8	disseminated neisserial infections, rheumatoid syndromes
C9	none
C1 inhibitor	hereditary angioedema

Fig. 7.24 Inherited human complement deficiencies. Deficiency in a particular complement component is associated with the conditions indicated.

INHIBITION OF C1 AND HEREDITARY ANGIOEDEMA

C$\overline{1}$ inhibitor (α_2-neuraminoglycoprotein or C1INH) is the only natural inhibitor of C$\overline{1}$r and C$\overline{1}$s. In this respect C$\overline{1}$r and C$\overline{1}$s are unique proteinases in not being inhibited by α_2-macroglobulin, α_1-antitrypsin or anti-thrombin III. C$\overline{1}$ inhibitor binds stoichiometrically to each molecule of C$\overline{1}$r and C$\overline{1}$s in the C$\overline{1}$qrs complex and in doing so dissociates a pair of C1r-C1s complexes from C1q. C$\overline{1}$ inhibitor is irreversibly bound to the complex, which is then catabolized (Fig. 7.25). C$\overline{1}$ inhibitor is also a stoichiometric inhibitor or plasmin, kallikrein, activated Hageman factor and factor XIa, and it can be assumed that a substantial part of its *in vivo* catabolism occurs by its combination with these proteinases. If this assumption

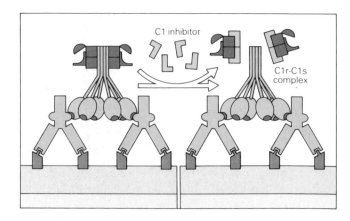

Fig. 7.25 C1 breakdown. C1 inhibitor binds to the C$\overline{1}$r and C$\overline{1}$s components of C$\overline{1}$qrs and removes from C1q a pair of C1r-C1s complexes, which are now inactive.

is correct, then it goes a long way in explaining the clinical disease of hereditary angioedema. The disease arises as sporadic attacks of deep tissue oedema, often starting around the mouth and spreading to the neck and face and sometimes arising in the gut. It is inherited as an autosomal dominant condition and so cases occur in every generation. The patients are heterozygously deficient in C$\overline{1}$ inhibitor and are assumed to have one normal structure gene. The blood levels of C$\overline{1}$ inhibitor are less that 35% of normal and often fall to zero during attacks of angioedema. An explanation for why the levels in the patients are less than the mean predicted 50% values, can be deduced from considering the nature of the catabolism of C1 inhibitor by its combination with active proteinases. If

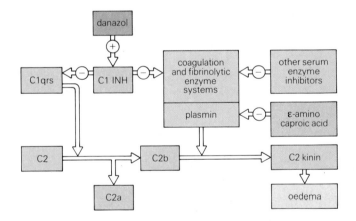

Fig. 7.26 Molecular pathways in angioedema. Classical pathway C2b is converted by plasmin into an abnormal peptide fragment, C2 kinin, which is responsible for the oedema. In patients with hereditary angioedema, the low levels of C$\overline{1}$ inhibitor may become exhausted by binding to proteinases of the coagulation and fibrinolytic systems, factors XI and XII (though note that other inhibitors of these systems are normally present in the serum). Since C1 INH is the only protein capable of inactivating C$\overline{1}$r and C$\overline{1}$s, its depletion leads to uncontrolled production of C2b, the substrate for the production of C2 kinin. Therapy of the disease is aimed either at increasing the level of C1 INH (by administering Danazol), or decreasing the activity of plasmin (with ε-aminocaproic acid).

the greater part of its natural catabolism is by this mechanism, then the plasma level will be a balance between this catabolism and the synthetic rate for two structural genes. Where only one structural gene is operating, the set plasma level will be much less than 50% since the system will be operating under stressed conditions with a half synthetic rate.

The relationship between C1 inhibitor deficiency and angioedema is still not full understood. During attacks C4 and C2 fall to zero and free C1 may appear in the plasma. No C4b2b enzyme is formed and little C3 is consumed, probably because the action of C1 on C4 and C2 occur in the fluid phase. The angioedema-producing peptide is thought to be derived from C2 and recent evidence suggests that it might be an abnormal cleavage product produced by the action of C1 on C2 followed by the action of plasmin on C2b. When hereditary angioedema is treated by Danazol, both C1 inhibitor and plasminogen rise, suggesting that the consumption of C1 inhibitor and the activation of plasminogen to plasmin are linked (Fig. 7.26).

COMPLEMENT AND THE MAJOR HISTOCOMPATIBILITY COMPLEX

Evidence for the localization of a structural gene for a given complement component derives from a study of the frequency of recombinants between the complement markers and HLA markers, and from the study of linkage disequilibria between complement and HLA alleles (eg. factor B and HLA-B). In general, allelic variation or polymorphism of a complement component has been demonstrated by finding fixed and reproducible charge differences for that component on high voltage electrophoresis or electrofocusing. Use of the allelic markers then allows linkage to HLA to be determined from family studies. In addition, linkage can be studied where there is a null complement allele expressed and detectable in a family as a complement deficiency. Using one or both of these techniques, no convincing recombinant has yet been demonstrated between C2, factor B, C4 and HLA-B. It therefore seems most probable that the gene cluster for these complement proteins lies close to the HLA-B locus. In contrast, complement components C3, C5, C,6, C7 and C8 are not linked to HLA.

A rather curious genetic phenomenon is seen in the inheritance of C4. C4 is coded for by tandem genes and most of the population possess two isotypes of C4. They are not allotypes since they are coded for at adjacent loci and must have arisen by unequal crossover. The result is that most individuals have both C4 (fast) and C4 (slow) isotypes. Furthermore, C4 is detectable on normal circulating red cells as the Chido and Rogers blood groups, which were determined and named from their reaction with rare alloantisera from either Chido or Rogers negative individuals. Thus Chido is almost certainly the slow isotype of C4 and Rogers is the fast isotype, while Chido negative or Rogers negative individuals lack the appropriate isotype and the corresponding tandem gene (Fig. 7.27). The principal actions of complement and its role in the acute inflammatory reaction are summarized in figure 7.28.

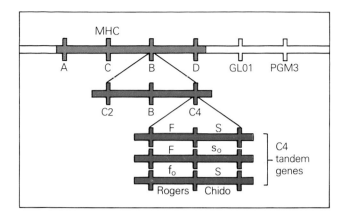

Fig. 7.27 Complement and the Major Histocompatibility Complex. The MHC region of the chromosome is shown in red and the position of the A, C, B and D alleles within this region indicated. Alleles outside of this region are also shown: these genes code for the enzymes glyoxylase (GLO1) and phosphoglucomutase (PGM3). The B allele region is expanded to show that it contains genes coding for C2, factor B and C4. Closer investigation of the area coding for C4 reveals a set of tandem genes. Two isotypes of each gene occur: a fast type (F) giving rise to the Rogers blood group through binding to red cells and a slow type (S), associated with the Chido blood group: f_o and s_o indicate non-functioning genes.

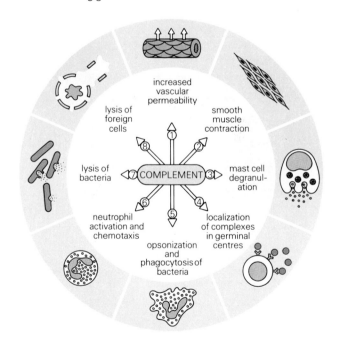

Fig. 7.28 Summary of the actions of complement and its role in the acute inflammatory reaction. Note how the elements of the reactions are induced: increased vascular permeability (1) due to the action of C3a and C5a on smooth muscle (2) and mast cells (3) allows exudation of plasma protein. C3 facilitates both the localization of complexes in germinal centres (4) and the opsonization and phagocytosis of bacteria (5). Neutrophils, which are attracted to the area of inflammation by chemotaxis (6) phagocytose the opsonized microorganisms. The membrane attack complex, C5-9, is responsible for the lysis of bacteria (7) and other cells recognized as foreign (8).

FURTHER READING

Boackle R.J., Johnson B.J. & Caughman G.B. (1979) An IgG primary sequence exposure theory for complement activation using synthetic peptides. *Nature* **282,** 742.

Borsos T. & Rapp H.J. (1965) Complement fixation on cell surfaces by 19S and 7S antibodies. *Science* **150,** 505.

Lachmann P.J. (1979) Complement.   In *The Antigens. Vol. V.* M. Sela (ed.) Academic Press, New York.

Lachmann P.J. (1979) An evolutionary view of the complement system. *Behring Inst. Mitt.* **63,** 25.

Ochs H.D., Wedgwood R.J., Frank M.M., Heller S.R. & Hosea S.W. (1983). The role of complement in the induction of antibody responses. *Clin. Exp. Immunol.,* **53,** 208.

Podack E.R., Biesecker G. & Muller-Eberhard H.J. (1979) Membrane attack complex of complement: generation of high-affinity phospholipid binding sites by fusion of five hydrophilic plasma proteins. *Proc. Natl. Acad. Sci.* **76,** 897.

Podack E.R. & Tschoop J. (1982) Polymerization of the ninth component of complement (C9). Formation of poly (C9) with a tubular ultrastructure resembling the MAC. *Proc. Natl. Acad. Sci.* **79,** 574.

Podack E.B., Tschoop J. & Muller-Eberhard H.J. (1982). The molecular organization of C9 within the membrane attack complex of complement. Induction of circular C9 polymerization by the C5b-8 assembly. *J. Exp. Med.* **156,** 268.

Porter R.R. & Reid K.B.M. (1978) The biochemistry of complement. *Nature* **275,** 699.

Tranum-Jensen J., Bhakdi S., Bhakdi-Lehnen B., Bjerrum O.J. & Speth V. (1978) Complement lysis: the ultrastructure and orientation of the C5b-9 complex on target sheep erythrocyte membranes. *Scand. J. Immunol.* **7,** 45.

8 The Antibody Response

When an individual first encounters an antigen the cells of the immune system recognize the antigen and either produce an immune reaction to it or become tolerant to it depending on the circumstances. The immune reaction can take the form of cell-mediated immunity or may involve the production of antibodies directed towards the antigen. Whether a cell-mediated immune response or an antibody response is elicited will depend on the way in which the antigen is presented to the lymphocytes: many immune reactions display both kinds of response. On second and subsequent encounters with the antigen the type of response is largely determined by the outcome of the first antigenic challenge, but the quantity and the quality of the response are different.

PRIMARY AND SECONDARY ANTIBODY RESPONSES

Following primary antigenic challenge with an antigen such as sheep erythrocytes injected into a mouse there is an initial lag phase when no antibody can be detected. This is followed by phases in which the antibody titre rises logarithmically to a plateau and finally declines again as the antibodies are naturally catabolized or bind to the antigen and are cleared from the circulation (Fig.8.1). Examination of the responses following primary and secondary antigenic challenge shows that the responses differ in four major respects:
1. Time Course. The secondary response has a shorter lag phase and an extended plateau and decline.

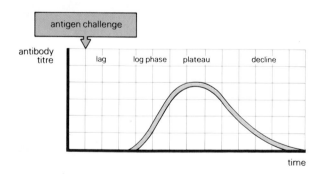

Fig. 8.1 The four phases of a primary antibody response.
Following antigen challenge the antibody response proceeds in four phases:
1. a *lag phase* when no antibody is detected.
2. a *log phase* in which the antibody titre rises logarithmically.
3. a *plateau phase* during which the antibody titre stabilizes.
4. a phase (*decline*) during which the antibody is cleared or catabolized.
The actual time course and titres reached will depend on the nature of the antigenic challenge and the responder.

2. Antibody titre. The plateau levels of antibody are much greater in the secondary response, typically ten-fold or more than plateau levels in the primary response.
3. Antibody Class. IgM antibodies form a major proportion of the primary response, whereas the secondary response consists almost entirely of IgG.
4. Antibody Affinity. The affinity of the antibodies in the secondary response is usually much greater. This is referred to as 'affinity maturation'.
The characteristics of primary and secondary antibody responses are compared in figure 8.2.

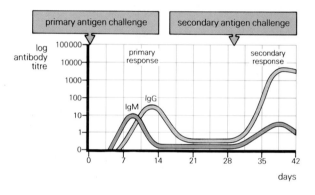

Fig. 8.2 Primary and secondary antibody responses.
In a typical immune response the antibody level following secondary antigenic challenge:
1. appears more quickly and persists for longer,
2. attains a higher titre,
3. consists predominantly of IgG,
by comparison with the antibody response following primary antigenic challenge. In the primary response the appearance of IgG is preceded by IgM.

ASSAYING ANTIBODY FORMING CELLS (AFCs) – THE PLAQUE ASSAY

In investigating antibody responses it is necessary to estimate both the level of antibody and the number of antibody forming cells (AFCs). The standard technique for identifying antibody forming cells is the plaque assay. In this assay the cells to be tested (usually spleen cells) are suspended with sensitized erythrocytes (erythrocytes chemically coated with antigen) in an immobile supporting medium or on assay plates. The plates are incubated, during which time antibody secreted by the test cells diffuses into the surrounding medium. If the antibody is of the correct specificity to bind the antigen on the erythrocytes subsequent addition of complement (an enzyme system which causes lysis of cells bound to some classes of antibody) causes lysis of the erythrocytes.

The zone of lysed erythrocytes around the antibody forming cell appears as a clear plaque, hence the name plaque forming cells (PFC) for antibody secreting cells (Fig. 8.3).

Using the plaque assay it is possible to compare the numbers of antibody forming cells in the spleen of an immunized animal with the titres of serum antibody. It is found that the rise in antibody forming cells in the spleen precedes the rise in serum antibody titres by about one day. The lag phase before the detection of IgG secreting cells is longer than for IgM secretors (Fig. 8.4).

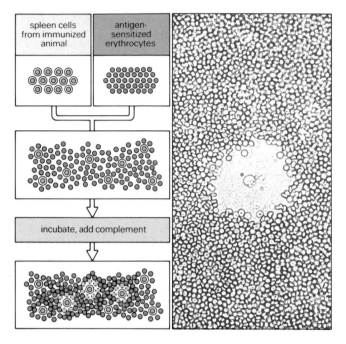

Fig. 8.3 Plaque forming cell assay. Antibody forming cells are assayed by taking spleen cells from an immunized animal and mixing them with antigen-sensitized erythrocytes in an immobile supporting medium. Following incubation the erythrocytes surrounding the cells secreting specific antibody become coated with the antibody. They may then be lysed by complement, producing a clear plaque of lysed cells around the antibody-secreting cell as shown in the photograph.

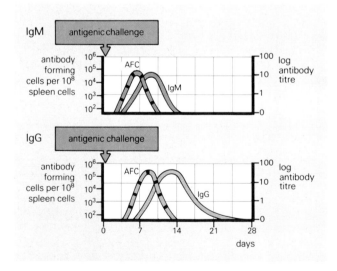

Fig.8.4 The kinetics of IgM and IgG antibody production. Specific serum antibody concentration is compared with the number of specific antibody forming cells (AFC) per 10^8 spleen cells in mice following antigenic challenge. The rise in serum antibody levels occurs approximately one day after the rise in antibody forming cells. IgM–producing cells appear before those producing IgG.

HAPTENS AND CARRIERS

To obtain the optimum secondary response to an antigenic determinant (eg. hapten, which is not immunogenic by itself) it is usually necessary to immunize the animal with the same antigen in both the primary and the secondary challenge. It is not sufficient that the antigens share a common antigenic determinant recognized by the B cells, the determinant must also be attached to the same carrier molecule. This is referred to as the carrier effect. (A carrier is a molecule which renders a hapten, linked to it, able to stimulate antibody production.) It implies that the cells involved in making the antibody response recognize at least two parts of the antigen. (Fig. 8.5).

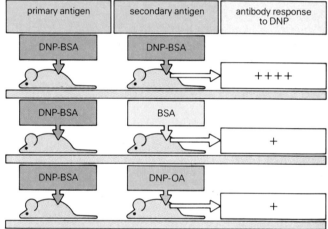

Fig. 8.5 The carrier effect. Three groups of mice were immunized (primary antigen) with dinitrophenylated bovine serum albumin (DNP-BSA) and rechallenged (secondary antigen) with either DNP-BSA, BSA or DNP-OA (dinitrophenylated ovalbumin). The antibody response to the DNP hapten was then measured. The optimal antibody response to DNP is obtained with animals immunized twice with the same antigen. The BSA acts as a specific carrier for the antibody response to DNP.

The requirement for priming lymphocytes to the carrier can be circumvented in the response to a hapten-carrier conjugate if the animal has been previously primed to the carrier alone, or receives spleen cells from a donor primed to that carrier (Fig. 8.6). Furthermore, it may be demonstrated, by removing T cells from the carrier-primed donor spleen cells, that the T cells are responsible for recognizing carrier determinants on the antigen and delivering help to the B cells which recognize the hapten (Fig. 8.7). In these two experiments antigen-primed cells are injected into irradiated recipient mice to determine their immunological activity – the irradiated mice act in this instance as 'living test tubes'.

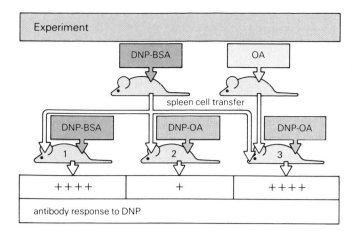

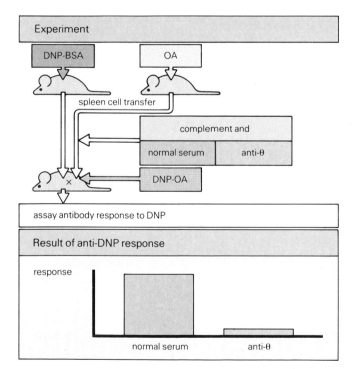

Fig. 8.6 Carrier priming. Three groups of X-irradiated mice were reconstituted with the antigen-primed spleen cells and challenged with antigen. Group one received DNP-BSA primed cells and when challenged with DNP-BSA produced a strong antibody response to DNP. Group two received DNP-BSA primed cells and were challenged with DNP-OA. This group produced a weak antibody response, demonstrating the carrier effect. Group three received cells primed to both DNP-BSA and to OA: they were then challenged with DNP-OA. This group made a strong response to DNP, demonstrating that the requirement for carrier priming can be circumvented by supplying carrier-primed spleen cells.

Fig. 8.7 T cell recognition of carrier (OA). An X-irradiated mouse, if reconstituted with spleen cells primed to the OA carrier and to DNP-BSA will, on subsequent challenge with DNP-OA produce a normal antibody response to DNP. This response is unaffected if the OA-primed cells were previously treated with normal serum and complement. However, if the OA-primed cells were treated with anti-T cell serum (anti-θ) and complement, which destroys T cells, the anti-DNP response is abrogated. This indicates that T cells recognize the carrier and give help to the hapten-primed B cells.

A more detailed analysis of the T cells responsible for this helper effect in the mouse shows that they carry Ly1 surface markers but do not carry the Ly2 or Ly3 markers, that is, they are Ly1$^+$23$^-$ cells.

These results have led to the basic scheme for cell interactions in the antibody response set out in figure 8.8. It is proposed that antigen entering the body is processed by antigen-presenting cells which present the antigen in a highly immunogenic form to the T-helper cells and B cells. The T cells recognize separate determinants on the antigen to those recognized by the B cells but they deliver help to the appropriate B cells which are stimulated to differentiate and divide into antibody forming cells. This has led to the concept that two types of signal are required to activate a B cell:

1. antigen interacting with B cell immunoglobulin receptors and crosslinking them,
2. a second signal(s) from T-helper cells. A variety of T cell stimuli are needed for optimal growth and differentation of B cells.

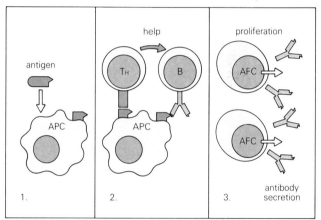

Fig. 8.8 Overview of the immune response.
1. Antigen encountering the immune system is processed by antigen-presenting cells (APCs) which retain fragments of the antigen on their surfaces.
2. T-helper cells (T_H) recognize the antigen via their surface receptors and provide help to B cells (B) which also recognize antigen by their surface receptors (immunoglobulin).
3. The B cells are stimulated to proliferate and divide into antibody forming cells (AFCs) which secrete antibody.

T-DEPENDENT AND T-INDEPENDENT ANTIGENS

According to the evidence presented so far the response to an antigen depends on both T cells and B cells recognizing that antigen. This type of antigen is called T-dependent (T dep). There are, however, a small number of antigens which are capable of activating B cells to produce antibody independently of T cell help and are therefore referred to as T-independent antigens (Tind). The T-independent antigens share a number of common properties, in particular they are all large polymeric molecules with repeating antigenic determinants, and many of them possess the ability, at high concentrations, to activate B cell clones other than those specific for that antigen, that is, *polyclonal* B cell activation.

At a lower concentration they activate only those B cells with specific antigen receptors for them. Many of the Tind antigens are particularly resistant to degradation. Some of the properties of commonly used T-independent antigens are listed in figure 8.9. It is found that the primary antibody responses to T-independent antigens *in vitro* are generally weaker than the responses to T-dependent antigens and that they peak fractionally earlier (Fig. 8.10).

antigen	polymeric	polyclonal activation	resistance to degradation
lipopolysaccharide (LPS)	+	+++	+
Ficoll	+++	–	+++
dextran	++	+	++
levan	++	+	++
poly-D amino acids	+++	–	+++
polymeric bacterial flagellin	++	++	+

Fig. 8.9 T-independent antigens. The major common properties of some of the main T-independent antigens are listed. (Note that both poly *L*-amino acids and *monomeric* bacterial flagellin are T-dependent antigens.)

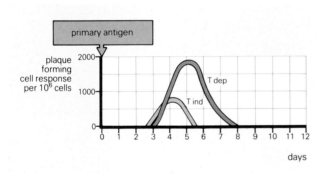

Fig. 8.10 Comparison of the primary immune responses to T dep and T ind antigens *(in vitro)*. The primary response, as assessed by plaque forming cell assay, to a T-dependent antigen and a T-independent antigen is shown here. The response to T ind antigens is weaker than to T dep antigens and peaks earlier.

The secondary response *in vitro* also differs between T-dependent and T-independent antigens. The secondary response to T-independent antigens resembles the primary response, by being weak and almost entirely confined to IgM production, whereas the secondary response to T dep antigens is far stronger and appears earlier (Fig. 8.11). It appears therefore that T-independent antigens do not usually induce the maturation of response involving class switching to IgG and increase in affinity seen with T-dependent antigens. Memory induction is also relatively poor. The mechanism by which T-independent antigens trigger B cells without the requirement for T-helper cells will be discussed later.

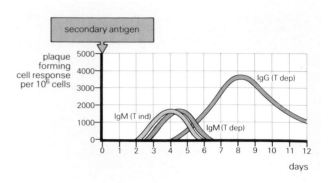

Fig. 8.11 Comparison of the secondary immune responses to T dep and T ind antigens *(in vitro)*. The IgM PFC response is similar for both T dep and T ind antigens but only T dep antigens produce an IgG PFC response.

AFFINITY MATURATION

It has been noted that the antibodies produced in a secondary response to a T-dependent antigen have higher average affinity than those produced in the primary response. Since individual lymphocytes do not change the specificity of their antigen receptors, it is evident that affinity maturation involves the selective expansion of clones of high affinity antibody producing cells. This is associated with the switch from IgM to IgG production, since there is no maturation in the affinity of the IgM response. Moreover, the degree of affinity maturation is dependent on the antigen dose administered. High antigen doses produce poor maturation and a lower affinity response than low antigen doses (Fig. 8.12). A plausible hypothesis to account for this observation is as follows: in the presence of low antigen concentrations only B cells with high affinity receptors bind the antigen and are triggered to divide and differentiate. However, in the presence of high antigen concentrations there is sufficient to bind and trigger both high and low affinity B cells (Fig. 8.13).

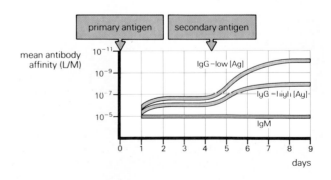

Fig. 8.12 Affinity maturation. The average affinity of the IgM and IgG antibody responses following primary and secondary challenge with a T-dependent antigen are shown. The affinity of the IgM response is constant throughout. The affinity maturation of the IgG response depends on the dose of the antigen. Low antigen does (low Ag) produce higher affinity immunoglobulin than high antigen does (high Ag).

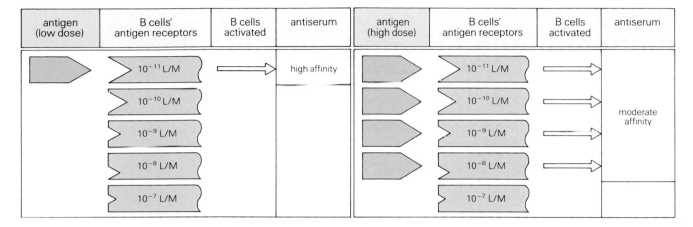

Fig. 8.13 Postulated mechanism of affinity maturation. Low antigen doses (left) bind to, and trigger only those B cells with high affinity receptors. High antigen doses (right) allow triggering of more B cell clones and therefore produce antibody responses with lower average affinity.

ANTIGEN PRESENTATION

The preceding section has described the course of events in the development of an antibody response and the evidence that both B and T cells are normally required for responses to T-dependent antigens, which constitute the majority of the antigens encountering the immune system. One of the crucial stages in the development of the immune response has so far been mentioned only briefly. This is the way in which antigen encountering the immune system is presented to the lymphocytes which react to it. *In vivo* this phase is complicated by the structural organization of the lymphoid tissue. Thus antigen from the periphery moves via the lymphatics to the local lymph nodes. The antigen may be carried free in solution or it may be carried on the surface of the antigen-presenting cells. On reaching the lymph node different antigens selectively move to different areas and are thus capable of stimulating different populations of lymphocytes. Some antigens remain within the lymph node for long periods providing a constant source of antigenic stimulation while others are fairly rapidly degraded or lost via the efferent lymphatics. This is illustrated in figures 8.14 and 8.15.

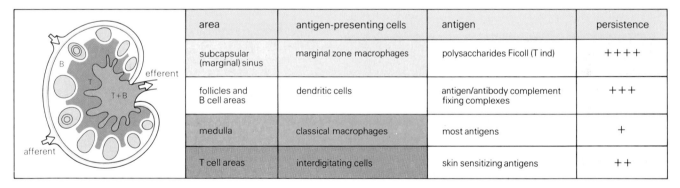

	area	antigen-presenting cells	antigen	persistence
	subcapsular (marginal) sinus	marginal zone macrophages	polysaccharides Ficoll (T ind)	++++
	follicles and B cell areas	dendritic cells	antigen/antibody complement fixing complexes	+++
	medulla	classical macrophages	most antigens	+
	T cell areas	interdigitating cells	skin sensitizing antigens	++

Fig. 8.14 Localization of antigen in lymph nodes. A lymph node is represented schematically (left) showing afferent and efferent lymphatics, follicles, the outer cortical B cell area and the paracortical T cell area. Different antigen-presenting cells predominate in these areas, although the demarcation is not absolute. The different antigen-presenting cells selectively take up different types of antigen which then persist on the surface of the cells for variable periods. Thus antigen/antibody complexes are preferentially taken up by follicular dendritic cells via their C3 and Fc receptors and may persist for months or years whereas antigens on recirculating (classical) macrophages (medulla) may only last for a few days or weeks. Note that recirculating 'veiled' cells (Langerhans cells) thought to arise from skin change their morphology to become interdigitating cells within the lymph node. Both these and the dendritic cells have long processes in intimate contact with lymphocytes. The persistence of the different antigens varies between species.

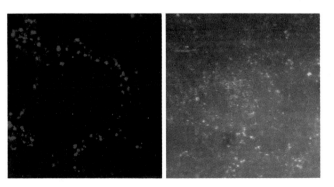

Fig. 8.15 Localization of antigen in the spleen. T ind antigens (here TRITC-Ficoll) preferentially locate on the marginal zone macrophages (red, left) while T dep antigens (FITC antigen/antibody complexes) locate on the follicular dendritic cells (green, right). Courtesy of Professor T. Humphrey.

8.5

With respect to antibody production the major antigen-presenting cells are follicular dendritic cells, macrophages and marginal zone macrophages. Langerhans cells of the skin appear to be more important in presenting antigen to T cells involved in delayed hypersensitivity reactions and they are discussed elsewhere ('Hypersensitivity – Type IV'). There is evidence that the presentation of antigen to responding lymphocytes is MHC restricted (see cytotoxic T cell killing of virally-infected target cells described in 'MHC'), that is to say that responding B cells only recognize antigen on the macrophage surface provided that both the B cell and the macrophage share determinants of the H-2 I region (in mouse) or its equivalent in other species (Fig. 8.16). The T cell receptor for antigen is described in 'Cell Mediated Immunity'.

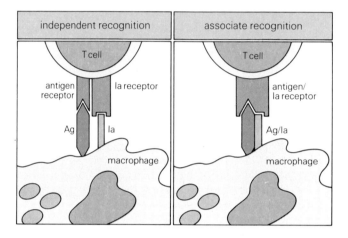

Fig. 8.16 Antigen presentation by macrophages. The way in which macrophages present antigen to T cells is MHC restricted. However, it is not certain whether the T cell recognizes antigen and MHC determinants separately (left) or as a combination of determinants (right) in which case the MHC/antigen combination on the macrophage may appear to the lymphocyte as 'altered self'. Receptors on the lymphocytes are responsible for recognition of MHC products on the macrophage and thus for the MHC restriction observed in antigen presentation. The exact MHC restriction observed is determined by the way in which lymphocytes are initially educated to discriminate self from non-self during their development in the thymus by association with cells bearing self MHC antigens.

There has been some doubt as to exactly what form the antigen presented to the T cells is in. The evidence suggests that the antigen on antigen-presenting macrophages has been extensively degraded and occurs in the form of small highly immunogenic peptides. These peptides are recognized in association with the H-2 I region gene products (or equivalent) but it is not known whether the antigen is intimately associated with the MHC products or whether the T cell recognizes antigen and MHC independently (dual recognition). Removal of surface antigen from macrophages does not lead to replenishment from an intracellular antigen pool. This finding is consistent with the view that phagocytosis of antigen and antigen presentation are two distinct functions. Some macrophages appear to lack MHC I region products and therefore are limited in function to phagocytosis.

MECHANISMS OF CELL COOPERATION

It is well established that the crucial event which determines the antigen specificity of an immune response is the triggering of particular clones of lymphocytes via their receptors for antigen (Fig. 8.17). In this sense the antigen selects the particular lymphocytes which will be involved in the response against it. As was shown earlier, the binding of antigen to particular lymphocytes is not necessarily sufficient to produce an immune response. B cells responding to a T dep antigen require T cell help to produce an optimum response, and in these immune responses the T dep antigen is recognized effectively via two different antigenic determinants. This allows the immune system greater specificity in discriminating foreign antigens than if only one antigenic determinant was recognized. Naturally, effective cooperation between the lymphocytes recognizing the different determinants is essential.

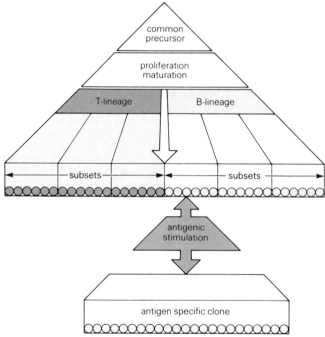

Fig. 8.17 Clonal expansion. T cells and B cells are derived from a single common precursor stem cell. The repertoire of B cells and T cells is generated before contact with antigen to produce a range of cells with different antigen binding specificities. Subsequent contact with antigen induces selective expansion of antigen specific clones.

It has been suggested that experiments with T ind antigens could throw light on the mechanisms of B cell activation. This assumes that the cells activated by the T ind and T dep antigens are essentially similar apart from the specificity of their antigen receptors, although this point is not proven. It is proposed that the T ind antigens have the inherent ability to deliver all necessary activating signals to the B cell. The properties of the T ind antigens suggest a number of ways in which they could themselves supply the second signal (Fig. 8.18).

1. Since the T ind antigens are polymeric they can cross-link the B cell's antigen receptors.

2. Since most T ind antigens are mitogenic, it is possible that the second signal is delivered via the B cell's mitogen receptor. In this scheme the antigen receptor serves to focus the mitogen onto the surface of the particular B cell. However, mitogen receptors of B cells have not yet been identified, and this effect may be due to IL–1 released from macrophages.

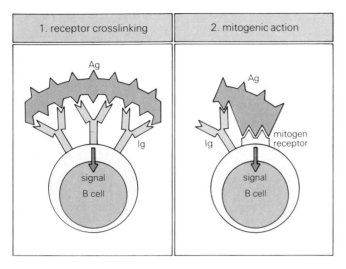

Fig. 8.18 Two possible mechanisms of B cell activation by T ind antigens:

1. polymeric antigens (Ag) crosslink the cell surface immunoglobulin of the B cells (Ig).

2. antigens with inherent mitogenic activity are bound to the B cell via the surface immunoglobulin and signal activation through a postulated mitogen receptor on the B cell.

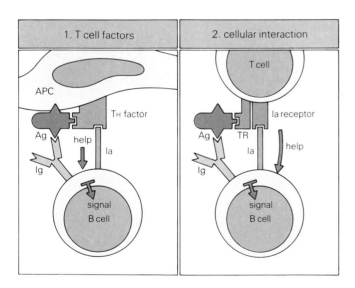

Fig. 8.19 Two possible mechanisms of antigen specific B cell activation by T dep antigens:

1. helper factors (TH) specific for carrier determinants on the antigen (Ag) and Ia molecules bind to the antigen and deliver a help signal, which, in conjunction with the signal from the B cell's antigen receptor triggers activation.

2. the T cell and B cell bind antigen via their receptors (TR and Ig) and help is delivered directly to the B cell. This requires cell/cell contact and recognition of Ia.

3. A third, though unlikely possibility, is that some of the T ind antigens fix complement by the classical or alternative pathways. Since B cells have complement receptors the second signal may be delivered in this way.

These hypotheses are not mutually exclusive, and it is possible that different mechanisms are valid for different antigens or B cells.

The way in which T cells activate B cells is still debated. There is evidence that some forms of interaction may be mediated by antigen specific T cell helper factors. These factors are released from the T cells and subsequently induce B cell activation (Fig. 8.19). There is also suggestive evidence that some forms of T cell help require direct cell/cell contact.

In all the mechanisms of B cell triggering so far mentioned it appears that failure to trigger the B cell in the correct way may lead to a state of unresponsiveness (tolerance) to that antigen. Thus, excessive mitogenic signal or excess receptor crosslinking apparently produces unresponsiveness in many cases. Similarly if a B cell encounters a T dep antigen but does not receive T cell help, specific tolerance may ensue.

T CELL FACTORS

The evidence for the existence of antigen specific T helper factors comes from culture systems in which the antigen-stimulated T_H cells are separated from the target B cells by a membrane permeable to molecules, but impermeable to cells (Fig. 8.20).

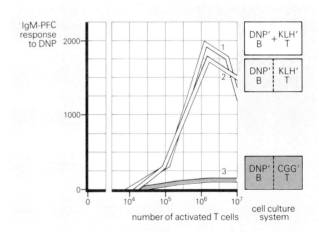

Fig. 8.20 Demonstration of antigen induced T cell helper factors. Cultures were set up containing DNP-primed (DNP') B cells and 1) KLH-primed T cells; 2) KLH-primed T cells separated from B cells by a protein-permeable membrane, 3) CGG (Chicken Gamma Globulin) primed T cells similarly separated from the B cells. All cultures contained KLH-DNP. The help given to the B cells was measured by plaque forming cell assay. The number of activated T cells initially introduced into the culture is varied and the B cell response depends on this. The response is unaffected by preventing direct cell/cell contact (2), implying the presence of helper factors. Also, the effect is antigen specific – T cells primed to CGG cannot substitute for KLH-primed T cells (3). The eventual decline in response may be due to T-suppressor cells.

It may be demonstrated (using either murine or human cells) for some types of antibody response, that separation of B cells and T cells does not affect cooperation, but it is notable that there is an optimum ratio of T:B cells to produce a maximum response. Initially the T-helper factors were not shown to be genetically restricted (ie recognize Ia antigens on their targets) but more recent work has

indicated that like T-helper cells themselves, they are restricted. There is also evidence for the action of antigen non-specific T cell helper factors. These factors are released during T cell activation and act on all clones of B cells. The factors may be demonstrated in supernatants from mixed lymphocyte cultures (MLC) consisting of allogeneic cells. In this system T cells are stimulated by contact with allogeneic lymphocytes (Fig. 8.21).

The cells stimulated in the MLC in figures 8.21 were participating in a cell-mediated immune response. The T cell factors produced are not antigen specific, that is, a T cell triggered by antigen X produces factors which can help a B cell produce antibody to antigen Y. The antigen non-specific factors only augment the response to some antigens, other antigens still require antigen specific help before an antibody response is generated. For example, the antibody to particulate antigens such as sheep red blood cells is enhanced by non-specific factors alone whereas the response to most protein antigens is not.

Although the systems used *in vitro* to detect the factors show that they have no antigen specificity, *in vivo* they may have some operational 'antigen specificity' due to the local organization of the lymphoid tissue. Thus it is possible that particular clones of B cells may be selectively stimulated by non-specific factors due to their close proximity to T cells releasing the factors. This situation might occur in an antigen stimulated lymph node.

Previously we have illustrated the helper factor interacting directly with the B cells but it has been shown that the factors can also have an affinity for macrophages and other antigen-presenting cells. It is likely that these factors act initially by binding to the antigen-presenting cell before exerting their effect on the target cell (Fig. 8.22). It is thought that suppressor T cells may exert their suppressive effects by releasing antigen specific T suppressor factors which act in a similar way to the helper factors.

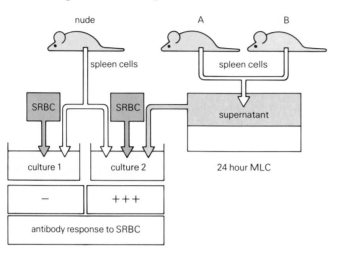

Fig. 8.21 Non-specific T cell helper factors. A mouse lacking T cells (known as a nude mouse) has its spleen cells removed. Two cultures of these spleen cells are set up.
1. to one culture are added sheep red blood cells (SRBCs), a T dep antigen, to which the spleen cells are unable to produce an antibody response,
2. to a second culture are added SRBCs and the supernatant of a mixed lymphocyte culture (MLC) produced by cultivating spleen cells from two different mouse strains for 24 hours. This supernatant stimulates the spleen cells to produce antibody against the SRBCs. It is concluded that the supernatant contains non-specific T cell helper factors.

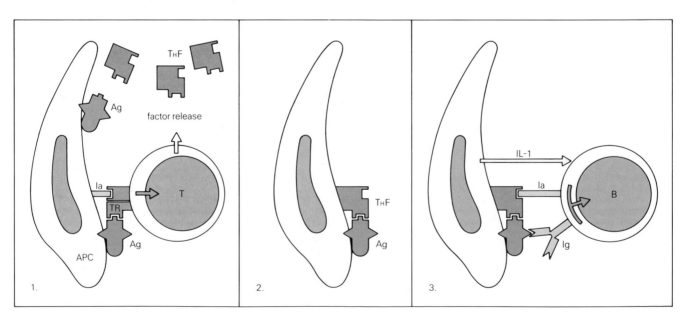

Fig. 8.22 The action of T cell helper factors.
1. T cells encountering antigen (Ag) on the APC recognize the antigen through their receptors (TR) and release antigen specific helper factors (THF).
2. Factors bind to the APC possibly in association with antigen.

3. Subsequently, a B cell encountering the APC is stimulated by the matrix of antigen and T helper factor and also possibly by interleukin 1 (IL-1) released from the activated APC (if a macrophage). The interaction is thought to be MHC restricted.

Some of the factors described here carry determinants of the H-2I region in mice or its equivalent in humans: their characteristics are summarized in figure 8.23. The nature of non-specific factors has recently been partly elucidated. Previously these factors had been defined by their effects in different assay systems, thus a single factor with several biological actions could be known by various names. These factors appear to fall into four groups and their properties are summarized in figure 8.24.

	GRF	helper factor	suppressor factor
source	macrophage	Ly1⁺ T cell	Ly23⁺ T cell
target	Ly1⁺ Ly123⁺ T cell	macrophage B cell	T cell
effect	induces TH cells	induces B cells	suppresses T cells
Ag specificity	?	+	+
mol.wt.	55 – 75K	55 – 80K	55 – 80K
serology V/C	–	+	+
MHC I	I-A	I-A (I-J)	I-J
MHC restriction	+	+ or –	+ or –

Fig. 8.23 Characteristics of factors carrying I-region determinants. The three factors described here are genetically restricted factor (GRF) produced by macrophages, helper factor produced by TH cells (carrying the Ly 1 marker) and suppressor factor produced by Ts cells (carrying the Ly2, Ly3 marker). The characteristic labelled serology V/C refers to their reactivity with antisera. These antisera appear to detect both variable and constant regions (not to be confused with, but analogous to immunoglobulin V and C regions) on T cell factors but not on macrophage factors. The factors also share determinants in common with MHC-I subregion molecules. MHC restriction refers to the possible requirement for the cells interacting through these factors to be matched with respect to the MHC molecules displayed on their surfaces.

	source	target	effect
Interleukin 1 (LAF)	macrophage and other cells	T and B cells	promotes multiplication and activation
Interleukin 2 (TCGF)	Ly1⁺, 23⁻ T cell in presence of macrophage	T cells	proliferation of activated T cells
T cell replacing factor (TRF)	Ly1⁺, 23⁻ T cell in presence of macrophage	B cells	B cell differentiation
B cell growth factor (BCGF)	Ly1⁺, 23⁻ T cell in presence of macrophage	B cells	synergizes with IL-1 in B cell activation

Fig. 8.24 Antigen non-specific factors. Interleukin 1 (Lymphocyte Activating factor – LAF) acts during antigen priming of lymphocytes. Interleukin 2 (T Cell Growth Factor – TCGF) is essential for long term growth of activated T cells. T Cell Replacing Factor (TRF) is required for optimal B cell differentiation in response to antigen. B Cell Growth Factor (BCGF) is a signal for B cell activation. Both TRF and BCGF are really groups of molecules and not necessarily single entities.

ADJUVANTS

Adjuvants are substances which non-specifically enhance the immune response to antigen. In certain circumstances it is possible to completely change the mode of response (tolerance vs immunity) by administering antigen together with adjuvant. For example, it is possible to break self tolerance to a large number of self antigens by injecting them into the host animal in an appropriate adjuvant. The most frequently used adjuvants are water-in-oil emulsions with the antigen in the aqueous phase (eg. Freund's Incomplete Adjuvant). The adjuvant properties are further enhanced by the addition of a microbial antigen to the mixture (eg. heat-killed *Mycobacterium tuberculosis* in Freund's Complete Adjuvant). Antibody responses to antigens in adjuvants are greater, more prolonged and frequently consist of different classes to the response obtained without adjuvant (Fig. 8.25).

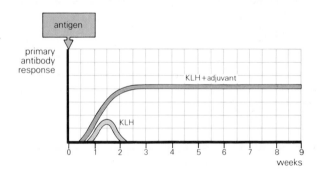

Fig. 8.25 Effect of adjuvants on the antibody response following injection of antigen (KLH). The response with adjuvant is greater and more prolonged.

Adjuvants are thought to work in a variety of ways. Firstly, the antigen in emulsion is resistant to dispersal, and it therefore acts as a depot for prolonged antigen stimulation. Secondly, microbial products activate macrophages thus leading to the production of antigen non-specific factors which will enhance the response. Thirdly, it is possible that the antigen somehow bypasses the requirement for the T cell signals in B cell differentiation leading to maturation of the response with class switching.

In summary, the antibody response is a coordinated reaction of B cells, T cells and antigen-presenting cells, communicating either directly or via antigen specific and non-specific factors. Communication between the cells involves products of the MHC and other gene products. Failure to produce a properly coordinated response may lead to tolerance.

FURTHER READING

Erb P., Vogt P., Cecka M. & Feldmann M. (1980) Activation of T cells by I region products released by macrophage. *Lymphokines* **2,** 125.

Feldmann M. & Kontiainen S. (1981) The role of antigen specific factors in the immune response. *Lymphokines* **2,** 87.

Howard M. & Paul W.E. (1983) Regulation of B cell growth and differentiation by soluble factors. *Ann. Rev. Immunol.* **1,** 307.

Inglis J. (1982) *B lymphocytes today.* Elsevier Biomedical.

Inglis J. (1983) *T Lymphocytes today.* Elsevier Biomedical.

Singer A. & Hodes R. (1983) Mechanism of T cell-B cell interaction. *Ann. Rev. Immunol.* **1,** 211.

Unanue E.R. (1984) Antigen-presenting function of the macrophage. *Ann. Rev. Immunol.* **2,** 395.

9 The Generation of Antibody Diversity

Antibodies are remarkably diverse; not only must they provide enough different combining sites to recognize the millions of antigenic shapes in the environment, but also each class of antibody has a different effector region such that, for instance, IgE can bind to Fc receptors on mast cells whilst IgG can bind similarly to phagocytes. It has been estimated that an individual produces more different forms of antibody than all the other proteins of the body put together. Looked at another way, we produce more types of antibody than there are genes in our genome. How then can all this diversity be generated? Ideas about the formation of antibodies have changed considerably over the years but it is, perhaps, surprising how close Ehrlich came with his side chain hypothesis at the beginning of this century (Fig. 9.1). His idea of antigen-induced selection is close to our present view of clonal selection except that he placed several different receptors on the same cell.

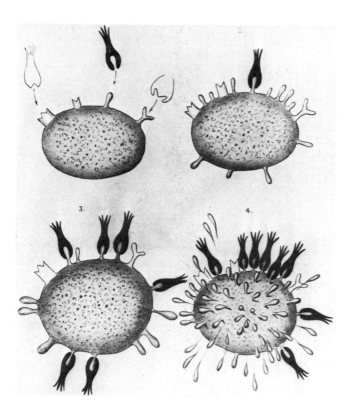

Fig. 9.1 Ehrlich's side chain theory. Ehrlich proposed that the combination of antigen with a preformed B cell receptor (now known to be antibody) triggered the cell to produce and secrete more of those receptors. Although the diagram indicates that he thought a single cell could produce antibodies to bind more than one type of antigen, it is evident that he anticipated both the clonal selection theory and the idea that the immune system could generate receptors before contact with antigen.

THEORIES OF ANTIBODY FORMATION

After Ehrlich the situation became complicated. The problem was that many new organic chemicals were now being synthesized and Landsteiner was showing that the immune system could react with the production of specific antibody for each new compound. It was simply not thought possible that the immune system could have maintained, by natural selection, genes for all these antibodies directed at novel, artificial compounds. This led to the development of the instructive hypothesis which suggested that a flexible antibody molecule is induced by antigen to form a complementary binding site (Fig. 9.2).

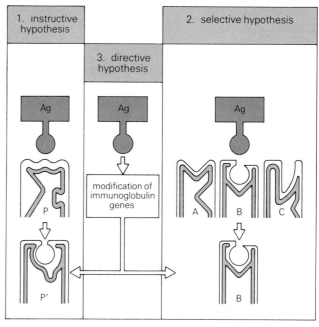

Fig. 9.2 Historical ideas of antibody formation. There have been three major hypotheses explaining the generation of antibody diversity. In the instructive hypothesis (1) antigen encounters a pluripotent immunoglobulin molecule (P) which assumes a shape complementary to the antigen (P'). In the selective hypothesis (2) the antigen encounters a variety of different immunoglobulins generated by the immune system (A, B, C) only one of which fits the antigen. Only the cells producing this type of antibody respond to the antigenic stimulus. The instructive hypothesis was discarded since it is now known that changes in protein structure cannot be translated into changes in the DNA, which is necessary to retain the alteration of P' during clonal proliferation. The directive hypothesis (3) also envisaged antigen generating the molecules necessary to recognize it, but suggested that this occurred directly at the DNA level. This hypothesis has also been discarded in favour of the selective theory.

With the spectacular progress in molecular biology in the 1950s and 60s the instructive hypothesis became untenable. The circle turned, and selective theories came back into favour with Jerne and Burnett independently putting forward the idea of clonal selection: each lymphocyte produces one type of immunoglobulin only, and the antigen selects and stimulates cells carrying that immunoglobulin type.

This still leaves the problem of antibody diversity. At its simplest we can propose the existence of a separate gene for each antibody specificity (Fig. 9.3). This immediately presents a problem: if we consider the structure of a light chain, half the chain is variable in amino acid sequence but the other half is constant. Similarly with heavy chains, a quarter of the chain is variable while the rest is constant. How, if there are many genes, is it possible to maintain this constancy of sequence in the constant regions? Dreyer and Bennett proposed a solution to this problem by suggesting that the constant and variable portions of the chains are coded for by separate genes with one or only a few genes coding for the constant region and many genes coding for the variable region. Thus the germ line theory now only had to account for the multiple variable regions! A second solution of the diversity problem was suggested by the idea of somatic mutation. A relatively few germ line genes would give rise to many mutated genes during the lifetime of the individual. Furthermore, it has been suggested that a number of gene segments could recombine to give a complete V gene.

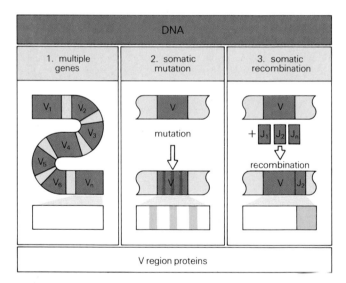

Fig. 9.3 **Generation of antibody diversity.** Three mechanisms are proposed by which the immune system could generate different V regions on the immunoglobulin H and L chains.
1. Multiple genes. There are a large number of separate genes (V_1-Vn) each encoding one V region domain.
2. Somatic mutation. A primordial V gene mutates during B cell ontogeny to produce different genes in different B cell clones.
3. Somatic recombination. A number of gene segments (J_1-J_n) recombine to join the main part of the V region gene. This occurs during B cell ontogeny and results in a protein containing elements coded for by different gene segments. It is now known that *all three* mechanisms are involved in the generation of antibody diversity.

IMMUNOGLOBULIN VARIABILITY

Immunoglobulins are composed of heavy and light chains, the light chains being either κ or λ. Since virtually any light chain can combine with any heavy chain the number of possible combining sites is the product of the number of heavy and light chains. Part of the variability in immunoglobulin structure is derived from the interaction of these separate polypeptide chains. For example, if there are 10^4 different light chains each capable of binding with any of 10^4 different heavy chains, then theoretically 10^8 different antibody specificities may be produced: separate diversification mechanisms exist for each of the chains as they are coded for on separate chromosomes (Fig. 9.4).

Polymorphic forms of immunoglobulins derive from variation in many parts of the molecule (Fig. 9.5).

peptide	mouse	human
IgH	12	14
λ	16	22
κ	6	2
MHC	17	6
β_2-microglobulin	2	15

Fig. 9.4 **Chromosome locations of immunoglobulin and MHC genes.** The numbers in this table refer to the chromosome on which the genes coding for the listed peptides are found. Note that in both mouse and man the genes for heavy chains and the two different light chains are on three different chromosomes, and all these are also on different chromosomes to the genes which form the major histocompatibility complex proteins.

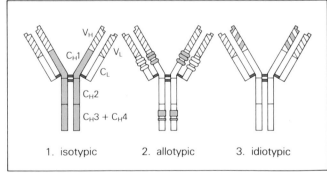

Fig.9.5 **Variability of immunoglobulin structure.** All immunoglobulins have the basic four chain structure. The variability of different immunoglobulins is of three types.
1. Isotypic variation is present in the germ line of all members of a species, producing the heavy (μ, δ, γ, ε, α) and light chains (κ, λ), and the V region frameworks (subgroups).
2. Allotypic variation is intraspecies allelic variability.
3. Idiotypic variation refers to the diversity at the binding site and in particular relates to the hypervariable segments of the antibody combining site (paratope).

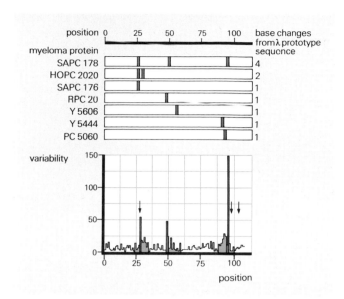

Fig. 9.6 **Variability of lambda light chains.** The amino acid sequences of seven λ1 myeloma proteins are represented. Positions in yellow indicate identity to the prototype sequence (MOPC 104E), positions in red indicate differences. The number of base changes in the DNA required to produce the given alteration in amino acid structure is given on the right. Below is a Kabat and Wu plot of light chain variability as described in 'Antibody Structure and Function'.

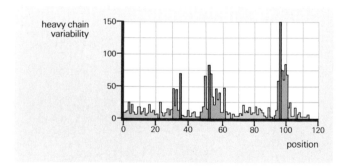

Fig. 9.7 **Variability of heavy chains.** This Kabat and Wu plot shows variability concentrated in three regions of the variable region of heavy chains.

It is the idiotypic variability, which pertains to the generation of the antigen combining site, with which we shall first be concerned. Kabat and Wu analysed the amino acid sequences of many light and heavy chains. When the variable regions from light chains derived from myelomas were compared it was clear that the variability in amino acid sequence was concentrated in three hypervariable regions which were surrounded by relatively invariant framework residues. (A myeloma is a monoclonal B cell tumour producing antibody.) These hypervariable regions were shown to be the areas which made contact with the antigen (complementarity determining regions, CDRs). In the mouse less than 5% of the antibodies possess λ light chains and diversity is correspondingly less. Out of 19 λ1 light chain sequences examined, 12 were found to be identical, with the other 7 differing from each other and the prototype sequence by only a few residues (Fig. 9.6).

The variability in the heavy chain is similarly concentrated in three hypervariable regions with background variability on each side of the complementarity determining regions (Fig. 9.7). The heavy chain frameworks can be arranged into groups on the basis of similarity and in some cases identity of framework sequences (Fig. 9.8).

LIGHT CHAIN GENE RECOMBINATION

With the advent of recombinant DNA techniques in the 1970s it became possible to attempt analysis of the genes responsible for coding for antibodies. Because of its lesser heterogeneity, work started on the λ1 system using restriction endonucleases to digest the DNA. It was revealed that not only were there two separate segments of DNA coding for the constant and variable regions but also, in cells not producing antibody these gene segments are arranged far apart on the chromosome, whereas in antibody forming cells these segments are brought much closer together. Even in a fully differentiated B lymphocyte these two gene segments do not join directly together but remain about 1500 base pairs apart. Between the V and C segments and joined onto the V segment in the rearranged chromosome is an extra short section of DNA known as the J segment.

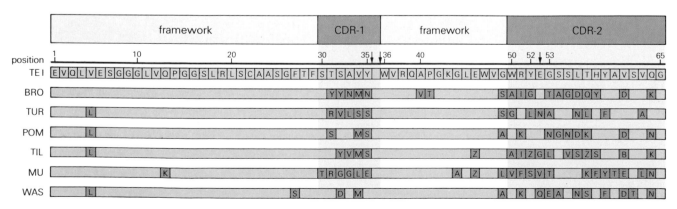

Fig. 9.8 **Heavy chain group V$_H$ III: human.** The 65 N terminal amino acids of six human myelomas falling into the V$_H$ III group are compared diagrammatically to the prototype sequence TEI. Amino acids identical to those in TEI are shown in yellow, amino acids which differ from those at the same position in TEI are orange. The majority of the differences within a single group occur within the complementarity determining regions CDR-1 and CDR-2.

Basically the V segment codes for the V region of the light chain up to and including amino acid 95 and the J segment gene codes for the rest of the V region (Fig. 9.9). In the mouse λ light chain system there are four C genes,

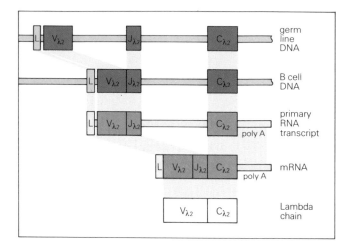

Fig. 9.9 Lambda chain production: mouse. During B cell differentiation one of the germ line V_λ genes ($V_{\lambda2}$) recombines with its J segment ($J_{\lambda2}$) to form a VJ combination. The V gene is preceded by an appropriate signalling leader sequence (L). The rearranged gene is transcribed into a primary RNA transcript complete with introns (DNA occurring between the genes), exons (which code for protein) and a poly-A tail. This is spliced to form messenger RNA (mRNA) with loss of the introns and is in turn translated into protein. Note that exons are indicated in a darker shade than introns, DNA in red, RNA in green and immunoglobulin peptides in yellow. The λ2 gene illustrated is only one of a small number of different λ genes arranged in tandem on the same chromosome.

each with its own J gene, and two V genes. Each V segment gene is preceded by a signal or leader sequence coding for a short hydrophobic sequence that is responsible for the transport of the antibody molecule through the membrane of the endoplasmic reticulum during translation. This leader sequence is then cleaved away after synthesis of the chain. Note that the J segments which form part of the V domains are completely different from the J chain present in IgM and dimeric IgA.

The κ chain system is more heterogeneous because there are more V segment genes but only one constant region gene (Fig. 9.10). In an embryonic or non-lymphoid cell the V segment genes, of which there are about 350, are again at some distance on the chromosome from the C gene. In the mouse these V segment genes appear to be organized in sets comprising about seven genes per set. In between and closer to the C gene are five J genes (one of the J genes is a pseudogene and is never expressed). During differentiation of lymphoid cells there is a rearrangement of the DNA such that one of the V segment genes is joined to a J segment gene. Thus the number of possible κ chain variable regions that can be produced is approximately 1400 (350×4). There is still a gap or intron between the J segment genes and the gene for the C region. This whole stretch of DNA, including introns, from the leader to the end of the C gene is then transcribed into heterogeneous nuclear RNA (ie. unprocessed mRNA). A process of RNA splicing then removes the introns, leaving messenger RNA which is finally translated into protein. This splicing out of introns can be revealed by heteroduplex analysis, where the mRNA is mixed with denatured single stranded DNA from the antibody forming cell, allowed to reanneal and then examined by electron microscopy. Hybridization of V and C regions readily occurs revealing the intron that lies between them (Fig. 9.11).

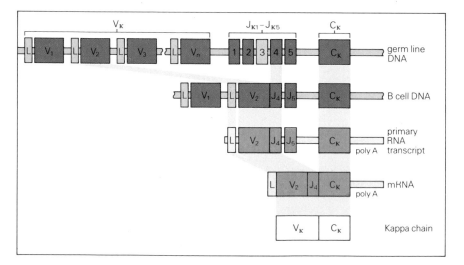

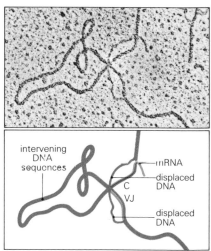

Fig. 9.10 Kappa chain production: mouse. During differentiation of the pre-B cell one of several V_K genes on the germ line DNA (V_1-V_n) is recombined and opposed to a J_K segment (J_{K1}-J_{K5}). Each V_K gene is preceded by a leader sequence (L). The B cell transcribes a segment of DNA into a primary RNA transcript which contains a long intervening sequence of additional J segments and introns. This transcript is processed into mRNA by splicing the exons together and is translated by ribosomes into kappa chains. (Note that the J3 gene lacks the necessary base sequences to allow it to recombine and is therefore effectively an intron.) The rearrangement illustrated is only one of the many possible recombinations.

Fig. 9.11 Heteroduplex analysis of a kappa VC region. The mRNA for a kappa gene is incubated with denatured single stranded germ line DNA of a plasmacytoma (plasma cell tumour) producing the heteroduplex above, as seen under the electron microsope. There is a large intron in the DNA between VJ and C but no intron between V and J in this active B cell.

HEAVY CHAIN GENE RECOMBINATION

The heavy chain is also encoded by V and J segment genes. Additional diversity is provided by a third gene segment, the D segment gene (Fig. 9.12).

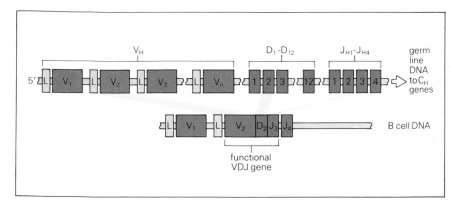

different V_H segments and four functional J segments. The combination of V, D and J segments in the heavy chain make up the third complementarity determining region, which forms an essential part of the antigen binding site. In fact in some systems, such as the family of anti-dextran antibodies, the differences between antibodies are nearly all situated in this region.

Fig. 9.12 VDJ recombination: mouse. The heavy chain gene loci combine three segments to produce the exon (VDJ gene) which will code for the V_H domain. One of several hundred V genes recombines with one of twelve D segments and one of four J segments to produce a functional VDJ gene, in the B cell. The rearrangement illustrated is only one of the many thousands possible.

If one examines the family of monoclonal antibodies which bind dextran, the gene segment for the V_H domain appears to end at codon 99 while the gene segment for the J_H segment starts at codon 102. This leaves two codons in between not accounted for either by V or J segments, and these form the additional D or diversity segment. This section is highly variable both in the sequences of the codons and in their number. In antibodies binding dextran this section comprises two amino acids but in those binding phosphoryl choline up to eight amino acids are inserted, while in anti-levan antibodies this section is completely missing. So far twelve germ line D segments have been identified together with 100-200

RECOMBINATION SEQUENCES

A key feature then of the generation of a functional gene for both light and heavy chain variable regions is the recombination of gene segments. The precise mechanism by which this recombination is brought about is unknown but specific base sequences that appear to act as joining signals have been identified (Fig. 9.13). On the J or downstream side of each V and D segment gene (in the direction of the J gene) are found two signal sequences, each of which is highly conserved.

Fig. 9.13 Recombination sequences. This diagram shows the sequences of introns next to the V and J genes (kappa light chains) and V, J and D genes (heavy chains) which are involved in recombination of these genes. The recombinational events involved in VJ splicing and VDJ splicing are facilitated by the base sequences of the introns following the 3' end of V and D matching up with the bases preceding the 5' end of J and D. Base pairing between these sequences apposes the exons. Note that individual base pair sequences may vary slightly from the stated ones but the heptamer/spacer/nonamer pairing patterns remain. It is thought that enzymes related to those involved in DNA repair effect the join.

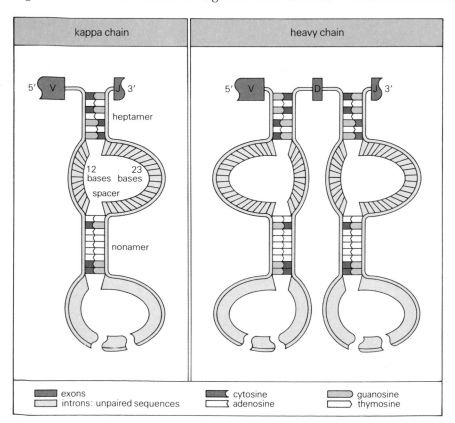

The first is composed of seven nucleotides, a heptamer CACAGTG or its analogue followed by a spacer of unconserved sequence and then a nonamer ACAAAAACC, or its analogue. Immediately preceding all germ line D and J segments are again two signal sequences, first a nonamer and then a heptamer, again separated by an unconserved sequence. The heptameric and nonameric sequences following a V_L, V_H or D segment are complementary to those preceding the J_L, D or J_H segments with which they recombine. All functional V_κ, J_λ and D spacers are twelve base pairs long, while all functional V_λ, V_H and J_H spacers are 22-24 base pairs long. This has led to the suggestion that the recombination may be brought about by a recombinase enzyme containing two DNA binding proteins, one recognizing the heptamer and nonamer with a 12 base pair spacer and the other recognizing them with a 23 base pair spacer. Alternatively, base pairing may occur directly between heptamers and nonamers, and the recombining enzyme(s) then recognize the overall paired structure.

ADDITIONAL DIVERSITY

Variable Recombination
As if the diversity generated by simple recombination were not enough, the precise place at which V and J segment genes join may vary slightly. The 95th residue of the κ light chain is coded for by the last codon of the V segment gene while the 96th is frequently coded by the first J_κ triplet. Sometimes, however, the 96th amino acid

is coded for by a composite triplet formed by the second and third, or third base alone, of the first J_κ triplet with the other bases of the triplet being supplied by additional bases from the intron 3' from the V segment gene (Fig. 9.14). This will lead to variations in amino acid sequence at this point. Obviously to produce a functional light chain the correct reading frame must be preserved but it is possible for the gene segments to join out of phase leading to non-functional lymphocytes.

Similar imprecision in joining occurs on the heavy chain chromosome between the D and J_H segment genes and can extend over as many as 10 nucleotides (Fig. 9.15). Furthermore, it has been suggested that a few nucleotides may be inserted between D and J_H and between V_H and D without the need for a template.

Somatic Mutation
The idea that somatic mutations during the lifetime of an individual could increase the diversity of antibodies has been strongly argued for many years. As seen earlier (Fig. 9.6) most V_λ sequences are identical, with a few variations in the complementarity determining regions giving eight sequences in all, but as only one $V_{\lambda 1}$ gene segment has been found per haploid genome and as this corresponds to the main shared prototype sequence, all the variant sequences must be generated by somatic mutations. All the variants could be produced by single base changes. Similar somatic mutants have been identified in κ light chains and in heavy chains.

The family of antibodies binding phosphoryl choline has been extensively investigated. Nineteen V_H segments from antibodies binding phosphoryl choline have

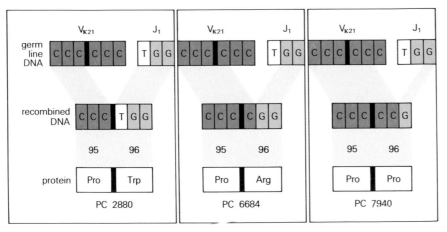

Fig. 9.14 Light chain diversity created by variable recombination.
The same V_{K21} and J_1 sequences of the germ line genes create three different amino acid sequences in the proteins PC 2880, PC 6684 and PC 7940 by variable recombination. PC 2880 has proline and tryptophan at positions 95 and 96, caused by recombination at the end of the CCC codon. Recombination one base further down produces proline and arginine in PC 6684 and recombination two bases down from the end of V_{K21} produces proline and proline in PC 7940.

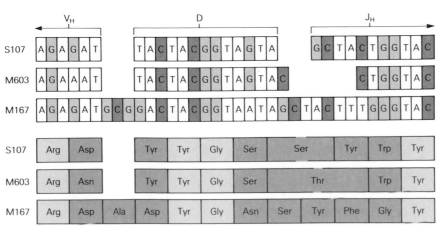

Fig. 9.15 Heavy chain diversity created by variable recombination.
The DNA sequence (above) and amino acid sequence (below) of three heavy chains of anti-phosphoryl choline are shown. Variable recombination between the germ line V, D, and J regions causes variation (red) in amino acid sequences. In some cases (eg. M167) there appear to be additional inserted codons, however, these additions do not alter the overall reading frame.

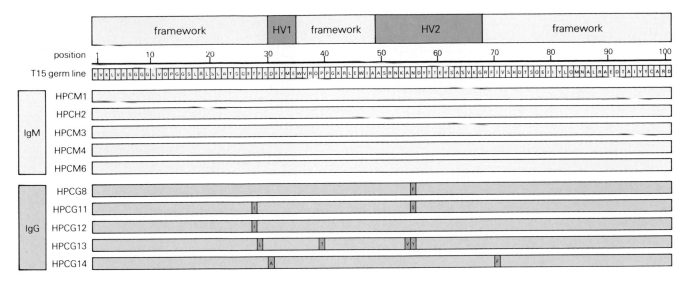

Fig. 9.16 Somatic mutation. The amino acid sequences of five IgM and five IgG hybridoma anti-phosphoryl choline antibody V_H regions are compared to the primary amino acid structure of the T15 germ line DNA, as identified by sequencing sperm cell DNA. Positions which correspond to the germ line sequence are shown in yellow; points at which different amino acids occur are shown in red. Areas of hypervariability (HV1, HV2) are also indicated. Mutations have only occurred in the IgG molecules and the mutations are seen in both hypervariable and framework segments.

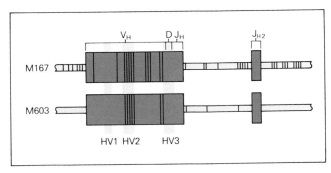

Fig. 9.17 Mutations in the DNA of two V_H, T15 genes. The DNA of two anti-phosphoryl choline antibodies with the T15 idiotype is shown (black lines indicate positions where the genome has mutated from the germ line sequence). There are large numbers of mutations in the introns and the exons of both genes, but particularly in the second hypervariable region, HV2. (By comparison, no mutations are detectable in the genes coding for the constant regions.)

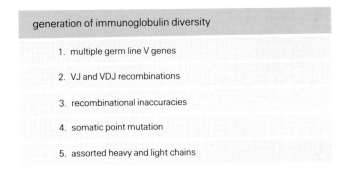

generation of immunoglobulin diversity

1. multiple germ line V genes

2. VJ and VDJ recombinations

3. recombinational inaccuracies

4. somatic point mutation

5. assorted heavy and light chains

Fig. 9.18 Five mechanisms for the generation of antibody diversity. Since each mechanism can occur with any of the others the potential for increased diversity multiplies at each step of immunoglobulin production.

been fully sequenced. Ten of these have an identical sequence while the other nine differ by one to eight residues. The germ line genome, from sperm, was examined to see if each of these sequences was coded for by a separate DNA sequence. In fact, only DNA coding for the main prototype sequence could be found, indicating that the other sequences must have arisen by somatic mutation (Fig. 9.16). Strikingly, all the mutated forms were in the IgA and IgG clases suggesting that the mutation event might be associated with immunoglobulin class switching. Presumably those somatic variants with a better fit for antigen are selected for, and certainly the somatic variants binding phosphoryl choline are of higher affinity than the germ line coded antibodies.

There is some evidence that the region of DNA encoding the variable region may be particularly susceptible to mutation. For example, examination of the nucleotide sequences of two anti-phosphoryl choline antibodies (T15 idiotype) shows them to have numerous mutations from the germ line sequence (3·8% of bases are mutated in the protein M167). These mutations occur in both introns and exons of the region implying that the whole region of DNA is particularly mutable, by comparison with adjoining regions of DNA, where mutations have not been found (Fig. 9.17).

Antibody diversity thus arises at several levels, first there are the multiple variable region genes recombining with J and D segments. Then above this the imprecision with which recombination occurs achieves further variation. At this level the structures of the first and second hypervariable regions are coded for entirely by germ line genes while the third complementarity determining region is largely the result of recombination. Additionally, point mutations are added throughout the variable region to give fine variations in specificity. As virtually any light chain may pair with any heavy chain the combinatorial binding of heavy and light chains amplifies the diversity enormously (Fig. 9.18).

HEAVY CHAIN CONSTANT REGION GENES

All the different classes of immunoglobulin use the same set of variable region genes. When the class is changed all that is switched is the constant region of the heavy chain. This has been shown by the sharing of heavy chain variable region subgroups on different immunoglobulin classes and by the analysis of double myelomas, where two monoclonal antibodies are present in the serum at the same time. On sequencing the IgM and IgG antibodies from a patient with multiple myeloma it was shown that they had identical light chains and V_H regions, only the constant regions were switched from μ to γ. Frequently IgM and IgD are found on the lymphocyte surface membrane at the same time. Capping these receptors with antigen has revealed that both the IgM and IgD have the same specificity for antigen, indicating similarity of V_H regions on the two classes (Fig. 9.19).

All the constant region genes are arranged downstream from the J segment genes (Fig. 9.20). Just upstream (5') to

the μ gene is a switch sequence (S) which is repeated 5' to each of the other constant region genes except δ. This S region is a recombination site which allows class switching to the other constant region genes (Fig. 9.21). Class switching is important in the maturation of the immune response and as earlier stated may be accompanied or preceded by somatic mutation. Initially a complete section of DNA, including the recombined V_H region through the δ and μ constant regions, is transcribed, then by differential splicing, two messenger RNA molecules are produced each with the same V_H but having either μ or δ constant regions. It is suggested that sometimes much larger stretches of DNA are also transcribed together, with differential splicing giving other immunoglobulin classes sharing V_H regions. This has been observed in cells simultaneously producing IgM and IgE. More often class switching appears to be mediated by a recombination between S recombination sites allowing a looping out and deletion of DNA and bringing another C region gene close to the VDJ gene (Fig. 9.22). A further possibility has been suggested involving exchange between sister chromatids.)

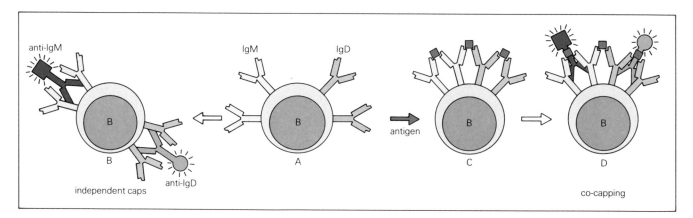

Fig. 9.19 Cocapping of IgM and IgD with antigen. Some B cells have both IgM and IgD on their surface (A). This can be demonstrated by treating the cells with rhodaminated anti-IgM (red) and fluoresceinated anti-IgD (green) in which case the conjugated antibodies separately aggregate the surface IgM and IgD causing a red and a green cap to occur on the cell (B). If the experiment is repeated by first treating the cells with antigen (blue) as in (C) and then with the anti-IgM and anti-IgD, both the red anti-IgM and green anti-IgD caps appear together on the cell, that is, they cocap. This implies that IgM and IgD on the cell surface were crosslinked by antigen (D). This can only occur if the IgM and IgD have the same antigen binding specificity and it is therefore evidence that different constant regions (μ and δ) can be linked to the same V region.

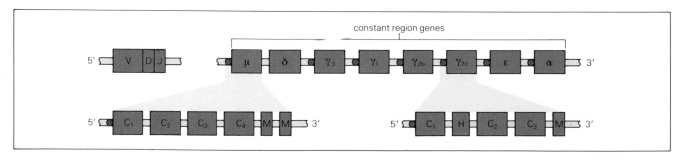

Fig. 9.20 Constant region genes: mouse. The constant region genes of the mouse are arranged 6.5 kilobases downstream from the recombined VDJ segment. Each C gene except that for δ has a switching sequence at its start (red circles) which corresponds to a sequence at the 5' end of the μ gene. This allows any of the C genes to recombine with VDJ. δ genes appear to use the same switching sequence as μ but the μ gene is lost in RNA processing to produce IgD. The C genes (expanded below for μ and γ_{2a}) contain introns separating the exons for each domain (C1, C2 etc.). The γ genes also have a separate exon coding for the hinge (H) and all the genes have one or more exons coding for membrane bound immunoglobulin (M). All the introns are lost during RNA processing.

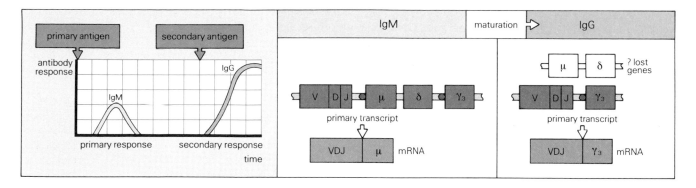

Fig. 9.21 Maturation of the immune response and class switching.

As shown in the graph, following a primary antigen injection there is an antibody response which consists mostly of IgM whereas the response following a secondary challenge is mostly IgG. The underlying cellular mechanism for this class switch is shown on the right. In the primary response the VDJ region is transcribed with a μ gene and, after removal of introns during processing, mRNA for secreted IgM is produced. During maturation, which involves T cell help, and possibly also the activation of a mutation mechanism for the VDJ segment, another C gene (here illustrated as Cγ3) is brought up to exchange with the μ gene at its switch region (red). The μ and δ genes are probably lost; transcription and processing produce mRNA for IgG3.

MEMBRANE AND SECRETED IMMUNOGLOBULIN

The membrane immunoglobulin produced by a cell as its antigen receptor and the immunoglobulin that it secretes are identical except for a stretch of amino acids at the C terminus of the heavy chains. Membrane immunoglobulins are larger than their secreted counterparts, their additional amino acids traverse the cell membrane to anchor the molecule. This can be seen in membrane IgM where a section of hydrophobic (lipophilic) amino acids are sandwiched between hydrophilic residues which lie on either side of the membrane (Fig. 9.23).

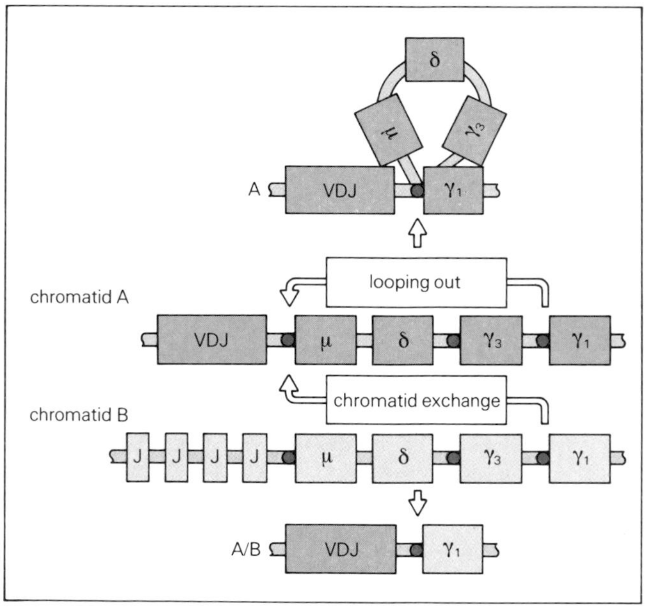

Fig. 9.22 Lost genes: hypothesis.

Two hypotheses explain the loss of genes during class switching (here illustrated as an IgM→IgG1 switch). A and B are chromatids of the chromosome section for the immunoglobulin genes. Chromatid A contains the rearranged VDJ segment. According to the looping out hypothesis, a section of C genes (μ, δ, γ₃) loop out and are lost. According to the chromatid exchange hypothesis the similarities in the switching sequences permit unequal somatic recombination between maternal and paternal chromatids. The A chromatid recombines with another part of the unrearranged B chromatid. The 'lost' intervening C genes are found on the other, non-functional chromatid (B) which now contains two copies of several C genes (ie. unrearranged V, D, J, μ, δ, γ₃, γ₁, etc.).

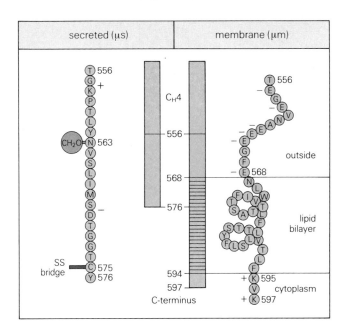

Fig. 9.23 Membrane and secreted IgM: mouse.

This diagram shows the C-terminal amino acid sequences of the IgM molecule for the secreted and membrane-bound molecules. The structures of both molecules are identical up to residue 556. Secreted IgM has twenty further residues. Residue 563 (asparagine) has a carbohydrate unit attached to it while residue 575 is a cystine involved in the formation of interchain disulphide bonds. Membrane IgM has forty-one residues beyond 556. A stretch of twenty-six residues between 568 and 595 contain hydrophobic amino acids sandwiched between sequences containing charged residues. It has been proposed that this hydrophobic portion traverses the cell membrane as two turns of alpha helix. A short, positively-charged section lies inside the cytoplasm.

The hydrophilic residues lie on either side of the membrane, and the section of hydrophobic residues is thought to form a stretch of alpha helix within the membrane. Membrane immunoglobulins do not form polymers of the basic four chain unit. The production of the two forms of immunoglobulin is brought about by differential transcription of the germ line C region gene which can be transcribed in two different ways (Fig. 9.24). It is thought that the poly A sequence is important in determining which RNA transcript is produced, but how this is controlled is uncertain. Evidently the way in which the cell regulates which immunoglobulin it produces is very complicated. The first step is the VJ and VDJ recombinations to produce light and heavy chain variable region genes. It is postulated that this occurs repeatedly until a functionally recombined gene is produced or the genetic material is exhausted and the cell is aborted. Once the V regions of that cell are determined they remain essentially unaltered thereafter (except for any somatic mutation). However there is still switching in the C_H genes to produce different isotypes and a change to production of secreted immunoglobulin following activation of the cell. A compilation of known facts and hypotheses is presented in figure 9.25.

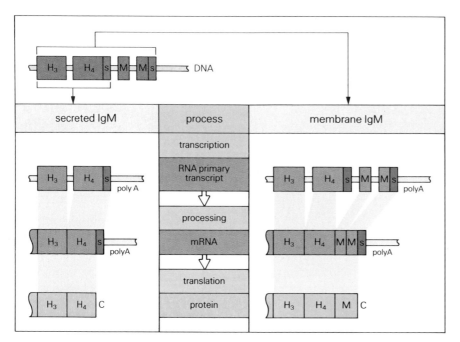

Fig. 9.24 Membrane and secreted IgM. Part of the DNA coding for IgM is shown diagrammatically. The exons for the µ3, and µ4 domains (H_3 and H_4) and the intramembranal segment of membrane IgM (M) are indicated. Translation stop sequences (s) are present at the end of the H_4 and second membrane segments. The DNA can be transcribed in two ways. If transcription stops after H_4 the transcript with a polyA tail is processed to produce mRNA for secreted IgM. If transcription runs through to include the membrane segments, processing removes the codons for the terminal amino acids and the stop signal of H_4 so that translation yields a protein with a different C terminus.

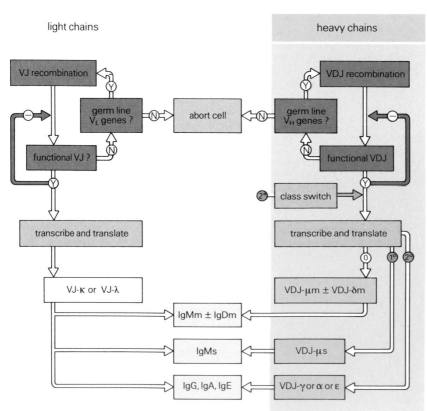

Fig. 9.25 Summary scheme of immunoglobulin production: fact and hypothesis. This diagram is based on a series of steps at which different outcomes may occur. Pre-B cells attempt to recombine a VJ from the germ line genes (left). If functional (Y) it is transcribed and translated to form a light chain. Once a cell has produced a functional recombination, feedback (−) prevents further rearrangements. If the VJ is not functional (N) the cell makes another attempt. If a cell exhausts its store of germ line gene segments then it is aborted. A similar process occurs for heavy chains (right) so that the early B cell (right) expresses IgMm±IgDm. This occurs with no antigen stimulation (0). After primary antigen stimulation (1°) the transcriptional process changes so that secreted IgM is released. After secondary antigen stimulation (2°) and with T cell help there is a DNA rearrangement, resulting in a class switch, possibly also with mutation in V_H and V_L. The end products are cells bearing and secreting IgG, IgA or IgE.

9.10

PRODUCTION OF IMMUNOGLOBULIN

The processes discussed so far concern recombinational events in the B cells' DNA and production of RNA transcripts. Before the antibody protein is synthesized it is first necessary to splice the introns out of the primary RNA transcript. It is found that the beginning and end of each intron have particular forms of RNA base sequences referred to as donor and acceptor junctions. It is thought that the junctions interact with each other and with ribonucleoproteins in the nucleus to remove the introns and splice the joins back together again to form mRNA (Fig. 9.26). It is, of course, essential that this is done accurately so that the reading frame of the mRNA is unaltered. Messenger RNA for immunoglobulins is translated across the membranes of the endoplasmic reticulum, after which the H and L chains associate (Fig. 9.27). Cellular immunoglobulins and secreted immunoglobulins are processed differently to arrive at their correct locations, by mechanisms which are unknown at present.

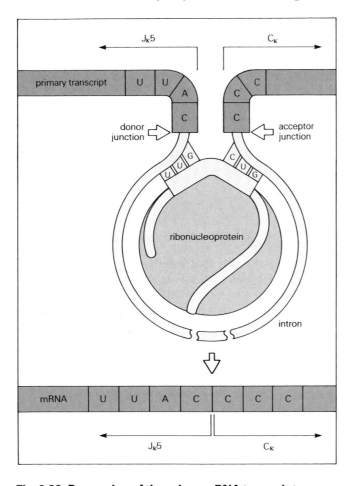

Fig. 9.26 Processing of the primary RNA transcript.
Processing is thought to occur as illustrated for the join between Jκ5 and Cκ. The bases on either side of the join are indicated. The two exons are brought together at the donor and acceptor junctions. The junctions are held together in the correct reading frame by base pairing with a small piece of RNA associated with a ribonucleoprotein particle. This particle cuts the RNA strands at the junctions and rejoins the ends to excise the intron. This scheme is based on mechanisms established in other transcriptional systems of eukaryotes.

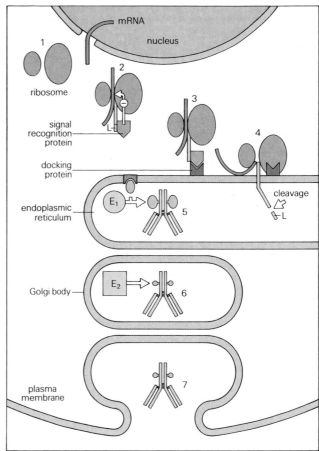

Fig. 9.27 Production of secreted immunoglobulin.
Messenger RNA for a secreted heavy chain leaves the nucleus and enters the cytoplasm where it is bound by a ribosome (1). The leading sequence (L) is translated and this binds to signal recognition protein (SRP) which blocks further translation (2). The signal recognition protein/ribosome complex migrates to the endoplasmic reticulum (ER) where the SRP binds to the docking protein at a vacant site on the ER (3). Translation may now proceed and the synthesizing chain traverses the membrane into the endoplasmic reticulum (4). The leader sequence is removed and the chain combines with other H and L chains to form the immunoglobulin subunit (5). Enzymes (E$_1$) add carbohydrate (blue) as the ER pinches off to form the Golgi body (6). In the Golgi body further enzymes (E$_2$) modify the carbohydrate before the completed molecule is secreted to the outside by reverse pinocytosis (7).

FURTHER READING

Baltimore D. (1981) Somatic mutation gains its place among the generators of diversity. *Cell* **26,** 295.

Brack C., Hirama M., Lenhard-Schuller R. & Tonegawa S. (1978) A complete immunoglobulin gene is created by somatic recombination. *Cell* **15,** 1.

Cushley W. & Williamson A. R. (1982) Expression of immunoglobulin genes. *Essays Biochem.* **18,** 1.

Gearhart P J. (1982) Generation of immunoglobulin variable gene diversity. *Immunol. Today* **3,** 107.

Gottlieb P. D. (1980) Immunoglobulin genes. *Mol. Immunol.* **17,** 1423.

Honjo T. (1983) Immunoglobulin genes. *Annu. Rev. Immunol.* **1,** 499.

Siu G., Clark S. P., Yoshikai Y., Malissen M., Yanagi Y., Strauss E., Mak T. W. & Hood L. (1984) The human T cell antigen receptor is encoded by variable, diversity, and joining gene segments that arrange to generate a complete V gene. *Cell* **37,** 393.

Tonegawa S. (1983) Somatic generation of antibody diversity. *Nature* **302,** 573.

10 Regulation of the Immune Response

Once an immune response is initiated the components of that response (eg. B cells) are capable of immense replication. Not only can this be seen in the classical secondary response, but even more so in experiments involving the transfer of lymphocytes into irradiated recipients. Here it can be demonstrated that, if given the opportunity, a clone of B cells will continue to expand indefinitely (Fig. 10.1). It is thus evident that immune responses must normally be subject to strict and specific controls. Moreover, these controls must be specific not only for the antigen but for the type of immune response elicited. This enables a choice to be made among such responses as T cell-mediated cytotoxicity and antibody responses of one or more of the several isotypes which are available. The control of humoral immunity is better understood than that of cellular immunity.

In an immune response the primary regulator is the antigen, but regulation by intrinsic components of the immune system is also important. Moreover, antigen itself can induce two different types of response, namely immunity to that antigen or tolerance to it, and generally speaking these two conditions are stable for each antigen. Whether an antigen will produce immunity or tolerance depends largely on the way in which it first encounters the individual's immune system.

THE REGULATORY EFFECT OF ANTIBODY

The simplest and longest-known mechanism for regulation of humoral immunity is that by which circulating antibody itself regulates the production of antibody. A direct demonstration of this is seen in the prompt increase in the rate of antibody synthesis which occurs in a long-term immunized rabbit when antibody is removed by replacing its serum with normal serum (Fig. 10.2).

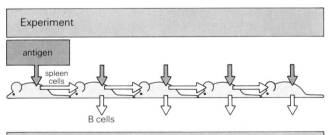

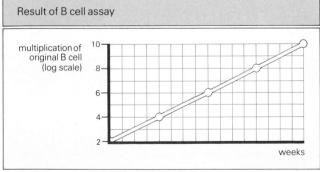

Fig. 10.1 Replicative potential of a B cell clone. A mouse was immunized with antigen and the antigen-primed spleen cells (5×10^6) transferred into irradiated (X) recipient mice, which were then injected with antigen. Some recipients produced homogeneous antibody indicating that a single clone had been transferred. Assay of these B cells after each transfer revealed that the clone continued to multiply through 3 further transfers as shown in the graph. The transferred cells of such a clone increased 100 fold between each transfer, therefore a B cell must have the potential to produce at least 10^{10} cells.

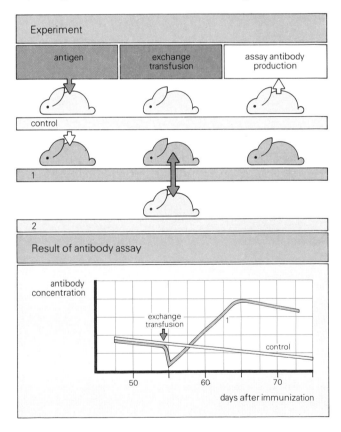

Fig. 10.2 Demonstration of the role of antibody in regulating its own production. Two rabbits (control, 1) are injected with antigen. Rabbit (1) has its serum exchanged with that of a non-immunized rabbit (2) in order to reduce the serum antibody concentration. The production of antibody by both the control and the exchange-transfused rabbits is then assayed. If the antibody is artifically reduced (1) then the rate of specific antibody production is increased causing the concentration to overshoot that expected without exchange transfusion. Exchange transfusion does not remove the antigen because it is fixed in the lymphoid tissues.

There are two ways in which antibody is known to suppress the production of further antibody. One is by simply combining with the antigen and thus competing with the antigen receptors of responding B cells. As might be expected this mechanism depends strictly on the concentration of the antibody and its affinity relative to the cellular receptors, and is independent of the Fc portion of the antibody. However, in many situations antibody can be shown to have a suppressive effect which is Fc-dependent. As a result of experiments *in vitro* (which overcome the problem that F(ab')$_2$ fragments are so rapidly cleared *in vivo*) the Fc-dependent effect has been shown to interfere with the *productive* response of T-dependent B cells, but to leave the *priming* of both T and B cells unimpaired. The whole antibody molecule is postulated to inhibit B cell differentiation by crosslinking the antigen-receptor with the Fc-receptor (Fig. 10.3). The F(ab')$_2$ fragment, on the other hand, has no effect at the low concentrations at which whole antibody works, but by its blocking activity at higher concentrations it is able to inhibit both T and B priming and the productive response. Doses of antibody which are insufficient to completely inhibit the production of antibody have the effect of increasing its average affinity (Fig. 10.4). For this reason antibody-feedback is thought to be an important factor driving the process of affinity maturation: it is thought that this process involves competition between the free antibody and the B cell antigen receptors. Antibody binds to the stimulating antigen, thus

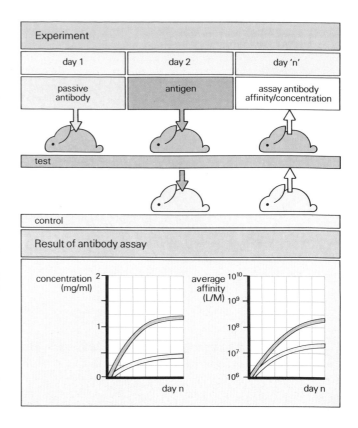

Fig. 10.4 Effect of passive antibody on the affinity and concentration of secreted antibody. One of two rabbits was injected with antibody (passive antibody) on day 1. Both rabbits were immunized with antigen on day 2 and the affinity and concentration of antibody raised to this antigen assayed at a later time (day n). The results of the antibody assay show that passive antibody reduces the concentration but increases the affinity of antibody produced.

reducing the free antigen concentration; consequently only those B cells with high affinity receptors bind to the antigen and are stimulated into division and maturation.

THE REGULATORY EFFECT OF IMMUNE COMPLEXES

It was seen in the preceding section that antibody, in its Fc-dependent mechanism, only regulates the B cell after first forming an immune complex with the antigen. Thus it is not surprising that pre-formed immune complexes often suppress B cell activation. Sometimes, however, they may augment the immune response. This tends to happen particularly when the ratio of antigen to antibody is high. This enhancing effect is also Fc-dependent, and may operate by encouraging fixation of the antigen on certain antigen presenting cells (APCs). Consistent with this is the fact that antigen shows greatly enhanced localization in germinal centres (where some APCs occur) when complexed to antibody. The postulated mechanisms for the action of immune complexes are illustrated in figure 10.5. In a more general sense it could clearly be useful for the early-appearing antibody to augment the response, and then later inhibit it when the antibody concentration exceeds that required to neutralize antigen.

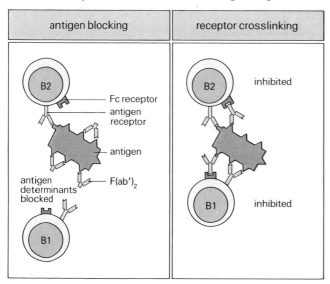

Fig. 10.3 Antibody-dependent B cell regulation — two ways in which antibody feedback can suppress the antibody response.
Antigen blocking. High doses of antibody (or its F(ab')$_2$ fragment) block the interaction between an antigenic determinant (epitope) and B cell receptors for that determinant, which are then effectively unable to recognize the antigen (B1). (This receptor blocking mechanism also prevents B cell priming.) B cells with receptors for different epitopes are unaffected (B2).
Receptor crosslinking. Low doses of antibody — but not F(ab')$_2$ — allow crosslinking between a B cell's Fc receptors and its antigen receptors. This inhibits the B cell from entering the phase of antibody synthesis but does not inhibit B cell priming. The effect is not determinant-specific.

The effect of antibody and of complexes is greatly influenced by the antibody's isotype. In general IgM antibodies have the strongest tendency to enhance the response, while IgG is more often suppressive. (While there are interesting differences among the IgG isotypes, it is not profitable to particularize in the present context.)

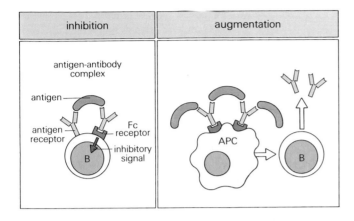

Fig. 10.5 Regulatory effects of immune complexes – inhibition and augmentation.
Inhibition. When the B cell's Fc-receptor is crosslinked to its antigen receptor by an antigen-antibody complex a signal is delivered to the B cell inhibiting it from entering the antibody production phase.
Augmentation. Antibody encourages presentation of antigen to B cells when it is present on an antigen presenting cell (APC), bound via Fc receptors. (Complexes can also activate complement and bind to APCs via their C3b receptors in an analagous way.)

IDIOTYPIC REGULATION

An antibody's variable and hypervariable regions may act as antigenic determinants. The experimental induction of anti-idiotype antibodies shows that lymphocytes exist which are capable of recognizing and responding to the combining sites of antibodies and receptors on other lymphocytes. The possibility is thus presented for regulatory interactions between the cells and antibodies of the immune system via their antigen combining sites. To facilitate discussion of this field, it is first necessary to define the structures which may be involved in these regulatory interactions (Fig. 10.6). The antigenic constitution of the V region of an immunoglobulin is known as its idiotype. The antigenic determinants of which the idiotype is made up are referred to as idiotopes. Finally, that part of the V region which forms its specific binding site is called its paratope. Some idiotopes will be found within the paratope, others outside it.

Anti-immunoglobulin sera do not normally contain a high concentration of antibody directed against a particular idiotype (anti-idiotype). This is because the normal immunoglobulin used for immunization is too heterogeneous in its V region to induce a particular anti-idiotype. Using a myeloma protein however, or homogeneous antibody, it is possible to produce an anti-idiotype serum which reacts with one or more idiotopes in the V region of the immunizing antibody (Fig. 10.7).

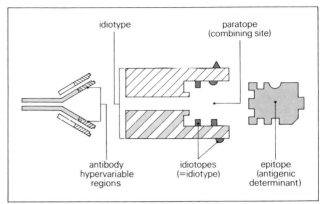

Fig. 10.6 Nomenclature in relation to the antibody variable domain. The determinants making up the antibody V region are termed idiotopes. Some idiotopes are located in the combining site (also referred to as the paratope), whilst others occur outside the paratope. The full set of V region determinants is termed the idiotype of the antibody molecule. Determinants on the antigen molecule are called epitopes.

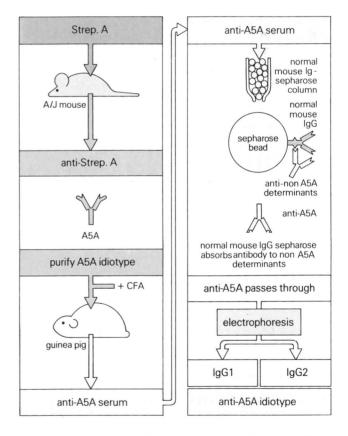

Fig. 10.7 Production of heterologous anti-idiotype. Mice of strain A/J, when immunized with streptococcal A (Strep. A) carbohydrate, make antibody consisting mainly of one idiotype – A5A. This is purified and injected (together with Complete Freund's Adjuvant – CFA) into a guinea pig tolerant to the constant region determinants of mouse immunoglobulin. The resulting anti-A5A serum is absorbed with normal mouse IgG on a sepharose column. Since normal IgG has negligible A5A idiotype the antibody to non A5A determinants binds to it and is removed while anti-A5A passes through the column. The anti-idiotype antibody can then be fractionated into subclasses by electrophoresis.

It is possible to distinguish between anti-idiotypes directed against idiotypes within the combining site and those directed against idiotopes outside the combining site: only those binding to the antigen combining site inhibit the interaction between that combining site and hapten (Fig. 10.8). The possibility is clear, then, for anti-idiotype to substitute for the original antigen (Fig. 10.9). Like antigen it may either stimulate or depress the immune response. The direction of its effect depends on a great many factors, most of which are unknown. It should be noted however that, unlike antigen, anti-idiotype

bears an Fc-region and so could interact with Fc-receptors, as in figure 10.5.

Knowing that such interactions between idiotypes and anti-idiotypes are possible, Jerne has built up a conceptual framework indicating how they may function in the maintenance of immunological homeostasis by forming a network with multitudinous connections (Fig. 10.10). This very general concept is currently undergoing more detailed investigation. The evidence that such a network may exist is mainly indirect, and is discussed in the next section.

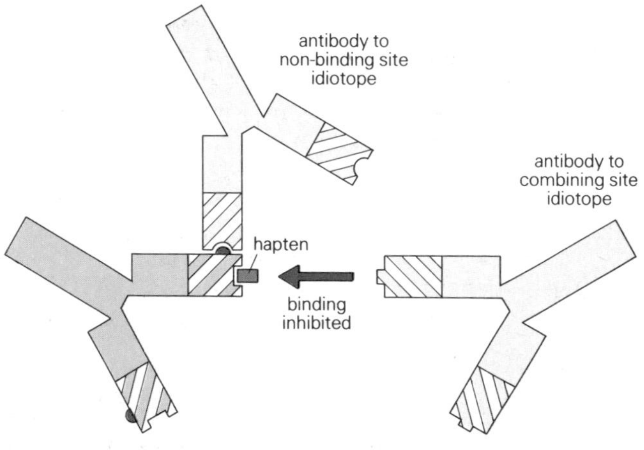

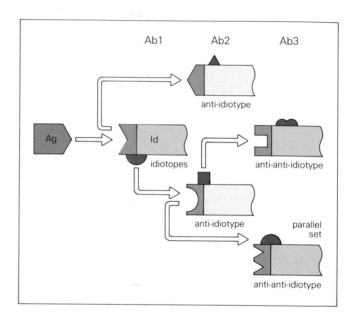

Fig. 10.10 Jerne's Network Hypothesis. Antigen (Ag) stimulates the production of an antibody (Id) which carries a number of idiotypes (orange and red). The Id stimulates anti-idiotypes which regulate production of the Id. The anti-idiotypes are in turn regulated by anti-anti-idiotypes. The sets of antibodies comprising these chains of recognition are sometimes referred to as Ab1, Ab2, Ab3 etc. Note that the upper anti-Id has an idiotope resembling the antigen (external antigen) and is known as the internal image of the antigen. Some antibodies share idiotopes with the original idiotype (Id) but do not share paratopes; these parallel sets of antibodies will be regulated in tandem. The hypothesis does not make specific predictions on the degree of regulation or even its direction (stimulation or inhibition).

Fig. 10.8 Distinction between idiotopes inside and outside the antibody combining site. An anti-idiotype serum may contain some antibodies directed to idiotopes associated with the combining site (site associated). The binding to these can be inhibited by hapten. Other antibodies, to non-binding site idiotopes (non-site associated) will not be inhibited by hapten.

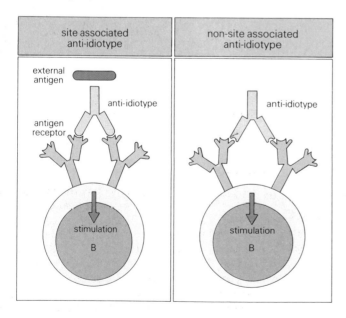

Fig. 10.9 Regulation by site-associated and non-site associated anti-idiotype.
Site-associated anti-idiotype mimics the external (original) antigen and crosslinks the B cell's antigen receptors. This delivers a stimulatory signal to the B cell.
Non-site associated anti-idiotype also crosslinks the B cell's antigen receptors and can also deliver a stimulatory signal.

EVIDENCE THAT IDIOTYPIC INTERACTIONS ARE IMPORTANT IN IMMUNOREGULATION

Very striking evidence has been obtained from the effects of anti-idiotype sera on the representation of the recognized idiotype in immune responses. Depending on the experimental conditions it is possible to produce either enhancement or suppression of antibody responses using anti-idiotype sera. Some of the clearest experimental studies of idiotype/anti-idiotype regulatory interactions have been performed in mice. For example some mouse strains, when challenged with the antigen phosphoryl choline (PC) produce antibodies of mostly one idiotype, T15. The effect of idiotypic interactions may be observed by injecting anti-T15 antibodies into the mice and observing the effect on the antibody response to PC. Injection of a high dose of anti-T15 into the adult produces transient suppression of the antibody response to PC. This appears to be due to a temporary blocking of T15 idiotype-bearing B cells. On the other hand the same antibody given to the neonate results in long-lasting inactivation of the T15 clones (Fig. 10.11).

In addition to the suppressive effect of anti-idiotype, a priming effect can also occur. This may be demonstrated in the antibody reaction to the Streptococcal A carbo-hydrate. The major idiotype to this antigen in A strain mice, which represents about 50% of the total serum anti-Strep. A, is the A5A idiotype. Anti-A5A raised in guinea pigs can prime or suppress the A5A response in exceedingly small doses (10-100ng). The different isotypes of the anti-idiotype antibody have different actions. The IgG1 isotype primes the A5A clone so that its product comes to represent a higher fraction of the total antibody to Strep. A, while the IgG2 isotype results in specific suppression of the A5A idiotype, while leaving other idiotypes unaffected (Fig. 10.12).

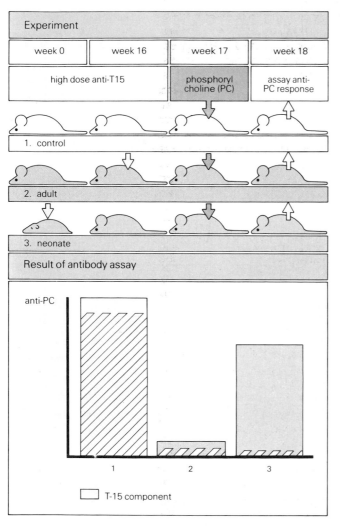

Fig. 10.11 Suppression of the antibody response by anti-idiotype. At week 0 a neonate was administered a high dose of anti-T15 (T15 is the major idiotype raised against the antigen, phosphoryl choline-PC), and at week 16 one adult mouse was similarly treated. At week 17 both anti-T15 treated mice and an untreated, control were immunized with PC, and a week later the antibody raised to PC (both the total anti-PC and the T15 anti-PC idiotype) was assayed. The results of the anti-PC assay are shown in the bar diagram. The T15 response to PC normally represents 90% of the total antibody response to this antigen (control). A high dose of anti-T15 given to the adult temporarily suppresses T15 (adult) whereas a high dose given to the neonate results in a long-term deletion of the T15 component of the antibody response to PC. However, since T15 is partly replaced by other idiotypes, the total anti-PC response is much less affected.

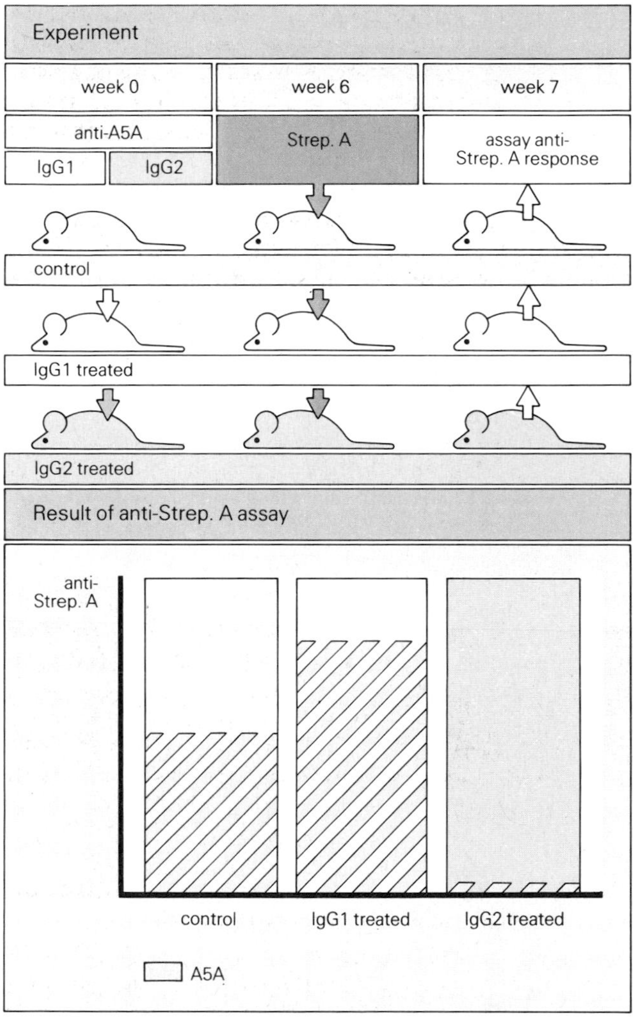

Fig. 10.12 Idiotype priming or suppression induced by different isotypes of an anti-idiotype serum. In this experiment at week 0 one group of mice is left untreated (control) and two others are administered 0.1mg of IgG1 anti-A5A or IgG2 anti-A5A. Six weeks later all three groups were immunized with Streptococcal A carbohydrate and the anti-Strep. A responses assessed one week later. The results of the anti-Strep. A assay are shown in the bar diagram. Normally the A5A idiotype represents 50% of the total antibody response to the Strep. A antigen. It was found that IgG1 anti-idiotype primes the A5A clone so that it makes the major contribution to the total antibody concentration while the IgG2 anti-idiotype suppresses the A5A clone so that it makes a very small contribution. Total levels of antibody to Strep. A are not markedly affected by the different anti-idiotype treatments.

The suppression is long-lasting and is maintained by an idiotype-related suppressor T cell, as shown by transferring the suppression to recipient animals with T cells. Of significance both for network theory and for the nature of T cell recognition is the finding that some anti-idiotypes also recognize receptors on helper T cells (Fig. 10.13).

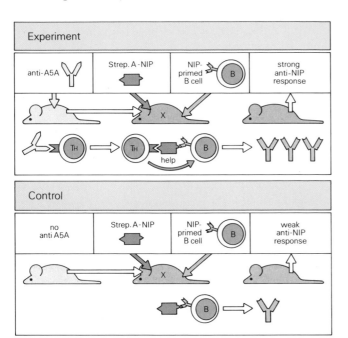

Fig. 10.13 Experiment suggesting that anti-idiotypes may recognize helper T cell receptors. A low dose of anti-A5A given to the adult mouse primes T-helper cells (TH). When these T-helper cells are transferred into an irradiated mouse, together with an immunizing dose of Strep. A linked to the hapten NIP (nitrophenylacetic acid), and NIP-primed B cells, a strong antibody response takes place. In this situation the Strep. A antigen is acting as a carrier for NIP. A similarly treated mouse, but lacking the T-helper cells primed by anti-idiotype produces a weak response to the NIP hapten.

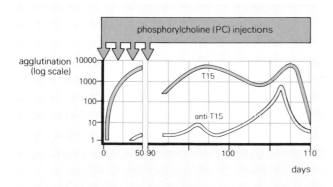

Fig. 10.14 Anti-idiotype production during the response to an antigen. Mice were repeatedly immunized with pneumococcal vaccine (bearing the phosphoryl choline determinant) for 90 days. The resulting antiserum was assayed both for T15 (anti-PC) and anti-T15 antibodies. As shown, anti-idiotype is produced during the course of the anti-PC response. T15 and anti-T15 production occur in synchronous waves, which lead to the suggestion that the anti-T15 acts as a feedback control on T15 production.

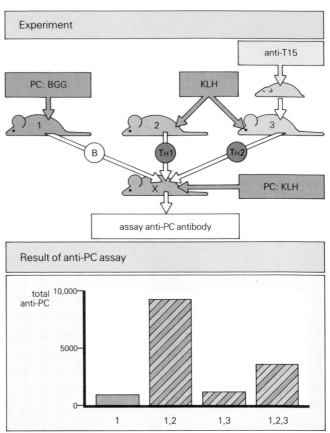

Fig. 10.15 Requirements for antigen-specific and idiotype-specific T-helper cells for a normal antibody response. Irradiated mice (X) were reconstituted with different combinations of T and B cells (spleen cell transfer):
1. B cells primed to phosphoryl choline from a mouse immunized with the conjugate, phosphoryl choline – bovine gamma globulin (PC-BGG),
2. T-helper cells from a mouse immunized with keyhole limpet haemocyanin (KLH). These mice normally have TH cells capable of expanding the B cell population carrying the T15 idiotype.
3. T-helper cells from a mouse primed with KLH but whose T15-bearing lymphocytes were suppressed with anti-T15 antibody soon after birth.

The recipient mice were then challenged with the PC-KLH conjugate and the resulting anti-PC response assayed. The antibody raised to phosphoryl choline for each combination of treatments (represented by the Plaque Forming Cells per spleen) is given in the bar chart. When the recipient mouse is reconstituted with B cells specific to PC (1) in the absence of any T cell help very little anti-PC antibody is raised. When T helper cells primed to the KLH determinant (2) are introduced the B cells are helped to generate a normal antibody response – most of this antibody carries the T15 idiotype. If, however, the mouse donating the T-helper cells is suppressed for T15 (3) the T15 response is suppressed. When spleen cells from mouse 2 are added the response is partly restored, presumably by the activity of T15-specific T-helper cells. In this system T15 forms over 80% of the total anti-PC antibody and there is little tendency for compensation by other idiotypes when it is suppressed, for example, in mouse 3.

Although the anti-idiotype in the foregoing experiments was produced by artificial means there is increasing evidence that anti-idiotypic antibodies are produced in the course of natural immune responses and coexist in serum with their specific idiotype presumably in the form of immune complexes (Fig. 10.14). It has been suggested that anti-idiotypic regulation is responsible for the waves of antibody production which are seen in certain immune responses, but it is more difficult to prove that this is actually the case. In favour of the view that idiotypic regulation is important in physiological immune responses, one may note that the amount of anti-idiotype which will experimentally modulate an immune response is similar to that normally found in serum.

The evidence so far discussed has been derived from the effects of anti-idiotype antibodies. However there is also evidence that regulatory cells, for example, helper and suppressor T cells may be idiotype- rather than antigen-specific and thus control the expression of different idiotypes in an immune response. It may be demonstrated by transferring primed T and B cells into irradiated recipients that the development of a normal immune response requires both antigen-specific T$_H$ cells and idiotype specific T$_H$ cells (Fig. 10.15). The antigen specific T$_H$ cells help B cells to produce antibodies to determinants on the antigen, while the idiotype specific T$_H$ cells amplify certain of the idiotype bearing B cell clones. In this scheme the antigen specific T$_H$ cells are MHC restricted while the idiotype specific T$_H$ cells are not (Fig. 10.16).

A further prediction of the network hypothesis in its original form was that the network was multiply branched, with each idiotype-producing cell being controlled by several anti-idiotypes. This implied that the whole network was dependent for its control on all other parts. Some experiments however (Urbain, 1979), imply that the branching of the network is less extensive than originally suggested (Fig. 10.17).

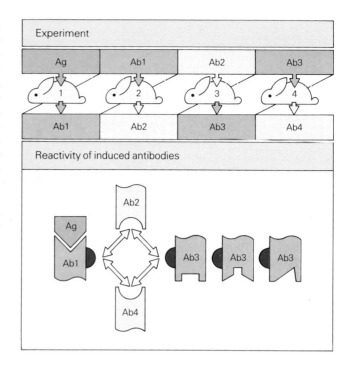

Fig. 10.17 Experiment demonstrating the limited nature of the idiotype control network. A rabbit (1) immunized with Streptococcal vaccine (Ag) produced a monoclonal antibody (Ab1). This was purified and used to immunize another rabbit (2), which produced an anti-idiotype antibody (Ab2). This anti-idiotype was used to immunize a third rabbit, and so on. The reactivity of each antibody with the antigen and the other antibodies was tested and the results are indicated below. Firstly, only Ab1 reacts with the antigen. Secondly, the pattern of reactivity between the antibodies shows them to alternate in specificity such that any odd numbered antibody reacts with the even numbered antibodies, but not other odd numbered antibodies. In the mechanism shown here, Ab1 has a non site-associated idiotope (red) which is also present on Ab3 and is recognized by Ab2 and Ab4. This simple control network is unbranched and may be more representative of the physiological control networks than the one originally postulated Jerne.

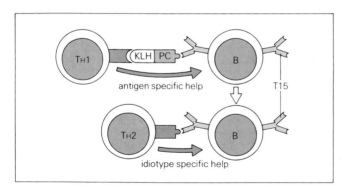

Fig. 10.16 Antigen specific and idiotype specific T-helper cells. Two varieties of T-helper cells have been postulated. **Antigen specific T help.** T$_H$1 is the classical T-helper cell: it has receptors which recognize both the antigen KLH and MHC antigens (Ia) on the antigen presenting cell (not shown). T$_H$1 helps B cells carrying receptors for the PC hapten attached to the antigen. T$_H$1 is obligatory for an immune response, and because it must interact with Ia antigens on the APC in order to help the B cell response, it is MHC-restricted. **Idiotype specific T help.** T$_H$2 is the idiotype specific T-helper cell. It has a receptor which recognizes the idiotype carried on the B cell, T15. It will help B cells carrying the T15 idiotype and has the effect of amplifying the B cell clones carrying this idiotype. T$_H$2 is not MHC restricted.

It was noted that the number of anti-idiotypes produced to a particular idiotype was limited, and that if anti-anti-idiotypes were raised a considerable proportion of these would resemble the original idiotype. This implies that a large proportion of antibodies may carry particular controlling idiotypes.

To summarize, the network hypothesis is still the subject of considerable controversy, but there is good evidence that idiotypic interactions can modulate the immune response, although the relative importance of these interactions in the resting state and the immune state have not been determined finally. On balance it appears that antigen is of prime importance in regulating the active immune state, but that idiotypic regulation may direct the antibody response towards a particular spectrum of idiotypes. In the resting state where antigen has not yet impinged on the immune system it is conceivable that idiotype/anti-idiotype regulation may be important in determining the initial state of the immune system in which it encounters antigen.

REGULATION BY CELLULAR MECHANISMS –
SUPPRESSOR T CELLS

While some lymphocytes either possess their own effector function (eg. cytotoxic T cells) or instruct non-specific cells to exert an effector function (eg. B cells, which instruct polymorphs and macrophages via antibody, and T cells which activate macrophages) others function purely as regulators of other lymphocytes. The best known of these is the helper T cell. Besides helpers, however, there exist T cells which specifically suppress immune responses – T suppressor (Ts) cells. These can become activated after certain procedures designed to induce immunological tolerance and can be demonstrated in cell transfer experiments by their effect in suppressing the response of normal cells (Fig. 10.18). T-suppressor cell activity can also be demonstrated during normal immune responses, suggesting that they play a continuous role in regulation.

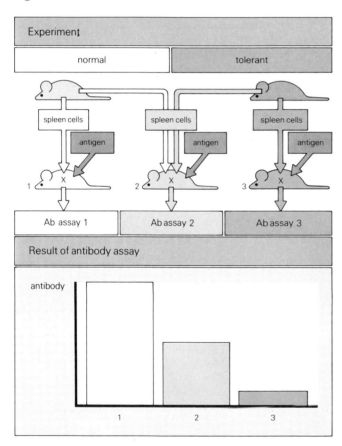

Fig. 10.18 Demonstration of suppressor cells. Three X-irradiated mice (1, 2, 3) are reconstituted with:
1. cells from a normal mouse only,
2. cells from both a normal mouse and a mouse rendered tolerant to the antigen sheep red blood cells,
3. cells from the tolerant mouse only.
All three mice are then immunized with antigen, and the antibody produced to the antigen assessed. Mouse 1 produces a normal response, mouse 3 produces a weak response and the response of mouse 2 is intermediate demonstrating that cells from the tolerant mouse can suppress the response of normal cells.

The mode of action of suppressor T cells is uncertain. As with helper cells, they have been found to release specific factors *in vitro*, but the usual failure to find these in serum suggests that they normally act over a very short range. These factors can often be shown to adhere to macrophages. Thus one reasonable suggestion is that lymphocytes (Ts or Th) migrating through lymphoid tissue leave their message behind as factors adhering to antigen presenting cells where they can serve to activate or suppress the next lymphocytes of appropriate specificity which come along (Fig. 10.19). The balance of helper

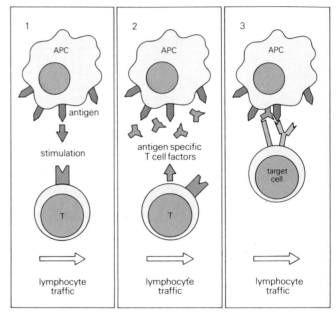

Fig. 10.19 Hypothetical action of antigen-specific T cell factors *in vivo*.
1. T cells (Th or Ts) passing through lymphoid tissue are stimulated by antigen on the antigen presenting cells to produce antigen-specific factors – helper or suppressor factors depending on the T cell's type.
2. These factors bind to the APC along with the antigen.
3. Later, target cells (B or T cells) passing through the tissue recognize both the antigen and the antigen-specific factors on the APC and are thereby directed into an appropriate state of immunity.

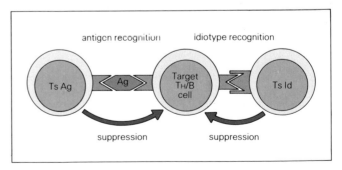

Fig. 10.20 Two types of T-suppressor cells. The antigen-specific T-suppressor cell (Ts Ag) binds to antigen and interacts with target B or Th cells by an antigen bridge. Alternatively, idiotype specific T-suppressor cells (Ts Id) bind directly to the receptors of the target cells and do not require antigen to produce suppression.

and suppressor factors on any particular APC may then determine whether it does or does not activate other lymphocytes. The action of T-suppressor cells may be directed at either the T-helper cell or the B cell, and the receptors of the Ts cells may recognize either antigen or idiotype. In the case of antigen recognition it requires the presence of antigen to act as a bridge between the Ts and its target before regulation can be exerted. In the case of idiotype recognition the Ts may produce direct suppression by binding to the receptors of its target (Fig. 10.20). This is an extension of the original network hypothesis to include the possible action of Ts cells, rather than anti-idiotypic antibody. A regulatory chain formed by idiotype-specific Ts cells is presented in figure 10.21.

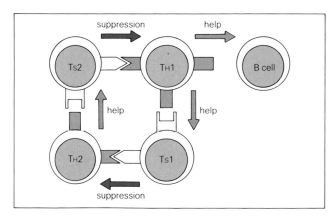

Fig. 10.22 A hypothetical regulatory circuit. The properties of this model are such that it can exist in either of two stable states:
1. T_H1 and $Ts1$ are active, resulting in help to the B cell, suppression of T_H2 and consequent lack of help to $Ts2$, or
2. T_H2 and $Ts2$ are active, resulting in lack of activity of T_H1 and $Ts1$ and lack of help to the B cell.
It is necessary that the interactions between the T helpers and T suppressors are directed only to the appropriate target cell, therefore this hypothesis requires a mechanism to ensure directionality in the regulatory loop, that is, that T_H1 helps $Ts1$ and not $Ts2$.

It is clear that the interactions of cells and antibodies in regulation of the immune response are exceedingly complex, and one can be certain only of the most broad generalities. A minimum model to include the elements so far discussed is set out in figure 10.23.

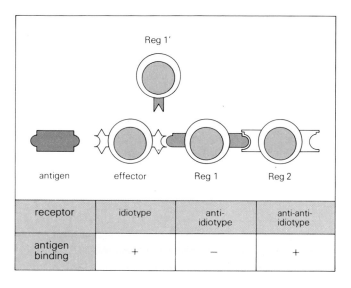

Fig. 10.21 A hypothetical regulatory chain. Effector cells (eg. T cells) are stimulated by antigen and are regulated, via their antigen receptors, by regulator cells (Reg 1, Reg 1'). These cells are in turn regulated by other cells via their surface receptors (eg. Reg 2). In the scheme illustrated here the effector cell carries idiotype, Reg 1 and Reg 1' are anti-idiotypic (Reg 1 carries a site-associated anti-idiotype and Reg 1' a non site-associated anti-idiotype), and Reg 2 carries the anti-anti-idiotype, which also binds antigen. Chains may be branched when regulator cells (eg. Reg 1') recognize idiotypes outside the combining site.

CELLULAR CIRCUITS

Various experiments have demonstrated the interaction of Ts, T_H and B cells. They have provided evidence for different models of immunoregulation although it is by no means certain which of these are important *in vivo*. On the theoretical side, there is a need to account for the tendency of the immune system, once triggered, to enter into a stable state of tolerance of immunity – or indeed into any of its modalities. It has been suggested that this might be achieved by means of a circuit (or circuits) of helper and suppressor cell interactions. An essential feature of such a circuit is that a cell being regulated ('regulatee') must not be capable of directly influencing its regulator. Such a circuit can be seen to behave in a 'flip-flop' manner, as explained in figure 10.22.

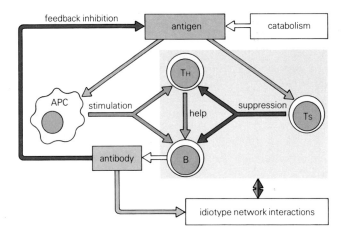

Fig. 10.23 Regulation of the immune response: a summary. This diagram outlines a minimum model for immunoregulation involving the feedback inhibition by antibody on antigen and through the idiotype network. Antigen is presented to T-helper and B cells by an APC which stimulates them. Furthermore, T-helper cells once activated, help their specific B cells to produce antibody. T-suppressor cells are also stimulated by antigen and regulate both T-helper cells and B cells. Antibody and idiotype-specific T cells interact with the antigen-specific cells (blue box) to regulate the response. The stimulating effect of antigen on the immune system is diminished by complexing with antibody and by its catabolism.

FUNCTION OF THE MHC IN REGULATION

It has been discussed above how some lymphocytes (eg. TH cells) recognize antigen only in association with MHC products. One consequence is that these lymphocytes must ignore antigen in the free state, and recognize it only after presentation or 'processing' by the special antigen-presenting cells which are capable of this. In this way the lymphocytes could be forced to take note of the message left on these APCs by other lymphocytes. These antigen-presenting cells now appear to be distinct from the true macrophages, which form part of the effector side of the response. Such a mechanism may account not only for regulation of the intensity of response, but of its modality as discussed in the next section.

REGULATION OF THE MODE OF RESPONSE

There are good reasons why different modes of response should be appropriate to cope with different infections. For example, cytotoxic cells may be appropriate for many virus infections, complement-fixing antibody for acute bacterial infections, and macrophage activation for those organisms which would normally resist the microbicidal powers of macrophages. Just how the response is directed into these different modes is unknown. The discovery that different types of APCs exist in different parts of the body offers a partial answer. For example, the Langerhans cells in skin seem particularly adapted towards mediation of delayed hypersensitivity and thus account for the tendency of antigens, on cutaneous application, to favour response in this mode. On the other hand the dendritic cells of lymphoid follicles probably mediate priming of B cells for antibody production.

It is also likely that the mode of response depends to a large extent on certain physical or chemical properties of the antigen or infective organism, which are perceived in a way which is not immunologically specific. Although these properties of the antigen can be either suppressive or stimulatory, it is convenient to lump them together as the 'adjuvanticity' of the antigen. It is well-known that different adjuvants injected in conjunction with the same antigen tend to favour different modalities of response. The available evidence often points to APCs as the immediate site of action of these adjuvant effects. It has been found for example that when lipids are coupled to protein antigens these tend to induce delayed hypersensitivity rather than antibody production and to localize in T-dependent rather than B-dependent areas of lymphoid tissues. This suggests that lipophilic properties direct the antigen to a different set of APCs, programmed to trigger a different modality of response.

How does an APC engage with the correct type of lymphocytes to bring about a particular mode of response? It is suggested that this is a function of MHC products or other cellular-interaction molecules. Examples already known are the associations of H-2K and D with the cytotoxic response, of the I-A subregion with Ia restricted helper cell activation, and I-J with suppression (Fig. 10.24). More associations such as these probably exist.

10.10

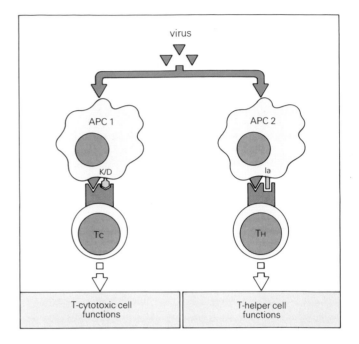

Fig. 10.24 Mode of response regulated by antigen presentation. This scheme shows how an antigenic stimulus, in this case a virus, may activate two different cell classes. The virus will activate cytotoxic T cells (Tc) if seen on the APC (APC 1) in association with the K or D MHC antigen (mice); or will activate helper T cells if seen in association (APC 2) with Ia antigens. Some T-helper cells will subsequently help cytotoxic reactions while others will help antibody production.

Cellular interaction molecules would also be required to guide circuits of the type shown in figure 10.22.

NON-SPECIFIC REGULATION

While so far the emphasis has been on the specificity of regulation, whether to antigen or idiotype, it is clear that there also exist non antigen-specific mechanisms of regulation. Certain T cells for example, when activated, release a factor previously termed T cell growth factor (TCGF) but now known as interleukin 2 (1L-2) which has a non-specific effect in amplifying the proliferation of other T cells. Both helper and cytotoxic T cells are affected. But it is important to note that interleukin 2 only amplifies the proliferation of cells already activated into blast transformation by antigen or other means (Fig. 10.25). Less well characterized are interleukin 1 (previously, lymphocyte activating factor – LAF) from macrophages, and T cell-replacing factor, both of which act on B cells. While regulation can be non antigen-specific it can still be specific for the mode of response. For example, factors have been described which suppress either total IgE or total IgG production independently. The requirement for antigen bridging in certain types of cell cooperation guides non-specific signals to specific cells. This is illustrated in figure 10.26, which also shows the uncertainty which exists over just how the bridge is made, by indicating three possible mechanisms.

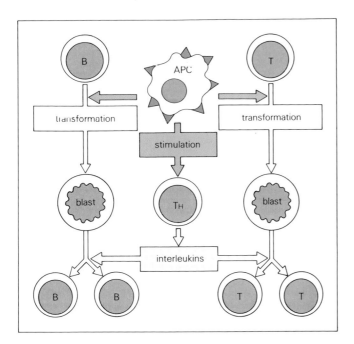

Fig. 10.25 Non-specific augmentation of immune responses by interleukins. Antigen presented to T and B cells causes them to transform into blast cells. T-helper cells are stimulated to release interleukins which amplify the proliferation of cells already activated into blast formation.

SELF/NON-SELF DISCRIMINATION

Although immunological tolerace is dealt with fully else-where, it is worth considering briefly here how the complex variety of regulatory mechanisms can lead either to full-scale immunity or profound tolerance. The direction taken determines whether an antigen is eventually accepted as self or rejected as non-self. To make such a discrimination a number of signals must be integrated. Pre-eminent amongst these is the time element: antigens are accepted as self provided that they persist long enough. In embryonic life it may be sufficient that the antigen is present throughout the maturation of the immune system. Tolerance could then be achieved by the simple mechanism of lymphocytes being tolerized at an immature stage and only developing the capacity to be immunized later. In the adult, however, such a mechanism cannot be sufficient because although mature lymphocytes are already present, tolerance can still readily be induced with certain antigens (such as foreign immunoglobulins) provided that no kind of adjuvant stimulus is present. Thus adjuvanticity, while yet poorly defined, is a vital factor influencing the tolerance/immunity decision. Most antigens contain sufficient adjuvanticity to produce a primary response, yet even these

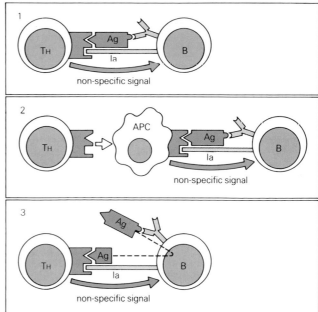

Fig. 10.26 Three possible mechanisms for T-B cooperation. Consider T-helper cells primed to antigen (Ag) associated with an MHC molecule (Ia) on antigen presenting cells as shown in figure 10.24. The primed T$_H$ cells then help B cells by:
1. using antigen as a direct bridge, or
2. releasing their receptors as 'helper factors', which then adhere to the APC and form an antigen bridge to the B cell.
3. A third possibility recently suggested is that the B cell internalizes the antigen, digests it and re-expresses a fragment in association with the Ia molecule.
In each case the B cell may receive a non-specific signal, which could also be delivered to other B cells. The exact physical relationship of the antigen and MHC receptors is unknown, though they have been depicted here as one unit. Cooperation between T cell and B cell is I region restricted. This is due to either a requirement for the same type of MHC on the T and B cells and/or a requirement for the same type of MHC on the T cell and the APC which primes the T cell. T-suppressor cells could operate by similar mechanisms, but with the difference that the T cell receptors ('suppressor factors') often do not need to recognize MHC together with antigen.

will eventually induce tolerance if injected in sufficiently large and frequent doses over a long enough time, whereas more intermittent doses over the same time only potentiate the response.

To elucidate how the system discriminates on the basis of so many signals, including their timing, is likely to be difficult and will require more detailed knowledge of the operation of immunological circuits.

FURTHER READING

Bach F., Bonairda B. & Vitetta E. (eds.) (1979) *T and B lymphocytes: Recognition and Function.* Academic Press, New York.

Eichmann K. (1978) Expression and function of idiotypes on lymphocytes. *Adv. Immunol.* **26,** 195.

Fabris N., Garaci E., Hadden J. & Mitchison N.A. (1983) *Immunoregulation.* Plenum Press, New York and London.

Katz D.H. (1977) *Lymphocyte Differentiation, Recognition and Regulation.* Academic Press, New York.

Klein J. (1982) *Immunology: The Science of Self-Nonself Discrimination.* Wiley, New York.

Moller G. (ed.) (1980) Regulation of the immune response by antibodies against the immunogen. *Immunol. Revs.* **49.**

Moller G. (ed.) (1982) Interleukins and lymphocyte activation. *Immunol. Rcvs.* **63.**

11 Cell-mediated Immunity

The term 'cell-mediated immunity' (CMI) was originally coined to describe localized reactions to organisms, usually intracellular pathogens, mediated by lymphocytes and phagocytes rather than by antibody (humoral immunity). However it is now often used in a more general sense for any response in which antibody plays a subordinate role.

It is not possible however to consider cell-mediated and antibody-mediated responses entirely separately. Cells are involved in the initiation of antibody responses, and antibody acts as an essential link in some cell-mediated reactions. Moreover no cell-mediated response is likely to occur in the total absence of antibody, which can modify cellular responses in numerous ways. For instance, antigen-antibody complexes may form during an immune response in which chemotactic molecules are released causing cellular aggregation and local inflammation. Antibody may block antigenic determinants which would otherwise be recognized by cells, or cause stripping or modulation of such determinants from target cell membranes. It may also be involved in linking antigens to T cells via their Fc receptors, thus modulating the cells' responses.

The various aspects of cell-mediated immunity are summarized in figure 11.1 which illustrates the most important functions of cells: individual cells may perform more than one function. This figure does not include secondary effects of the activities of these cell types, such as delayed hypersensitivity or granuloma formation.

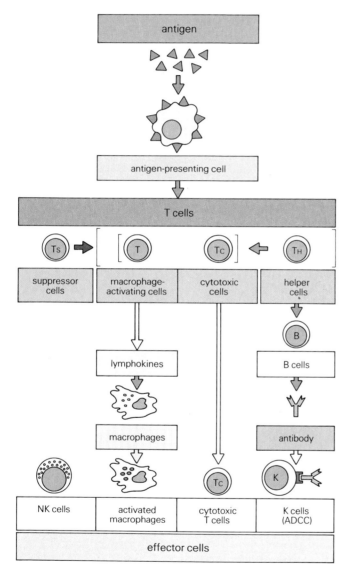

Fig.11.1 Scope of cell-mediated immunity. Cell-mediated immune responses follow antigen presentation and activation of T cells. Activation is regulated by suppressor and helper cells. Certain T cells (macrophage activating cells) elaborate lymphokines which activate macrophages to enhance their phagocyte and bactericidal functions. Cytotoxic T cells are activated by antigen and receive help from helper T cells. Helper cells also cooperate with B cells in the production of antibody which may arm cells (eg. K cells) carrying Fc receptors. NK cells act non-specifically, particularly against cellular targets.

RECOGNITION OF ANTIGEN BY T CELLS

The specificity of T cell clones has dispelled any lingering doubts about the existence of antigen specificity at the level of individual T cells. However, the specificity differs from that of antibodies, which may discriminate between antigens not distinguished by T cells, and vice versa.

Helper and cytotoxic T cells do not bind free antigen: they appear to recognize antigen only in association with MHC products, expressed on cell membranes. This need for simultaneous recognition of antigen and self MHC products has led to two major hypotheses:

1. the *dual receptor hypothesis* suggests that the MHC product and the antigen are recognized by separate receptor molecules on the lymphocyte surface. Some authors supplement this hypothesis with the suggestion that the separate antigen-recognition receptor is not expressed until MHC-recognition has occurred (the 'flasher' hypothesis). This could explain the failure of cells to bind free antigen,

2. the *associative recognition hypothesis* proposes that antigen, possibly modified by antigen-presenting cells, associates with the MHC products, and is recognized by a single T cell receptor. This hypothesis has been modified to give the *altered self hypothesis* according to which the self-MHC on the antigen-presenting cell is somehow modified by the presence of antigen. It is proposed that a single T cell receptor recognizes both antigen and altered self.

These hypotheses are illustrated in figure 11.2. There are clearly other theoretical possibilities which combine aspects of both major hypotheses. For convenience, the MHC and antigen-recognition functions are considered separately below. Suppressor T cells can bind free antigen and there are numerous reports that they secrete antigen-binding factors (described in 'Regulation of the Immune Response').

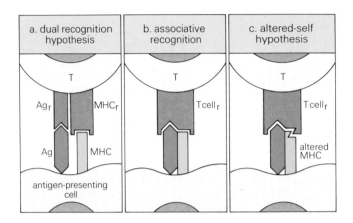

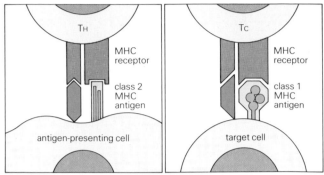

Fig.11.3 Antigen recognition by T cells II. T-helper cells and T-cytotoxic cells recognize antigen in association with different types of MHC molecules expressed on different kinds of cells. Tн cells recognize antigen in association with class 2 molecules while Tc cells use class 1 MHC molecules. It is probable that the T cells' receptors have different molecular structures: here they are shown to be different.

Fig.11.2 Antigen recognition by T cells I. T cells recognize antigen in association with self-MHC molecules. This could occur in one of three ways: either a) the T cell separately recognizes antigen with one receptor (Ag_r) and self-MHC with another, (MHC) or b) a single T cell receptor (T cell $_r$) recognizes antigen associated with self-MHC. A modification of this hypothesis c) states that the antigen alters the self-MHC in some way and the T cell thus recognizes altered self. This idea is based on the observation that T cells recognize and react to non-self MHC on foreign cells very efficiently.

MHC RESTRICTION

Although most T cells recognize antigen in relation to MHC products on cell surfaces, not all T cells use the same MHC products: each T cell is 'restricted' to either class 1 or class 2 glycopeptides. For instance, cytotoxic T cells usually recognize antigen in association with class 1 MHC products, which are expressed on all nucleated cells, while helper T cells and most of the T cells which proliferate in response to antigen *in vitro,* recognize antigen in association with class 2 products, which are expressed mostly on antigen-presenting cells, and some lymphocytes (Fig.11.3).

There are several ways of demonstrating this MHC restriction experimentally. Thus cytotoxic T cells which kill virus-infected autologous cells, will not kill cells infected with the same virus, if the infected cells do not also express the same class 1 glycopeptides, even if the class 2 products are identical. Moreover, antibody to class 1, but not to class 2 glycopeptides can block killing of infected autologous cells. The reverse results can be obtained in proliferative, or helper T cell assays. The relationship between function and the class of MHC glycopeptide to which T cells of that function are usually restricted 'makes sense' from an evolutionary point of view. Thus cytotoxic T cells may be required to kill virus-infected cells in any tissue, so they must 'see' antigen in relation to something

expressed in all tissues. On the other hand, proliferation, or help for antibody production, are regulatory 'decisions' within the lymphoid system, and are restricted by MHC products which are unique to that system and to specialized antigen-presenting cells (discussed later). However, some exceptions to this relationship between function and MHC restriction are mentioned below.

T cell function	T cell clone phenotype	antibody		
		anti-T3	anti-T4	anti-T8
cytotoxity	T4	↓	↓	–
	T8	↓	–	↓
antigen proliferation	T4	↓	–	–
	T8	↓	–	–
IL-2 induced proliferation	T4	↑	–	–
	T8	↑	–	–

Fig.11.4 T cell surface antigen. The effect of antibody to three cell surface antigens of T cells (T3, T4 and T8) on different T cell functions was noted. Two cloned cell lines were used: one expressed the T4 antigen (and recognized antigen in association with MHC class 2 molecules), and the other expressed the T8 antigen (and recognized antigen in association with MHC class 1 molecules). The effect of the antisera is expressed as increase (↑), decrease (↓) or no change (–) in reactivity by comparison with controls without antibody. Anti-T4 and anti-T8 reduced the cytotoxicity of T cells carrying the appropriate cell surface antigen but did not affect antigen- or IL-2 induced T cell proliferation. Anti-T3 recognizes a 20 KD protein present on all mature T cells and blocks functions which require antigen stimulation of cells (cytotoxicity and antigen proliferation) but increases the susceptibility to IL-2 induced proliferation, possibly by causing the cells to express more IL-2 receptors. The data suggest that T3 is associated with the T cells antigen receptor and that T4 and T8 are associated with their MHC restriction.

T CELL RECEPTORS FOR MHC GLYCOPEPTIDES

Human T cells can be divided in two major subpopulations on the basis of their cell membrane glycoproteins, which can now be defined with monoclonal antibodies. The T4$^+$ subset express a 62 KD (kilodalton) glycoprotein (T4), while the T8$^+$ subset express a 76 KD glycoprotein (T8). There is a very strong correlation between:
1. expression of T4 and class 2 restriction
2. expression of T8 and class 1 restriction
This has led to the suggestion that T4 and T8 are the receptors for class 2 and class 1 MHC glycopeptides respectively. This hypothesis is supported by the observation that monoclonal antibodies against T4 will block killing of appropriate target cells by class 2-restricted cytotoxic T cells, while anti-T8 will block killing by class 1-restricted cells. Evidence is presented in figure 11.4 that T4 and T8 are the receptors for MHC glycopeptides of class 2 and class 1 respectively and that a third glycoprotein, T3, forms part of the antigen receptor, as discussed in the next section.

T CELL RECEPTORS FOR ANTIGEN

It is logical to assume that whatever the nature of the molecule which gives T cells their antigen specificity, it must contain a constant, or 'framework' segment, and a variable region (cf. antibody structure) (Fig. 11.5).

Monoclonal antibodies specific for the T3 glycoprotein on T cell membranes recognize all mature T lymphocytes. Other properties of this antibody include:
1. blockage of induction and effector phases of T cell responses,
2. blockage of T cell proliferative responses to soluble antigen,
3. blockage of cytotoxicity of both class 1 and class 2 restricted cells,
4. enhancement of responsiveness to IL-2,
5. mitogenicity for resting T cells.
These findings are compatible with the possibility that anti–T3 binds to a constant part of the T cell receptor for antigen. The simplest hypothesis to explain the receptor's antigen specificity would involve immunoglobulin V_H genes. Does the T cell antigen receptor contain immunoglobulin? There have been numerous attempts to demonstrate immunoglobulin-related molecules on the T cell membrane, using fluorescein or ^{125}I labelled antibodies to various parts of immunoglobulin chains, or immunoprecipitation of extracts of T cell membrane surface labelled with ^{125}I. Such studies are open to several types of error. False positive results can be due to:
1. contamination of T cell preparations with immunoglobulin from other sources,
2. the existence on T cell membranes of other molecules with segments homologous to immunoglobulin (eg. Thy-1, β_2–microglobulin, MHC glycopeptides).
A further complication is the fact that most T cells do not bind free antigen and may not therefore express their antigen-specific receptor under resting conditions, or without interaction with self-MHC products.

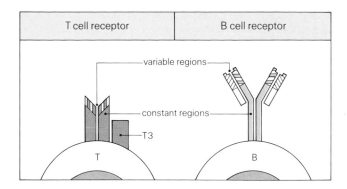

Fig. 11.5 The nature of the T cell's receptor for antigen– surface protein analysis. By analogy with B cells, which have immunoglobulin as their antigen receptor, it has been shown that the T cell's receptor has a constant and a variable (antigen binding) portion. Earlier hypotheses proposed that the T cell could use some immunoglobulin genes in its structure, however, attempts to identify immunoglobulin on T cells have failed. Immunoglobulin may have been incorrectly identified as a T cell synthesized surface protein when in fact it is cytophilic antibody bound to T cells' Fc receptors or cross-reacting with homologous molecules such as MHC glycoproteins or β_2–microglobulin. Recent data indicates that the T cell's antigen receptor has two chains which carry the idiotype (presumably the antigen binding site) and which are associated with the T3 molecule.

It has now been shown that the T cell's antigen receptor has structural homologies with immunoglobulin domains. It also has a V region and a C region, but it is encoded by genes which are wholly separate from the immunoglobulin genes.

A hypothesis to explain the MHC restriction of T cells and what is known about the receptor for antigen is set out in figure 11.6.

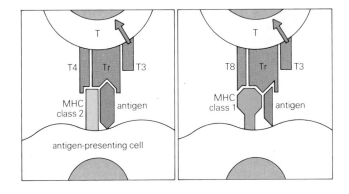

Fig. 11.6 Hypothesis to explain the T cell recognition of antigen. It has been proposed that the MHC class 2 restricted cells (eg. T_H) possess a molecule, T4, which recognizes MHC class 2 antigens. The T cell receptor, Tr recognizes the MHC protein and the antigen. The activation signal is transmitted to the T cell via the T3 peptide, which is associated with the T cell receptor. Class 1 restricted cells have a molecule, T8, which recognizes MHC class 1 antigens. The cell receptor, Tr recognizes MHC and antigen. Both classes of MHC molecule have four globular domains and it is proposed that the T4 and T8 molecules recognize different domains to those recognized by the T cell receptor.

Gene Arrangement and Structure of the T Cell Receptor

The T cell receptor consists of two disulphide-linked polypeptides, termed α and β, each of molecular weight 40-50 KD. Gene clones are available for the mouse β chain gene segments. The gene arrangement is very similar to that of immunoglobulin, and so the same style of nomenclature is used. The region contains a number of V_T sequences and D_T segments. This is followed by tandem sets of J_T genes (six functional and one pseudogene) and a C_T gene. The tandem arrangement of these J_T and C_T genes resembles the tandem alleles of the λ light chains. The C_T gene is made up of four exons, one of which resembles an Ig constant domain gene, the next encodes a short hinge-like section, while the third and fourth exons encode the transmembrane and intracytoplasmic portions. The V, J and D segments have flanking sequences similar to the analogous immunoglobulin segments, permitting recombination to occur similarly (see Fig.9.13). Early data suggest that the α chain is structurally similar to the β chain.

Immunoglobulin Idiotypes

There is still controversy about the presence on T cells of immunoglobulin idiotypes. The evidence for their presence is particularly difficult to interpret. For instance, Thy-1, a surface protein found on all T cells, is homologous to antibody variable (V) domains, and anti-idiotypes can show other bizarre 'cross-reactivities'. Consider for instance, an anti-idiotype which mimics the antigen for which the idiotype-bearing immunoglobulin is specific. The anti-idiotype could theoretically be bound to a T cell receptor for the same antigen, even if that T cell receptor were of a totally different molecular type from immunoglobulin. In this context, it must be emphasized that anti-idiotype recognizes a particular receptor shape, which may occur on different types of molecule.

ANTIGEN-PRESENTING CELLS

B cells and some T cells, in particular T-helper cells, cannot recognize free antigen; for recognition to occur it must be presented together with MHC class 2 products. This function is performed by cells termed antigen-presenting cells.

Some of the monocyte/macrophage series express class 2 glycopeptides (Ia antigens) and can act as antigen presenting cells for T cells or B cells. Other cell types, for instance vascular endothelial cells, may also act as antigen-presenting cells, and it has been recently shown that certain stimuli in vitro will cause class 2 glycopeptide expression on cells such as thyroid follicular cells which do not normally do so. However it is not clear whether this automatically correlates with the antigen-presenting function.

Dendritic cells found in blood, lymph and other tissues are non-phagocytic Fc-receptor negative cells which strongly express class 2 glycopeptides. Their relationship to the monocyte/macrophage series is doubtful. They are very efficient presenters of antigen to T cells in several in vitro and in vivo systems. They may be related to the strongly Ia positive Langerhans cells found in the epidermis. It should be remembered that other cell types, possibly variants of the macrophage lineage, may be involved in antigen presentation to B cells. These cell types probably do not express class 2 glycopeptides and therefore presumably do not present antigen to T cells. For example, some T-independent antigens localize in the marginal zone macrophages, which may be involved in the induction of T-independent antibody responses. Ia (class 2) negative follicular dendritic cells (not to be confused with the Ia positive dendritic cells discussed above) express receptors for Fc and complement C3 and appear to pick up immune complexes via these receptors and present for B cell memory (T-dependently). The important characteristics of these different antigen-presenting cells are tabulated in figure 11.7.

antigen-presenting cell		characteristics			
		phago-cytosis	Fc/C3 receptors	class 2 MHC expression	present to:
marginal zone macrophages	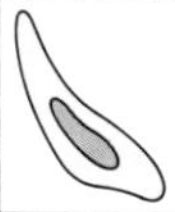	+	+	−	B
follicular dendritic cells	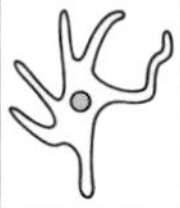	−	+	−	B
dendritic cells	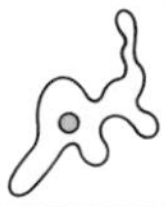	−	−	+	T
monocytes/macrophages	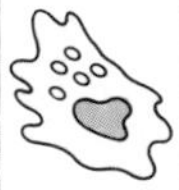	+	+	+/−	T + B
Langerhans cell	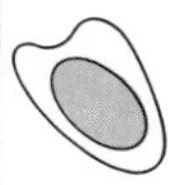	−	+	+	T

Fig.11.7 Chief characteristics of different antigen presenting cells. Those cells which present antigen to T cells have class 2 MHC molecules. B cells do not need to recognize antigen in association with MHC but can be stimulated by free antigen or complexed antigen which has bound to APCs with Fc and C3 receptors.

ACTIVATION OF T CELLS BY ANTIGEN PRESENTING CELLS

The initiation of T cell proliferation involves not only recognition of antigen and MHC determinants as already discussed but also signals passing between the APC and lymphocytes via interleukins. Figure 11.8 illustrates this diagrammatically as a three step process.

Macrophages are known to be able to release IL-1 but it is not known whether dendritic cells can also do so. The generation of lines of T cells involves exploitation of the third step of this sequence where antigen-specific cells are driven into continuous division by the appropriate antigen and IL-2.

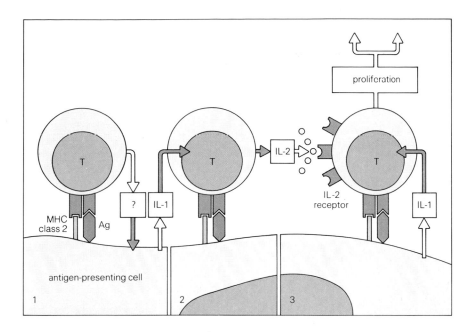

Fig.11.8 Activation of T cells by antigen-presenting cells. The activation of T cells is thought to occur in three phases. Following binding of the T cell to the antigen-presenting cell an unknown factor (?) from the T cell induces the APC to produce IL-1(1). This, in association with antigen stimulation induces IL-2 receptors on the T cells (3, possibly a separate subset from that which induced IL-1 production) and stimulates T cells to release IL-2 (2) which drives antigen activated cells into proliferation (3).

CELL-MEDIATED CYTOTOXICITY

Certain subpopulations of lymphoid, and under some circumstances, myeloid cells can lyse target cells to which they are sufficiently closely bound. This binding can be due to:
1. MHC-restricted T cell receptors (cytotoxic T cells),
2. determinants recognized by NK cells,
3. antibody/Fc receptors (K cells, antibody-dependent cell-mediated cytotoxicity),
4. lectins (experimental models)

These possibilities are illustrated in figure 11.9. There are other cell-mediated cytotoxic mechanisms which involve the secretion of cytotoxic molecules, or activation of macrophages, and these will be considered in later sections.

The first three types of (physiological) cell-mediated cytotoxicity will now be described. It should be noted that they are *functional* categories and more than one type may be manifested by a particular morphological cell type.

MHC RESTRICTED CYTOTOXIC T CELLS

Cytotoxic T cells bind to target cells bearing the correct MHC products and antigen. No antibody is required to achieve this binding. The T cells involved are often T8 positive (in humans) and MHC class 1 restricted. After binding there are changes in membrane permeability of the target cell followed by swelling and disruption. Following lysis of the target cell the T cells survive, and may go on to kill more targets. It is likely that the most important physiological role of these cytotoxic T cells is the elimination of virally-infected target cells.

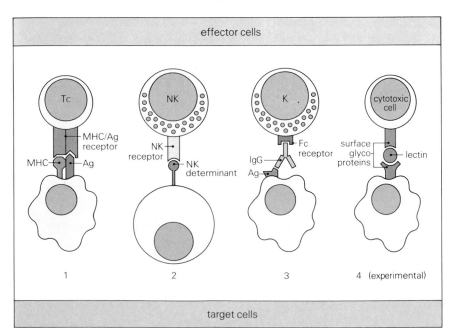

Fig.11.9 Cell-mediated cytotoxicity. Four different types of cell binding in cell-mediated cytotoxicity.
1. Cytotoxic T cells (Tc) bind their target while recognizing antigen and MHC determinants.
2. NK cells recognize determinants expressed on neoplastic cells.
3. K cells recognize the Fc of IgG antibody bound to antigen on the target cell surface.
4. Experimentally, glycoproteins on the surface of effector and target can be crosslinked by lectins.

NATURAL KILLER CELLS

Natural killer (NK) cells are so called because they are found in normal animals, which appear not to have been exposed to relevant antigens. They can kill a variety of transformed, virus-infected, or embryo-derived cells *in vitro* in the absence of antibody.

The Identity of NK Cells
It is important to distinguish between the *functional* property of natural killing and the *morphological* cell type responsible for this function, which is currently undetermined. NK activity is usually enriched in preparations of Large Granular Lymphocytes (LGL) (Fig.11.10). They express some markers shared by T lymphocytes (OKT3, OKT4, OKT8, in man, and Thy 1 in mice) but may also express determinants more often associated with other cell types, such as OKM1, (a monocyte/granulocyte marker). They also express Fc receptors but they are found with a different tissue distribution to macrophages (see 'Immunity to Tumours') (Fig.11.11).

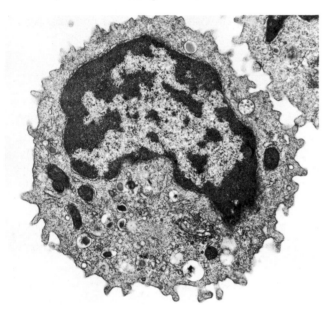

Fig. 11.10   A large granular lymphocyte. Large granular lymphocytes isolated by density gradient centrifugation contain the majority of serum NK effector activity.

NK cells are heterogeneous, and different clones may vary both in their sensitivity to regulatory effects of interferon and interleukins and possibly also in the range of targets they will lyse.

Thus it is not yet clear whether NK cells are:
1. a single distinct cell lineage, with or without a clonally distributed diversity of receptors,
2. several distinct lineages,
3. a function which can be expressed by an assortment of cell types.

Relationship of NK Cells to K Cells and Cytotoxic T Cells
Some large granular lymphocytes will bind to NK-susceptible targets via their NK receptor and to antibody

	NK cells	macrophages
thymus	−	−
spleen	+++	+++
bone marrow	±	+++
peritoneal exudate	+++	+++
lymph node	±	++
thoracic lymph duct	−	−
blood	+++	+++

Fig.11.11   Distribution of NK cells and cytolytic macrophages in lymphoid tissues. The distribution reveals that the two cell types are distinct, despite their common possession of Fc receptors.

coated NK-resistant cells via their Fc receptors. Observation of single cells has shown that both targets can be lysed. Thus K and NK activity can be properties of the same cells. There are also reports that some MHC-restricted cytotoxic T cell lines may express NK activity.

Mechanism of NK Cell-Mediated Lysis
It has been suggested that there are three distinct phases:
1. binding to the target,
2. a Ca^{++} dependent phase, involving vesicular secretion, which modifies the target cell so that it is 'programmed' for lysis,
3. a late phase which is independent of the NK cells, during which the 'programmed' cell undergoes lysis.

A soluble cytotoxic factor, with a target range similar to NK cells themselves, has been demonstrated in NK cell supernatants. This raises the possibility that two receptors on the target cell are involved – one for the NK cell and one for the NK cytotoxic factor.

ANTIBODY-DEPENDENT CELL-MEDIATED CYTOTOXICITY (ADCC)

Cells with cytotoxic potential, which also possess Fc receptors for IgG, may bind to and lyse target cells coated with antibody of the relevant class (Fig.11.12). The models most frequently studied involve antibodies to viral antigens expressed on the target cell membrane; to tumour, or MHC-associated determinants; to haptens such as TNP conjugated onto the membrane, or to the membranes of nucleated (Avian) erythrocytes.

The cells most active in ADCC in these models are poorly defined, and of uncertain lineage. They may resemble NK cells, as suggested previously, and both functions can be expressed by the same cells, that is, the 'classical' K cells. However monocytes, and according to some controversial reports, polymorphonuclear cells, may also be active against antibody-coated tumour targets. Myeloid cells (monocytes and eosinophils) are certainly important effectors of damage to antibody-coated schistosomulae (see 'Immunity to Protozoa and

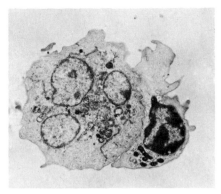

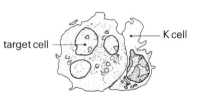

target cell — K cell

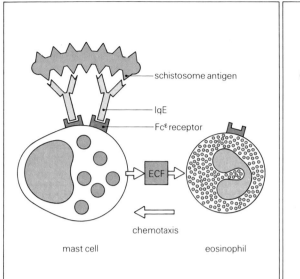

schistosome antigen

IgE

Fcε receptor

ECF

chemotaxis

mast cell

eosinophil

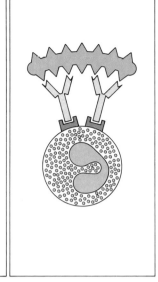

Fig. 11.12 Electron micrograph of a K cell engaging a target cell. × 2500. Courtesy of Mr. P. Penfold.

Fig.11.13 Dual role for antibody in the immune reaction to schistosomes. Mast cells sensitized with IgE anti-schistosome release eosinophil chemotactic factor (ECF)

following contact with antigen (left). The arriving eosinophils attach to the antibody-coated worm via their Fc receptors and are important effectors in damaging the parasites (right).

Worms'). In this system (which may apply also to other parasites), the important antibody classes appear to be the anaphylactic ones (IgE in all species, IgG in mice, and IgG2a in rats). This raises the intriguing possibility that IgE acts by first triggering release of Eosinophil Chemotactic Factors from mast cells, and then binding the arriving eosinophils onto the target (Fig.11.13).

The mechanism of killing by these meloid ADCC effectors may differ from that of the NK/K cell group.

THE CENTRAL ROLE OF MACROPHAGES

Macrophages play a central role in cell-mediated immunity, because they are involved both in the initiation of responses as antigen-presenting cells, and in the effector phase as inflammatory, tumoricidal and microbicidal cells, in addition to their regulatory functions (Fig.11.14).

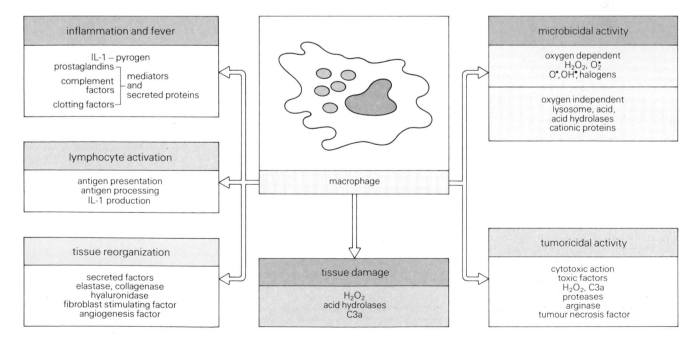

inflammation and fever

IL-1 – pyrogen
prostaglandins ⎤
complement factors ⎥ mediators and secreted proteins
clotting factors ⎦

lymphocyte activation

antigen presentation
antigen processing
IL-1 production

tissue reorganization

secreted factors
elastase, collagenase
hyaluronidase
fibroblast stimulating factor
angiogenesis factor

macrophage

tissue damage

H_2O_2
acid hydrolases
C3a

microbicidal activity

oxygen dependent
H_2O_2, $O_2^{\bullet}$
$O^{\bullet}$, $OH^{\bullet}$, halogens

oxygen independent
lysosome, acid,
acid hydrolases
cationic proteins

tumoricidal activity

cytotoxic action
toxic factors
H_2O_2, C3a
proteases
arginase
tumour necrosis factor

Fig.11.14 The central role of macrophages. Macrophages and their products listed here are important in both the induction phases of inflammation and tissue reorganization

and repair (left) as well as performing their effector functions (right). The effector functions may also cause tissue damage as in delayed hypersensitivity reactions.

Macrophage Activation by T Lymphocyte-Derived Mediators

Many of the macrophage functions are enhanced by a process known as 'activation'. The destruction of intracellular parasites and, *in vitro*, of some tumour cells at least requires activation of macrophages by signals derived from lymphocytes (Fig. 11.15). The classical experiment demonstrating this involved BCG (attenuated *Mycobacterium tuberculosis* used in vaccines against tuberculosis) and *Listeria monocytogenes* (Fig. 11.16). From these experiments it was concluded that the activation of macrophages involved antigen-specific triggering by a mechanism, which subsequently led to an enhanced microbicidal activity which was not specific for that antigen. Antigen-specificity was known to be a property of lymphocytes, and Listericidal activity, a property of macrophages. The next step was to demonstrate *in vitro* that immune lymphocytes (eg. derived from a BCG-immunized mouse) when cultured with appropriate antigen (PPD) would release mediators which non-specifically enhanced the ability of macrophages to kill the above microorganisms, and often also unrelated organisms. However, as will be made clear below, macrophage activation is a complex phenomenon and enhanced ability to kill one microorganism is *not* always accompanied by the ability to kill all others.

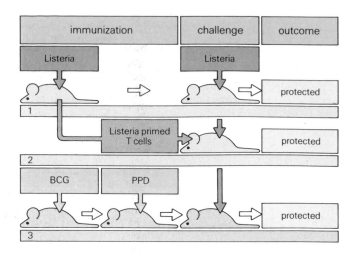

Fig.11.16 Macrophage activation II. Animals immunized with Listeria parasites are protected against a subsequent challenge with viable bacteria (1). This effect is due to antigen-specific T cells since the immunity can be transferred with T cells from immunized animals (2). However, protection can also be induced by immunization with BCG followed by PPD (antigen of BCG) a few hours before challenge with Listeria. This implies that specific antigen triggering (T cells) can produce activation of antigen non-specific immune mechanisms (macrophages).

Figure 11.17 shows macrophages infected with *Leishmania enriettii,* and incubated with or without mediators derived from lymphocytes illustrating the difference between activated and non-activated cells.

LYMPHOKINES

The experiments described above have led to the acceptance of the model whereby mediators released from antigen-activated T cells can then activate macrophages: these mediators are termed lymphokines.

This raises a number of questions:

1. which lymphocytes can release lymphokines?
2. how many lymphokines are there?
3. does the effect of a lymphokine depend on the stage of maturation of the macrophage on which it acts?
4. can different functions of activated macrophages be dissociated from each other?
5. what is the relationship of this activation to immunopathological cell-mediated immunity (described in 'Hypersensitivity-Type IV')?

Some of the answers to these questions presented below suggest that this macrophage-activation pathway should not be regarded as a single pathway, but as a family of related ones.

The Nature of Lymphokines and the Cells of Origin

Lymphocyte-derived mediators which modify macrophage function (lymphokines) are released by both B cells and T cells. However, cell transfer experiments show that it is T cells which are important for classical cell-mediated responses, described above, and lymphokines from B cells have received little attention.

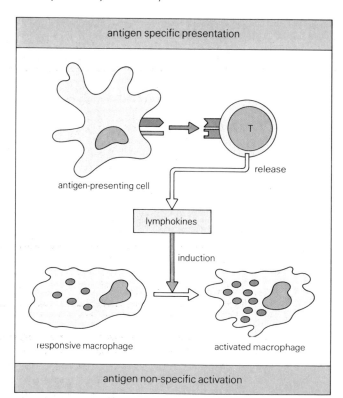

Fig.11.15 Macrophage activation I. When antigen is presented to T cells they are stimulated to release factors termed lymphokines. Lymphokines released by antigen-activated T lymphocytes act (primarily) on macrophages, causing them in turn to become activated. Note that T cell activation is antigen specific whereas subsequent macrophage activation is not antigen specific. Thus, lymphokines released in response to one microorganism's antigens may bring about the destruction of a different microorganism residing in the activated macrophage.

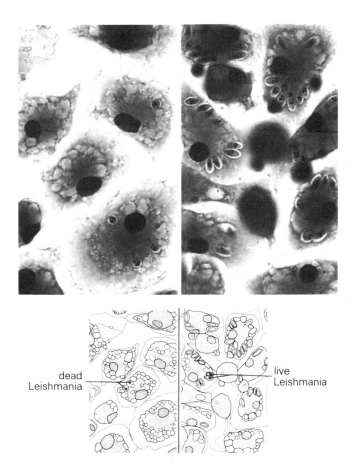

Fig. 11.17 Killing of Leishmania by activated macrophages.
The destruction of *Leishmania enrietti* by C57 strain mouse
macrophages is enhanced by lymphokines. Parasites within the
macrophages are destroyed during 48 hours culture with
lymphokine (macrophage activating factor) (left) by comparison
with control cultures containing no lymphokine (right). Giemsa
stain, ×800. Courtesy of Dr. J. Mauel.

Numerous activities have been attributed to lymphokines but few of these can yet be attributed to single
molecules. Some of the better characterized activities are
listed in figure 11.18.

Many of the studies which have been undertaken on
lymphokines have identified the factors by their activity
in different biological assays, without isolating the molecules responsible; in many cases the cell supernatants
used as a source of mediators contain a large number of
different lymphokines. For these reasons it is not always
known whether an activity is due to one molecule or
several, or whether there is overlap between the lymphokines. For example, it has recently been demonstrated
that one macrophage activating factor (MAF) is lymphocyte produced interferon (IFNγ).

Since there are clearly many lymphokines, each with
a distinct function, it is important to know whether they
are all released together, acting functionally as one en-
tity, or whether different lymphokines are released under
different circumstances, or by different T cell subpopulations. In an attempt to answer these questions cloned
T cells (that is, the progeny of a single T cell, or T cell hy-
bridomas formed by fusing a normal T cell with an
immortal T cell) are being studied. Both of these
approaches are unphysiological however, and it is possible that they selectively and artificially induce or suppress secretion of some mediators. Thus the interpretation of the data is difficult and controversial. Some
authors deny that there is any correlation between cell
phenotype, MHC restriction, function (eg. cytotoxic, or
non-cytotoxic) and the type of lymphokine secreted,
which may vary from all, to none of those which can be
assayed. Others suggest that cytotoxic (class 1 MHC-
restricted) cells tend to release macrophage activating
factor and interferon, while class 2 restricted T cells tend
to release colony stimulating factor and interleukin 2.
Thus it is not yet clear whether different T cells release
different 'blends' of lymphokines.

1. regulation of other lymphocytes (non-antigen specific factors)		4. modulation of the function of phagocytes	
interleukin-2	(IL-2)	migration inhibition factor	(MIF)
interleukin-3	(IL-3)	macrophage activation factor	(MAF)
interferons α + γ	(IFN)	leucocyte migration inhibition factor	(LIF)
soluble immune response suppressor	(SIRS)	chemotactic factor	(CF)
inhibitor of DNA synthesis	(IDS)	interferons (α + γ)	(IFN)
allogeneic effector factor	(AEF)	colony stimulating factor	(CSF)
T cell replacing factor	(TRF)	macrophage fusion factor	(MFF)
2. regulation of other lymphocytes (antigen specific factors)		**5. regulation of other tissues**	
assorted antigen specific helper factors	(ThF)	colony stimulating factor	(CSF)
assorted antigen specific suppressor factors	(TsF)	osteoclast activating factor	(OAF)
3. induction of inflammation and mononuclear cell infiltration		**6. destruction of non-leucocyte target cells**	
skin reactive factor	(SRF)	lymphotoxins (heterogenous)	(LT)

**Fig. 11.18 A complete list of lymphokines and their
activities.** There may be overlap between these
lymphokines, for example, MAF activity is partly due to IFNγ.
There may also be heterogeneity within a category, for
example, TRF is a mixture of lymphokines causing B cell
proliferation and maturation to the antibody forming, plasma
cells. (Note that only colony stimulating factor, IFNγ and IL–2
are available in a pure form.)

The Complexity of Macrophage Activation

Macrophage activation is a complex phenomenon and the various effector functions can be dissociated from one another. Thus it is possible to activate murine macrophages so that they have an increased ability to kill *Listeria monocytogenes* without increased ability to kill tumour cells, or mycobacteria.

There are two reasons for this complexity. First, the monocyte/macrophage series is very heterogeneous and cells taken from different sites differ in such relevant characteristics as expression of class 2 MHC glycopeptides, Fc receptors, lymphokine responsiveness and production of peroxidase. Most authors nevertheless believe that there is only one lineage of macrophages and that these differences are due to environmental and maturational effects.

Secondly, as hinted in the previous section, the functions activated may depend not only on the pre-existing functional and maturational stage of the macrophage, but also on the precise 'blend' of lymphokines and inflammatory stimuli to which it is exposed. Figure 11.19 shows some of the changes which can be induced by inflammation alone as well as by lymphokine treatment *in vitro*.

It is suggested that activation occurs in stages, and requires sequential stimuli, which include lymphokines, endotoxin, various mediators and regulators of inflammation (*in vitro*, plastic or glass surfaces and tissue culture media are important). Different effector functions may be expressed at each stage.

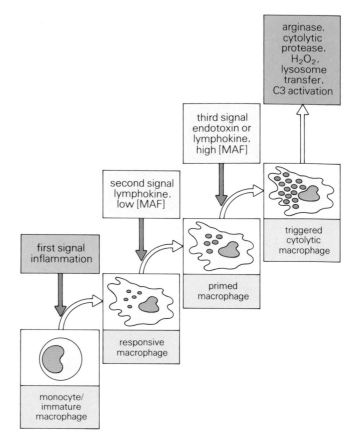

Fig.11.20 A hypothetical scheme for the activation of murine peritoneal macrophages to destroy tumour cells. It is thought that macrophage activation occurs in a series of steps. Note how the scheme is somewhat analogous to the three step activation of T cells illustrated in figure 11.8.

characteristic		inflammatory	lymphokine-treated *in vitro*
cell volume		↑	↑
spreading		↑	↑
pinocytosis		↑	?
phagocytosis	via Fc receptor	↑	?
	via C3 receptor	↑	?
secretion of O₂-reduction products (O₂• and H₂O₂)		↑	↑
secretion of neutral proteases	plasminogen activation	↑	↑
	collagenase	↑	↑
hydrolase content of lysosomes		↑	↓?
plasma membrane 5'- nucleotidase		↓	↓

Fig.11.19 Changes occurring in inflammatory, or lymphokine-activated macrophages. Some of the changes may be due to recruitment of monocytes. It is difficult to study purely lymphokine mediated effects without any contribution from inflammatory or environmental ones, such as culture plates, or synthetic media. These findings are based on mouse peritoneal macrophages. The common decrease in plasma membrane 5'–nucleotidase is shown to indicate that the activation has some specificity and that not everything increases.

There is also evidence that activated macrophages can be de-activated. It has been suggested that prostaglandin E may have this effect.

Figure 11.20 shows a scheme for the activation of the tumoricidal function of murine peritoneal macrophages. Binding to the tumour cells occurs via a receptor for an unknown feature of tumour membranes, or via Fc-receptors and antibody. There may be distinct slow, and rapid mechanisms for tumour cell damage.

When foreign antigenic material cannot be degraded, T cells accumulate and release lymphokines. This leads to the aggregation and proliferation of macrophages and the characteristic appearance of a nodular mass called a granuloma which consists of multinucleate giant cells epithelioid cells and activated macrophages. The granuloma isolates the focus of the infection (Fig.11.21). A granuloma can be produced experimentally using soluble antigen conjugated covalently onto an insoluble particle, such as a sepharose bead. Antigen-coated beads will evoke T cell-dependent granulomata in appropriately immunized mice, whereas control beads will not (Fig.11.22). If such granulomata are explanted *in vitro* they can be shown to release mediators, presumably lymphokines, with macrophage-activating and chemotactic properties. Thus the T cell plays a dual role in granuloma formation by causing both accumulation and activation of phagocytes.

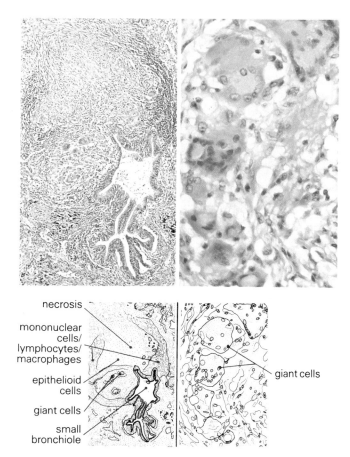

Fig.11.21 **A granulomatous reaction in pulmonary tuberculosis.** The central area of caseous necrosis is surrounded by a ring of epithelioid cells and mononuclear cells. Multinucleate giant cells are also present (left, ×170). Giant cells are illustrated at a higher magnification (right, ×270). Haematoxylin and Eosin stain. Courtesy of Dr. G. Boyd.

necrosis

mononuclear cells/ lymphocytes/ macrophages

epithelioid cells

giant cells

small bronchiole

giant cells

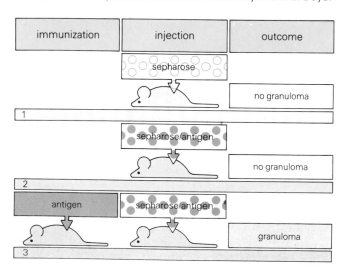

Fig.11.22 **Artificial production of a granuloma.** Mice injected with either normal sepharose beads (1) or sepharose beads coupled to antigen (2) do not develop any local granulomatous reaction, but if the animal is previously immunized to the antigen (3) they do. If the granulomatous tissue and beads are recovered from animal 3 they release into culture factors with macrophage chemotactic and activating properties.

Such granulomata are characteristic of infections with organisms which live at least partly intracellularly (eg. *Mycobacterium tuberculosis, M. leprae,* Leishmaniasis, *Listeria monocytogenes*) or which are large and persistent, (Schistosome ova). They are both a site of localization and destruction of organisms by activated macrophages, and a component of the immunopathology of the diseases. Analysis of the phenotype of the T cells in granulomatous foci indicate that T4$^+$ cells are located at the centre of the reaction and T8$^+$ cells around the periphery suggesting that T4$^+$ cells are of prime importance in antigen recognition and accumulation of other lymphocytes and macrophages (Fig.11.23). In mice the activity of T cell dependent granulomata eventually wanes, under the influence of suppressor T cells.

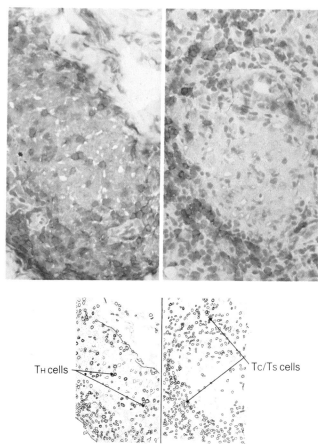

TH cells

Tc/Ts cells

Fig.11.23 **OKT4 and OKT8 staining of a granuloma.** Shown here is a dermal granuloma from a patient with borderline tuberculoid leprosy stained (red) with peroxidase-coupled antibodies to Leu 3 (equivalent to T4) (left) and Leu 2 (equivalent to T8) (right). Leu 3 T-helper cells are present in and around the lesion while Leu 2 cytotoxic/suppressor T cells occur mainly on the periphery. Courtesy of Drs. R. L. Modlin and T. H. Rea.

FURTHER READING

Adams D. (1982) Molecules, membranes, and macrophage activation. *Immunology Today* **3,** 285.

Bloom B.R. (1982) Natural killers to rescue immune surveillance? *Nature* **300,** 214.

Carrick L. & Boros D.L. (1980) The artificial granuloma 1. *In vitro* lymphokine production by pulmonary artificial hypersensitivity granulomas. *Clin. Immunol. & Immunopathol.* **17,** 415.

Eckels D.D., Lamb J.R., Lake P., Woody J.N., Johnson A.H. & Hartzman, R. (1982) Antigen-specific human T lymphocyte clones. Genetic restriction of influenza virus-specific responses to HLA-D region genes. *Human Immunology* **4,** 313.

Kaufmann S.H.E. & Hahn H. (1982) Biological function of T cell lines with specificity for the intracellular bacterium, *Listeria monocytogenes in vitro* and *in vivo. J. Exp. Med.* **155,** 1754.

Kohl S. & Loo L.S. (1982) Protection of neonatal mice against *Herpes simplex* virus infection: probable *in vivo* antibody-dependent cellular cytotoxicity. *J. Immunol.* **129,** 370.

Lachman L.B. & Maizel A.L. (1983) Human immunoregulatory molecules: Interleukin 1, interleukin 2, and B cell growth factor. *Contemp. Top. Mol. Immunol.* **9,** 147.

McMichael A.J., Gotch F. & Noble G.R. (1983) Cytotoxic T cell Immunity to Influenza. *New Engl. J. Med.* **309,** 13.

Nathan C.F., Murray H.W., Wiebe M.E. & Rubin B.Y. (1983) Identification of interferon-γ as the lymphokine that activates human macrophage oxidative metabolism and antimicrobial activity. *J. Exp. Med.* **158,** 670.

Oppenheim J.J. & Gery I. (1982) Interleukin 1 is more than an interleukin. *Immunology Today* **3,** 113.

Robertson M. (1984) Receptor gene rearrangements and ontogeny of T lymphocytes. *Nature* **311,** 305.

Robertson M. (1984) T cell antigen receptor. The capture of the snark. *Nature* **312,** 16.

Rosenstein M., Eberlein F.J. & Rosenberg S.A. (1984) Adoptive immunotherapy of established syngeneic solid tumours: role of T lymphoid subpopulations. *J. Immunol.* **132,** 2117.

Steinman R. M. & Nussenzweig M.C. (1980) Dendritic cells: features and functions. *Immunological Reviews* **53,** 127.

Unanue E.R. (1984) Antigen-presenting function of the macrophage. *Ann. Rev. Immunol.* **2,** 395.

Warner J.F. & Dennert G. (1982) Effects of a cloned cell line with NK activity on bone marrow transplants, tumour development, and metastasis *in vivo. Nature* **300,** 31.

Zinkernagel R.M. & Doherty P.C. (1979) MHC-restricted cytotoxic T cells. Studies on the biological role of polymorphic major transplantation antigens determining T cell restriction specificity, function and responsiveness. *Adv. Immunol.* **27,** 51.

12 Immunological Tolerance

Immunological tolerance is the acquisition of non-reactivity towards particular antigens (referred to in this context as tolerogens), and as such it is the converse of immunity. The importance of tolerance to self-antigens was appreciated very early in the development of immunology by Ehrlich and is fundamental to the normal functioning of the immune system. However, in the 1920's, it was discovered that tolerance could also be induced in animals to non-self antigens. For example, it was noted that sufficiently large doses of diphtheria toxoid would suppress the immune response, which would normally be elicited by smaller antigen doses.

A major breakthrough in understanding the mechanisms by which tolerance can be induced was made in 1945 when it was discovered that dizygotic cattle twins (developed from two fertilized ova and therefore, non-identical) became tolerant to each others tissue antigens, if they had exchanged embryonic blood following placental fusion (Fig. 12.1). These non-identical animals would normally be expected to reject tissue grafts from the other twin, but having exchanged embryonic blood it was found that the animals were stable chimaeras (composed of cells of two genetically different tissue types) with respect to their haemopoietic tissue and could mutually exchange skin grafts. This phenomenon was examined experimentally by Billingham, Brent and Medawar who injected spleen cells of adult mice into newborn mice of a different strain.

Upon maturation the recipient mice were tolerant to skin grafts of the donor strain but rejected grafts of unrelated strains (Figs. 12.2 & 12.3).

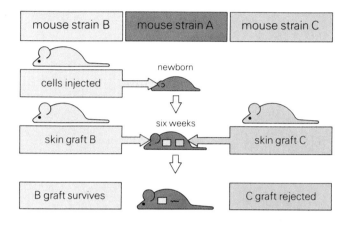

Fig. 12.2 Billingham, Brent and Medawar's neonatal grafting experiment. This demonstrates the induction of specific tolerance to grafted skin in mice by neonatal injection of spleen cells from a different strain. Mice of strain A normally reject grafts from strain B. However, if newborn mice of strain A receive cells from strain B mice and 6 weeks later are grafted with skin from mice of strains B and C, the mice show tolerance towards skin grafts from the donor strain B, but reject grafts from other strains (C).

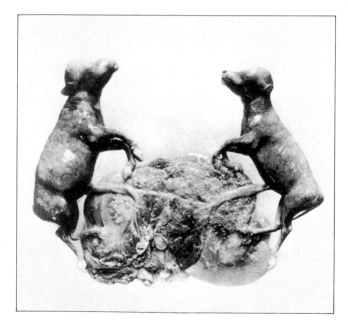

Fig. 12.1 Dizygotic cattle twins fused at the placentae. Fusion of the placentae leads to exchange of blood cells in foetal life. Following separation the animals permanently retain the cells of the other twin, and are permanently tolerant to grafts of that twin's tissue type.

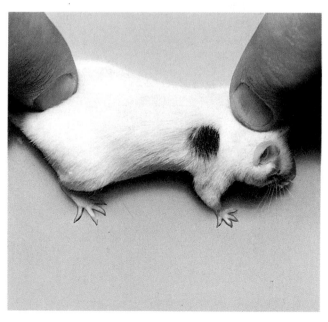

Fig. 12.3 A healthy brown hair graft growing on a tolerant white mouse 45 days after grafting.

The historical development of the concept of tolerance may be summarized under three headings:

1. high doses of antigen in adult life leading to specific unresponsiveness: antigens observed include –
    1924 protein (diphtheria toxoid)
    1927 polysaccharide (pneumococcal)
    1929 simple chemical (neoarsphenamine)

2. exposure of antigen in embryonic life leading to specific unresponsiveness
    1945 stable haemopoietic chimaerism in dyzygotic cattle twins (see Fig. 12.1)
    1949 natural or artificial exposure to antigen (non-self) in embryonic life creates tolerances (as for 'self')
    1951 skin grafts exchanged reciprocally in chimaeric cattle twins found to survive
    1953 chimaerism induced in neonatal mice which accepted skin grafts from each other in adult life
    1959 maturation of lymphocytes involves a stage where exposure to an antigen leads to an alteration in the lymphocyte's development, which involves the loss of its immune function – that is, the lymphocytes become tolerant to that antigen.

3. in the early 1960s it was appreciated that tolerance and immunity could be induced with all classes of antigens in neonatal and adult animals – whether it is immunity or tolerance which is produced depends upon the dose. Although a single mechanism accounting for the generation and maintenance of the tolerant state has not been discovered, many studies have defined important characteristics of the phenomenon. This chapter will summarize some of the experimental work which has been performed in this area.

PATHWAYS TO TOLERANCE

By 1960 it had become evident that there were several pathways to immunological tolerance, and recent data suggests that both B cells and T cells may become tolerized under particular circumstances and that they are affected independently and differently.

This section examines the different ways in which B cells and T cells may become tolerized in vivo or in vitro. Not only do B cells and T cells differ in the ways in which they can be tolerized, they also vary in their susceptibility to tolerance throughout their clonal ontogeny. Immature B cells are particularly susceptible to tolerization by contact with antigen, but following development into mature B cells and subsequently into antibody forming cells (AFCs) they become increasingly resistant to tolerization. T cells, by contrast do not vary in their susceptibility during ontogeny to such a marked extent. During foetal development of the immune system, and in the first weeks of neonatal life, none of the cells of the immune system have reached maturity, and for this reason the entire immune system of an animal is particularly susceptible to tolerance induction at this stage of development.

It is now recognized that fundamentally different mechanisms for establishing tolerance may lead to similar effects on the overall action of the immune system; indeed several mechanisms may operate simultaneously in a single animal.

PATHWAYS TO B CELL TOLERANCE

Four pathways leading to the tolerization of B cell function will be described here and these are summarized below in fig. 12.4.

Clonal Abortion
Immature B cells encountering antigen for the first time are particularly susceptible to tolerization in the presence of low concentrations of antigen. In these circumstances the normal maturation of the B cell is aborted, so that it is not able subsequently to respond normally to antigenic challenge.

Clonal Exhaustion
Repeated antigenic challenge with immunizing doses of a particular T-independent (T-ind) antigen may cause clonal exhaustion. In this form of tolerance, all the mature B cells capable of responding to the antigen are stimulated to differentiate into short-lived antibody producing cells (terminal stage for B cell differentiation). If all mature responding B cells undergo this exhaustive terminal differentiation, there will be no cells left capable of responding to a subsequent challenge with the antigen.

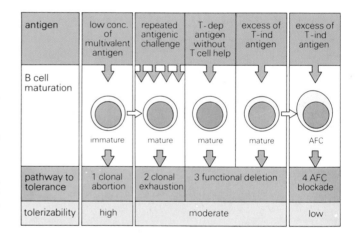

Fig. 12.4 Pathways to B cell tolerance. As an immature B cell matures into an antibody forming cell it becomes increasingly resistant to tolerization (tolerizability, the susceptibility to tolerization, decreases). At the same time, the form of antigen presentation which will produce tolerance also varies. The type of tolerance induced therefore, is dependent on the maturity of the cell, the antigen, and the manner in which the antigen is presented to the immune system.

1. Clonal Abortion. Low concentrations of multivalent antigen may cause the immature clone to abort. Tolerizability of immature B cells is high.

2. Clonal Exhaustion. Repeated antigenic challenge with a T-ind antigen may remove all mature functional B cell clones. Tolerizability of mature B cells is moderate.

3. Functional Deletion. Absence of T cell help, concurrent with the presence of T-dep antigen (or with T-suppressor cells) or an excess of T-ind antigen prevents mature B cells from functioning normally.

4. AFC blockade. Excess of T-ind antigen interferes with the secretion of antibody by the AFC. Tolerizability of AFCs is low.

Functional Deletion

1. By T-dependent (T-dep) antigens. These antigens require the help of specific T cells in order for the B cell to respond normally. Normal B cell responses to T-dep antigens require that the B cell binds to one determinant on an antigen and receives T specific help directed to another determinant. If the T help is not available the B cell may be unable to respond normally and is therefore, functionally deleted.

2. By T-independent (T-ind) antigens. These are high molecular weight polymers with repeating antigenic determinants capable of forming multiple bonds to the B cells, thus circumventing the requirement for T cell help. If, however, a T-ind antigen is presented to a B cell in excess or in a non-immunogenic form, the B cell will not give a normal response and will again therefore be functionally deleted.

Antibody Forming Cell (AFC) Blockade

Although it is very difficult to tolerize antibody forming cells, it is noted that very large doses of T-independent antigens can sometimes lead to an effective tolerization. In these circumstances it appears that the high concentrations of antigen are blockading the surface receptors of the cell and thereby interfering with antibody secretion.

PATHWAYS TO T CELL TOLERANCE

The pathways to T cell tolerance are superficially similar to those for B cell tolerance, for example, there is some evidence that immature T cells may be clonally aborted in a manner similar to that noted above. However, whereas all B cell clones have identical cellular functions, ultimately leading to antibody synthesis, there are several subsets of T cells performing very different functions. The T-helper (T_H) T-delayed hypersensitivity (T_D) and T-cytotoxic (T_C) subsets may all be deleted under different circumstances leading to tolerization with respect to only one of the T cell functions. For example, precursors of mouse T_C cells may be tolerized by exposure to mouse H-2 K and D antigens, whereas T_H cells are tolerized only by I region antigens. Evidently, T cell subsets may only be tolerized to those antigenic determinants which they normally recognize. One other T cell subset is particularly important in the development and maintenance of tolerance – the T-suppressor cell (T_S).

T-Suppressors

This T cell subset possesses the ability to suppress the function of B cells or other T cell subsets. Although it has been suggested that they act by bringing about deletion of either T or B cell clones, they probably directly suppress T and B cells. T-suppressors are antigen specific cells and can be generated experimentally under certain injection schedules. The action of T_S cells in these experimental systems can be demonstrated by transferring tolerance to a recipient by T cells. In this case the tolerance is temporary and is only maintained by the continued presence of T_S cells. Experimental systems of this type in which tolerance may be transferred display 'infectious tolerance'. The pathways to T cell tolerance are summarized in figure 12.5.

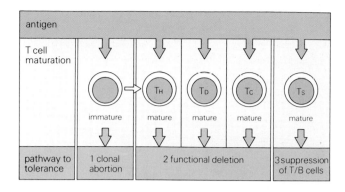

Fig. 12.5 Pathways to T cell tolerance. T cells do not show marked differences in their tolerizability at different stages of maturation. The antigen required to produce tolerance (not specified here) and the circumstances of its presentation, is particular to each individual T cell subset.

1. Clonal Abortion. Immature T cell clones may be aborted in a similar manner to B cells.

2. Functional Deletion. The subsets of mature T cells (T_H, T_D and T_C) may be individually deleted leading to the loss of only one of the functions of the T cell group.

3. T suppression. T-suppressors actively suppress the actions of other T cell subsets or B cells.

GENERAL CHARACTERISTICS OF T CELL AND B CELL TOLERIZATION

B and T cells differ in their susceptibility to *in vivo* tolerization with respect to the time course of tolerance induction, its duration and also the levels of antigen required to tolerize the cells (Fig. 12.6).

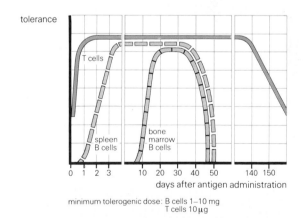

Fig. 12.6 Relative susceptibilities of T and B cells to tolerization *in vivo*. A mouse is administered antigen (human gammaglobulin – a T-dependent antigen) at a dose to produce tolerance (a tolerogenic dose), and the duration of tolerance measured. T cell tolerance is more rapidly induced and more persistent that B cell tolerance. This is true whether the B cells are derived from the spleen or bone marrow, although bone marrow B cells may take considerably longer than splenic B cells to tolerize. Typically, much lower antigen doses are sufficient for T cell tolerization: 10 µg as opposed to 1-10 mg ie. a thousand-fold difference.

Induction Time

T cells from the spleen and thymus are tolerized rapidly with T-dependent antigens within hours of challenge. Such antigens tolerize adult splenic B cells within 4 days, but tolerization of bone marrow B cells may require up to 15 days. On the other hand T-independent antigens tend to tolerize B cells more quickly. This may be related to the higher avidity of these multivalent antigens for the B cells, or to the preferential handling of these antigens by different B cell classes.

Antigen Dose

Although B cells vary in their susceptibility to tolerance induction as they mature, the levels of antigen required to tolerize B cells are usually 100 to 1000 fold larger than those needed to tolerize T cells. The B cell requirement for high doses of antigen is reduced when high avidity binding between the B cell and tolerogen occurs as in reactions involving high affinity B cell receptors or multivalent antigens. Although it was initially observed that tolerance was best induced with high doses of antigen (referred to as high zone tolerance) subsequent research showed that some weakly immunogenic antigens would also induce tolerance if administered in minute quantities, typically several orders of magnitude less than would produce high zone tolerance. It has been determined that this form of tolerance is maintained by the action of T-suppressor cells, which are triggered at much lower antigen doses than the T-helper cells. This form of tolerance (termed low zone tolerance) is partial however, and only affects some of the immunocytes.

Antigen Persistence

Generally speaking it seems that antigen must be continually present to maintain the state of tolerance, therefore tolerance to slowly catabolized antigens (such as a D-amino acid polymer) is altogether more persistent following a single injection (up to 1 year in mice) than tolerance to rapidly catabolized antigens. The particular ways in which antigens are handled *in vivo* is a major cause of discrepancy between *in vivo* and *in vitro* studies in this field.

Specificity

Experiments have shown that tolerance is developed for particular antigenic determinants, and not for particular antigens (Fig. 12.7). This can lead to tolerance to a variety of different antigens when T cells become tolerized to a single antigenic determinant which is shared by all the antigens. This tolerance can be maintained by just one of the mechanisms described above.

Duration

Since the persistence of antigen plays a major role in maintaining tolerance, the duration of tolerance is best studied by transferring cells from tolerant animals into recipients whose immune system has been rendered non-functional by X-irradiation. It is then found that T cell tolerance is more persistent than B cell tolerance.

When tolerance is due to clonal deletion, recovery is related to the time required to regenerate mature lymphocytes from the stem cell population. If on the other hand tolerance is due to blockade of antibody forming cells (an example is the tolerance produced by high doses

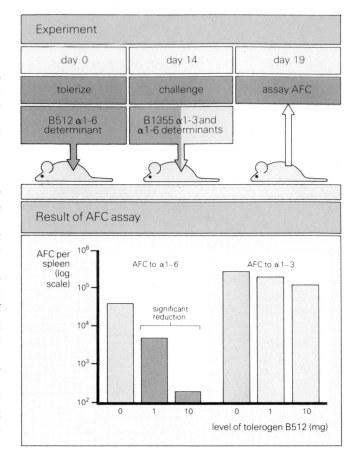

Fig. 12.7 Specificity of tolerance to one determinant, but not another on the same antigen. The tolerogen used in this experiment was the dextran B512 polysaccharide which possesses the α 1-6 glucosyl determinant. Three groups of mice were used: the first group received no tolerogen (control), the second received 1 mg, and the third received 10 mg. On day 14 all mice were challenged with an immunogenic dose of another polysaccharide, dextran B1355, possessing both the α 1-6 and the α 1-3 determinants. The antibody produced to these determinants was estimated on day 19 (by assaying AFCs per spleen). The results of the assay are shown in the bar charts. The left hand chart shows the antibody response to the α 1-6 determinant: the response is significantly reduced and, moreover, the tolerance produced increases as the tolerogenic dose rises. The right hand chart representing the response to the α 1-3 determinant shows no significant reduction.

of lipopolysaccharide) transfer of the tolerant cells to an environment free of antigen leads to a rapid loss of tolerance.

The duration of tolerance may also be studied experimentally by thymectomizing an animal, tolerizing it to a particular antigen and then comparing its recovery from tolerance with that of a similarly treated non-thymectomized individual. It is found that when a T-independent antigen (such as levan) is used, the profile of the thymectomized individual's recovery is identical to that of the non-thymectomized animal (Fig. 12.8). Both immunity and tolerance to T-ind antigens are B cell functions therefore the lack of a thymus does not affect the development of tolerance or recovery from it.

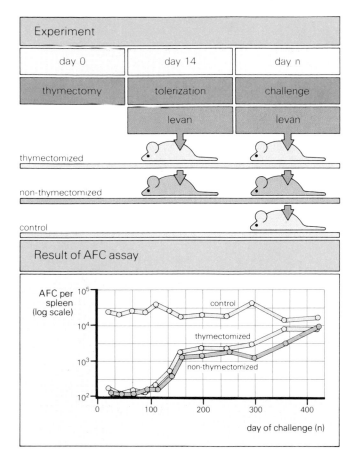

Fig. 12.8 Duration of tolerance — recovery from levan tolerance is similar in both thymectomized and non-thymectomized animals. On day 0, one of three groups of mice was thymectomized. On day 14 both the thymectomized group and a non-thymectomized group were tolerized with levan. At a later day (day n) both these two groups and a control group were challenged with an immunogenic dose of levan. The antibody response (AFCs per spleen) was then assayed and plotted against the day of levan challenge. The antibody response increases with the time interval between tolerization and antigen challenge. This recovery from tolerance shows a similar pattern for both thymectomized and non-thymectomized groups indicating that T cells are not responsible for the tolerance to this antigen.

INCOMPLETE TOLERANCE

The tolerance to an antigen need not necessarily be complete, but rather involve the deletion of some aspects only of the immune response.

Affinity and Isotype Maturation
Under normal circumstances the antibody response to a second challenge with an antigen will lead to a shift in the isotype of antibody produced from IgM to IgG, with an associated increase in the overall affinity. The antibody response may however, fail to mature in the normal way following tolerance induction with the result that second challenge with an antigen leads to a response marked by an altered spectrum of immunoglobulin isotypes or antibodies of lower affinity than normal. This may be due

to the preferential tolerization of high affinity B cells, blockade of AFCs of a particular isotype and/or the selective action of suppressor T cells. The order of susceptibility of B cell isotypes to tolerization is $B^\varepsilon > B^\gamma > B^\mu$ (with T-independent antigens) and $B^{\gamma 2} > B^{\gamma 1}$ (with some T-dependent antigens).

Humoral and Cell-Mediated Responses
Antigens in particular forms or doses may preferentially tolerize particular populations of lymphocytes (B cells or T cell subsets). Thus it is possible for an antigen to produce an antibody (humoral) response to an antigen but fail to produce sensitization when applied to the skin (T cell mediated response). In these circumstances the T_D cells responsible for delayed hypersensitivity (see 'Hypersensitivity-Type IV') are tolerized while T_H cells and B cells are not. This response difference may be due to the effects of cells regulating the immune response according to the antigen's dose, chemical modification or manner of presentation.

Determinants
The phenomenon in which tolerance to one determinant on an antigen may be induced independently of any other determinants on that antigen has been discussed (see figure 12.7). In this case the determinant's size and density or differences in B cell receptor affinity may provide the basis for the discrimination observed (see 'The Antibody Response').

Tissue Specifity
It may occur that an animal (strain A) tolerized to *tissue* antigens of another strain (B) by neonatal injection of haemopoietic cells is not tolerant to *skin* cells of strain B. This is due to the host (A) recognizing foreign alloantigens on the strain B skin cells which are not expressed on the strain B haemopoietic cells to which the strain A animal has become tolerant. These different types of incomplete tolerance are summarized in figure 12.9.

level	phenomenon	basis
affinity and isotypes	antibody secretion impaired in quantity and affinity maturation, selective tolerization of isotype precursor B cells	preferential tolerance in high affinity B cells, AFC blockade, order of susceptibility $B^\varepsilon > B^\gamma > B^\mu$ (T ind Ag) $B^\mu / B^{\gamma 2} > B^{\gamma 1}$ (some T-dep Ag)
humoral/CMI responses	suppression of one response independently of the other	regulatory cell interactions involving critical dosage or chemically modified antigen
determinants	different determinants on an antigen may be tolerized independently of one another	determinant size and density B cell receptor affinity
tissue specificity	animal tolerized to haemopoietic cells may not be tolerant to skin from donor strain	epidermal alloantigens not expressed by haemopoietic cells

Fig. 12.9 Incomplete tolerance. This table summarizes the types of incomplete tolerance which may be independently established and suggests the bases for the resulting phenomena observed.

MECHANISMS OF TOLERANCE INDUCTION

Antigen Induced Tolerance
This section covers experiments performed to investigate the mechanism of tolerance induction by antigen.

B cell tolerance B cells may be tolerized to a variety of T-independent antigens. Generally speaking these antigens are slowly metabolized *in vivo* and tend therefore to promote relatively long lasting tolerance. The response of B cells to T-independent antigens is dependent on the dose of antigen injected (Fig. 12.10).

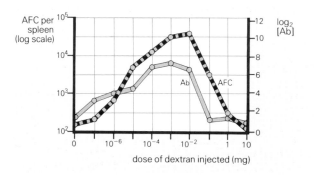

Fig. 12.10 The immune response to a T-independent antigen, dextran B512, depends upon the dose. Different groups of mice were injected with different doses of dextran and the resulting levels of antibody (Ab) and antibody forming cells (AFCs) per spleen assessed and plotted against the different antigen doses. The dose of dextran required for tolerance induction appears lower with the Ab assay than with AFC counts. This is attributable to peripheral neutralization of antibody by higher antigen doses. The AFC curve thus represents tolerance at the B cell level.

Despite their higher avidity for the B cells, T-independent antigens are required in higher doses than T-dependent antigens, to act as effective tolerogens. T cells play no role in the tolerance to T-ind antigens, hence tolerization to these antigens is still seen in nude (athymic) mice. It can also be shown that humoral factors are not involved in the development of this form of tolerance since serum transfer from suppressed to normal mice does not transfer the tolerance (Fig. 12.11). Studies demonstrating the lack of any humoral factor in the induction of tolerance in mature B cell clones suggests that clonal deletion or AFC blockade are the mechanisms responsible. The requirement for a large antigen dose supports this conclusion. Indeed it might be expected that the large doses of antigen used in some experiments (such as in figure 12.10) would be capable of producing AFC blockade. However, the phenomenon of tolerance by B cell deletion or AFC blockade displays different characteristics in respect of the doses required to produce tolerance and in the degree of antibody suppression produced, which in turn is related to the difficulty encountered in trying to suppress the fully differentiated AFCs. AFC blockade and B cell clonal deletion are dissociable phenomena (Fig. 12.12).

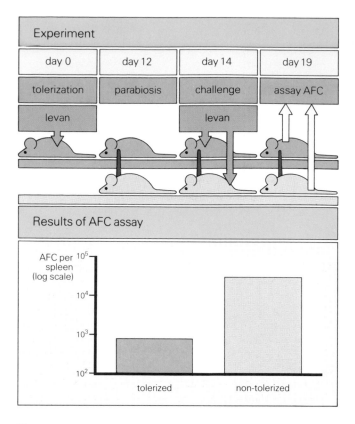

Fig. 12.11 Induction of tolerance to a T-independent antigen (levan) is not due to a humoral factor. On day 0 one of two mice was tolerized with levan and then parabiosed (fused circulation) with a second mouse 12 days later. Both mice were challenged with levan on day 14. AFC assay was performed on day 19 and the results are shown in the bar diagrams. The finding that the non-tolerized mouse produces a normal immune response implies that there is no role for a soluble factor in the tolerance induced in the first mouse.

		B cell functional deletion	AFC blockade
		deletion	inhibits Ab secretion
minimum effective tolerogenic doses (mg)	dextran(5×10⁵M.W.)	1	0.01
	levan (6×10³M.W.)	10	inactive
isotype susceptibility		IgG >IgM	IgM >IgG
tolerance attainable		complete	partial

Fig. 12.12 Different characteristics of B cell clonal deletion and AFC blockade. Binding of the T-ind antigen to the B cell's receptors may cause functional deletion of the B cell clone. Alternatively, antigen binding to the AFC reduces antibody production by interfering with processes involved in antibody secretion. These two mechanisms of tolerance induction may be distinguished by the minimum dose of tolerogens which are effective, their molecular weight, the relative susceptibility of different classes of antibody affected and the level of tolerance attainable.

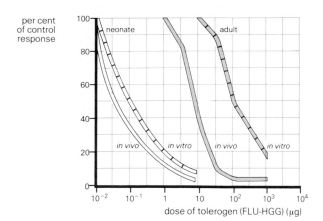

Fig. 12.13 Tolerance susceptibility of neonatal B cells to a T-independent antigen (FLU-HGG) *in vivo* **and** *in vitro.* The antibody response is represented as a percentage of the normal response. The dose required to achieve a tolerant state in the neonate is about 100-fold smaller than that required in the adult, since in the neonatal period, all B cells are at an early stage of their clonal ontogeny and are relatively easily tolerized. It is easier to tolerize B cells *in vivo* than *in vitro,* a phenomenon which is probably related to the different methods of antigen presentation in the lymphoid tissue *in vivo*

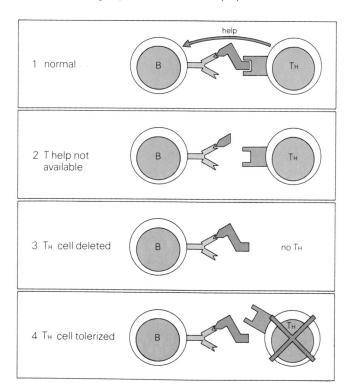

Fig. 12.14 Induction of B cell tolerance in adults to T-dependent antigens. Normally the T-helper cell delivers help to a responding B cell via an antigen bridge, thus activating antibody formation (1). The strategy for inducing tolerance in the adult is based on preventing the delivery of T help to the B cell. If the T-helper cells fail to recognize the antigen (eg. univalent deaggregated globulin) no help will be delivered to the B cell (2); the T cells may be deleted eg. in nude mice (3), or the T-helper cells may be tolerized, thus preventing activation of the B cell clone (4).

In contrast with mature B cells, neonatal B cells are much more susceptible to tolerance induction. It is found that the levels of antigen which will produce B cell tolerance in neonates are approximately 100 fold smaller than those in adults. (Fig. 12.13). The production of B cell tolerance to T-dependent antigens in the adult is a more difficult procedure to study since T-helper cells will normally supply help directed to determinants on the antigen (carrier determinants) enabling them to trigger B cells into a response. Thus, tolerance to these antigens can only be produced where this mechanism is circumvented such as when the animals lack T cells (nude mice) or the T cells are effectively tolerant to the carrier determinants (Fig. 12.14).

T cell tolerance Mature T cell tolerance may either be due to functional deletion of T cells or be related to the induction of suppressor T cells. Some of the ways of distinguishing the two types of tolerance were briefly mentioned earlier.
It is found that:
1. T-helper cell deletion occurs more rapidly than T-suppressor cell generation
2. T-helper cell deletion can be induced by stimuli that do not induce Ts cell generation (eg. the drug cyclophosphamide, whose action is discussed later)
3. tolerance due to T-helper cell deletion may not be transferred to recipient animals by cells of a tolerized animal (see Fig. 12.11)
4. tolerance due to deletion of T-helper cells persists even after the loss of T-suppressor cells.
These points are summarized in figure 12.15.

> Evidence for clonal deletion in antigen-induced T cell tolerance (1) dissociability from suppressor T cell generation:–
>
> rapid onset of Tн cell deletion preceeds Ts cell generation
>
> induced when Ts cell generation is suppressed (eg. cyclophosphamide)
>
> tolerance broken *in vivo* by normal lymphocytes (parabiosis)
>
> tolerance persists after loss of Ts cells

Fig. 12.15 Evidence for clonal deletion in antigen-induced T cell tolerance: dissociability from T-suppressor generation. These four experimental findings favour the view that the tolerance produced in the experiments that were performed is due to T cell deletion rather than the induction of suppressor T cells.

In practice, the evidence for the deletion of T cell classes is strongest in some transplantation systems, which cannot be explained by the presence of Ts cells:
1. in neonatally produced chimaeras fully tolerant to a foreign donor H-2 haplotype it is impossible to find any T cells capable of recognizing the foreign tissue type, nor are any Ts cells found, in spite of the chimaera being permanantly in contact with potentially antigenic cells.
2. when irradiated F1 mice are repopulated with donor cells of both parental strains (the mice now become

radiation chimaeras) the donor cells do not react against one another as would be normal, and a stable chimaera is produced. Since no Ts cells are found it is concluded that the tolerance is due to deletion of the donor *cytotoxic* T cells, which recognize and destroy cells carring allotypic markers of the other parental strain.

3. although neonatally induced tolerance can be broken by the immunological termination of chimaerism, this breaking of tolerance does not occur in thymectomized animals, since they are unable to produce new mature T cells capable of reacting with the foreign tissue type. Such thymectomized animals will still accept tissue grafts of donor type despite procedures which would normally break their neonatally induced tolerance. The evidence for T cell deletion derived from transplantation systems is summarized in figure 12.16.

Evidence for clonal deletion in antigen-induced T cell tolerance (2) evidence from transplantation models:—

fully H-2 tolerant neonatal chimaeras lack anti-donor T cells and Ts cells

radiation chimaeras possess reciprocally tolerant donor cells, no Ts cells

loss of tolerance by terminating chimaerism is prevented by thymectomy — implying that recovery involves recruitment

Fig. 12.16 Evidence for clonal deletion in antigen-induced T cell tolerance: evidence from transplantation models. The tolerance produced in these experimental models cannot be due to suppressor T cell activity. It is concluded that T cell clones have been deleted.

T cells are much more susceptible to tolerization than B cells, particularly in adult life. Additionally, it appears that tolerance due to T cell deletion differs from B cell deletion in its initial stages, particularly in respect of the dose and form of the antigen needed. For example, T cells may be tolerized by the monomeric form of the protein, flagellin, whereas B cells require polymerized flagellin. Thus, it seems that it is not necessary to cross-link the T cells' receptors with high doses of multivalent antigens to induce tolerance; the implication is that T cell tolerance can be induced by a single signal to the T cell. It is also observed that it is virtually impossible to tolerize T$_H$ cells *in vitro* whereas it is perfectly possible to tolerize B cells in similar systems.

There are a number of instances where it has been shown that tolerance is maintained by Ts cells. Generally these are cases where suppression is generated in adult life and they contrast with the normal self-tolerance induced in neonatal life which is maintained by T$_H$ cell deletion. There is evidence that in different conditions Ts cells may act in different ways. In some cases they interfere with the process of T/B cooperation, in others they act directly on functioning T$_H$, T$_C$ and other Ts populations. Some antigens are so immunogenic that they can induce tolerance only if administered along with potent immunosuppressive measures such as irradiation or the drug cyclophosphamide. These forms of suppression are maintained by Ts cells (Fig. 12.17).

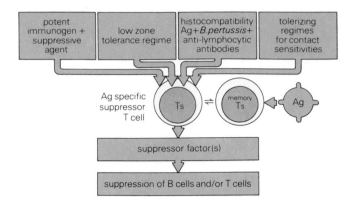

Fig. 12.17 Tolerance induced in adult life attributable to suppressor T cells. Antigen may be presented in a number of special ways to induce suppressor T cells specific to that antigen. Examples include the combination of a potent immunogen with a suppressive agent (eg. the drug cyclophosphamide); sufficiently low levels of tolerogen to produce low zone tolerance; suppression of immunity to histocompatibility (MHC) antigens by administering the antigen together with a microorganism (eg. *B. pertussis*) and anti-lymphocytic serum. Certain tolerizing regimes for contact sensitivities selectively activate Ts cells when the antigen is introduced via a different route to that which induces skin sensitization. Ts cells may become memory cells in the same way as all other types of T cell. Memory Ts cells are reactivated following a subsequent contact with antigen. Suppressor cells release factors responsible for suppressing the activity of B cells or other T cells.

Tolerance Enhanced by Immunosuppressive Drugs

Immunosuppressive drugs administered alone cannot produce antigen specific tolerance since they act equally on all susceptible clones. Certain immunosuppressive drugs such as cyclosporin A act preferentially against different lymphocyte subsets — cyclosporin A for example acts preferentially on T cells. Immunosuppressive drugs can only be rendered antigen specific by including an antigen specific element in the tolerizing regime, thus the drugs act as cofactors in tolerogenesis. An experiment demonstrating the effect of cyclophosphamide in promoting antigen-induced tolerance is described in figure 12.18. There is evidence that these drugs may act in one of two different ways:

1. lowering the threshold for tolerance induction
2. blocking differentiation sequences in cells triggered by antigen.

The commonly used immunosuppressive drug cyclophosphamide acts both on T and B cells. Its action on B cells is to increase B cell sensitivity to tolerogenesis by the normal mechanisms, and its action may be related to the inability of B cells treated with cyclophosphamide to regenerate their cell surface immunoglobulin receptors (for antigen) at the normal rate. It is noteworthy that neonatal B cells are also unable to regenerate their surface receptors after contact with antigen, and following capping. Capping is a procedure in which surface immunoglobulin aggregates when coated with anti-immunoglobulin. The cap so formed is internalized by the cell, leaving the membrane free of immunoglobulin receptors (Fig. 12.19).

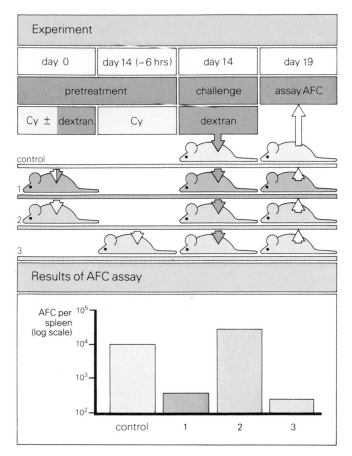

Fig. 12.18 Promotion of antigen-induced tolerance by cyclophosphamide (Cy). Four groups of mice are used. One group is a control and the three others receive different pretreatments: (1) cyclophosphamide and a normally immunogenic dose of antigen (dextran) on day 0, (2) cyclophosphamide only on day 0, and (3) cyclophosphamide only, six hours prior to antigen challenge, which occurs on day 14. The immune response was assessed on day 19 by AFC assay, and the results are shown in the bar diagram. Cyclophosphamide administered together with antigen promotes long-lasting antigen-specific tolerance, but if administered immediately prior to antigen challenge it will lead to a temporary generalized unresponsiveness.

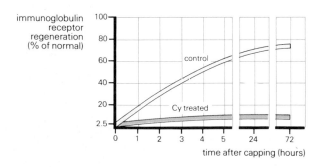

Fig. 12.19 Effect of cyclophosphamide on the ability of B cells to regenerate their immunoglobulin receptors. B cells are capped using anti-immunoglobulin, either in the presence (Cy-treated) or absence (control) of cyclophosphamide, and the time taken to regenerate the receptors is measured: Cy-treated cells regenerate their receptors very slowly.

Antibody-Induced Tolerance

The antibody combining site may itself act as an antigen and induce the formation of specific antibody. Such antibodies, directed to the combining sites (idiotypes) of other antibodies, are termed anti-idiotypic antibodies (see 'Regulation of the Immune Response'). This type of antibody will bind specifically to the particular idiotypes which induced their formation, and if they bind to cell surface idiotypes, leading to cross-linking of the surface immunoglobulin receptors, they are effectively mimicking the action of antigen, and so may produce specific tolerance (or immunity in appropriate circumstances). These anti-idiotypic antibodies act only on the cells bearing the idiotype.

In some animals the immune response to particular antigens produces antibodies of which the majority carry a particular idiotype. Suppression of this idiotype by blocking cell surface receptors with anti-idiotype can fundamentally alter the character of the immune response to that antigen. In this case tolerance to the antigen is partial, and other antibodies to this antigen carrying a different idiotype are still present. Furthermore, administration of an anti-idiotype in the neonate seriously impairs the response of that idiotype resulting in prolonged tolerance. The effect of anti-idiotype on adult and neonate mice is illustrated in figure 12.20.

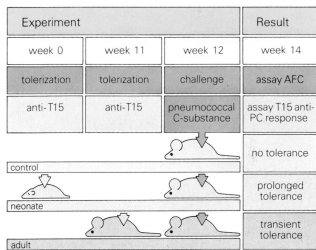

Fig. 12.20 Passive induction of tolerance by anti-idiotype. Three groups of BALB/c strain mice were used in this experiment: two adult and one neonate. BALB/c mice normally produce a particular antibody carrying the T15 idiotype, to the phosphoryl choline (PC) determinant on the antigen, pneumococcal-C-substance (control). In the first week (week 0) the neonates were administered antibody to the T15 idiotype (anti-T15). A group of adults were similarly treated in week 11. In week 12 all mice were challenged with pneumococcal-C-substance and the production of anti-PC antibody of the T15 idiotype was assayed in week 14. It is found that exposure of neonates to the anti-idiotype produces prolonged tolerance of the T15 anti-PC response, whereas exposure in adults leads to transient tolerance. It is presumed that the prolonged tolerance is due to clonal abortion, and the transient adult tolerance to AFC blockade and B cell exhaustion. The tolerance is passively induced in this example since the tolerizing agent (anti-T15) is not actively generated by the individual but received passively by injection.

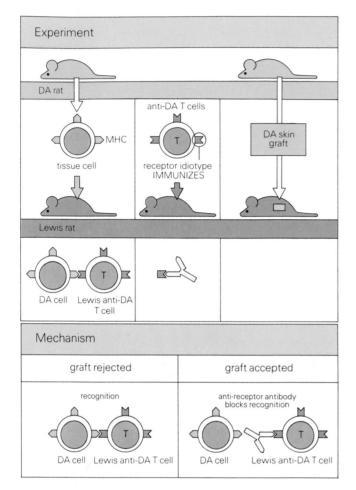

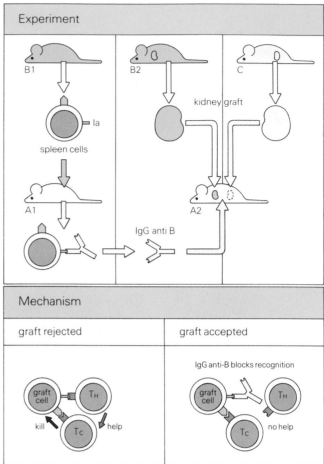

Fig. 12.21 Active induction of tolerance by anti-idiotype.
In this experiment Lewis strain rats receive a tissue implant
from rats of a different strain, DA. The Lewis rat's T cells (T$_H$
and T$_C$) recognize the MHC antigens carried on the DA rat
cells, by anti-DA receptors (anti-DA idiotype). These receptors
may be isolated and administered to the Lewis rat in an
immunogenic form. Antibody is raised to the receptor idiotype
and it is then found that Lewis rats will accept skin grafts from
a DA rat. According to the normal mechanism of graft
rejection, Lewis rats' T cells recognize DA tissue antigens (by
their anti-DA receptor idiotype) to initiate an immune
response. In the experimental situation however, antibody
raised against the receptor idiotype blocks recognition of the
DA cell by Lewis T cells, thereby preventing them from
recognizing and rejecting DA tissue grafts.

In other conditions animals can themselves be induced to
generate anti-idiotypes (auto-anti-idiotypes) leading to
tolerance by blockade of the animal's own idiotype. If the
idiotype is on a receptor involved in the recognition of
foreign tissue antigens the blockade of this receptor
idiotype will lead to the animal becoming tolerant of
tissue grafts from animals of that tissue type (Fig. 12.21). A
similar mechanism operates in the phenomenon termed
passive enhancement. Alloantisera raised to H-2I region
antigen determinants of a foreign tissue interfere with
graft rejection in a recipient animal. The anti-I region
antibodies bind to the graft I region determinants and
block recognition of these determinants by the recipient's
T$_H$ cells involved in graft rejection (Fig. 12.22).

**Fig. 12.22 Passive enhancement of graft survival by
donor strain-specific alloantisera.** Spleen cells are
transferred from a B strain mouse (B1) to an A strain mouse
(A1) where an antiserum is raised against these cells' Ia
antigens. The antibody produced (IgG anti-B) is transferred to
a second strain A mouse (A2). When kidneys from another
individual of strain B (B2) and an individual of a third strain (C)
are grafted into the A2 mouse, the C graft is rejected but the B
graft survives. According to the normal mechanism of graft
rejection the host T$_H$ cells recognize the graft cell antigens and
help the host T$_C$ cells kill the graft cell. In this experiment
however, alloantisera blocks the normal T$_H$ recognition of the
graft and consequently no help is given to the T$_C$ cell.

SELF TOLERANCE

The fundamental basis of the immune system is tolerance
to self tissues and lack of tolerance to foreign antigens,
marked by an appropriate immune response. Failure of
the appropriate response may be marked by a failure to
respond against foreign antigens, or a hypersensitivity
reaction. The original hypothesis of Burnet and Fenner,
dealing with unresponsiveness to self-antigens, stated
that all anti-self lymphocytes were eliminated before
maturity. This view is untenable since anti-self B cells are
found in normal adult animals. At present it is believed
that anti-self B cells are normally present, but quiescent
due to lack of associative recognition of the self-antigens
by T$_H$ cells (functional deletion).

In this hypothesis the Ts cell system is seen as a backup mechanism to the primary mechanism of deletion of anti-self TH cells in maintaining self-tolerance. Although tolerance due to the action of Ts cells is known to operate, whether it constitutes a major mechanism depends upon its importance with respect to the TH cell deletion mechanism — the two are not mutually exclusive.

	maintenance of self-tolerance	breakdown of self-tolerance
historical	self antigen — TH ✗ B ✗	self antigen — help → mutant TH, mutant B
TH Deletion	self antigen — TH ✗ B	foreign antigen — help → TH, B
suppression	self antigen — TH, B, Ts suppression	self antigen — help → TH, B, Ts ✗

Fig. 12.23 Self-tolerance: three alternative explanations. Historical. The original hypothesis of Burnet and Fenner, that all self-antigens induce the elimination of anti-self T and B lymphocyte clones in the neonate, is untenable. Loss of self-tolerance leading to autoimmunity would occur by mutation in adult life, producing new clones of anti-self lymphocytes.
TH deletion. According to the second possibility, B cell clones are unable to respond to antigens due to lack of T help against these antigens resulting from the clonal deletion of anti-self TH cells. One way of circumventing this tolerance is by a foreign antigen cross-linking the B cells with TH cells of a different specificity, which are able to substitute for the deleted TH clone. (Alternatively, adjuvants and B cell mitogens circumvent the requirement for T cell help.)
Suppression. This does not propose clonal deletion but the continuous suppression of TH and B cell function by suppressor T cells. Loss of the Ts cells means the loss of the tolerance. This third possibility may be considered as a failsafe mechanism suppressing any autoantibodies that are produced following the failure of clonal deletion.

However, it seems that the immune system relies primarily on TH cell deletion (effective from neonatal life onwards), and secondarily, Ts cell generation, which is required particularly to deal with self-antigens encountered later in life (eg. antigens appearing at puberty). Ts cells are also probably involved in immuno-regulation of normal immune responses. These three possible mechanisms of maintaining self tolerance are summarized in figure 12.23.

TOLERANCE IN AREAS OF POTENTIAL THERAPEUTIC APPLICATION

It is sometimes desirable to promote a patient's tolerance to a foreign tissue graft, or to control an inappropriate

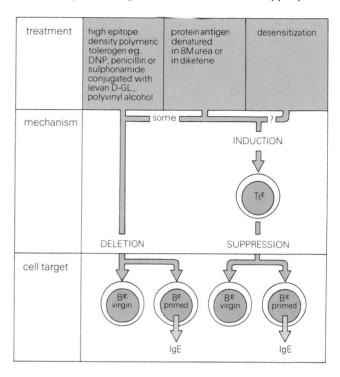

Fig. 12.24 Immunosuppression of the allergic response. An overvigorous IgE response to the antigen (allergen) by the hypersensitive individual is responsible for the allergic response. The aim of treatment is either to delete the B cells that are producing IgE specific to the allergen, or to promote IgE class specific T-suppressors. The treatments in the box on the left delete both newly formed, virgin IgE – producing B cells (Bε) and primed B cells (ie. which have already responded to the allergen). Some of these agents, as well as denatured protein antigen, can induce suppressor T cells (Ts), which specifically suppress Bε cells. It is also possible to desensitize an allergic individual (to specific allergens) by administering the allergen under a carefully controlled regime to limit the danger of anaphylactic reaction. This may operate by inducing suppressor T cells. The mechanism of this diagram is based on animal studies only.

hypersensitivity reaction. Suppression of transplant rejection can either be aimed at mimicking self tolerance (eg. by inducing tolerance in perinatal life) or at activating the Ts population. Unfortunately, perinatal tolerance induction, which offers the best hope of success, cannot by its very nature be performed on adult graft recipients. Suppression of allergic responses (see 'Hypersensitivity Type I') is aimed primarily at causing a switch in the antibody isotype produced by the B cell's response, rather than in blocking recognition of the sensitizing agent (Fig. 12.24). A better understanding of the mechanism of isotype switching will lead to improved approaches to the therapy of these ailments.

FURTHER READING

Howard J.G. (1979) Immunological Tolerance. In *Defence and Recognition* Vol. 22 – Cellular Aspects E.S. Lennox (ed.) University Park Press, Baltimore, USA.

Howard J.G. & Mitchison N.A. (1975) Immunological Tolerance. In *Progress in Allergy.* **18, 43**. Waksman B.H. (ed.) Karger, Basel.

Humphrey J.H. et al (1976) Immunological Tolerance. *British Medical Bulletin,* **32**, 99.

13 Genetic Control of Immunity

There are many potential sites at which genetic factors could play a role in the generation of an immune response. It was in the latter half of the nineteenth century that Jacobi noted that genetic factors influenced the susceptibility to disease. The observation that diphtheria tended to occur in families prompted the tentative proposal that resistance or susceptibility of an individual to the infectious agent, *Corynebacterium diphtherii*, might be an inherited trait. This proposal was supported by the finding that different strains of guinea pigs displayed different resistance patterns to diphtheria and that the characteristic was inherited. Fjord-Scheibel demonstrated in 1943 that the production of diphtheria anti-toxin was controlled by a gene, inherited in a Mendelian dominant fashion, by selective breeding of high and low responder guinea pig strains. This study was the first demonstration of the dominance of high responsiveness since ninety percent of the offspring of the two high responder strains were anti-toxin producers in the first generation whereas it took five generations of inbreeding non-producers to achieve ninety percent of the offspring as non-producers.

In the 1920's and 30's Webster noted that in a stock of outbred Swiss mice there was variation in the susceptibility to infection by *Bacillus enteritidis*. By selective inbreeding Webster was able to obtain two lines of mice; one resistant to bacteria (BR) and the other susceptible (BS). Studies on the susceptibility of these lines to *virus* infection allowed development of further lines which were either susceptible (BSVS and BRVS) or resistant (BSVR and BRVR) to these viral infections: the BSVS line was therefore highly susceptible to both bacterial and viral infections. Once again, breeding studies demonstrated that responsiveness was a dominant trait since F_1 hybrid mice derived from parental lines BSVR and BRVS were resistant to both bacterial and viral infections. These experiments laid the groundwork for further studies on the role of immune response genes.

GENES CONTROLLING THE IMMUNE RESPONSE

By using inbred strains of animals and employing antigens of a more defined composition it became possible to subject the genetic regulation of immune responsiveness to a finer analysis. Therefore, instead of using complex antigens like bacteria or red blood cells researchers used small proteins such as insulin or synthetic polypeptides like poly-L-lysine (PLL) or (T,G)-A--L, (H,G)-A--L and (P,G)-A--L. These have an alanine-lysine copolymer backbone substituted with glutamic acid and tyrosine, histidine, or phenylalanine branches.

Benacerraf and his colleagues found that outbred guinea pigs either made a delayed hypersensitivity response and antibodies to the antigen DNP-PLL or failed to make either a delayed hypersensitivity response or anti-

bodies. By selective inbreeding it was possible to show that such responses were inherited, the dominant trait being attributable to a single gene. If DNP-PLL were coupled to another antigen, for example ovalbumin, the resulting immunogen was found to induce antibodies to DNP-PLL in the non-responder strain, but it did not induce delayed hypersensitivity.

MHC LINKED IMMUNE RESPONSE GENES

In the 1960's McDevitt and Chinitz followed the observation of John Humphrey that sandy lop rabbits differed from the Himalayan in their responses to synthetic branched amino acid copolymers. Using inbred strains of mice and the antigen (T,G)-A--L, McDevitt and colleagues demonstrated that the response to (T,G)-A--L was under the control of a single autosomal dominant gene or gene cluster. This gene was termed immune response 1 (Ir-1) and was found to be linked to the mouse major histocompatibility complex (H-2) (Fig. 13.1).

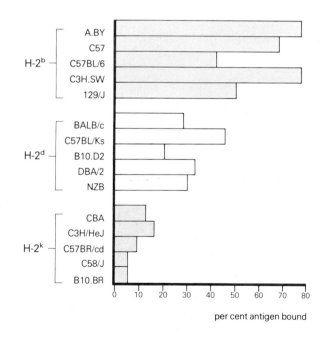

Fig. 13.1 Strain differences in the antibody response to (T,G)-A--L. Fifteen strains of mice were given a standard dose of the synthetic antigen (T,G)-A--L. Antibody responses are expressed as the antigen-binding capacity of the antisera. Animals with the H-2^b haplotype are high responders, H-2^d are intermediate and H-2^k are low responders. Note that there is some overlap between the level of response in the different haplotypes indicating that the H-2 linked genes are not the only ones to control the response.

Using another synthetic antigen, (H,G)-A--L genetic mapping localized the Ir1 gene to the I-A subregion of the mouse MHC (Fig. 13.2). After this first demonstration of an MHC-linked immune response gene the responses to a large number of T-dependent antigens have been found to be under the control of genes located in this part of the MHC. These antigens include linear and branched chain synthetic amino acid copolymers, other antigens, such as for example alloantigens, the male antigen H-Y, and protein antigens including insulin, hen egg lysozyme, cytochrome C and myoglobin. It is notable however, that a high responder strain for one antigen is a low responder for other antigens, while other strains have the opposite high and low response patterns, as tabulated in

figure 13.3. Thus the MHC-linked Ir genes act in an antigen specific fashion. But not all the immune response genes are linked to the MHC. Most of these non-MHC immune response genes do not seem to have the degree of antigen specificity which MHC linked Ir genes have. It is likely that Ir genes play a role in determining the level of a response to any T-dependent antigen. Since an Ir gene may control the recognition of a given epitope on an antigen, antigens which are antigenically complex will provide many determinants subject to Ir gene control. This was demonstrated by Berzofsky's studies on sperm whale myoglobin in which separate determinants on the molecule are shown to be under control of distinct Ir genes (Fig. 13.4).

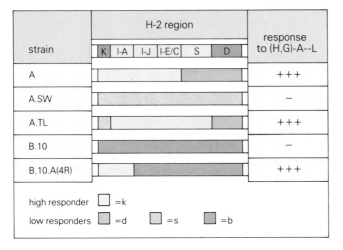

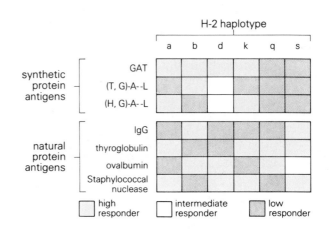

Fig. 13.2 Mapping of the ir gene controlling responses to (H,G)-A--L. The H-2 regions of 5 strains of mice are illustrated, three strains are high responders to (H,G)-A--L and two are low responders. All three high responder strains have only the H-2^k I-A region in common, indicating that the gene present in H-2^k mice controlling the immune response to (H,G)-A--L is in the I-A region. Colours represent haplotypes.

Fig. 13.3 High and low responder haplotypes. This table shows the response of six inbred strains of mice, with different H-2 haplotypes, to seven different antigens. High responders to some antigens produce low responses to others, the pattern of response is quite unsystematic. Even with very closely related antigens such as (T,G)-A--L and (H,G)-A--L the response is different in H-2^a and H-2^b strains.

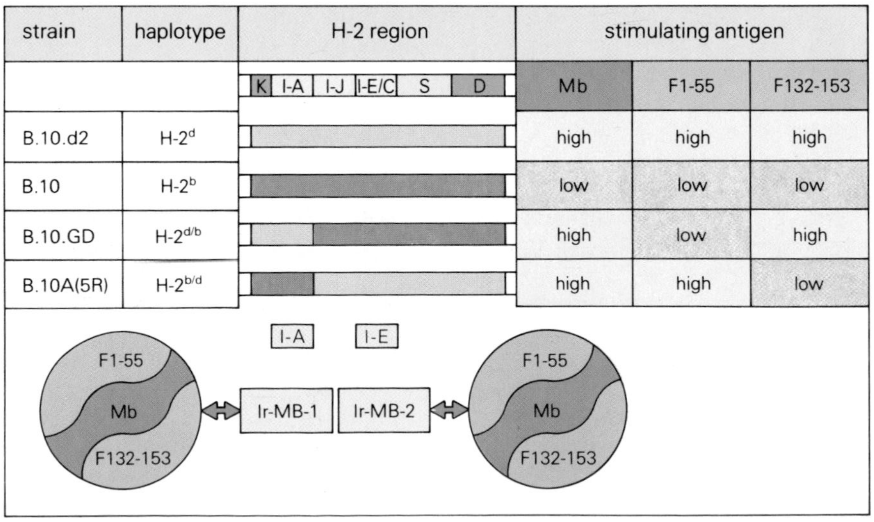

Fig. 13.4 Genetic control of the response to myoglobin. Mice of four different strains were immunized with myoglobin (Mb). The different strains were genetically identical except at the H-2 locus, where they were either H-2^d (purple), H-2^b (pink) or recombinants containing part b and part d (pink and purple). The spleen cells from the immunized animals were set up in cultures containing either whole Mb antigen or fragments of the antigen, consisting of amino acids 1-55 (f1-55) or amino acids 132-153 (f132-153). Proliferation of T cells in response to the antigen or fragments was measured and the strains showed either high responses or low responses. H-2^d mice show high responses to the whole antigen and fragments whereas H-2^b mice show low responses. B.10. GD mice which have a high responder I-A region make a high response to the whole antigen and to f132-153

strain	haplotype	H-2 region						stimulating antigen		
		K	I-A	I-J	I-E/C	S	D	Mb	F1-55	F132-153
B.10.d2	H-2^d							high	high	high
B.10	H-2^b							low	low	low
B.10.GD	H-2$^{d/b}$							high	low	high
B.10A(5R)	H-2$^{b/d}$							high	high	low

while B10. A(5R) mice, which have a high responder I-E/C region respond to f1-55 but not f132-153. This implies that a gene in I-A (Ir-MB-1) controls the response to f132-153 while

a gene in I-E/C (Ir-MB-2) controls the response to f1-55 in H-2^d mice. H-2^b mice lack these genes. These conclusions are summarized in the lower part of the diagram.

LEVEL OF ACTION OF IMMUNE RESPONSE GENES

MHC-linked Ir gene control is very specific, in many cases a single amino acid substitution will affect responsiveness. For example in figure 13.3 it was shown that

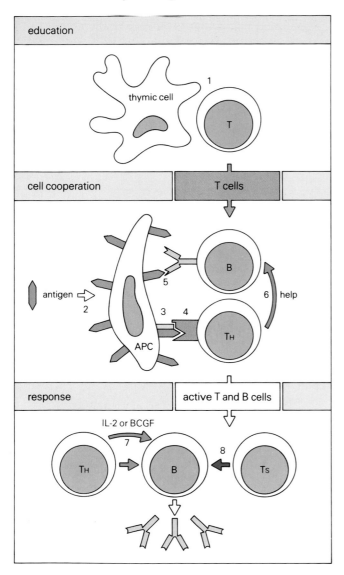

Fig. 13.5 Levels of action of Ir genes. A great number of genes can affect the outcome of the immune response; this diagram indicates their most likely points of action.
Education. During T cell development T cells are educated in the thymus to discriminate self from non-self (1).
Cell cooperation. Antigen entering the immune system is processed by antigen-presenting cells (2) and is presented in association with MHC class 2 molecules to the T_H cells (3). T cells and B cells can only recognize the antigen if they have a suitable repertoire of receptors (4 and 5). T and B cells cooperate optimally if they share haplotypes (6).
Response. Following activation the T cells and B cells proliferate, a function partly dependent on lymphokines from T cells (IL-2) (7) and macrophages. The strength of the response is also dependent on whether the antigen induces T_S cells (8), which in turn depends on the repertoire of T_S cells as well as processing and presentation of the antigen.

whereas H-2^b mice are high responders to (T,G)-A--L but not to (H,G)-A--L, H-2^k mice are the opposite, being high responders to (H,G)-A--L but not (T,G)-A--L. However, both H-2^k and H-2^b mice respond to (P,G)-A--L. This pattern of responsiveness is not what would be predicted in terms of antibody specificity since substantial cross-reactivity is observed between the antibodies to (H,G)-A--L (T,G)-A--L and (P,G)-A--L. This has led to the proposal that MHC-linked Ir genes exert their control at the level of T cell recognition of antigen and not at the level of B cells. The possible levels at which Ir genes may exert their control are outlined in figure 13.5

Antigen Presentation and T/B Cooperation
Analysis of the levels at which Ir genes exert their control on cellular interactions has focused on Ir genes controlling antigen presentation between macrophages and the T cells and Ir genes regulating T/B cooperation.

Rosenthal and Shevach clearly demonstrated that a T cell proliferative response to antigen only occurred if the T cells and APC were derived from guinea pigs of the same strain (Fig. 13.6).

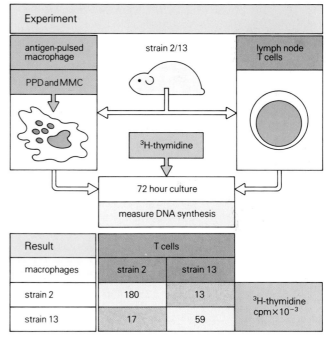

Result	T cells	
macrophages	strain 2	strain 13
strain 2	180	13
strain 13	17	59

³H-thymidine cpm × 10⁻³

Fig. 13.6 Genetic restriction in macrophage/T cell cooperation. Peritoneal macrophages and T cells were isolated from antigen-primed strain 2 and strain 13 guinea pigs. The macrophages were pulsed with antigen (PPD) and mitomycin C (MMC – to prevent the macrophages proliferating). The T cells and antigen-pulsed macrophages were cocultured and DNA synthesis by the T cells measured by incorporation of tritiated thymidine (³H-thymidine). The incorporation is given in the table below. Lymphocytes of both strains respond well when the antigen is presented on syngeneic macrophages, but poorly when presented on allogeneic macrophages.

A similar requirement for MHC I region compatibility was demonstrated for T/B collaboration, in the immune response of mice to hapten-carrier conjugates.

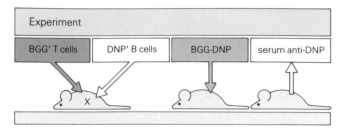

Experiment			
BGG' T cells	DNP' B cells	BGG-DNP	serum anti-DNP

Result				
experiment	T cells	B cells	recipient	response
1	C	C	CxD	+
2	D	D	CxD	+
3	C	D	CxD	−
4	D	C	CxD	−
5	CxD	D	CxD	+

Fig. 13.7 Genetic restriction in T/B cooperation. Mice were irradiated (X) and reconstituted with T cells primed to bovine gamma globulin (BGG') and B cells primed to the hapten dinitrophenyl (DNP'). The animals were challenged with BGG-DNP and the anti-DNP response measured. This experiment was performed using different combinations of strain C and D, B cells and T cells with hybrid mice (CxD) as with recipients. The responses obtained with different combinations of T and B cells are shown. Strain C T cells cooperate with strain C B cells (1) and strain D T cells also cooperate with strain D B cells (2). However, strain C T cells cannot cooperate with strain D B cells and vice versa (3 and 4). Sharing of *one* haplotype between T cells and B cells is sufficient to produce a response, as demonstrated by using T cells from hybrid (CxD) mice (5).

T cells recognizing carrier cooperate with B cells recognizing hapten if they are the same H-2 type as demonstated *in vivo* in figure 13.7. This has also been demonstrated *in vitro* in a T-dependent antibody response, in which responsiveness could only be restored to a macrophage-depleted population by the addition of the macrophages of a responder genotype (isolated by adherence to a plastic plate). In the response to TNP-(TG)A-L this ability to restore the response was mapped to the I-A subregion of the mouse MHC. In F_1 animals it can be shown that T cells are genetically restricted to one or other of the two parental strains. An elegant *in vitro* demonstration of this is shown in figure 13.8. This phenomenon can also be demonstrated *in vivo*. It has been shown that cells from F_1 hybrid mice can transfer delayed hypersensitivity to only one of the two parental strains if the F_1 mouse is primed only with antigen-pulsed APCs of that parental strain. Using T cell *lines* or *clones* this restriction of recognition between APC and T cells has been fully substantiated. Interestingly the use of such T cell clones has allowed Sredni and Schwarz to demonstrate that T cells also exist in F_1 animals which are restricted to unique elements on F_1 APCs, that is to say, elements which are absent from either of the parental strains.

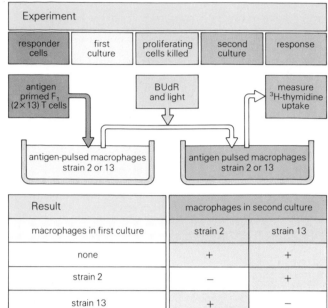

Experiment				
responder cells	first culture	proliferating cells killed	second culture	response
antigen primed F_1 (2×13) T cells	BUdR and light			measure ^{3}H-thymidine uptake
	antigen-pulsed macrophages strain 2 or 13		antigen pulsed macrophages strain 2 or 13	

Result	macrophages in second culture	
macrophages in first culture	strain 2	strain 13
none	+	+
strain 2	−	+
strain 13	+	−

Fig. 13.8 Demonstration of two types of genetically restricted T cell in F_1 animals. T cells (responders cells) from an F_1 (strain 2×strain 13) guinea pig were cultured on an antigen-pulsed layer of macrophages (antigen-presenting cells – from a strain 2 or strain 13 animal). The T cells were harvested and exposed to bromodeoxyuridine (BUdR) and light which killed the responding, proliferating cells. The surviving, non-responding cells were then cultured with a second layer of antigen-pulsed macrophages and their response was measured by the uptake of ^{3}H-thymidine. The results tabulated below show that F_1 cells with no first culture can respond to antigen presented on macrophages of either parental strain in the second culture. If the T cells are first cultured on strain 2 macrophages and the proliferating cells killed, there are no cells available to proliferate in a second culture containing strain 2 antigen-presenting cells, but there are cells still present which can respond to antigen on strain 13 cells. The converse occurs with preculture on strain 13 macrophages. This implies there are two sets of T cells in the F_1 animal. One responds to antigen presented by cells of one parental haplotype, the other responds to antigens presented by cells of the other haplotype.

Cytotoxic T Cells

The need for MHC compatibility is also noted in the activity of specific cytotoxic T cells which are directed against virally-modified targets, chemically modified self antigens or a variety of minor histocompatibility antigens, including the male antigen H-Y, for which expression is determined by genes on the Y chromosome. The requirement for compatibility is primarily restricted to the H-2K or H-2D regions of the mouse MHC (that is, class 1 antigens). Thus specific cytotoxic T cells can only lyse virally-infected cells or TNP-modified target cells if they are matched with the targets at the H-2K or H-2D regions (Fig. 13.9). The way in which viral proteins are associated with the MHC class 1 products has been examined by precipitating the surface proteins of virally-infected cells with specific antisera. It is found in some cases that precipitation of the surface MHC antigens with antibody

Fig. 13.9 Genetic restriction of cytotoxic cells. The cytotoxic cells of virus-infected adult mice of different strains were tested for their ability to kill virus-infected target cells of different H-2 haplotypes (k, s and d).

The strain A.TL is H-2K^s, H-2I^k and H-2D^d and its cells kill target cells infected with lymphocytic choriomeningitis virus (LCM) only if the targets share the H-2K^s or the H-2D^d haplotypes. Haplotype identity between the cells and targets at the H-2I locus does not produce cytotoxicity.

Note that the cytotoxicity is determined mostly by the H-2D locus. By comparison, in A.TL mice infected with Sendai virus the cytotoxicity is principally determined by the H-2K locus. Infection of CBA mice with LCM confirms the importance of genetic restriction in these responses, while the

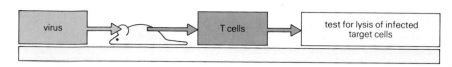

virus	mouse strain	H-2 region				percent lysis of infected targets of haplotype		
		K	I	S	D	H-2^s	H-2^k	H-2^d
LCM	A.TL					25	1	64
Sendai	A.TL					63	4	24
LCM	CBA					2	34	1
LCM	A/J					0	30	64

infection of A/J mice with LCM confirms the finding that cytotoxicity to LCM is strongest to the H-2D-matched infected targets. It is thought that different viruses may associate preferentially with particular H-2K or H-2D MHC molecules to present a target for cytotoxic cells.

Fig. 13.10 Education of cytotoxic T cells. Recipient mice (type A and B) were irradiated (X) and reconstituted with donor lymphocytes (bone marrow or spleen cells). This produced chimaeric animals, in which the lymphocytes were of the donor type and other tissues were of the recipient type. The chimaeras were then challenged with vaccinia virus and the spleen cells removed and assayed for cytotoxicity against either type A or type B cells infected with vaccinia (A-vaccinia and B-vaccinia). Five experiments using different combinations of donor cells and recipient mice were conducted. Experiment 1 demonstrates that type B bone marrow (BM) cells maturing in a type A mouse cannot kill infected targets. Experiments 2 and 3 demonstrate that mice reconstituted with A×B bone marrow cells can only kill infected targets of the same type as the recipient. Experiments 4 and 5 show that mature adult A×B spleen cells can kill both A and B infected targets. The interpretation is that immature stem cells (BM) are educated to recognize antigen only in association with the recipient's MHC haplotype, whereas mature cells (spleen) have already been educated. In most cases the education process requires that donor and recipient share at least one I region haplotype.

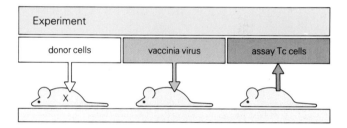

Results			cytotoxicity to:	
experiment	donor cells	recipient	A-vaccinia	B-vaccinia
1	B(BM)	A	−	−
2	A×B(BM)	A	+	−
3	A×B(BM)	B	−	+
4	A×B(spleen)	A	+	+
5	A×B(spleen)	B	+	+

specific for class 1 products coprecipitates viral proteins and vice versa, implying that the class 1 antigens are physically associated with viral antigens on the membrane. It is notable that the presence of virus in these cells modifies the β$_2$-microglobulin-dependent transport of the class 1 MHC antigens to the golgi apparatus. The mechanism by which MHC restriction of cytotoxic cell activity occurs has been broadly established by using radiation-induced bone marrow chimaeras (Fig. 13.10). It can be seen that an irradiated parental type A mouse reconstituted with F$_1$ (A×B) bone marrow develops T cells which can only respond cytolytically to virally-infected parental type A cells but not to B cells infected with this virus. This experiment demonstrates the critical role played by the environment in which the T cell matures. The educative function performed by the thymus has also been demonstrated by placing parental type B or

A thymus grafts in a thymectomized and lethally-irradiated F$_1$ mouse reconstituted with T cell-depleted bone marrow: T cells from such mice are restricted to the parental thymus MHC type. These experiments illustrate the principle that MHC restriction manifesting itself in mature T cells may be an outcome of T cell education.

Although at one time it was thought that cytotoxic T cells were restricted to class 1 MHC antigens only, this is not wholly true since clones of Tc cells have been isolated which are restricted to class 2 antigens (see 'Cell-mediated Immunity'). It is still uncertain to what extent this may occur in vivo. The use of mice with mutant alleles coding for the H-2K antigens has greatly facilitated the studies on the fine specificity of cytotoxic T cells. For example, mutant animals spontaneously arising in the wild type C57BL/6 mouse strain (H-2K^b) have been studied extensively at the functional and structural levels.

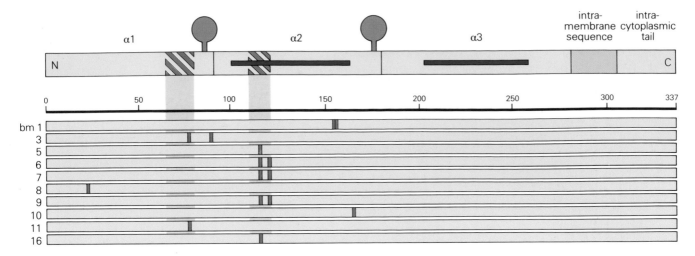

Fig. 13.11 Mutation in the MHC. In this representation of an H-2K molecule, blue=carbohydrate, red=intradomain disulphide bonds and hatching=proposed allotypic sites. Mutations in the H-2K locus of mice in the bm series were identified by skin grafting between a very large number of mice of a single strain (H-2^b). The mutations in the H-2K locus of 10 animals are clustered in the α1 and α2 domains with particular sites being especially mutable. These findings indicate that MHC genes have the highest mutation rate of any germ line genes yet studied.

These mice are referred to as the bm series and have haplotypes designated H-2K^{bm} (Fig. 13.11). The H-2K glycoproteins of the mutant mouse H-2K^{bm1} is serologically almost indistinguishable from the wild type. However, cytotoxic T cells can discriminate between the H-2K^b and the H-2K^{bm1} virally-infected targets.

ANTIGEN RECOGNITION BY T CELLS AND B CELLS

T cells and B cells have different receptors for antigen and it appears that they recognize a different repertoire of antigens. This can be demonstrated in the response to hapten-carrier combinations. For example, high affinity antibody to DNP can react with the similar hapten TNP, indeed, it has been estimated that approximately 80% of anti-DNP antibodies also bind TNP. On the other hand effector T cells sensitized by TNP-modified stimulator cells and cytotoxic for TNP-modified target cells do not crossreact with DNP-modified target cells and vice versa indicating differences in the repertoire of B cells and T cells. Further examples are shown in figure 13.12. This

idea raises the possibility that an animal's unresponsiveness may be due to a gap in the antigen-recognizing repertoire of either B cells or T cells (Fig. 13.13). Furthermore, T-helper cells and T-suppressor cells may recognize different determinants on an antigen as indicated in the well-studied system of the immune response to hen egg white lysozyme (HEL).

Immune Response to HEL
In an immune response against an antigen many factors determine the outcome of the antigenic challenge. Not only does the ability of the APC to process and present the antigen or of T-helper cells to recognize carrier determinants determine the level of response but also the amount of T-suppressor cell activity generated by priming influence the amount, allotype and possibly the idiotype of the antibody produced. This is illustrated by studies on HEL and its peptides, N-C, LII and LIII. The response to HEL is under Ir gene control and it is possible to demonstrate T cell proliferation and generation of T$_H$ cells to HEL in responding strains following priming by either the N-C peptide, or the LII peptide. When intact HEL is used for priming, it is found that T$_H$ activity is triggered

Fig. 13.12 Antigen recognition by B cells and T cells. Animals were immunized with the hapten 2,4 DNP coupled to mycobacteria (Myc-2,4 DNP). Their T and B cell responses to four related antigens was assessed. Myc-4-NP and Myc-2,4,6 TNP are recognized by both T and B cells. Myc-2,6-DNP is recognized poorly by T and B cells, indicating the importance of the 4-NP group in recognition. Using a spacer molecule, ala.gly.gly between the carrier and 2,4-DNP hapten allows antibody binding but does not stimulate T cells.

antigen	Myc-2, 4 DNP	Myc-4NP	Myc-2,4,6 TNP	Myc-2,6 DNP	Myc-spacer 2,4 DNP
T cell response	++++	+++	+++	weak	–
B cell response	+++	+++	+++	weak	++++

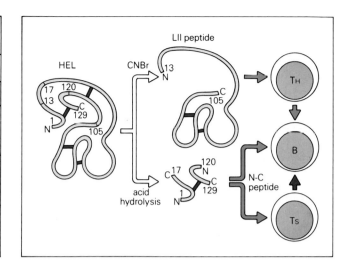

	delayed hyper-sensitivity to		antibody to	
	PLL		DNP	
	strain 2	strain 13	strain 2	strain 13
1 PLL-DNP → normal	+	−	+	−
2 BSA-PLL-DNP → normal	+	+	+	+
3 BSA-PLL-DNP → BSA tolerant	+	−	+	−

Fig. 13.13 Holes in the repertoire of T cell responses.
Strain 2 and strain 13 guinea pigs were immunized with the antigens shown and the T_D cell response measured by delayed hypersensitivity to poly-L-lysine (PLL), and the T_H cell response measured by the ability to cooperate with B cells in the production of antibody to DNP. 1. Strain 13 animals do not respond to PLL or DNP whereas strain 2 do, suggesting a hole in the functional T cell repertoire. 2. The lack of antibody response can be bypassed for the T_H cells by adding a BSA carrier to the PLL-DNP. 3. If the animal is tolerant to BSA the BSA-PLL-DNP no longer stimulates the T_H cells, confirming that bypass is via the new BSA carrier. It is not certain whether the hole in the T cell repertoire is at the point of education, presentation or in the antigen receptor.

predominantly by epitopes on the LII peptide (Fig. 13.14). Mice of the $H2^b$ haplotype do not develop this pattern of reactivity indicating a hole in the functional T cell repertoire. Studies by Sercarz and colleagues have revealed that the non-responsiveness of certain mouse strains to HEL is due to the development of overriding antigen-specific T suppression. These T-suppressors are generated by the N-C peptide region of HEL. Responder strains primed by N-C peptide develop some T_H for HEL while non-responder strains subjected to the same immunization develop T-suppressors. Therefore the pattern of overall responsiveness in a particular mouse strain may reflect selective induction of either T_H or T_S.

Cross-Reactive Idiotypes

Another interesting feature of the response to HEL is that following priming with HEL in appropriate strains, 70-95% of the antibody appears to be directed against the N-C peptide and is of a predominant idiotype. This form of dominant idiotype expression has been noted in response to many antigens and are called cross-reactive idiotypes. Figure 13.15 shows the distribution patterns of responsiveness to simple antigens which suggests that idiotype expression is linked to the Ig heavy chain haplotype. However, it is clear that the association between haplotype and idiotype is not complete: cross-reactive idiotype can be expressed on antibodies directed against different epitopes. In other words, the presence of a cross-reactive idiotype on an antibody does not necessarily reflect amino acid sequence identity at the antigen binding site.

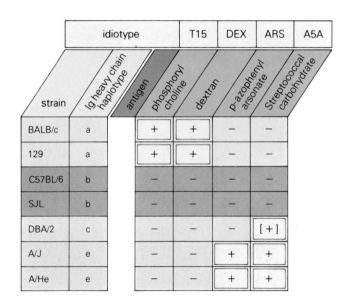

Fig. 13.14 Immune response to hen egg white lysozyme (HEL). The structure of HEL is shown with disulphide bonds in red. Certain amino acids are marked. The molecule can be cleaved by acid hydrolysis to yield an N-C peptide or by CNBr to yield a large peptide, LII. The LII peptide is recognized by T_H cells which give help to B cells. B cells recognize a determinant on the N-C peptide. T_S cells also recognize the N-C peptide so that the antibody response results from the balance between help and suppression. (Incidentally H-2^a high responder animals have T cells which recognize LII but no T_S recognizing N-C, whereas H-2^b low responders have high numbers of T_S and few T_H.)

strain	Ig heavy chain haplotype	T15 — phosphoryl choline	DEX — dextran	ARS — p-azophenyl arsonate	A5A — streptococcal carbohydrate
BALB/c	a	+	+	−	−
129	a	+	+	−	−
C57BL/6	b	−	−	−	−
SJL	b	−	−	−	−
DBA/2	c	−	−	−	[+]
A/J	e	−	−	+	+
A/He	e	−	−	+	+

Fig. 13.15 Cross-reactive idiotypes. The four main idiotypes to four different antigens in different strains of mice. These idiotypes appear to be linked to the Ig heavy chain locus. In general, each idiotype is present in mice of only one heavy chain haplotype. Sometimes however, the idiotype may be found in a different haplotype strain also, such as the A5A idiotype detectable in DBA/2. The A5A idiotype is present in lower amounts than in Ig^e strains and it is thought that either (a) the shape of the A5A idiotype has been generated on a protein with a different sequence to that of the A/J strain or (b) mutation and recombination generated the A5A amino acid sequence from a different germ line gene than in the Ig^e haplotype strains.

The occurrence of particular cross-reactive idiotypes in particular strains may represent a genetic disposition to make particular antibodies and as such is the opposite of a hole in the repertoire. The function of cross-reactive idiotypes is unclear but they may play a role in immunoregulation perhaps by being sites on antibody molecules or B cell immunoglobulin receptors which are recognized and modulated by idiotype-specific T-helper cells or idiotype-specific T-suppressor cells.

NON-MHC IMMUNE RESPONSE GENES

The responses to many antigens are under polygenic control. High or low responsiveness to a complex antigen could arise in many ways; through macrophages, T cells or B cells. Biozzi noted that within an outbred mouse colony some mice were high responders, in terms of antibody production, to erythrocyte antigens whereas other mice were low responders to these antigens. Following selective inbreeding of high responder mice and separate inbreeding of low responder mice Biozzi had, after twenty generations, established two strains of mice; one producing a high response to erythrocyte antigens the other producing a low response. The differences between the two strains is attributed to at least ten genes, some of which affect macrophage functions. The high responder Biozzi mice present the antigen on the surface of the presenting cell for a longer time than the low responder strain. The macrophages of the low responders appear to

be highly efficient at taking up the antigen and degrading it within the lysosomes (Fig. 13.16). This high lysosomal activity in the low responder mice also renders them less susceptible to intracellular parasites.

Resistance or susceptibility to *Leishmania donovani*, *Salmonella typhimurium* and *Mycobacterium bovis* appears to map to a gene locus on chromosome 1 of the mouse. Thus the genes Lsh, Ity and Bcg, which determine innate responsiveness to these respective infectious agents, may be identical. Resistance to *Leishmania donovani* appears to be linked to macrophage function.

Therefore although the MHC has been shown to play a role in determining the course of viral and some bacterial infections it is apparent that resistance to some parasites and some bacteria is either wholly controlled by some non H-2 linked genes or by H-2 and non-H-2 linked genes.

GENETICALLY IMMUNODEFICIENT MOUSE STRAINS

B Cell Defects
CBA/N mice carry an X-linked B cell defect manifested in the inability to respond to certain T-independent antigens such as TNP-Ficoll. These mice may have a B cell maturational defect and lack a subset of B cells bearing all three of the Lyb antigens (cell surface markers specific for B cells). B cells bearing Lyb 3, 5, 7 alloantigens have been shown to be those that respond to TNP-Ficoll. CBA/N mice have also been shown to lack a clonable B cell population (Fig. 13.17). Interestingly, Wiskott-Aldrich patients (an X-linked disease) are also incapable of responding to some polysaccharide antigens and they may also lack a B cell subset. Therefore, non-responsiveness to a given antigen could in some cases be attributed not only to overriding T_S, or lack of T_H, but also to lack of a relevant B cell subset.

There is some evidence which suggests that B cells are sensitive to some non-specific T cell factors. A T cell replacing factor (TRF) has been found in the supernatants

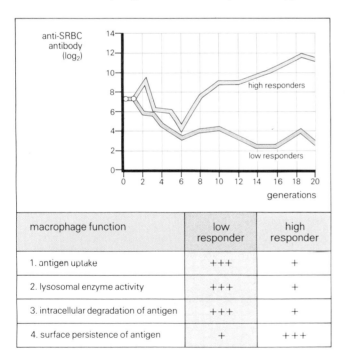

macrophage function	low responder	high responder
1. antigen uptake	+++	+
2. lysosomal enzyme activity	+++	+
3. intracellular degradation of antigen	+++	+
4. surface persistence of antigen	+	+++

Fig. 13.16 Macrophage functions in high and low responder mice. Mice giving high responses and low responses to sheep red blood cells (a complex multideterminate antigen) were inbred over twenty successive generations to produce separate high and low responder strains – Biozzi mice. As shown in the table, the low responder strain processes antigen in the macrophages faster than the high responder strain.

		CBA/N	normal
antibody response	poly I:C	–	+
	poly I:C-BSA	+	+
spleen (B) cell colony formation from 5×10^4 cells	spontaneous	0	49
	LPS	0	248
Lyb5 positive spleen cells		0%	30%

Fig. 13.17 Genetic defects of CBA/N mice.
Antibody response. CBA/N mice are unable to respond to the Tind antigen, poly I:C, but can recognize the antigen when it is coupled to a T-dependent carrier, BSA.
Spleen cell colony formation. CBA/N spleen cells (5×10^4) fail to produce colonies in culture spontaneously, or when stimulated with LPS. They appear to lack a subset of B cells carrying the Lyb5 allogeneic marker.

of suitably stimulated murine spleen cell cultures. TRF can be shown to overcome the usual MHC-restricted interaction of T and B cells. Recently a mouse strain DBA/2Ha has been described which is unable to respond to TRF since its B cells lack a receptor for it. This has been shown to be an X-linked disorder (Fig. 13.18). Another mouse strain which expresses a B cell function abnormality is the C3H/Hej mouse. These mice do not respond to the lipid A extract of LPS but do respond to the lipoproteins. Functionally this defect results in a greater than 1000-fold reduction in the number of B cell precursors which respond to LPS. The lack of responsiveness to LPS has been attributed to the lack of a relevant receptor for LPS on the surface of the C3H/Hej B cell.

	♂ response		♀ response	
BALB/c		+		+
DBA/2Ha		−		−
BALB/c(♀)×DBA/2Ha(♂)		+		+
DBA/2Ha(♀)×BALB/c(♂)		−		+

Fig. 13.18 TRF receptor defect in DBA/2Ha mice. Male and female mice were assayed for their response to T cell replacing factor (TRF). Male (XY) and female (XX) BALB/c mice respond to the factor, whereas neither male nor female DBA/2Ha mice do. Offspring of crosses between these responder and non-responder strains were tested. If BALB/c females are crossed with DBA/2Ha males both male and female offspring respond, whereas in the reciprocal cross only the females respond. This implies that a gene on the DBA/2Ha X chromosome is defective. In the F_1 mice those animals which have at least one normal BALB/c X chromosome can respond.

Models of Autoimmune Disease

Several animal models of autoimmunity exist which partly mimic human diseases. The obese strain chicken is perhaps the best available animal model of Hashimoto's thyroiditis in man (see 'Autoimmunity and Autoimmune

defect	strain(s) affected
thymic epithelium	NZB × NZW (F_1)
thymic hormone levels	NZB
pre-T cells	NZB
T cell immunoregulation	NZB, MRL/lpr
IL-2 levels	MRL/lpr
generation of non-specific suppression	NZB × NZW (F_1)
tolerance induction	NZB, NZB × NZW (F_1)
B cells	NZB
DNA repair	NZB

Fig. 13.19 Defects in genetically autoimmune mice.

Disease') and a rat strain has been described which develops a disease resembling juvenile onset diabetes.

Perhaps the best studied models of autoimmunity have been those spontaneously arising in mice. The NZB, NZB×NZW F1 and MRL/lpr mice are animal models of Coomb's positive haemolytic anaemia, systemic lupus erythematosus and rheumatoid arthritis respectively. These animals have a variety of disorders and regulatory disturbances due to the spontaneous occurrence of autoimmunity (Fig. 13.19). However, no single convincing cause or genetic characteristic has yet been identified and studies in recombinant inbred strains derived from one NZB parent and one normal parent have clearly shown that there is no direct linkage of the disease to the MHC.

DEVELOPMENT OF THE GENES OF THE IMMUNE SYSTEM

The immune system of vertebrates has apparently evolved more rapidly than the defence systems of invertebrates although nearly all multicellular animals show at least some ability to recognize self and non-self. These developments have been accompanied by, and based on, radiation within the different groups of molecules serving immunological functions, namely the immunoglobulins, the complement system and the MHC antigens. It was suggested in 'Complement' that the classical pathway complement system arose from the more primitive system ('The Archaeo-complement System') in response to the need for antigen-antibody reactions to activate inflammatory reactions. This idea is based on the overall similarity of the classical and alternative reaction pathways and in structural similarities between their components (Fig. 13.20). The components seem to have arisen by duplication followed by divergence of the two copies. Divergent pairs of proteins can lie on the same chromosome as is the case with C2 and factor B or on different chromosomes as occurs with C3 and C4.

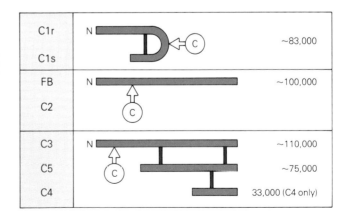

Fig. 13.20 Molecular families: complement. Three families of complement molecules are shown. Cleavage points (C) and approximate molecular weights of each type of chain given. Members of each family are activated by cleavage at the same points and structural homologies imply that they have arisen by gene duplication. FD, a serine esterase, may be related to C1r and C1s. (It is thought that C6 and C7 are related and form another family.)

Fig. 13.21 Products of H-2 loci.
Families of molecules are associated with the H-2 complex. This diagram shows chromosome 17 which contains the H-2 and Qa loci. The products of the genes are shown inserted in a cell membrane. Class 1 molecules (K,D,L,R,Qa,Tla) are 44K MW peptides and are associated with β_2-microglobulin (β_2M, the 12 K MW protein which is encoded on chromosome 2). Class 2 molecules (I-A, I-E) have two peptides, both of which traverse the membrane. Class 3 molecules – a term used for MHC-associated complement components – include the tandem alleles for C4 (Ss, Slp) and FB and C2 (not shown).

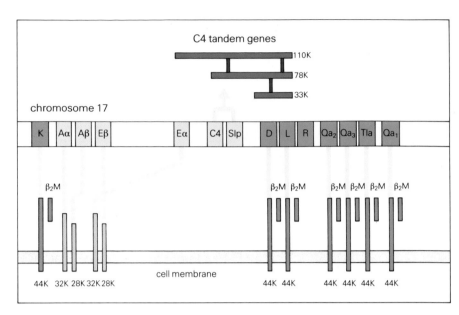

The immunoglobulins present evidence of a different kind of gene duplication. Here it is supposed that gene duplication in a single primordial domain gene led to the development of the first immunoglobulin chain, with further duplication on the separate chromosomes to produce heavy chains, kappa chains and lambda chains. This has permitted independent diversification of heavy and light chains with the advantages of higher antigen combining site diversity which this entails. All the different genes involved in the formation of the variable and constant regions provide excellent examples of gene replication and diversification on a grand scale. The primordial domain gene was presumably involved in functions of recognition since β_2-microglobulin, which also has amino acid and structural homology with immunoglobulin domains, is associated with all MHC class 1 antigens, the other major recognition arm of the immune system (See 'MHC' Fig. 4.23). It is easy to see the advantages inherent in the great diversity of immunoglobulins but it is more difficult to envisage what advantages arise from the enormous polymorphism and diversity of the MHC gene products. Here again the different classes of MHC antigen have probably arisen by gene duplication (Fig. 13.21). Even between different species there has been no change in the overall structure and length of the MHC class 1 molecules while there have been a large number of amino acid changes (Fig. 13.22).

Evidence of the rate of diversification of the MHC can be derived from the bm mutants mentioned earlier. By estimating the amount of mutation required to generate this number of mutants in the number of mice tested it appears that the MHC has the greatest rate of mutational diversification of any set of genes so far studied. If the T cell's antigen receptor were coded for by genes of the MHC as was once suggested one could see the advantages of polymorphism within this region by analogy with the diversity of the immunoglobulin genes, but this is not the case.

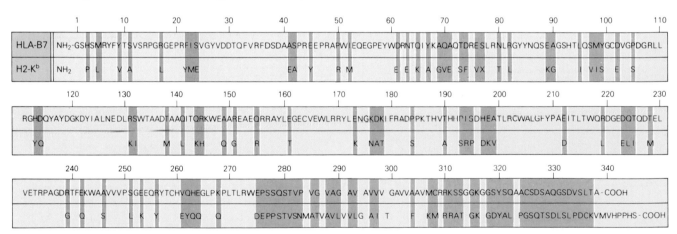

Fig. 13.22. Comparison of HLA and H-2 class 1 molecules. The amino acid sequences of HLA-B7 and H-2K^b are given. The amino acids are represented by single letters with the NH$_2$-terminal on the left. Positions at which the amino acids differ are shown in red. There is a great degree of structural homology between these molecules: in particular the finding that few gaps need be introduced into either sequence to demonstrate homology is significant. There appears to be greater constraints on the evolutionary development of the extracellular, N terminal portion of the molecule than on the C terminal portion. (Residues are in the single-letter code: A,Ala; B,Asx; C,Cys; D,Asp; E,Glu; F,Phe; G,Gly; H,His; I,Ile; K,Lys; L,Leu; M,Met; N,Asn; P,Pro; Q,Gln; R,Arg; S,Ser; T,Thr; V,Val; W,Trp; Y,Tyr; and Z, PCA).

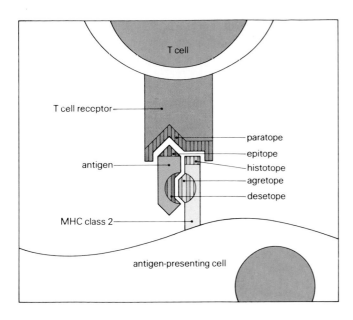

Fig. 13.23 Antigen presentation – a hypothesis. T cells recognize antigen in association with MHC class 2 antigens. The advantages of having different MHC Class 2 antigens, that is, polymorphism can be explained by assuming that the part of the MHC antigen (the agretope) which combines with the antigen (the part termed the desetope) associates preferentially with some antigens.

What then is the advantage of polymorphism within the MHC? Although MHC genes do not form the T cell's antigen receptor they are still associated with T cell mediated recognition. This has led to the suggestion that there is an advantage in having a diversity of MHC products: different MHC proteins might be better than others at presenting different antigens to T cells since in the associate recognition theory the T cells recognize an MHC/Ag combination. This could occur in one of two ways; either (a) a particular MHC/Ag combination is recognized more effectively by T cells or (b) a particular MHC protein associates more effectively with particular antigens (Fig. 13.23). A similar explanation could be advanced for polymorphism in the MHC class 1 antigens. However, another theory considers the advantages of MHC polymorphism at a population level. The idea is that with a polymorphic MHC, self/non self recognition systems are based on different molecular structures in different individuals. This means that 'the perfect pathogen' cannot exist since an organism which evades the immune system in one individual will not do so in another (see 'MHC'). The polymorphism of the immune system is represented schematically in figure 13.24.

One consequence of this great diversity of molecules is that the MHC and other systems can be used to identify individuals genealogically and demographically, a point at which immunology starts to impinge on a number of other scientific disciplines.

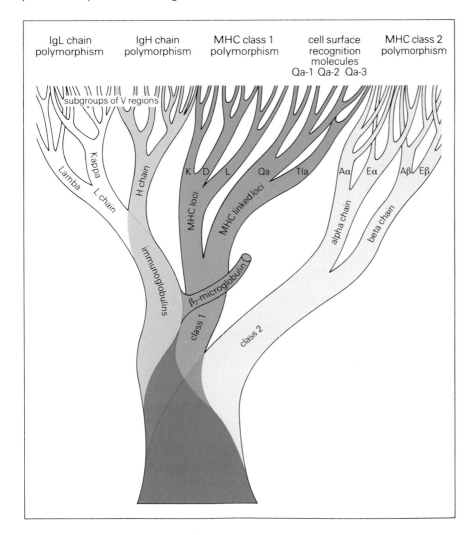

Fig. 13.24 Polymorphism of immune recognition molecules. This diagram provides a schematic analogy for the generation of the molecules involved in immune recognition and cellular interactions. Note the associations of β_2-microglobulin with MHC class 1 molecules and the association of the alpha and beta chains which go to make up the class 2 molecules (Ig heavy and light chains also associate of course.) The enormous degree of polymorphism ensures that in an outbred population every individual's immune system is different.

FURTHER READING

Benjamin D.C. & Berzofsky J.A. et al (1984) The antigenic structure of proteins: a reappraisal. *Annu. Rev. Immunol.* **2,** 67.

Heber-Katz E., Hansburg D. & Schwartz R.H. (1983) The Ia molecule of the antigen-presenting cell plays a critical role in immune response gene regulation of T cell activation. *J. Mol. Cell. Immunol.* **1,** 3.

Jareway C.A. (1983) Immune response genes, the problem of the non-responder. *J. Mol. Cell. Immunol.* **1,** 15.

Krco C.J. & David C.S. (1981) Genetics of the Immune Response: a survey. *C.R.C. Critical Reviews in Immunology* **1,** 211.

Longo D.L., Matis L.A. & Schwartz R.H. (1981) Insights into immune response gene function from experiments with chimeric animals. *C.R.C. Critical Reviews in Immunology* **2,** 83.

Marchalonis J.J., Vasta G.R., Warr G. & Barker W.C. (1984) Probing the boundaries of the extended immunoglobin family of recognition molecules: jumping domains, convergence and minigenes. *Immunol. Today* **5,** 133.

14 Development of the Immune System

An efficient immune system depends upon the interaction of many cellular and humoral components which develop at different rates during foetal and early life. Many of the cells involved in the immune response are derived from undifferentiated, haemopoietic stem cells (HSC) and are thought to differentiate into the various cell lineages under the influence of different microenvironmental factors (Fig. 14.1). In birds the stem cells originate from blood islands within the yolk sac and embryo and later in the bone marrow. In mammals the adult bone marrow is thought to provide a continuous source of stem cells and most, or all of the other cells involved in the immune response.

LYMPHOID CELLS

Lymphocytes develop in the primary lymphoid organs, T cells in the thymus and B cells in the bursa of Fabricius or mammalian equivalent. They then migrate to the secondary lymphoid tissues where they can respond to antigen.

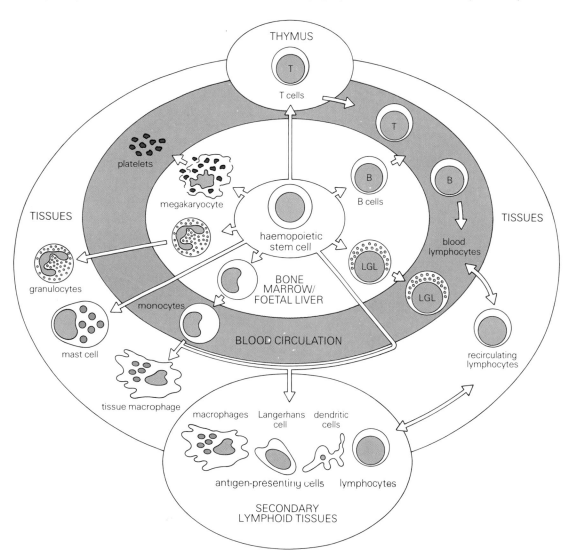

Fig. 14.1 Origin of cells of the immune system. All of these cells arise from the haemopoietic stem cell. Platelets produced by megakaryocytes are released into the circulation, granulocytes pass from the circulation into the tissues. Mast cells are identifiable in all tissues. B cells mature in the foetal liver and bone marrow in mammals while T cells mature in the thymus. The origin of the large granular lymphocytes (LGL) is uncertain. Both lymphocytes and monocytes (which develop into macrophages) can recirculate through secondary lymphoid tissue. Langerhans cells and dendritic cells act as antigen-presenting cells in secondary lymphoid tissue.

T Cells

The thymic rudiment develops from the third (and in some species fourth) pharyngeal pouch as an outpushing of the gut endoderm and then becomes seeded with blood-borne lymphoid stem cells. Few stem cells appear to be needed to give rise to the repertoire of the mature T cells with diverse antigen binding specificities. Migration of stem cells into the thymus is not a random process. In birds, at least, it has been shown that they enter in two or possibly three waves. This has been demonstrated using chicken and quail chimaeras (Fig. 14.2). Attraction factors released by the thymus have been proposed to explain the immigration of thymic stem cells. Once there the stem cells begin to differentiate into thymocytes under

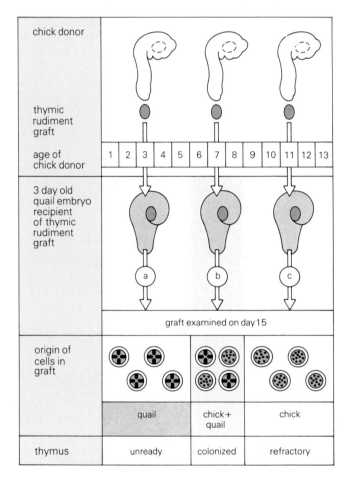

Fig. 14.2 Stem cell colonization of the chick thymus. The thymic rudiment from a chick embryo of different ages was grafted onto a 3 day old quail embryo and examined later to determine the origin of cells in the thymus. Quail cells can be distinguished from chicken cells by the appearance of condensed chromatin in the resting cell. If the graft was less than 6 days old it had not yet become colonized with chick stem cell pre-T cells and on subsequent examination was found to contain quail cells only (a). If the graft was older than 8 days it had already been colonized with chick lymphocytes (c). Grafts transferred between day 6 and day 8 contain both chick and quail cells (b). The interpretation is that before 6 days the chick thymus is unready to receive stem cell pre-T cells. There follows a window of colonization after which (from day 8) the thymus becomes refractory to further colonization. Further studies indicate that there may be additional windows later in embryogenesis.

the influence of the thymic epithelial microenvironment. Whether or not the stem cells are precommitted to becoming T cells, that is, pre-T cells before they arrive in the thymus is controversial.

The thymocytes become organized into well-defined lobules forming a cortex and a medulla (see 'The Lymphoid System') where epithelial cells and bone marrow derived dendritic cells rich in MHC class 2 antigens are important in differentiation of the T lymphocytes (Fig. 14.3). Cortical cells represent 85 to 90% of the thymocytes whilst the remainder are medullary cells. Studies of their function and cell surface markers have indicated that cortical thymocytes are less mature than medullary thymocytes. It has been found that cortical cells are more sensitive to high levels of steroids *in vivo* and this may be reflected by the decrease in this cell population during pregnancy. Some cortical cells migrate to, and mature in, the medulla whilst others enter the circulation directly. These circulating thymus-derived cells (T lymphocytes) migrate to, and function in, the secondary lymphoid tissues.

T cell markers including enzymes, surface glycoproteins and receptors have been useful in defining the pathways of T cell differentiation both within the thymus and in the periphery. Some markers are lost while others are gained during differentiation. For example, Tdt (terminal deoxyribonucleotidyl transferase) is present in the stem cell (or pre T cell) and cortical cells, but cannot be detected on thymus medullary and peripheral lymphocytes. The classical marker for a human T cell, that is the receptor for sheep erythrocytes, develops early in the pathway of differentiation but is present on mature T cells. Like these receptors, the T3 glycoprotein is acquired relatively early in differentiation and maintained during maturation. It is likely that the T3 surface glycoprotein is involved in antigen recognition by T cells and their subsequent activation. Two other markers, T4 and T8, occur simultaneously on T cells expressing T3 but one or the other is lost during thymic differentiation. This irreversible loss of T4 or T8 may result in commitment of each cell to a particular function in the secondary lymphoid tissues (Fig. 14.4). Similar differentiation events occur in the mouse thymus (see 'Cells Involved in the Immune Response').

Thymic hormones or factors may play a role in the development of T cells in the thymus and their maintenance within the secondary lymphoid tissues. Figure 14.5 lists some of the better studied preparations and their properties. It seems likely that different hormones or factors act on T cells at different stages of their development. Whereas some may act within the thymus and induce thymic cell maturation, others could act at peripheral sites (ie. as true hormones). They have, in fact, been found in thymic epithelial cells and in the circulation where they decrease with age concomitantly with thymic atrophy. Many of the thymic factors or hormones have now been sequenced and synthesized. Since a number of endogenous pharmocologically active agents have been shown to have similar effects to thymic factors/hormones eg. cyclic AMP and epinephrine, their exact physiological relevance needs to be established. Addition of these factors to T lymphocytes *in vitro* causes maturation as determined by marker analyses and increased functional ability.

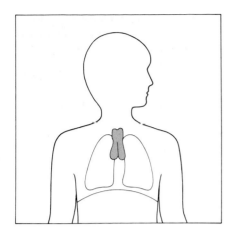

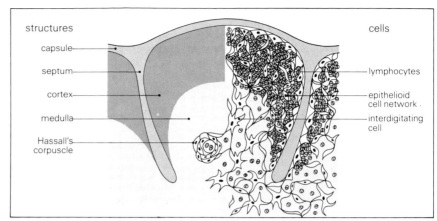

Fig. 14.3 The structure of a thymus lobule.

The thymus is an encapsulated organ divided into lobules by septa. The cortex contains densely packed dividing lymphocytes in a network of epithelioid cells which extends into the medulla. The medulla contains fewer lymphocytes, but there are more bone marrow-derived interdigitating cells. Note the close association of the developing lymphocytes with epithelial and interdigitating cells.

The function, if any, of the whorled structures termed Hassall's corpuscles is unknown.

Fig. 14.4 Human T cell differentiation.

The development of identifiable markers on human T cells is shown, including receptors (brown), enzymes (purple) and cell surface antigens (turquoise). The events which occur before the cells enter the thymus are less well defined. Receptors for IgM appear on some medullary cells and many peripheral T cells, whereas receptors for IgG are found only on some peripheral T cells. These receptors might be important in antibody-mediated immune regulation. Tdt (terminal deoxynucleotidyl transferase) is an enzyme present in pre T or thymic stem cells and is present in cortical but lost in medullary and peripheral cells. Acid phosphatase- a lysosomal enzyme (see 'Cells Involved in the Immune Response') is present in T cells throughout their differentiation. Several surface glycoproteins have been detected

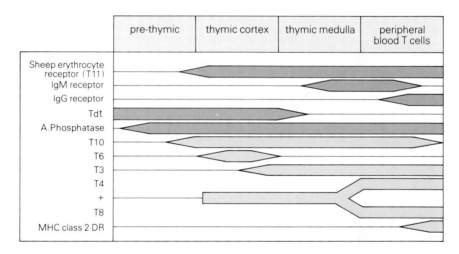

during differentiation. For example, the sheep erythrocyte receptor, T11, is one of the first surface antigens to appear during human T cell differentiation and is present on mature T cells. However, T6 appears to be restricted to cortical thymocytes. Mature peripheral T cells either have the T4 marker (helper cells) or the T8 marker (cytotoxic and suppressor cells), whereas thymocytes initially have both and lose one as they develop. T3 is thought to be associated with the T cell antigen receptor. DR is present on mature activated T cells.

Fig. 14.5 Thymic hormones and factors.

All preparations, except FTS, were originally extracted from bovine (cattle) thymus. FTS was derived from pig serum but has now been shown to be present in the thymus. (Ubiquitin, a 74 amino acid protein with a molecular weight of 8457, has similar properties to the other factors and at one time was thought to be a thymic hormone; however it is present not only in thymus but in many other animal and plant tissues, bacteria and yeasts). Preparations marked (*) have been synthesized artificially.

name	chemistry	comment
Thymosin (fraction 5)*	α, β and γ polypeptides α-1-sequenced- 28 amino acids MW −3,108	some produced in thymic epithelial cells
Thymopoietin 1 and 2	sequenced: 49 amino acids MW −5,562	produced only in thymus, activity in pentapeptide (TP-5) *
Thymic humoral factor (THF)	31 amino acids MW 3,220	partially sequenced
Thymostimulin (TP-1)	group of peptides	least well characterized
Facteur thymique serique (FTS)*	9 amino acids	present in serum, disappears after thymectomy

B Cells

In the chicken, primary B cell lymphopoiesis occurs in a discrete lympho-epithelial organ, the bursa of Fabricius. The bursal rudiment develops as an outpushing of the hindgut endoderm and becomes infiltrated with blood-borne stem cells. Studies on chicken/quail chimaeras have indicated that there is a window for the immigration of cells between days 10 and 14 (see 'Evolution of Immunity'). Pyroninophylic cells, the putative stem cells, are seen in contact with epithelial cells. Bursal cell proliferation gives rise to the cortex and the medulla in each bursal follicle, which, like the thymus lobules, may be seeded by one or a few stem cells (Fig. 14.6).

Mammals do not have a specific discrete organ for B cell lymphopoiesis, instead these cells develop directly from lymphoid stem cells in the haemopoietic tissue of the foetal liver (Fig. 14.7) from eight to nine weeks of gestation in man and by about fourteen days in mice. The function of the foetal liver as a site of B cell production wanes and the site of production transfers into the bone marrow where it is continued into adult life. This is also true of the other haemopoietic stem cells. The microenvironment of the foetal liver may be important in the differentiation of B cells. The characteristic marker of the B lymphocyte lineage is the possession of immunoglobulins which act as the cell surface antigen receptor. Lymphoid stem cells (probably expressing Tdt) proliferate and differentiate and following immunoglobulin gene rearrangements (see 'The Generation of Antibody Diversity') pre-B cells emerge which express new heavy chains in the cytoplasm (Fig. 14.8). Allelic exclusion of maternal or paternal immunoglobulin genes has already occurred by this time. The proliferating pre-B cells are thought to give rise to smaller pre-B cells which may be found in the foetal spleen. On synthesis of light chains, which may be either of κ or λ type but not both, the B cell assembles surface immunoglobulins (sIg) and each B cell is then committed to the antigen binding specificity of the sIg for the rest of its life. Thus one B cell can only ever make one specific antibody and this forms the basis of the clonal selection theory for antibody production. Following their production in the foetal liver B cells migrate and function

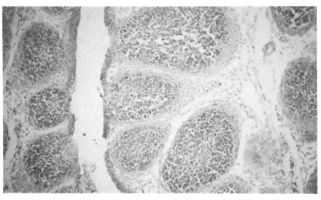

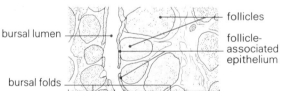

Fig. 14.6 Section of a bursa showing B lymphocytes developing in follicles. Like the foetal liver, the bursa is a site of haemopoiesis as well as myelopoiesis. H&E stain, ×50.

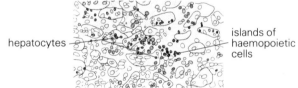

Fig. 14.7 Section of foetal liver showing islands of haemopoietic cells. These cells include those giving rise to B lymphocytes. H&E stain.

Fig. 14.8 B cell differentiation: expression of immunoglobulins. B cells differentiate into plasma cells from lymphoid stem cells. Only the final stage is antigen driven. The cellular location of immunoglobulin is shown in yellow. The genes coding for antibody are rearranged in the course of stem cell differentiation into pre-B cells. Pre-B cells express cytoplasmic μ chains only. The immature B cell has surface IgM and the mature B cell other classes of Ig. On antigen stimulation the B cell proliferates and develops into a plasma cell. The occurrence of Tdt, Ia, DR antigens and the receptors (R) for Fc of IgG and C3 are shown.

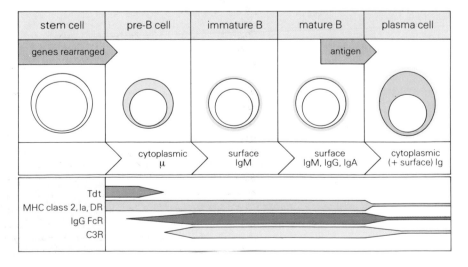

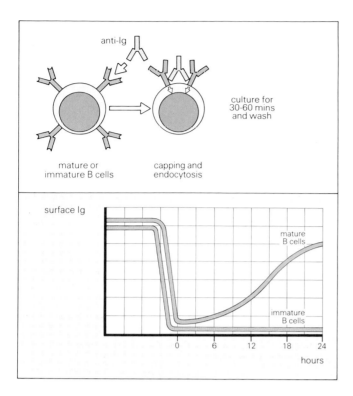

Fig. 14.9 Differentiation of B cells:differential modulation of sIg on mature and immature B Cells. Mature (adult) and immature (neonatal) B cells are incubated (at 37°C) together with antibody to their surface immunoglobulin (anti-Ig) for 30-60 mins; this causes capping of the surface immunoglobulin and its internalization by endocytosis. The cells are then washed free of anti-Ig. As shown in the graph, mature B cells resynthesize their surface immunoglobulin over the following 24 hours, but immature B cells do not.

in the secondary lymphoid tissues. Early immigrants into foetal lymph nodes (17 weeks in man) are sIgM +ve and also carry a T cell marker (T1 – 69KD) (Ly1 +ve and sIgM +ve in mice). This B cell phenotype is present in small numbers in secondary follicles of adult lymph nodes. Following maturation, the B cells, on antigen stimulation, can develop into antibody forming plasma cells. Surface Ig is usually lost by this stage since its function as a receptor is finished. Immature B cells acquire Fc receptors for IgG and C3 receptors which decrease in quantity during differentiation. Immature B cells respond differently to antigens than mature B cells. Treatment of both mature and immature B cells with anti-Ig antibodies or antigen results in loss of the surface Ig by capping and endocytosis. After washing the B cells to remove anti-Ig, mature, but not immature, cells resynthesize surface Ig in culture (Fig. 14.9). This property of surface Ig modulation explains why immature B cells can be easily switched off resulting in central tolerance.

DEVELOPMENT OF CLASS DIVERSITY

It is presumed that class diversity in the antibody response evolved to cope in different ways and at different anatomical sites with the multitude of non-self antigens.

Mature plasma cells produce only one class of antibody thus immature B cells making only IgM are switched to other classes before reaching terminal differentiation as a plasma cell. A model for class switching within one clone is shown in figure 14.10. Some of the progeny of the immature B cells synthesize antibodies of other Ig classes including IgG and IgA. Further differentiation results in synthesis of surface IgD – an antibody class that is almost exclusively found on B cell membranes. All three classes of surface Ig on the same cell will have the same antigen specificity, that is to say that they express the same V region genes. From this point on in clonal differentiation antigen drives the cell into a fully mature plasma cell and/or a memory cell. Since there is a similar sequence of sIg expression on B cells of vertebrates raised in gnotobiotic (with a known and limited microbial flora) environments it seems likely that class diversity develops independently of extrinsic antigen. Furthermore, it is probable that class switching can occur independently of T cells, although these may play a significant role in switching to IgA and IgE. It is probable that all class switching events have already taken place before the B cell matures into a plasma cell. The occurrence of different classes of Ig on the surface of a single cell is probably related to the persistence of the different antibodies on their surface and the existence of long lived messenger RNA for the different classes within the cell.

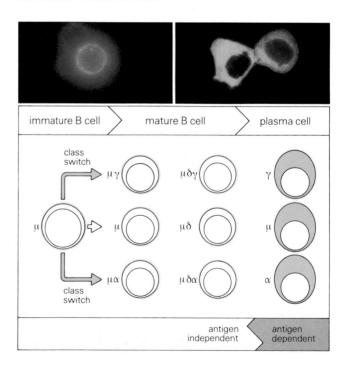

Fig. 14.10 B cell differentiation: class diversity. Immature B cells produce IgM only, but mature B cells can express more than one cell surface antibody, since mRNA and cell surface immunoglobulin remain after a class switch. IgD is also expressed during clonal maturation. Maturation can occur in the absence of antigen , but the development into plasma cells, which have little cell surface, but much cytoplasmic immunoglobulin requires antigen and (usually) T cell help. The photographs show B cells stained for surface IgM (green, left) and plasma cells stained for cytoplasmic IgM and IgG (green and red, right). IgM is stained with fluorescent anti-μ chain, and IgG with rhodaminated anti-γ chain.

The sequence of appearance of immunoglobulin classes on the cell surface is reflected in detection of serum immunoglobulin in the human foetus and neonate. Figure 14.11 shows that IgM is synthesized before birth whilst IgG and IgA begin to appear around birth. Serum IgG does not reach adult levels until one to two years after birth, whilst IgA takes even longer.

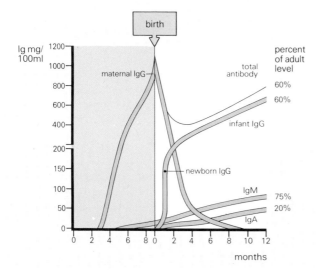

Fig. 14.11 Immunoglobulins in the serum of the foetus and newborn child. IgG in the foetus and newborn infant is derived solely from the mother. This maternal IgG has disappeared by the age of 9 months when the infant is synthesizing its own IgG. The neonate produces its own IgM and IgA: these classes cannot cross the placenta. By the age of 12 months the infant produces 60% of its adult level of IgG, 75% of its adult IgM and 20% of its adult IgA level.

DEVELOPMENT OF ANTIBODY DIVERSITY

There are tens of thousands of natural antigenic shapes to which antibodies are made and since one B cell can make only one antigen-specific antibody many B cells with specific antibody receptors have to be generated from B lymphocyte stem cells during development. Thus multiple V_H and V_L genes have to be expressed on different cells. It is thought that antigen-specific B cells appear in a programmed sequence (presumably through initial expression of germ-line genes) and that later specificities are due to the expression of different hypervariable region genes with other, diversity genes. Figure 14.12 shows the sequential appearance of antigen binding cells with specificity for keyhole-limpet haemocyanin, (T, G)-A--L and sheep erythrocytes in the chicken bursa of Fabricius. The same temporal sequence is found in chickens of different strains and occurs after the sIgM-positive B cells appear, when they are proliferating within the bursa. The development of antibody responses in the neonatal rat as assessed by the measurement of serum antibodies to different antigens also shows a sequential appearance of responsiveness (Fig. 14.13). Antibody production, as distinct from antigen recognition by B cells, is dependent on both T cells and macrophages.

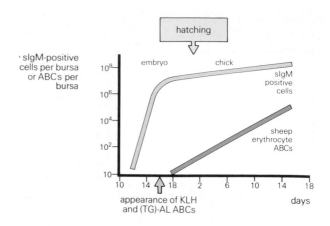

Fig. 14.12 Sequence of appearance of B cells and antigen binding cells (ABCs) in the avian bursa of Fabricius. Cells carrying surface IgM (sIgM positive) are detectable by day 12 of incubation and increase at a exponential rate consonant with a generation time of about 10 hours. An abrupt change in growth rate occurs near the time of hatching corresponding to the onset of substantial seeding to the periphery. Cells binding keyhole-limpet haemocyanin (KLH) and (T,G)-A--L appear by day 16. Cells binding sheep erythrocytes are not detectable in significant numbers before the 18th day of incubation, after which they increase at a rate significantly different from the total sIgM-positive population. This chronological appearance of sIgM positive and antigen binding cells is consistent with a programmed sequence of appearance of B cells with different antibody specificities during embryogenesis.

age (days)	Brucella	SRBC	DRBC	KLH	SSS$_{111}$
0	4.7	0	0	0	0
1	5.3	0	0	0	0
2		0	0		
3	7.3	2.9	0	0	0
4		5.4	0		
7			0.6	0	0
10-11			3.0	7.7	0
14-15			4.3	10.4	16%
20-22					70%
28					88%

Fig. 14.13 Development of immune responsiveness. The antibody responses to five different antigens, *Brucella abortis,* sheep red blood cells (SRBC), donkey red blood cells (DRBC), keyhole limpet haemocyanin (KLH) and type III pneumococcal polysaccharide (SSS$_{III}$) were measured after injection into neonatal rats of different ages. Responses to the first four antigens are expressed as $\log_2$ antibody titres. The response to SSS$_{III}$ is expressed as a percentage of animals responding. Blank boxes indicates not tested.

DEVELOPMENT OF MONONUCLEAR PHAGOCYTES AND ANTIGEN PRESENTING CELLS

Mononuclear phagocytes develop from haemopoietic foetal tissues in the liver, spleen and bone marrow and later in the adult bone marrow. Monoblasts differentiate into promonocytes and finally into blood-borne monocytes which are thought to represent a replacement pool for tissue fixed macrophages. Whereas the phagocytic function of the reticular endothelial system develops early in foetal life, the antigen presentation function develops somewhat later. For example, neonatal rats fail to make a normal antibody response to sheep red blood cells, unless they are also injected with adult macrophages (Fig. 14.14).

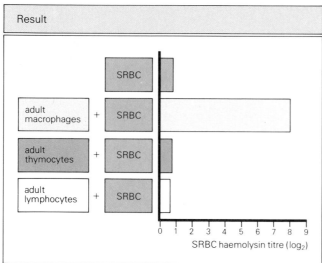

Fig. 14.14 Development of macrophage function: antigen processing and presentation. In this experiment neonatal rats are injected with sheep red blood cells and cells (macrophages, thymocytes or lymphocytes) from an adult of the same strain. The antibody response following each injection schedule is assayed and the results shown in the bar diagram. Neonatal rats injected with sheep red blood cells (SRBC) do not make an antibody response to this antigen. If the animals were given adult macrophages with the antigen, they could make a response. Neither adult thymocytes nor adult lymphocytes can perform this function. Thus neonatal macrophages are unable to present this antigen effectively.

THE COMPLEMENT SYSTEM

The complement system plays a role in protection against microorganisms and is particularly important as a

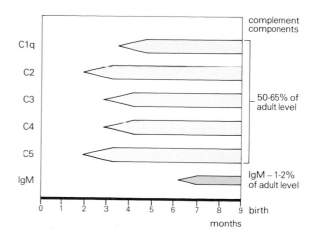

Fig. 14.15 Development of the complement system. The bar diagram shows the earliest times at which the components of the complement system can be detected in human foetal tissue. Most complement components reach more than 50% of their adult value by birth. By comparison endogenously produced immunoglobulin develops later.

mediator of antigen-antibody reactions. At least twenty distinct plasma proteins have been identified as belonging to this system. They appear during the development of the foetus, and are detected before circulating IgM antibodies (Fig. 14.15). They are present in the neonate at 50-60% of adult serum levels. The appearance of complement components before IgM synthesis probably reflects the fact that complement together with phagocytic cells provided the main protection of animals before the evolutionary development of antibodies. Thus ontogeny recapitulates phylogeny.

DEVELOPMENT OF NEUTROPHIL FUNCTIONS

Polymorphonuclear neutrophils (PMNs) are myeloid cells which develop from haemopoietic stem cells (as do other haemopoietic lineages). Myelopoiesis commences in the foetal liver from about six weeks of gestation in man and later in the spleen and bone marrow. After birth the normal bone marrow becomes the site of myelopoiesis. Stem cells develop into myeloblasts, myelocytes and finally blood-borne neutrophils, basophils and eosinophils. There is some evidence that neutrophil function as measured by phagocytosis and chemotaxis is lower in foetal life compared with adult life. This may be partly due to the lower opsonizing ability of the foetal serum (when measured using adult neutrophil phagocytes) as well as the intrinsically poorer phagocytic capabilities of the foetal PMNs.

In conclusion, we have described the development of many of the functional components of the immune system during foetal and neonatal life. Maternal IgG transmitted across the mammalian placenta and through suckling in some animal species plays an important role in protecting the developing animal until it acquires full immunological maturity.

14.7

FURTHER READING

Blaese R.M. (1975) Macrophages and the development of immune competence. In *The phagocytic cell in host resistance,* Bellanti J.A. & Dayton D.H. (eds.). Raven Press.

Forum on B cell ontogeny (1984) *Ann. Immunol.* (Inst. Pasteur) **135,** 220.

Le Douarin N.M., Dieterlen-Lievre F. & Oliver P.D. (1984) Ontogeny of primary lymphoid organs and lymphoid stem cells. *Am. J. Anatomy* **170,** 261.

Owen J.J.T. & Jenkinson E.J. (1984) Early events in T lymphocyte genesis in the fetal thymus. *Am.J. Anatomy* **170,** 301.

14.8

15 Evolution of Immunity

The study of the evolution of immune systems has been made possible by advances in comparative immunobiology, that is, comparison of the immune reactions occurring in different phylogenetic groups. This discussion will review the essential features of the immune systems of different phyla. The information provided so far (c. 1982) by phylogenetic studies has not revealed in great detail how the features of the sophisticated immune systems, exhibited in advanced creatures, have evolved from their primitive ancestors. What has become clear is the similar organization of different aspects of the immune response between phyla and the steadily increasing complexity and potentiality of the response, which attains its zenith in the vertebrates.

The evidence from comparative immunobiology has led to the abandonment of the notion that poikilothermic ('cold-blooded') vertebrates and invertebrates lack immune capabilities.

Figure 15.1 presents a simplified evolutionary tree of the animal kingdom and summarizes the immunopotentialities of the major vertebrate and invertebrate phyla. This shows that specific immune competence is not the prerogative of endothermic ('warm-blooded') vertebrates.

Coelomate animals are divided into two main evolutionary lines based principally on embryological differences. One line, embracing molluscs, annelids and arthropods, called the Protostomia, diverged early in evolution from the pathway (the Deuterostomia) that led to the echinoderms, tunicates and the vertebrates. It is somewhat paradoxical, therefore, that immunobiologists have until quite recently tended to concentrate on protostome phyla in searching for the origins of vertebrate immunity.

INVERTEBRATE IMMUNITY

The suggestion in figure 15.1 that immunocytes with functional similarities to mammalian T and B lymphocytes exist in several invertebrate phyla is speculative, but this approach does serve to focus attention on possible evolutionary origins of vertebrate cells possessing immunological activity.

Immunocytes
A variety of immunocyte types are found in the invertebrates, from the primitive amoebocytes of acoelomate phyla, through the blood leucocytes (haemocytes) and coelomocytes found in molluscs, annelids and arthropods (and also in early deuterostome groups), to the more lymphocyte-like cells seen for the first time in some echinoderms and tunicates. There is an early evolutionary trend of phagocytes, and other cells associated with the circulation, to aggregate into tissues.

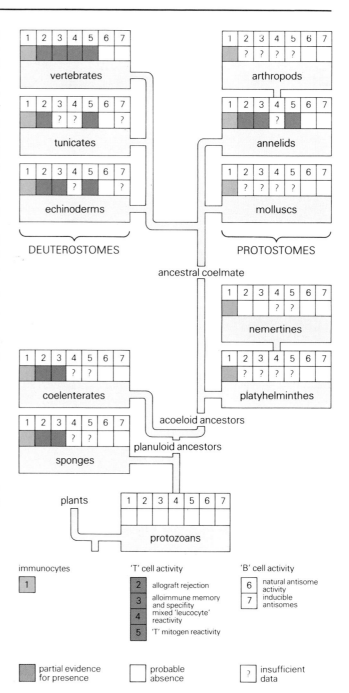

immunocytes

'T' cell activity

2	allograft rejection
3	alloimmune memory and specifity
4	mixed 'leucocyte' reactivity
5	'T' mitogen reactivity

'B' cell activity

6	natural antisome activity
7	inducible antisomes

partial evidence for presence   probable absence   insufficient data

Fig. 15.1 Immunopotentialities of vertebrate and invertebrate phyla. The numbered boxes represent immunocyte activity (1), aspects of 'T' cell activity (2-5) and antisome (similar to vertebrate opsonins eg. antibody and complement (C3b)) activity of 'B' cells (6, 7), all of which are observed in vertebrates. Because lymphocytes conforming to the type acting in vertebrate species do not occur in all phyla, 'T', 'B' and 'leucocyte' are apostrophied to emphasize that it is the functional activity which is being represented rather than the presence or absence of T and B cells per se.

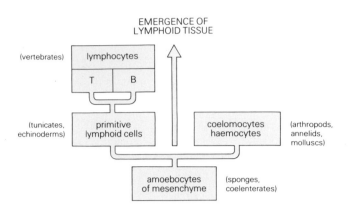

Fig. 15.2 Immunocyte evolution. The primitive defence cell of acoelomate creatures (eg. sponges, coelenterates) is the amoeboid mesenchymal cell. These evolved into the coelomocytes and haemocytes of arthropods, annelids and molluscs. A separate line of divergence for the amoebocytes can be traced to the primitive lymphoid cells of tunicates and echinoderms. These eventually developed, in vertebrate species, into T and B lymphocytes. Simple 'lymphoid' tissues can be seen to have emerged some time during the appearance of coelomate animals and to have developed into the multipotential tissues of vertebrates, comprised of T and B lymphocytes.

These tissues are here loosely termed 'lymphoid', although (certainly in lower forms) there is no firm evidence for homology with vertebrate lymphoid tissues (Fig. 15.2). The immunological potential of protostome leucocytes has been studied in more detail than has that of primitive amoebocytes of acoelomate phyla. For example, it has been found that annelid coelomocytes can transfer transplantation immunity and respond to putative T cell mitogens *in vitro*.

'Lymphoid' Tissues

Already at the protostomal level of evolution there is a tendency for immunocytes to develop within special cellular aggregations (eg. the haemal glands of earthworms, the white bodies and branchial spleens of certain molluscs, and the haemopoietic tissues of certain arthropods). Deuterostome invertebrates also possess aggregations of immunocytes within haemopoietic centres, such as the axial organ of echinoderms and the gill-associated lymph nodules of tunicates. Furthermore, immunocytes closely resembling vertebrate lymphocytes both morphologically and functionally are found in these creatures (eg. tunicate lymphocytes display mitogen and possibly mixed lymphocyte reactions). Within vertebrates the lymphoid system undergoes further differentiation, giving rise to distinct T and B cell subsets and to a variety of lymphoid tissues, all with specialized immune functions.

Cell-Mediated Immunity

Although there are still many gaps in our knowledge of invertebrate immunoevolution, primordial cell-mediated immunity, characterized by cytotoxic reactivity following allograft sensitization and by specifically inducible memory (defined as altered reactivity on secondary contact with the same alloantigens), has now been demonstrated in

parazoans (sponges), coelenterates, annelids and echinoderms. Allogeneic incompatibility, but isograft survival, has recently been demonstrated in the tropical sponge, *Callyspongia* (Fig. 15.3). Furthermore, in both this sponge and in the coelenterate, *Montipora*, second-set grafts applied within a few weeks of a primary reaction are destroyed in accelerated fashion, whereas third-party ('unrelated') grafts are often not. Whether alloimmune destruction and such short-term memory in these colonial invertebrates represent the presence of primordial T-equivalent functions, or simply reflect a capability analagous to T cell function related purely to the maintenance of colony specificity, remains uncertain.

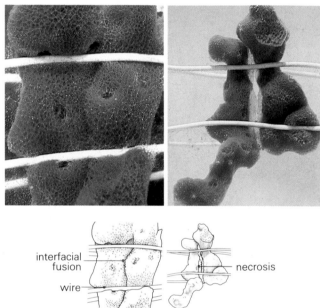

Fig. 15.3 Demonstration of cell-mediated immunity in sponges: allogeneic incompatibility and isogeneic compatibility. Two intact fingers of sponge *(Callyspongia)* from different colonies and two from the same colony are parabiosed (fused circulation) by being held together with vinyl-covered wire. The interfacial fusion between isogeneic parabionts (intracolony) persists indefinitely (left, ×0.5). Incompatibility between allogeneic parabionts (intercolony) results in a cytotoxic interaction: the soft tissue necrosis is clearly seen after 7-9 days (at 24-27°C) (right, ×0.25). Courtesy of Dr. W. H. Hildemann.

Allograft rejection has to date not been demonstrated in nemertines, molluscs or arthropods, presumably because members of each species tested express similar histocompatibility antigens. However, the ability of these phyla and also of the annelids to eliminate non-self material has been documented in xenograft experiments: all groups eliminate such foreign transplants although autografts survive indefinitely (Fig. 15.4). Echinoderms and tunicates have also been shown capable of rejecting body wall allografts (Fig. 15.5). Furthermore, second-set and third-party graft application has demonstrated short-term alloimmune memory in annelids and echinoderms, but the issue of specific versus non-specific amplification of cell-mediated immunity in these invertebrates is still unresolved.

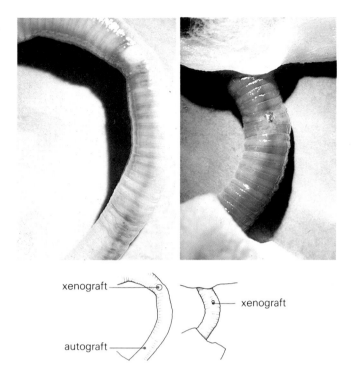

xenograft

xenograft

autograft

Fig. 15.4 Demonstration of transplantation immunity in annelids: graft rejection in the earthworm *Lumbricus*. Body wall tissue from the earthworm *Eisenia* is grafted onto the body wall of *Lumbricus*. This xenograft shows complete blanching, swelling and oedema 20 days later (15°C) (left): an autograft in the same worm persists indefinitely. At 50 days the xenograft has been destroyed, leaving a collagen pad overlain by dead pigment (right). Coelomocytes effect graft rejection in earthworms. Courtesy of Dr. E. L. Cooper.

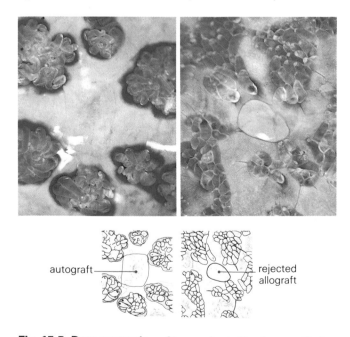

autograft

rejected allograft

Fig. 15.5 Demonstration of transplantation immunity in echinoderms: allograft rejection in starfish *(Dermasterias)*. An autograft remains in perfect condition at 300 days post transplantation (left). An allograft rejected at 287 days (14-16°C) is blanched and contracted (right). Rejection involves lymphocyte-like cells and larger phagocytic cells. ×4. Courtesy of Dr. W. H. Hildemann.

Non-Specific Defence

Important non-specific components of defence occurring throughout invertebrate phylogeny include phagocytosis (engulfment of small particles) and encapsulation (walling off of large particles) by amoeboid cells (Fig. 15.6). In many invertebrate phyla phagocytosis is augmented by coating of antigen with humoral factors (eg. agglutinins and bactericidins) present in the body fluids of non-immunized animals. Because of their role in antigen clearance these factors bear superficial resemblance to vertebrate opsonins (eg. antibody) and have been called 'antisomes'. However, it is important to stress that immunoglobulin molecules have not yet been found in any invertebrate. The extent to which invertebrate humoral factors can be induced by antigen administration is currently receiving considerable attention. To date, inducible antisomes have been demonstrated in all protostome coelomate phyla: indeed humoral immunity has recently been shown to be an important protective mechanism in the Arthropoda.

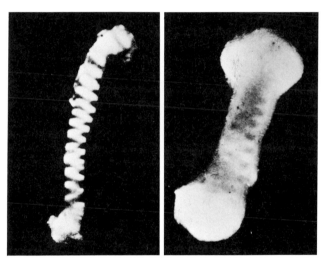

Fig. 15.6 Encapsulation response to a xenogeneic material in insects. Mouse tendon (left) is implanted in the haemocoel of a cockroach *(Periplaneta americana)*. Recovery of the tendon 24 hours later shows encapsulation with the tendon's striations just visible through the capsule (right). ×10. Courtesy of Dr. M. T. Scott.

In some invertebrate species, for example, the horseshoe crab (Arthropoda) and sipinculid worms (Annelida) haemolymph factors have been found that resemble the terminal components of the mammalian complement system, which can be activated *without* the involvement of antibody. A C3 proactivator has been demonstrated not only in these protostome invertebrates, but also in the starfish (Echinodermata). It therefore appears that genes coding for terminal complement components appeared early in evolution.

Insight into the molecular and genetic basis of non-self recognition by invertebrate immunocytes, and the role of humoral factors in defence is now urgently required. This should allow a much better comprehension of the origins of vertebrate T and B lymphocyte functions and the evolution of histocompatibility antigens and immunoglobulins.

Compared with the immense variety of forms seen within the panorama of invertebrate phyla, all vertebrates possess a fairly uniform basic plan of organization, being members of just one phylum – the Chordata. It is therefore to be expected that the basic cellular and molecular components of immunity will be common throughout vertebrate evolution, although increasing specialization of lymphoid tissues, T and B cell functions, histocompatibility antigens and immunoglobulins are likely to be associated with more complex grades of organization. The current (c. 1982) state of knowledge with respect to aspects of vertebrate immune systems indicates that these expectations are realized.

T and B Cell Functions

The evolutionary relationships amongst vertebrates are illustrated in figure 15.7, which also summarizes experimental findings (*in vivo* and *in vitro*) of responses to allogeneic cells ('T cell functions'). Acute graft rejection and strong mixed lymphocyte reactions are two of the

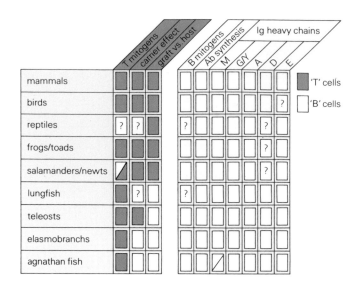

Fig. 15.8 Evolution of T and B cell activities, and immunoglobulin classes (Ig heavy chains) in vertebrates.

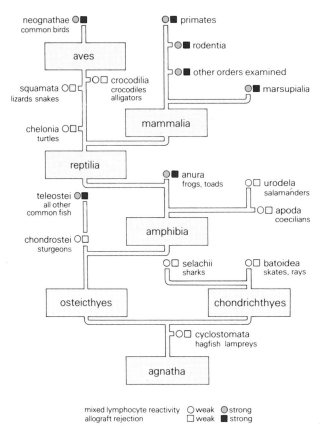

Fig. 15.7 Evolutionary tree illustrating the immunological relationships amongst vertebrates. This tree shows the development of acute allograft rejection and mixed lymphocyte reactivity (MLR) in the vertebrates. These two aspects of MHC function are present in anurans, teleostei, birds and mammals, but absent in the phyla from which they evolved, suggesting either that the MHC evolved independently on four separate occasions, or that the system has been lost from the primitive phyla which have evolved from the common ancestor of vertebrates.

functional markers of disparity between individuals, associated with the major histocompatibility complex (MHC). The presence of these markers in 'advanced' amphibians (anurans), 'advanced' fishes (teleosts), birds ('advanced' reptiles?) and mammals, but their absence in 'primitive' amphibians (urodeles and apodans) 'primitive fishes' (eg. agnathans, chondrichthyans and chondrosteans), and reptiles, suggests that the MHC may have evolved independently on four separate occasions during vertebrate phylogeny, and may reflect convergent gene evolution. It seems likely, however, that components of the MHC also exist in some of the 'primitive' forms, but allelic polymorphism may be minimal in these.

Functionally-equivalent T and B cells, specific immunologic memory and immunoglobulins exist in all vertebrates, even in agnathan fishes which possess a very limited array of lymphoid tissues and which probably lack a thymus (Fig. 15.8). A much greater variety of T cell functions and the beginnings of immunoglobulin class diversity are seen in anuran amphibians. Furthermore a full complement of lymphoid tissues, including bone marrow, 'lymph nodes' and nodular gut-associated lymphoid tissue, is found for the first time in these tetrapods (Fig. 15.9). The more sophisticated immune systems of anuran amphibians compared with fishes and urodeles may well be related to physiological and morphological changes (eg. improved circulation of body fluids) necessary for the emergence of frogs and toads onto land. Immunoglobulin and lymphoid tissue diversity persists in the reptiles, but the origins of B-equivalent lymphocytes in these (and other) poikilotherms remain uncertain. In contrast, birds possess a unique site for the differentiation of B cells; – the cloacal bursa of Fabricius (see Fig. 15.29). Although germinal centres are seen for the first time in avian peripheral lymphoid tissues, the most complex structural and functional immune systems are undoubtedly seen amongst the mammals.

With the exception of the agnathan fishes, which may possess only the terminal complement components, both classical (antibody mediated) and alternative pathways of complement activities have been demonstrated in all

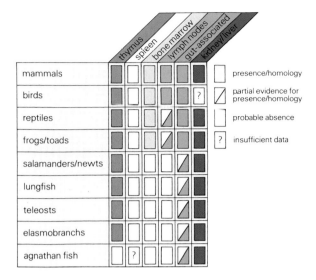

	thymus	spleen	bone marrow	lymph nodes	gut-associated	kidney/liver
mammals	■	■	■	■	■	□
birds	■	■	■	■	?	■
reptiles	■	■	■	▨	■	■
frogs/toads	■	■	■	▨	■	■
salamanders/newts	■	■	□	□	▨	■
lungfish	■	■	□	□	▨	■
teleosts	■	■	□	□	▨	■
elasmobranchs	■	■	□	□	▨	■
agnathan fish	□	?	□	□	▨	■

□ presence/homology
▨ partial evidence for presence/homology
□ probable absence
? insufficient data

Fig. 15.9 Evolution of lymphoid tissues in vertebrates.

vertebrate classes. Genes coding for the full complement system and the 2H-2L immunoglobulin molecule therefore appear to have arisen at about the same time in evolution. Basic properties of mammalian complement (thermolability, requirements for Ca^{++}, Mg^{++}) are shared by fish and amphibian complement, although the temperature ranges over which poikilotherm complement remains active is greater (activity remains at 4°C) and heat-inactivation can be achieved by lower temperature (eg. *Xenopus* serum is completely decomplemented by 45°C treatment for 40 mins). Guinea pig complement may be used successfully in *in vitro* haemolytic antibody assays in adult amphibians, whereas in most fish species isologous serum, or serum from a closely-related species, must be used.

MORPHOLOGY OF LYMPHOID TISSUES IN LOWER VERTEBRATES

Thymus

Two anuran amphibian species – the leopard frog, *Rana pipiens* and the clawed toad, *Xenopus laevis* – are used to illustrate general histological features of lymphoid tissues found in poikilothermic vertebrates. The adult frog thymus lies just under the skin, posterior to the middle ear (Fig. 15.10). Detachment of the thymus from the pharyngeal epithelium occurred early in development, as is the case in most other vertebrates except teleost fish. There is considerable evidence that the poikilotherm thymus produces lymphocytes with T cell functions, like its counterpart in endotherms. The ultrastructure of thymic lymphocytes and neighbouring (educating?) epithelial cells is shown in figure 15.11. Several other cell types are found within the thymic medulla. Myoid cells have been found in the thymus of mammals, reptiles and several amphibian species. It has been suggested that they are involved in promoting circulation of tissue fluids within the thymus or that they may provide a source of self antigen, which might be involved in the development of self tolerance and MHC restriction of T lymphocyte reactivity.

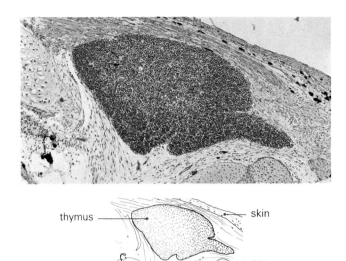

Fig. 15.10 Thymus section of the adult leopard frog, *Rana pipiens*. The thymus lies just below the skin and is differentiated into an outer cortex and central (paler staining) medulla. The cortex is the site of rapid lymphocyte proliferation. The medulla contains fewer lymphocytes, but large numbers of epithelial cells and a variety of other cell types, including Hassal's corpuscles and myoid cells. The organ is enclosed in a thick connective tissue capsule from which septal projections extend inwards to the parenchyma. H&E stain, ×20.

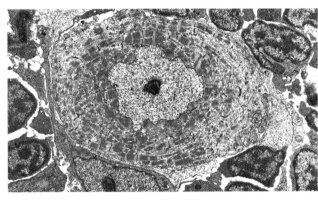

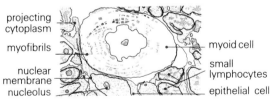

Fig. 15.11 Electron micrograph of thymus medulla of larval *Xenopus laevis* shows ultrastructure of a myoid cell, small lymphocytes and epithelial cell. Myoid cell: the nucleus is surrounded by concentric rings of striated myofibrils resembling those of skeletal muscle. Small lymphocytes: nuclear chromatin organized into a series of electron-dense zones with a thin margin of dense chromatin adjacent to the nuclear membrane; cytoplasm is scant with few organelles. Epithelial cells: nuclei possess evenly-dispersed chromatin and prominent nucleoli; cytoplasm is extensive and projections extend in an interdigitating fashion between lymphocytes and other cell types to form a supportive network. ×700. Courtesy of Dr. J. J. Rimmer.

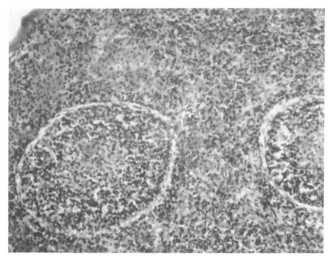

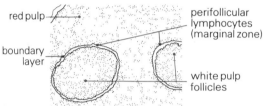

red pulp

boundary
layer

perifollicular
lymphocytes
(marginal zone)

white pulp
follicles

Fig. 15.12 Spleen section of adult *Xenopus* showing
thymus-dependent (perifollicular red-pulp) and thymus-
independent (white-pulp) areas. In *Xenopus* (unlike many
other poikilotherms) the white pulp is clearly separated from
the surrounding red pulp by lightly-staining boundary layer
cells. Concentrations of lymphocytes are also seen in the red
pulp. H & E stain, ×80.

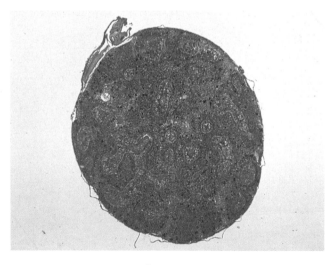

red pulp

white pulp

India ink
particles

marginal
zone

Fig. 15.13 Adult *Xenopus* spleen showing India ink
particles (black) concentrated in the perifollicular zone and
splenic red pulp 7 days after injection via the dorsal lymph sac
H&E stain, ×15.

Spleen

The spleen is a major peripheral lymphoid organ in all
jawed vertebrates. Together with 'lymph nodes' and
kidney it traps antigen, houses proliferating lymphocytes
following their stimulation by antigen and provides for
the appropriate release of these cells and their products.
Thymus-dependent (perifollicular red pulp) and thymus-
independent (white pulp follicles) zones within the
spleen have been demonstrated in *Xenopus* (Fig. 15.12).
Blood vessels enter the spleen through the white pulp
from where capillaries leave and empty into the surrounding red pulp. Experimental studies with India ink
and fluoresceinated antigens reveal that it is the red pulp
that initially receives material circulating in the blood
(Fig. 15.13). Circulating antigens are later trapped within
the white pulp follicles (ie. closely associated with potential antibody-producing cells) as illustrated in figure 15.14.

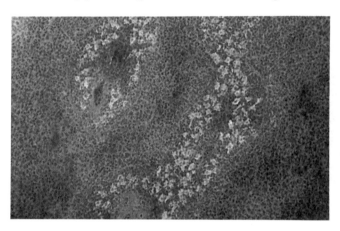

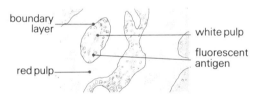

boundary
layer

red pulp

white pulp

fluorescent
antigen

**Fig. 15.14 Immunofluorescence of adult *Xenopus* spleen
showing antigen trapping.** The toad has been injected with
a soluble protein antigen (human IgG), three weeks prior to
the preparation of frozen sections and their incubation with
fluorescein-labelled antiserum (anti-human IgG). The bright,
apple green fluorescence indicates the presence of antigen
within white pulp follicles. The antigen is trapped in a dendritic
pattern which is similar to that seen in mammals and birds
where it appears to be held on reticular cell surfaces. ×35.

Lymphomyeloid Nodes

Lymphomyeloid nodes bearing superficial functional resemblance to endotherm lymph nodes are seen for the
first time in vertebrate evolution in certain anuran amphibians. Histologically these anuran nodes are very
different from their mammalian counterpart (Fig. 15.15).

The lymphomyeloid nodes are mainly blood-filtering
organs (cf. mammalian lymph nodes) although trapping
of material from surrounding lymph is also believed to
occur. In the adult frog, 'lymph nodes' of similar structure
to the larval lymph gland are found in the neck and axil-
lary regions.

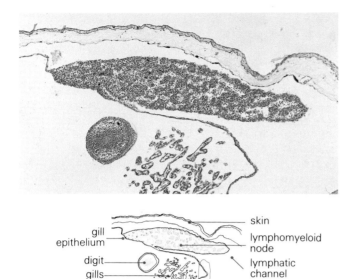

Fig. 15.15 Lymph gland section of larval *Rana.* The elongated (paired) lymphomyeloid node is seen attached ventrally to the epithelium of the gill chamber and projects into a large lymphatic channel. Gills, and a digit of the anterior limb lying in the gill chamber are seen medially, the larval skin lies laterally. The lymph gland consists of an extensive lymphoid parenchyma with phagocytes and intervening sinusoids (pale staining). H&E stain, ×25.

Gut-Associated Lymphoid Tissue

The nodular gut-associated lymphoid tissue (GALT) occurs throughout the small intestine in frogs (Fig. 15.16). Smaller accumulations of lymphocytes loosely associated with the gut are found throughout vertebrate evolution. GALT is conveniently situated to form a first-line of defence against antigens in the gut. Interestingly IgA, which is secreted into the gastrointestinal tract, is found only within endothermic vertebrates.

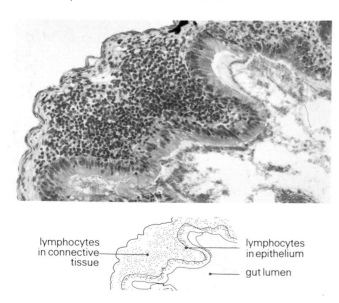

Fig. 15.16 Section of nodular gut-associated lymphoid tissue in adult *Rana.* Lymphocytes are seen in the subepithelial connective tissue and in the overlying gut epithelium. H&E stain, ×50.

Kidney

The kidney is a major lymphoid organ in fishes and amphibians, but this function wanes in the kidneys of amniotes. The kidney is currently believed to be the source of both T and B lymphoid stem cells in amphibians and may be the initial site of B lymphocyte development in ontogeny, prior to the liver. A section of *Rana* kidney, seen in figure 15.17 shows the haemopoietic tissue. Recent experiments suggest that the avian kidney may also be an important primary site of lymphoid stem cells.

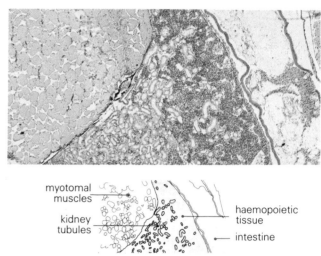

Fig. 15.17 Kidney section in larval *Rana* showing haemopoietic tissue. Haemopoietic tissue is extensive in the intertubular regions, where lymphocytes, granulocytes and other developing blood cell types are found. Myotomal muscles and a loop of the intestine lie adjacent to the mesonephros. H&E stain, ×25.

Bone Marrow

Although bone marrow makes its first appearance in amphibians, its immunological role at this level of evolution still awaits clarification (Fig. 15.18). It is an important site of lymphopoiesis and haemopoiesis in the adult anuran.

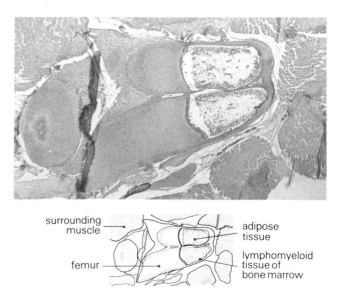

Fig. 15.18 Bone marrow section in *Rana.* H&E stain, ×20.

ASPECTS OF AMPHIBIAN IMMUNOLOGY

Anuran amphibians are proving to be excellent models for studying lymphocyte development and differentiation, and the ontogeny of immunity and tolerance induction. For example, frog larvae have been shown capable of displaying specific antibody responses when they possess less than one million lymphocytes. This finding must be taken into consideration when thinking about the generation of antibody diversity.

Thymus Development: *Xenopus laevis*

The clawed toad, *Xenopus laevis,* is ideally suited for investigating the role of the thymus in the development of the immune system, since the free living larva can be thymectomized very early in life (when the thymus is still extremely undifferentiated morphologically) without the animal runting (Figs.15.19 & 15.20). Different pairs of gill pouches yield the thymic buds in different vertebrates: in anurans the paired thymus develops from the dorsal epithelium of the second pharyngeal pouches. Recent evidence suggests that stem cells invade this epithelial bud (during the fourth day in *Xenopus*) and later develop

Fig. 15.19 *Xenopus* thymus at 3 days and 7 days. At 3 days (left, H&E stain, ×100) the developing thymus is still attached to the pharyngeal epithelium and comprised mostly of epithelial cells. At 7 days (right, EM, ×500) the thymus consists of less than 1000 cells which are of two major types.

The epithelial cells have a prominent nucleolus, dispersed chromatin and pale-staining cytoplasm.

Lymphoid cells possess large amounts of densely-staining cytoplasm with an abundance of free ribosomes and mitochondria. No small lymphocytes are found at this stage when thymectomy can be performed.

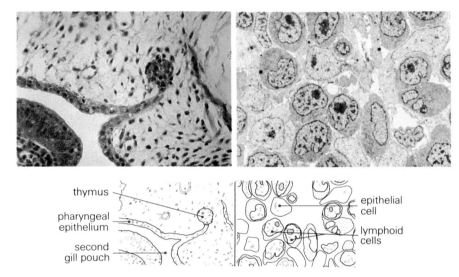

Fig. 15.20 The *Xenopus* thymus at 38 days. The pigmented paired thymus lies posterior to the eyes (left) but its absence is readily apparent in the sibling thymectomized at 7 days (right).

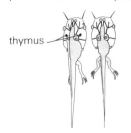

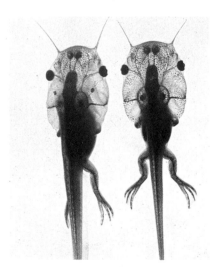

antibody response		cell mediated response	mitogen response	
	T-independent	T-dependent		T-independent	T-dependent
normal	LPS	SRBC	'T' — foreign graft cell rejected rapidly	LPS	PHA
thymectomized	LPS	SRBC	? — foreign graft cell rejected slowly	LPS	PHA

Fig. 15.21 Effect of thymectomy in *Xenopus*. Thymectomized *Xenopus* are assessed for antibody response, cell-mediated response and mitogen response *(in vitro)*. Treatments may be classified as T-dependent or T-independent according to whether or not thymectomy impairs the response to the treatment.

Antibody Response: *E. coli* lipopolysaccharide (LPS – a T ind antigen and B cell mitogen) induces antibody production in a T-independent manner, whereas the normal antibody

response to sheep red blood cells (SRBC) is impaired in the absence of T (T-helper?) cells.

The normal Cell-mediated Response is T-dependent, but chronic allograft rejection still occurs in thymectomized *Xenopus*.

Mitogen Response: lymphocytes may be stimulated by mitogens in two ways. LPS stimulates B cells polyclonally. A second group of mitogens, including phytohaemagglutinin (PHA) stimulates T lymphocytes polyclonally.

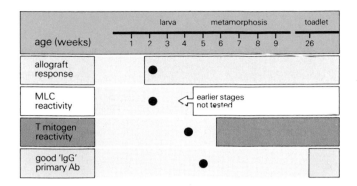

age (weeks)	larva				metamorphosis					toadlet
	1	2	3	4	5	6	7	8	9	26
allograft response		●								
MLC reactivity		●		earlier stages not tested						
T mitogen reactivity			●							
good 'IgG' primary Ab				●						

Fig. 15.22 Ontogeny of immune reactivity and the effect of sequential thymectomy in *Xenopus*. The allograft response and mixed lymphocyte reactivity appear early and are followed by T mitogen reactive cells and helper cells, particularly helper cells involved in the 'IgG' primary antibody response. ● Indicates the age until which thymectomy still impairs function.

into lymphocytes. Thymectomy of *Xenopus* from 5-7 days of age has demonstrated the existence of T-dependent and T-independent components of immunity (Fig. 15.21). However, the abrogation of both 'IgG' *and* 'IgM' antibodies to T-dependent antigens by thymectomy and the regular occurrence of plaque-forming ('B') cells and LPS mitogen-reactive cells in the anuran thymus suggest the presence of B-equivalent cells within the thymus. Thymectomy of anuran larvae at different times reveals that the different T-equivalent cell functions develop sequentially during larval maturation (Fig. 15.22). Thus the allograft response and mixed lymphocyte reactivity develop early, in contrast to the slower emergence of T mitogen-reactive and helper cells.

Alloimmunity: *Rana pipiens*

Delicate surgical manipulations can be achieved on amphibian embryos well before any components of the immune system have developed. This feature has been utilized to examine the ontogeny of alloimmunity in the leopard frog (Fig. 15.23). The onset of the alloimmune response observed correlates with lymphoid maturation of the thymus and, presumably, the appearance in the periphery of certain T-equivalent subsets. Later in development a more vigorous response is witnessed, concomitant with a rapid phase of lymphoid organ differentiation. Experiments on *Rana pipiens* and other amphibians show that embryonic transfer of large amounts of allogeneic material leads to tolerance rather than rejection.

One of the shortcomings of using amphibians for immunological research has been the absence of histocompatible animals, but histocompatible strains of several species are now becoming available. One approach has been the creation of isogeneic *Xenopus*. Hybrid females developing from *X. laevis/X. gilli* matings produce some diploid eggs: gynogenetic development of these eggs results in a clone, members of which are all identical to each other (and to the mother) as tested by ploidy, allograft responsiveness and mixed lymphocyte reactivity (Fig. 15.24). Several different clones, that are either MHC compatible (an ancestral homologue of the

mammalian MHC – the XLA locus – exists in *Xenopus*) or which possess one or two MHC haplotype differences, now exist. These animals are proving invaluable for cell transfer studies, experiments on MHC restriction of T lymphocyte reactivity and transplantation experiments in general. Individuals of a clone of isogeneic *Xenopus* make identical antibodies (measured by isoelectric focussing), a finding which argues in favour of a germ-line origin of antibody diversity.

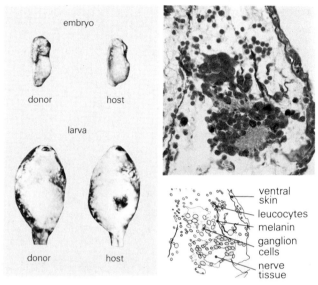

Fig. 15.23 Transplantation of embryonic tissue in *Rana* – ontogeny of alloimmunity. A piece of neural fold removed from one embryo (tail-bud stage, top left) is transplanted to the mid-ventral surface of another embryo (host). Intimately associated with the neural folds are the neural crest elements which are precursors of diverse cell types, including pigment cells The pigment cells that differentiate provide an externally visible means of following the progress of the embryonic transplant. The host larva has developed a distinctive mass of graft-derived pigment cells. The section on the right shows differentiated graft elements (large ganglion cells with prominent nucleoli, other nervous tissue and melanin), 15 days after transplantation. Despite the earliness of the transplantation, lymphocytes and granulocytes are invading the graft. H&E stain, x100. Courtesy of Dr. E. P. Volpe.

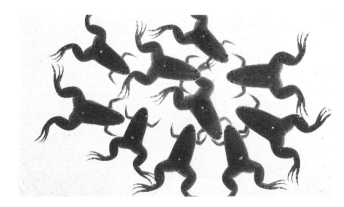

Fig. 15.24 A 'family' of genetically identical *Xenopus* The white spot on the back of each animal is a piece of belly skin grafted from another animal of the same family or clone. Courtesy of Dr. L. Du Pasquier.

Immunoglobulin Production

Studies using anti-Ig antibodies (prepared in mammals) on fishes and amphibians have, in general, revealed the presence of a high percentage of surface Ig-positive thymocytes ('T' cells). Furthermore capping and resynthesis of surface Ig *in vitro* suggest that thymic lymphocytes produce this membrane-bound Ig themselves. Although some reinterpretation of these experiments is in progress, these findings have supported the concept that the T cell receptor for antigen is Ig or a component of the Ig molecule. The immunofluorescence 'spot' test reveals that thymocyte surface Ig expression falls dramatically at the end of anuran metamorphosis (Fig. 15.25). This is ontogenetically correlated with the emergence of high affinity 'IgG' antibody production in the adult toad. Membrane Ig can still be detected on adult frog thymocytes by the more sensitive technique of 'capping'.

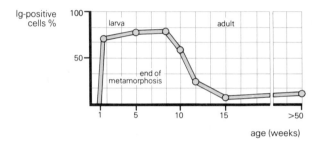

Fig. 15.25 Graph showing variation in membrane-bound immunoglobulin on *Xenopus* thymocytes with age.

Membrane-bound immunoglobulin was assessed throughout maturation by immunofluorescence (immunofluorescence 'spot' test) using anti-immunoglobulin. The dramatic fall in surface immunoglobulin at the end of metamorphosis may be correlated with the appearance of 'mature' T lymphocyte populations that can help B cells produce high affinity IgG antibody in adult *Xenopus*.

Metamorphosis and Immunoregulation

Amphibian metamorphosis is an extremely interesting period immunologically. During this period an internal histoincompatibility, in the form of the emergence of new adult-specific antigens, is presented to an immunocompetent animal. Thus the larva can recognize both these adult antigens and histocompatibility alloantigens as foreign. Immunologists wonder how amphibians escape the risk of dying from an autoimmune disease at the time of metamorphosis. Experiments designed to look into the mechanism of self-tolerance have revealed that metamorphosis in anurans is a priveleged period for the induction of tolerance to both minor *and* major histocompatibility antigens, as measured by impaired skin allograft rejection and MLC reactivity. The mechanism of this tolerance is still unclear, but is associated with a decrease in thymus cell number and is effected, in part, by an active alloimmune suppression mediated by lymphocytes of metamorphosing frogs.

It has also recently been suggested that during metamorphosis histoincompatible larval and adult lymphocytes may reciprocally stimulate T cells to secrete a factor that can substitute for T cell help. This would allow humoral responses to be effected at metamorphosis, when T helper cell numbers are diminished. Metamorphosis presents a unique opportunity for examining immunoregulatory T cell populations, which may have significance outside of purely phylogenetic considerations.

Models for the Study of Lymphocyte Development

Amphibian and avian experiments have yielded invaluable information concerning the embryonic origins of 'T' and 'B' lymphocytes. Embryonic transplantation of ploidy-marked gill buds in *Rana pipiens* and *Xenopus laevis* has revealed that thymic lymphocytes develop from stem cells which have colonized the thymus rather than from transformed epithelial cells as was originally suggested in the mid 1970's (Fig. 15.26). Ultrastructural observations on these and other amphibians lend support to these new findings. In anurans the lymphoid stem cells apparently originate from developing kidney rather than from the anuran equivalent of the endotherm yolk sac. There is some evidence for a similar pathway in birds, which possess an organ called the bursa of Fabricius: it appears to cause the differentiation of circulating stem cells into immunoglobulin-producing (bursa-derived or 'B') cells (Fig. 15.27). By transplanting quail bursal precursors into chickens it has been shown that the bursal precursor is receptive to colonization by stem cells for a

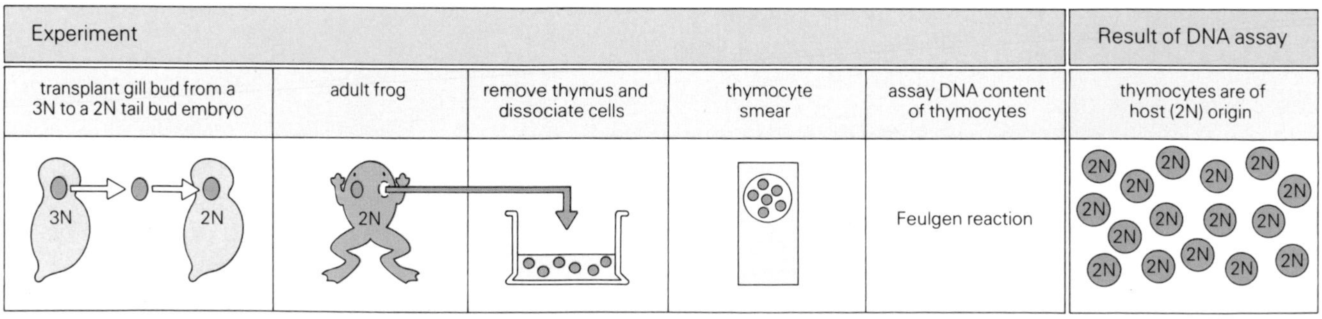

Experiment					Result of DNA assay
transplant gill bud from a 3N to a 2N tail bud embryo	adult frog	remove thymus and dissociate cells	thymocyte smear	assay DNA content of thymocytes	thymocytes are of host (2N) origin
				Feulgen reaction	

Fig. 15.26 Experimental demonstration of the extrinsic (stem cell) origin of thymic lymphocytes in amphibians. A
gill bud (containing the thymus precursor tissue) of an artificially induced triploid (3N) embryo (tail-bud stage) was transplanted into a normal, diploid (2N) tail-bud stage embryo. When the embryo developed into a normal adult frog the transplanted thymus was removed, and the thymus cells dissociated. A cell smear was prepared and the cell's DNA content determined by the Feulgen reaction. As a result the thymus cells were found to be diploid, that is, of host cell origin. The conclusion is that amphibian thymocytes are derived from cells external to the thymus.

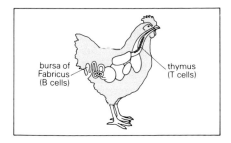

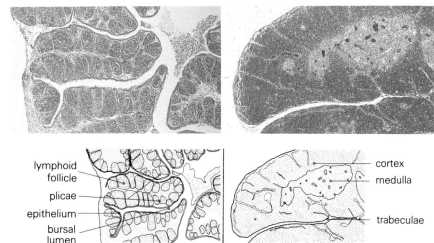

Fig. 15.27 The bursa of Fabricius. The two central organs in the avian immune system are the thymus (right) and the bursa of Fabricius (left). Lymphocytes passing through the thymus are termed T cells and those through the bursa, B cells. H&E stain, ×20.

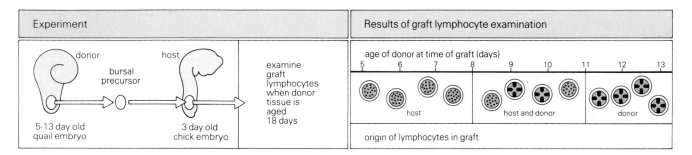

Fig. 15.28 Experimental demonstration of bursal lymphocyte origin by the colonization of stem cells. The bursal precursor of 9 quail embryos aged between 5-13 days were each transplanted into the somatopleure of 3 day old chick embryos. When the donor tissue was 18 days old the type of lymphocyte to develop in the graft was assessed. This is made possible by the distinct chromatin differences between the interphase lymphocyte nuclei of the two species. Grafts performed when the quail embryo donor was aged 5-8 days had developed, by day 18, into a bursa containing lymphocytes wholly of host (chick) origin, which had colonized the graft. Grafts performed between 9-11 days developed into chimaeric tissues. Grafts performed after 11 days developed into tissue composed completely of the donor cell type. It is concluded that the quail bursa is normally colonized by stem cells at 8-11 days. After 11 days and before 8 days, stem cells fail to colonize the bursa.

limited period only. This period occurs early in embryonic development and the bursa is subsequently (temporarily) refractory to colonization by host stem cells (Fig. 15.28). These experiments are possible because quail and chicken lymphocytes differ structurally, but are functionally identical. Similarly the embryonic thymus also appears to be receptive to stem cells for limited periods or 'windows of development'. The salient features of immunological phylogeny in vertebrates and invertebrates are summarized in figure 15.29.

invertebrates	vertebrates
1. phagocytosis/encapsulation important in eliminating non-self material	1. all display cell mediated/humoral immunity
2. primordial cell-mediated immunity evident early in evolution	2. all have IgM with 'higher' forms possessing different heavy chains
3. humoral immunity (inducible antisomes) in some coelomate forms, but no phyla possess immunoglobulins	3. all possess T and B lymphocytes/lymphoid tissues: these tissues become more complex in 'higher' forms
4. immunocyte types include amoebocytes, haemocytes, coelomocytes and primitive lymphoid cells	4. functional lymphocyte heterogeneity demonstrated in fish/amphibians *and* birds/mammals
5. nature of immunocyte receptor for antigen unknown	

Fig 15.29 Summary of the immune responses found in invertebrate and vertebrate phyla.

FURTHER READING

Borysenko M. (1976) Phylogeny of Immunity: an overview. *Immunogenetics* **3,** 305.

Cohen, N. (1977) Phylogenetic emergence of lymphoid tissues and cells. In *The Lymphocyte: Structure and Function.* J. J. Marchalonis (ed.) Marcel Dekker.

Cohen N. & Sigel M.M. (eds.) (1982) *The Reticuloendothelial System. Vol. 3. Ontogeny and Phylogeny.* Plenum Press, New York.

Cooper E.L. (1976) *Comparative Immunology.* Prentice-Hall, New Jersey.

Cooper E.L. (ed.) *Developmental and Comparative Immunology.* Pergamon Press.

Du Pasquier L. (1976) Phylogenesis of the vertebrate immune system. In *Mosbacher Colloquim* Melchers F. & Rajewsky K. (eds.) Springer-Verlag, Berlin.

Gershwin M.E. & Cooper E.L. (eds.) (1978) *Animal Models of Comparative and Developmental Aspects of Immunity and Disease.* Pergamon Press, New York.

Hildemann, W. H. & Benedict A.A. (eds.) (1975) *Immunologic Phylogeny.* Plenum, New York.

Horton J.D. (ed.) (1980) *Development and Differentiation of Vertebrate Lymphocytes.* Elsevier, Amsterdam.

Manning M.J. (ed.) (1980) *Phylogeny of immunological Memory.* Elsevier, Amsterdam.

Manning M.J. & Turner, R.J. (1976) *Comparative Immunobiology.* Blackie, Glasgow and Halsted Press, Wiley, New York.

Ratcliffe N.A. & Rowley A.F. (eds.) (1981) *Invertebrate Blood Cells. Vols. 1 & 2.* Academic Press, London.

Solomon J.B. (ed.) (1981) *Aspects of Developmental and Comparative Immunology I.* Pergamon Press, Oxford.

Solomon J.B. & Horton J.D. (eds.) (1977) *Developmental Immunobiology.* Elsevier, Amsterdam.

Wright R.K. & Cooper E.L. (eds.) (1976) *Phylogeny of Thymus and Bone Marrow-Bursa Cells.* North Holland, Amsterdam.

15.12

16 Immunity to Viruses, Bacteria and Fungi

IMMUNITY TO VIRUSES

The viruses are a group of organisms which must enter a host cell to proliferate, since they lack the necessary biochemical machinery to manufacture proteins and metabolize sugars. Some viruses also lack the enzymes required for nucleic acid replication, and are dependent on the host cell for these functions also. The number of genes carried by different viruses may be as few as 3 or as many as 250, but this is still much less than even the smallest bacteria. The course of a generalized virus infection is illustrated in figure 16.1.

The illnesses produced by virus infections are as varied as the viruses themselves. Illness may be acute, recurrent, latent (ie. dormant infection where the virus is not readily detectable but may recur), or subclinical (ie. acute or chronic symptomless infection where the virus is demonstrable). The immune response may range from the apparently non-existent, (eg. Kuru, Creutzfeld-Jacob) to lifelong immunity, or chronic immunopathology, (eg. hepatitis B) (Fig. 16.2).

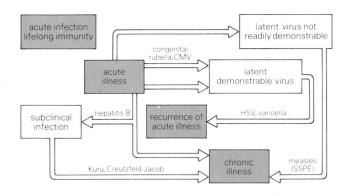

Fig. 16.2 Illness and virus infection. The varied pathology of different virus infections is indicated in the red boxes. While many viruses produce an acute illness followed by sterile lifelong immunity, some are followed by later recurrence, due to virus remaining latent within cells. Examples of different types are given.

This discussion will concentrate on those acute virus infections, which usually evoke obvious immunity, since these are the only ones about which there is reliable immunological data. It must therefore be remembered that apart from an assortment of clinical and clinico-immunological observations, we have little understanding of the immunological mechanisms underlying the recurrent or latent, or lifelong subclinical virus infections. Even the data relating to the acute virus infections must be interpreted with caution. A number of mechanisms can be shown to destroy viruses, or virus-infected cells *in vitro*, but it is much more difficult to be sure which ones are important *in vivo*. It may be possible to answer these questions in the near future, using clones of T cells from immune animals, grown *in vivo* in the presence of interleukin-2 and antigen. The protective efficacy of such clones in transfer experiments could then be correlated with their function (eg. T_C, T_H, T_D etc.) and phenotype.

This problem is also crucial to vaccine design. Since we do not know which effector functions constitute the normal protective mechanisms against individual human viral infections, the design of vaccines is a matter of trial and error. There is therefore the constant danger of priming inappropriate effector functions, leading to disease of enhanced severity, and immunopathology in later life. Moreover, even if we knew which effector functions to prime, we would not at present know how to modify the vaccine so as to prime the chosen cells.

In conclusion, what follows is a list of mechanisms, the relative importance of which in any one human infection, remains uncertain.

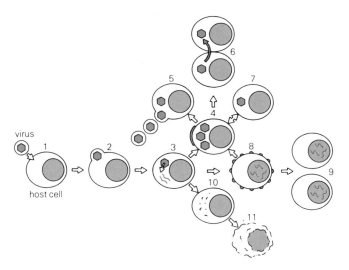

Fig. 16.1 A generalized viral life cycle. The virion becomes adsorbed by its receptors to a host cell (1). The virus then penetrates the cell and becomes uncoated (2 & 3). Infection may take several courses depending on the viral species. Some viruses replicate their components, which then assemble in the host cell (4) and are released by budding from the cell membrane (5). Alternatively the virus can spread by cell to cell contact (6) without being released. Viruses also remain dormant within cells, to be reactivated at a later date (7). Some viruses are capable of inserting their genetic material into the host cell genome, where they remain latent (8). Subsequently the cell may become productive (4) or in certain circumstances can undergo neoplastic transformation (9). Some virus infections may be abortive (10), either because the host cell is non-permissive for infection or because the virus is defective. Nevertheless both abortive infections or productive infections can lead to cell death (11).

Viral Infection

A typical viral infection starts with local invasion of an epithelial surface, and then after one or more viraemic phases, results in infection of the target organ, (eg. skin, or nervous system). Since different immunological mechanisms are effective against different forms of antigen (eg. intracellular or extracellular), the relevance of any particular mechanism will depend on the way the viral antigens and virion (a single infective virus unit) are encountered. This in turn depends on the species of virus and phase of the infection. The relevance to protection or immunopathology of the various effector systems of the immune response therefore depends on the phase of the infection and on the biology of the virus (fig. 16.3).

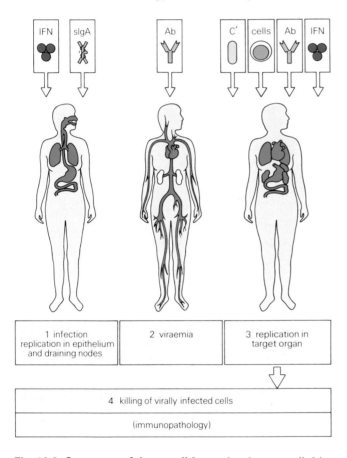

Fig. 16.3 Summary of the possible mechanisms available to combat the different phases of a generalized virus infection. The first line of defence is the interferon (IFN) and secretory IgA of epithelial surfaces (1). Some viruses which replicate entirely on these surfaces may be checked at this stage. Other viruses have one or two viraemic phases, susceptible to serum antibody (2). Virus in cells is attacked by a variety of cellular and humoral mechanisms (3). Generally the killing of virally infected cells is beneficial, but if the immune mechanisms produce greater damage than the original infection this may be regarded as immunopathological (4).

Antibody is only capable of directly binding to extracellular viruses: IgG and IgM antibodies are limited in their actions to plasma and tissue fluids, whereas secretory IgA may protect epithelial surfaces, and therefore is particularly important in protecting against viruses which lack a viraemic phase.

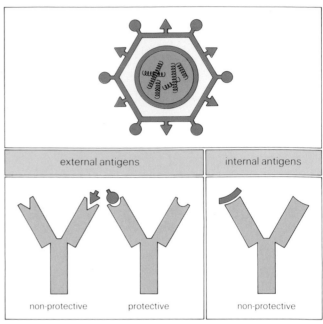

Fig. 16.4 Diagrams of a virus showing internal and external antigens surrounding the viral genetic material. Although antibody may be produced to all the antigens, only that which is produced to particular external antigens is usually protective.

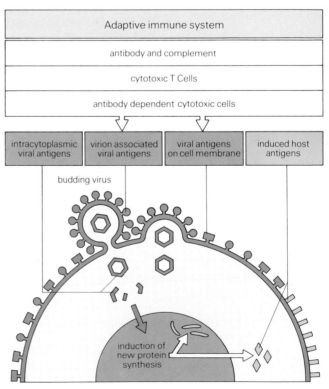

Fig. 16.5 Viral antigens associated with infected cells. An infected cell is shown diagrammatically carrying virally-encoded antigens (blue) which may be internal, associated with assembling virions or virus metabolism, or on the plasma membrane. Viruses often induce new host proteins (light blue) expressed in the nucleus, cytoplasm or plasma membrane. The actions of the adaptive immune system are only effective against antigens expressed on the cell surface.

16.2

Antibody in association with complement (C1-C9) can cause lysis of cells carrying viral antigens, or directly damage enveloped viruses.

The cell-mediated immune reaction (cytotoxic T cells, antibody dependent cytotoxic cells) are potentially effective against intracellular viruses which they recognize by the presence of viral antigens in the membrane of the infected cell.

Interferon acts in a protective capacity before the virus penetrates a cell, by inducing a state of resistance to viral multiplication.

The elements of the adaptive immune response recognize specific antigens on the virus and virally-infected cells. It is important to make the differentiation between viral antigens, which are coded for, at least in part by the viral genome, and those antigens induced in the cell by the presence of virus and coded for by the host genome. Although these 'host-coded' antigens are potentially useful as markers of virus infection, they are of little use in producing protective immunity.

Viral antigens are largely proteins or glycoproteins. The glycoproteins are often glycosylated by the host cell during the budding process. The internal antigens of the virion are not usually relevant to protective immunity. Antigens which are expressed on the surface of the virion may be potential targets for the immune response and so may antigens expressed on the membranes of infected cells (Figs. 16.4 & 16.5).

The response to viral antigens is almost entirely T cell dependent. Even the antibody response requires T cell help. Thus susceptibility to a virus is particularly associated with T cell dysfunction though this tells us little about the effector mechanisms involved, since T cells are required both for antibody production and some cytotoxic reactions.

Effects of Antibody

Antibody may upset the virus-cell interactions which lead to adsorption, penetration, uncoating, or replication. For instance, following entry into the phagocytic vacuole, some viruses have envelopes which interact with the vacuolar membrane and cause its dissolution. The viral nucleic acid is liberated into the cytoplasm. However, the essential interaction with the vacuolar membrane can be blocked if the virion is coated with antibody.

Antibody to some components of the virus surface (critical sites, eg. haemagglutinin of the influenza virus) neutralizes more effectively than antibody to other components (non-critical sites, eg. neuraminidase of the influenza virus) (Fig. 16.6). Complement assists neutralization, by coating the virus or by lysing those with lipid membranes. *In vitro*, neutralization is never complete. The 'persistent fraction' may be due to aggregates, or blocking by non-neutralizing antibody (ie. antibody to non-critical sites).

Antibody can lyse a variety of human cell lines infected with the virus responsible for measles, influenza or mumps. The *alternative* complement pathway is required to amplify the triggering of the lytic sequence by the classical pathway, which is not by itself sufficient to cause damage. Antibody may also result in modulation, or stripping of viral antigen from the cell surface allowing the infected cell to avoid destruction by cytotoxic cells. The effects of antibody are summarized in figure 16.7.

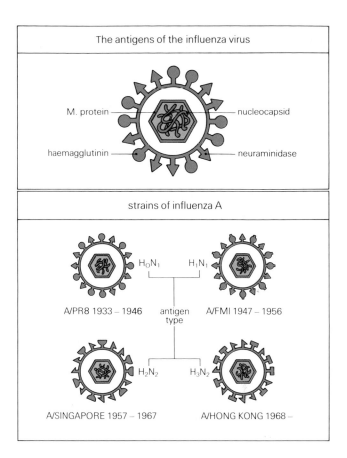

Fig. 16.6 The antigens of the influenza virus: antigenic shift and drift. The major surface antigens are haemagglutinin and neuraminidase. The haemagglutinin is involved in attachment to cells, and antibodies to haemagglutinin are protective (critical site). Antibodies to neuraminidase are much less effective, and those to the internal components are ineffective (non-critical sites). The influenza virus can change its surface slightly (antigenic drift) or radically (antigenic shift). Alterations in the structure of the haemagglutinin antigen render earlier antibodies ineffective and thus new virus epidemics break out. The diagram indicates the new strains which have emerged by antigenic shift since 1933. The official flu antigen nomenclature is based on the type of haemagglutinin (H_0, H_1 etc.) and neuraminidase (N_1, N_2 etc.) molecule. New strains replace old strains but the internal antigens remain unchanged.

	advantages		disadvantages
antibody only	blockage of critical sites	⇨ neutralization	persistent fraction
Ab + complement	lysis of virus with lipid membranes	⇨ neutralization	
Ab + complement	coating	⇨ removal via C3 receptors	may infect the phagocyte
Ab + alternative complement pathway	lysis of infected cell		may 'strip' virus and protect cell from other mechanisms

Fig. 16.7 Summary of the antiviral effects of antibody.

The relative importance of antibody and cellular mechanisms remains unclear. Thus in the intensively studied influenza model passive transfer of antibody to nude mice does not result in clearing of the virus, though it suppresses shedding, the release of infective viruses from cells, and hence infection. On the other hand, mice artificially made agammaglobulinaemic, which produce no detectable antibody to haemagglutinin, recover and are subsequently immune. Thus T cell responses appear to be important.

There is no doubt that passively administered antibody can protect humans against measles, hepatitis A and B, varicella, and possibly mumps and rubella, if given before, or sufficiently soon after exposure.

Antibody Dependent Cell-Mediated Cytotoxicity

K cells may be involved in some virus infections. These cells act by binding specific antibody on virus-infected target cells via their surface Fc receptors. They can then specifically kill the virus-infected cells.

The characteristics of the cytotoxic activity against vaccinia virus-infected cells are presented in figures 16.8. These characteristics indicate that K cells mediate immunity to vaccinia virus rather than cytotoxic T cells since cells carrying Fc receptors are essential – most Tc cells do not have Fc receptors. The importance of this mechanism clinically is unknown, but it may be more significant in man than in mice.

effector cells	fibroblast target cells	effect on target
1. leucocytes	infected	killed
2. leucocytes	non-infected	–
3. non T cells	infected	killed
4. leucocytes	allogeneic infected	killed
5. cells lacking Fc receptors	infected	–
6. leucocytes with blocked Fc receptors	infected	–

Fig. 16.8 K cell involvement in immunity to vaccinia virus infection. Human volunteers who had been vaccinated in childhood were revaccinated with vaccinia virus. Peripheral blood leucocytes (effector cells) taken 7 days after vaccination killed virus-infected HLA matched target cells (1) but not uninfected cells (2). This was not apprently due to Tc cells, since the effect is mediated by non-T cells (3) and the killing was not restricted to HLA matched targets (4). (In this and the next figure HLA difference between target and effector cells is indicated in red.) It was due to K cells since removal of cells with Fc receptors removed the effect (5), and blocking of antibody binding to Fc receptors (with F(ab')$_2$ anti-IgGFc) also blocked killing (6).

Cytotoxic T Cells and MHC Restriction

There is evidence for cytotoxic T cells in some virus infections. Figure 16.9 illustrates an experiment which demonstrates that vaccination of man with killed whole

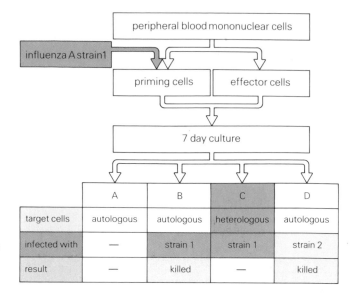

Fig. 16.9 Experiment to show cytotoxic T cell activity to influenza A in man. Peripheral blood lymphocytes from a person vaccinated 28 days previously with killed influenza A virus (strain 1) were harvested and divided into two aliquots. One aliquot (10% of the total) was incubated with influenza A strain 1 for 90 minutes. These were then mixed with uninfected (effector) cells and cultured for 7 days. The aim is to keep the effector cell population free from infection. Cytotoxic T cells generated in the culture were tested on either autologous HLA identical cells (yellow) or heterologous HLA mismatched cells (red) infected with strain 1 or strain 2 virus. The effector cells kill HLA matched infected targets (B) but not uninfected (A) or mismatched infected targets (C). The cytotoxic T cells are not virus-strain specific (D). Tc cells are implicated in these experiments since the cytotoxicity is restricted to infected autologous cells only.

influenza A results in increased ability to mount an *in vitro*, HLA-restricted, cytotoxic T cell response against cells infected with the same, or *different* strains (a virus subunit vaccine had little effect). The lack of strain specificity is in agreement with several reports that in mice, Tc cells generated by one variant can protect against serologically distinct variants. This may prove important because the influenza A virus avoids the antibody response by changing its surface haemagglutinin and neuraminidase glycoproteins every few years. Antibodies to these glycoproteins are type-specific and so do not block infection with antigenic variants. Note also that HLA restriction implies that Tc cells are involved (cf. 'MHC') unlike the K cell activity described previously.

Immunity in man appears to be virus strain specific but this does not rule out a role for cross-reactive Tc cells in the *recovery* phase of influenza infection. Although rapid boosting of cytotoxic T cell memory during an established infection may be essential for rapid recovery, this boosted response is short-lived and may not be able to block re-infection with another strain.

Other evidence for T cell activity is provided by studies involving human volunteers, in which it is found that high cytotoxic T cell activity before challenge with live influenza, correlates with low or absent subsequent shedding of virus.

Delayed Hypersensitivity to Viral Antigens

In the murine influenza model delayed type hypersensitivity responsiveness (or DTH, a measure of T cell sensitization) can be transferred to syngeneic recipients by either Ly1+ I-region restricted T cells, or by Ly2,3+, K- or D-region restricted T cells (Ly1+ cells are usually regarded as containing the T-helper cell population while Ly2,3+ cells contain the cytotoxic T cell and suppressor T cell populations). However only the Ly2,3+ are protective in transfer experiments. Indeed the Ly1+ cell type results in accelerated death following challenge with live virus (Fig. 16.10).

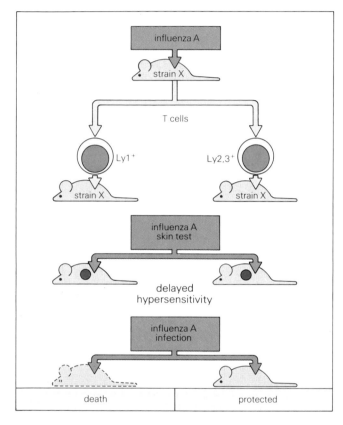

Fig. 16.10 Lack of correlation between delayed hypersensitivity and protection in murine influenza. A strain X mouse is infected with influenza A virus. T cells are later removed and divided into those carrying the Ly1 surface phenotype (Ly1+) and those carrying Ly2 and Ly3 (Ly2,3+). These are injected into other strain X mice. A delayed hypersensitivity response is then induced in both mice by skin testing with influenza A. Subsequent infection of the mice with virus results in the accelerated death of the mouse which received Ly1+ T cells. The mouse which received Ly2,3+ T cells is protected from the virus. Thus the capability to produce a delayed hypersensitivity response to a virus does not necessarily imply protective immunity.

This result illustrates the heterogeneity of the phenomena included under the 'umbrella' term 'delayed hypersensitivity'. Thus the presence of a positive delayed skin test response to viral antigen is unlikely to prove a reliable correlate of any one mechanism. Since T cells can have several actions, DTH responsiveness is not necessarily a corollary of protective immunity.

Interferon

The interferons are a family of related cell-regulatory glycoproteins produced by many cell types in response to virus infection, double stranded RNA, endotoxin and a variety of mitogenic and antigenic stimuli. Human and mouse interferons have recently been re-classified as IFNα, IFNβ, (previously type I, leucocyte and fibroblast respectively) and IFNγ, (previously type II, or 'immune'). There are heterogeneities within these groups, and considerable species specificity.

Interferon released from virus-infected cells binds to receptors on neighbouring cells and induces an anti-viral state which helps to isolate infective foci (Fig. 16.11). The mechanism may involve inhibition of viral protein or nucleic acid synthesis. IFN also powerfully inhibits cell growth, (suggesting a possible anti-tumour activity) and exerts selective effects on protein synthesis and the immune response. Thus interferon may contribute to the decrease in cell-mediated responses seen early in virus infections.

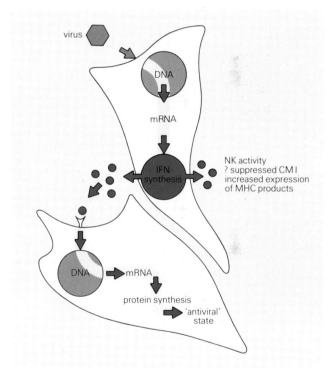

Fig. 16.11 The action of interferon. Virus infecting a cell induces the production of interferon. This is released and binds to interferon receptors on other cells. (Interferons are species specific and this is probably determined by the receptor specificity.) The interferon induces production of anti-viral proteins which are activated if virus enters the second cell. Interferon also has other actions, which may be effected by common molecular pathways.

Several workers have suggested common underlying biochemical pathways for these diverse effects, though none of these has yet gained universal acceptance. A particularly attractive idea is that interferon may influence the degree of saturation of certain membrane lipids, and so influence any biological activity dependent on membrane function.

16.5

There is also evidence that interferon causes cells to produce proteins which cause breakdown of RNA and block the initiation of protein synthesis. These proteins only become active when activated by the presence of viruses within the cell. The most effective inducers of interferon production are polyribonucleotides and particularly double stranded RNA. These polynucleotides are present in the replicative cycle of some viruses, but are not involved in normal cell metabolism.

The clearest evidence for the antiviral efficacy of interferons *in vivo* comes from experiments which show that mice treated with antibody to murine interferons can be killed by several hundred times less virus than needed to kill control animals.

Immunopathology

The immune response to viruses can cause damage to the host via the formation of immune complexes, or by direct damage to infected cells. Complexes can form in the fluid phase, or following capping and stripping of virus expressed on cell surfaces. Chronic immune complex glomerulonephritis can occur in mice infected neonatally with lymphocytic choriomeningitis virus (LCM) as shown by the experiment described in figure 16.12.

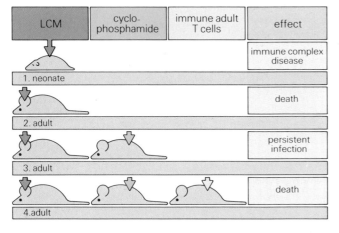

Fig. 16.12 Effects of lymphocytic choriomeningitis virus (LCM) in mice. The different effects of LCM are related to differences in immune status. Infection of neonatal mice (1) produces chronic virus shedding and immune complex disease, manifesting itself as glomerulonephritis and vasculitis. Intracerebral infection of adult mice (2) results in death. This is due to a T cell reaction, since suppression of immunity with cyclophosphamide (3) leads to persistent infection, but prevents death. The effect produced by cyclophosphamide can be reversed by T cells from an immune animal (4).

Direct damage to infected cells by a T cell dependent mechanism is responsible for most of the tissue damage in lymphocytic choriomeningitis virus infection of adult mice. A similar mechanism has been postulated for chronic active hepatitis in man. Thus the *in vitro* 'correlate' of cell-mediated immunity, leucocyte migration inhibition, is positive in a proportion of patients with chronic active hepatitis, but negative in asymptomatic carriers.

Viruses may also evoke autoimmunity, possibly by release of sequestered antigens, derepression of

delayed hypersensitivity reactions decreased

allograft rejection prolonged

in vitro lymphocytic reactivity decreased

increased or decreased antibody production

suppression of tolerance induction

? destruction of T cells (measles) or B cells (EB virus)

? alteration of lymphocyte traffic

? induction of suppressor cells

Fig. 16.13 Effects of virus on the host's immune response.

developmental antigens, inhibition of suppressors, or proliferative stimulation of autoreactive cells.

Virus infection may have profound effects on the immune system (Fig. 16.13). The classical observation is the loss of tuberculin test positivity during measles infections. The tuberculin test is a DTH reaction and in this instance is used as a marker of T cell reactivity.

Some of these effects may be due to infection of the lymphoid and phagocytic cells, while others may be secondary to the release of mediators with powerful non-specific activities, for example, interferon.

IMMUNITY TO BACTERIA

The body's defence against pathogenic bacteria consists of a variety of specific and non-specific mechanisms. Thus the skin and exposed epithelial surfaces have protective systems which limit the entry of potentially invasive organisms (Fig. 16.14). Very few organisms can breach intact skin, and the effectiveness of this barrier is made evident when considering the infections which frequently occur following skin loss (eg. by burns). Therefore, only a minute proportion of the huge numbers of potentially pathogenic organisms ever gain access to the body.

Bacterial Cell Walls

When bacteria do gain access to the tissues the mechanisms involved in immunity to them depend on the particular species involved: the effectiveness of an immune response depends to a large degree on the host's ability to damage the components of the bacterial cell wall. From the pathological point of view there are four major basic types of bacterial cell wall (Fig. 16.15), namely:
1. gram-positive
2. gram-negative
   (based on their uptake of Gram's stain)
3. Mycobacterial
4. Spirochaetal
The outer surface of the bacterium may also contain fimbriae or flagellae, or be covered by a protective capsule. Proteins and polysaccharides in these structures can act as targets for the antibody response.

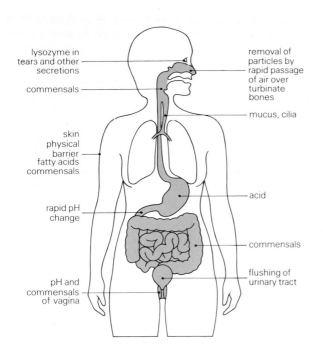

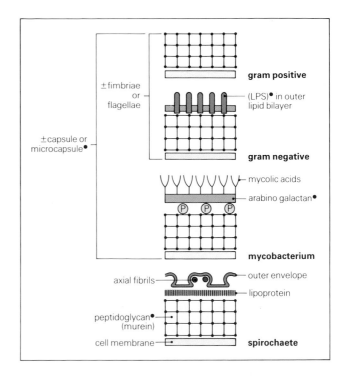

Fig. 16.14 Non-specific barriers to infection, before entry into the tissues. Invasion by potentially pathogenic organisms is limited by a variety of non-specific mechanisms:
1. the intact skin is impenetrable to most bacteria. Additionally fatty acids produced by the skin are toxic to many organisms. The pathogenicity of some strains correlates with their ability to survive on the skin.
2. epithelial surfaces are cleansed, for example, by ciliary action in the trachea or by flushing of the urinary tract.
3. pH changes in the stomach and vagina lead to destruction of many bacteria – both are acidic. In the case of the vagina, the epithelium secretes glycogen which is metabolized by particular species of commensal bacteria producing lactic acid. This also limits pathogen invasion.
4. commensals occupy particular ecological niches and so stop pathogens gaining access to it. Thus Candida or *Clostridium difficile* can occur when the normal flora is disturbed by antibiotics.

Fig. 16.15 Bacterial cell walls. The cell wall structure of the different groups of bacteria predetermines the type of mechanism which is able to destroy them. All types have an inner cell membrane and a peptidoglycan wall. Gram-negative bacteria also have an outer lipid bilayer in which lipopolysaccharide (LPS) is sometimes found. Lysosomal enzymes and lysozyme are active against the peptidoglycan layer, while cationic proteins and complement are effective against the outer lipid bilayer of the gram-negative bacteria. The compound cell wall of mycobacterium is extremely resistant to breakdown, and it is likely that this can only be achieved with the assistance of the bacterial enzymes working from within. The different types may also have fimbriae or flagellae, which can provide targets for the antibody response. Some bacteria have an outer capsule which renders the organisms more resistant to phagocytosis. The components indicated with a black spot (●) all have adjuvant properties.

However, although antibodies may interfere with bacterial functions and interact with other systems in the development of the immune response, ultimately destruction of the bacteria requires synergistic action with phagocytic cells.

Adjuvanticity and Other Non-Specific Mechanisms

The cell walls of most bacteria and the capsular substances of some of them have adjuvant properties. These probably represent phylogenetically ancient 'broad spectrum' recognition mechanisms for common microbial components, which evolved before antigen-specific T cells and immunoglobulins. The response to a pure bacterial antigen, without adjuvant is, for some bacteria an artefact created in the laboratory. Although adjuvanticity is therefore an adaption of the host, some organisms mayn 'exploit' it to disturb immunoregulation. The non-specific effects of the mycobacterial cell wall are given as an example in Figure 16.16.

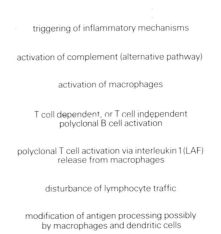

Fig. 16.16 Some known effects of the adjuvant-active components of the mycobacterial cell wall.

16.7

Many organisms, such as non-pathogenic cocci, are probably removed from the tissues without the need for a specific immune component (Fig. 16.17).

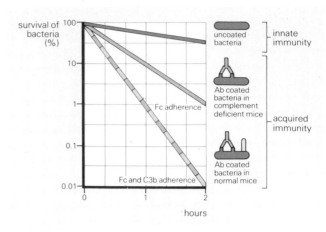

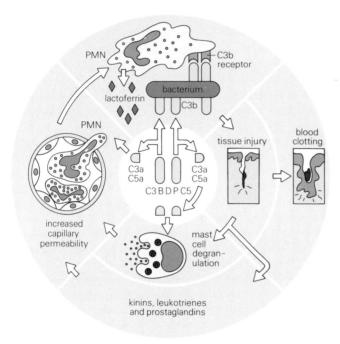

Fig. 16.17 Some non-specific mechanisms involved in immunity. Activation of the alternative complement pathway (Factors C3, B, D, P, C5) by components of the bacterial cell surface produce complement deposition (C3b) on the bacterial surface, which promotes opsonization by polymorphonuclear neutrophils (PMN) via C3b receptors. Polymorphs are also stimulated to release free lactoferrin which takes up available iron and thus inhibits bacterial growth: it is noted that the ability of many bacteria to grow depends on the availability of free iron. C3a and C5a act as chemotactic agents for polymorphs and macrophages as well as triggering mast cell degranulation. Tissue injury caused by the bacteria activates the clotting system and fibrin formation, which limits bacterial spread. Kinins, leukotrienes, prostaglandins and products of mast cell degranulation produce increased blood flow in the local capillary beds and increased capillary permeability. Prostaglandins also induce chemokinesis in phagocytes.

Antibody, if present, may enhace opsonization. However, the triggering (by 'procidins') of intracellular killing by phagocytes appears to be a separate event from opsonization. C3 at the concentrations likely to be achieved in inflammatory exudates is an effective procidin *in vitro*, as well as producing opsonization by alternative pathway activation.

The Role of Antibody
Some organisms, such as Group A streptococci, and some gut pathogens have receptors for epithelial surfaces. These can be blocked by antibody.

The effects of streptococcal M-proteins, which inhibit phagocytosis, can be neutralized by antibody, giving type-specific immunity. The same is true for many capsules (eg. meningococcal).

Fig. 16.18 Effect of opsonizing antibody and complement on rate of clearance of virulent bacteria from the blood. The uncoated bacteria are phagocytosed rather slowly (innate immunity) but on coating with antibody, adherence to phagocytes is increased many-fold (acquired immunity). The adherence is somewhat less effective in animals temporarily depleted of complement.

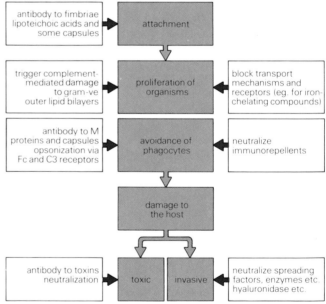

Fig. 16.19 The antibacterial roles of antibody. This diagram lists the stages of bacterial invasion (blue) and indicates the antibacterial effects of antibody that operate at different points (yellow). Antibody to fimbriae, lipoteichoic acid and some capsules block attachment of the bacterium to the host cell membrane. Proliferating bacteria trigger complement-mediated damage to gram-ve outer lipid bilayers. Antibody directly blocks bacterial surface proteins which pick up useful molecules from the environment and transport them across the membrane. Antibody to M proteins and capsules opsonizes the bacteria via Fc and C3 receptors for phagocytosis. Immunorepellents – factors which interfere with normal phagocytosis and may be toxic for leucocytes – are neutralized. Following host cell damage the bacterial toxins may be neutralized by antibody, as may be bacterial spreading factors, which facilitate invasion, for example, by the destruction of connective tissue or fibrin.

Opsonization can be more rapid in the presence of antibody, even when the organism activates the alternative pathway, since phagocytes have Fc as well as C3b receptors (Fig. 16.18). Classical pathway complement activation can also prime the alternate pathway amplification loop.

Antitoxin antibodies can neutralize toxins of tetanus, diphtheria, and so on, thus preventing the major damaging effect of the bacteria. The effects of antibody are summarized in figure 16.19.

Interaction with Phagocytes

Ultimately almost all bacteria are killed by phagocytic cells (Fig. 16.20). Pathogens have evolved ways of blocking this interaction at every point in the pathway, from the initial attraction of the phagocyte, to the final intracellular killing (Fig. 16.21). It should be noted that blockage of phago-lysosome fusion is only important if such fusion is necessary for the killing mechanism concerned.

There is a rare congenital disease, called Chediak Higashi syndrome in which macrophages and polymorphs are weakly active. In particular, there is a reduced ability of the lysosomes to fuse with the phagosome. Patients suffer from recurring bacterial infections involving organisms with normally low pathogenicity. The observation emphasizes the importance of the phagocytic mechanisms in defence against normally nonpathogenic bacteria. The defect is thought to involve the cytoskeletal elements of the cell.

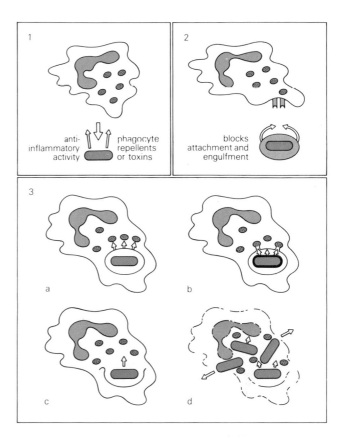

Fig. 16.21 Evasion of phagocytic killing mechanisms.
Different species of bacteria have evolved ways of evading the different phases of phagocytosis. 1. Some bacteria prevent the arrival of phagocytes by secreting toxic molecules or molecules which block inflammatory activity and chemotaxis. 2. Other organisms resist phagocytosis by having surface coats which resist phagocyte attachment (eg. capsules of Neisseria and the M protein of the microcapsule of *S. pyogenes*). 3. Once phagocytosed, different organisms can still resist killing by (a) preventing fusion of the lysosomes with the phagosome (eg. *M. tuberculosis*) (b) intrinsic resistance of the cell wall or the ability to neutralize the antibacterial proteins, H_2O_2 or superoxide (c) escape from the phagosome into the cytoplasm, where they are immune to lysosome attack. Any of these mechanisms may permit the bacteria to survive and multiply which may result in killing of the phagocyte (d).

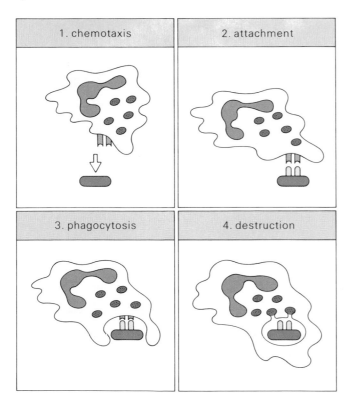

Fig. 16.20 The main stages of bacterial killing by phagocytes (polymorphs and macrophages). Phagocytes are attracted chemotactically to a bacterial infection. The phagocytes attach to the bacteria via C3b receptors and other receptors. The organism is phagocytosed. Finally lysosomes fuse with the phagosome to release microbicidal chemicals and proteins into the phagolysosome.

The Killing Mechanisms of Polymorphs and Macrophages – Non-Oxygen-Dependent

It is clear that not all organisms are killed by the same mechanisms. There is increasing interest in the cationic proteins. These bind to the bacterial cell and kill it. It now appears that there may be a transient phase during which the pH of the phagosome rises before it falls to become acid. The cationic proteins known to be present in polymorphonuclear cells and some macrophages are most toxic under alkaline conditions, when they damage the outer lipid bilayer of gram-negative bacteria.

Some organisms may be killed by the acidification itself which occurs within 10-15 minutes, though this is more likely to be related to the pH optima of lysosomal enzymes, which may themselves kill some species. Certain gram-negative organisms with readily exposed peptidoglycan may be killed by lysozyme.

A variety of other substances, such as lactoferrin (neutrophils) have been implicated. Lactoferrin can bind iron even at acid pH, and render it unavailable to bacteria; thus the ability of polymorphs to kill some bacteria is lost if they are loaded with iron. The above mechanisms may all require phagolysosome fusion (Figs. 16.22 & 23).

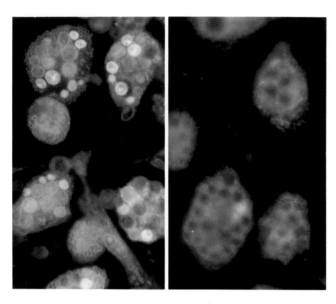

Fig. 16.22. Inhibition of fusion of secondary lysosomes with yeast-containing phagosomes by the addition of ammonium chloride. Mouse peritoneal macrophages were incubated in acridine orange which concentrates in secondary lysosomes. Live baker's yeast was then added – this assumes the appearance of 'holes' in the cell. In the absence of ammonium chloride the secondary lysosome fuses normally with the phagosome, into which the acridine orange enters and fluoresces green, yellow or orange depending on the concentration (left). However, in the presence of ammonium chloride fusion does not occur and the 'holes' remain dark (right). Such blocking of lysosomal fusion may be employed by M. tuberculosis and some leishmania which secrete ammonia. Some polyanions such as polyglutamic acid or suramin can also do this. Courtesy of Mr. R. Young and Dr. P. D. Hart.

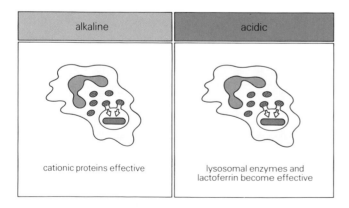

Fig. 16.23 Mechanisms involved in bacterial killing. After phagocytosis there is a transient increase in pH when cationic proteins may be effective. Subsequently the pH falls and lysosomal enzymes become effective. Lactoferrin acts by chelating free iron. Lysozyme digests the peptidoglycan of bacterial cell walls.

Oxygen-Dependent Killing Mechanisms

There may have been too much emphasis in the past on the oxygen-dependent pathways, which may be partly side-effects of an energy-generating electron transport chain (Fig. 16.24). However, cells from patients with chronic granulomatous disease lack this pathway, and are unable to kill some microorganisms. The disease is characterized by chronic inflammatory lesions involving pyogenic organisms (eg. staphylococci).

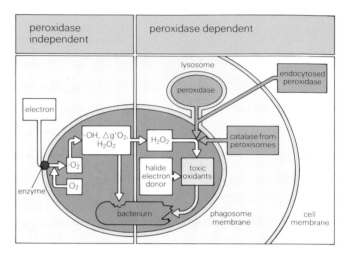

Fig. 16.24 Oxygen-dependent microbicidal activity. An enzyme in the phagosome membrane (possibly an oxidase, or a cytochrome b), reduces oxygen to superoxide anion ($.O_2^-$). This can give rise to hydroxyl radicals ($\cdot OH$), singlet oxygen ($\triangle g \cdot O_2$) and hydrogen peroxide (H_2O_2), all of which are potentially toxic. Lysosome fusion is not required for these parts of the pathway, and the reaction takes place spontaneously following internalization of the phagosome. If lysosome fusion occurs, myeloperoxidase may enter the phagosome. In the presence of peroxidase (or under some circumstances, catalase from peroxisomes) plus halides, additional toxic oxidants such as hypohalite are generated. The monocytes of individuals with congenital myeloperoxidase deficiency may show defective microbicidal activity. However, it remains unclear whether sufficient halide (preferably iodide) is available in phagosomes *in vivo*. Tissue macrophages do not contain peroxidase.

Defence Mechanisms in Bacterial Infection

The major defence mechanisms in a bacterial infection can be related to the nature of the organism, and the disease caused (Fig. 16.25). The pathogenicity of some non-invasive infections of epithelial surfaces (eg. C. diptheriae and V. cholerae) depends on toxin production, and neutralizing antibody is probably sufficient for immunity, though antibody blocking adhesion to the epithelium may also be important.

The pathogenicity of most invasive organisms does not rely so heavily on a single toxin, so that immunity requires killing of the organism itself. Organisms with an outer lipid membrane (gram-negative) may be killed by antibody and the lytic pathway of complement (eg. N. meningitidis). Gram-positive organisms (eg. S. aureus) are killed by phagocytic cells, and the role of the specific immune response is opsonization by antibody and complement. The lytic pathway is probably irrelevant.

Organisms which are resistant to the killing mechanisms of polymorphs and monocytes (eg. *M. tuberculosis)* or are obligate intracellular parasites (eg. *M. leprae)* are killed by additional poorly understood mechanisms which are induced in macrophages by T cell products.

infection	pathogenesis	major defense mechanisms
Corynebacterium diphtheriae	non-invasive pharyngitis. Toxin	neutralizing antibody
Vibrio cholerae	non-invasive enteritis. Toxin	neutralizing and adhesion-blocking antibodies
Neisseria meningitidis	nasopharynx → bacteraemia → meningitis	opsonized and killed by antibody and lytic complement
Staphylococcus aureus	locally invasive and toxic in skin etc.	opsonized by antibody and complement. Killed by phagocytes
Mycobacterium tuberculosis	invasive, locally toxic. Hypersensitivity	macrophage activation by T cells
Mycobacterium leprae	invasive, space-occupying and/or hypersensitivity	

Fig. 16.25 The major mechanisms of immunity in some important bacterial infections.

IMMUNITY TO FUNGI

Little is known about the precise mechanisms involved in immunity to fungal infections, but it is thought that they are essentially similar to those involved in resistance to bacterial infections. The fungal infections of man fall into four major categories:

1. Superficial mycoses. Dermatophytes usually restricted to the non-living keratinized components of skin, hair and nails.
2. Subcutaneous mycoses. Saprophytic fungi which can cause chronic nodules or ulcers in subcutaneous tissues following trauma (eg. chromomycosis, sporotrychosis, mycetoma).
3. Respiratory mycoses. Soil saprophytes which produce subclinical or acute lung infections, rarely disseminated or producing granulomatous lesions (eg. histoplasmosis, coccidioidomycosis).
4. *Candida albicans.* Ubiquitous commensal causing superficial infections of skin and mucous membranes, rarely systemic.

The cutaneous fungal infections are usually self-limiting and recovery is associated with a certain limited resistance to reinfection. Resistance is apparently based on cell-mediated immunity since patients develop DTH reactions to fungal antigens, and the occurrence of chronic infections is associated with lack of these reactions. T cell immunity is also implicated in resistance to other fungal infections, since resistance can sometimes be transfered with immune T cells. It is presumed that T cells release lymphokines which activate macrophages to produce destruction of the fungi (Fig. 16.26). In respiratory mycoses, spectra of disease activity, somewhat similar

to the spectrum of activity in leprosy can be seen (see 'Hypersensitivity Type IV'). Disturbance of normal physiology by immunosuppressive drugs or of the normal flora by antibiotics can predispose to invasion by Candida. Candida infections are also commonly seen in immunodeficiency diseases (Swiss, DiGeorge syndrome etc) implying that the immune system is involved in confining the fungus to its normal commensal sites.

There is also evidence for neutrophil involvement in immunity to some respiratory mycoses such as mucor mycosis (Fig. 16.27). As with bacterial infections different mechanisms are active against different organisms.

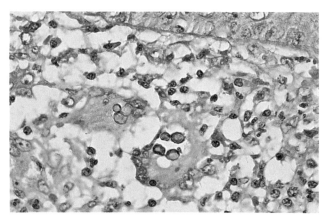

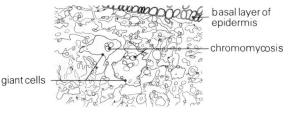

Fig. 16.26 Evidence for T cell immunity in chromomycosis. Pigmented cells of chromomycosis (a subcutaneous mycosis) are visible in giant cells in the dermis of a patient. The area is surrounded by a predominantly mononuclear cell infiltrate. Haematoxylin & eosin stain, ×400. Courtesy of Dr. R. J. Hay.

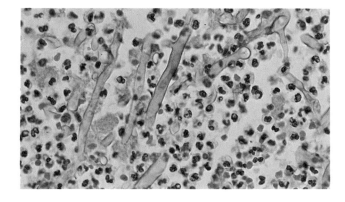

Fig. 16.27 Evidence for neutrophil-mediated immunity to mucormycosis. Section through a lung of a patient suffering from mucor mycosis – an opportunistic infection in an immunosuppressed subject. The inflammatory reaction consists almost entirely of neutrophil polymorphs around the fungal hyphae. The disease is particularly associated with neutropenia. Silver stain, ×400. Courtesy of Dr. R. J. Hay.

FURTHER READING

Viruses

Eckels D.D., Lamb J.R., Lake P., Woody J.N., Johnson A.H. & Hartzman R.J. (1982) Antigen-specific human T lymphocyte clones. Genetic restriction of influenza virus-specific responses to HLA-D region genes. *Human Immunology* **4,** 313.

Denman A.M. (1983) Viruses and Immunopathology. In *Immunology in Medicine* Holborow E.J. & Reeves W.G. (eds.). Grune & Stratton.

Mandel B. (1979) Interaction of viruses with neutralising antibodies. In *Comprehensive Virology*. Fraenkel- Contrat H. & Wagner R.R. (eds.). Vol. 15, Plenum Press, New York.

McMichael A.J., Gotch F. & Noble G.R. (1983) Cytotoxic T Cell Immunity to Influenza. *New Engl. J. Med.* **309,** 13.

Mims C.A. & White D.W. (1984) *Viral Pathogenesis and Immunology*. Blackwell Scientific Publications, Oxford.

Sehgal P.B., Pfeffer L.M. & Tamm I. (1982) Interferon and its inducers. In *Chemotherapy of viral infections*. Camc P.E. & Caliguiri L.A. (eds.) Springer-Verlag, Berlin.

Sissons J.G. & Oldstone M.B.A. (1980) Antibody-mediated destruction of virus-infected cells. *Adv. Immunol.* **31,** 1.

Stroop W.G., & Baringer J.R. (1982) Persistent, slow, and latent viral infections. *Progr. Med. Virol.* **28,** 1.

Smith, G.L. & Moss B. (1984) Uses of Vaccinia virus as a vector for the production of live recombinant vaccines. *BioEssays* **1,** 120.

Wiley D.C.. Wilson I.A. & Skehel J.J. (1981) Structural identification of the antibody binding sites of Hong Kong influenza haemagglutinin and their involvement in antigenic variation. *Nature* **289,** 373.

Zinkernagel R.M. & Doherty P.C. (1979) MHC-restricted cytotoxic T cells. Studies on the biological role of polymorphic major transplantation antigens determining T cell restriction, specificity, function and responsiveness. *Adv. Immunol.* **27,** 51.

Bacteria

Easmon C.S.F. & Jeljaszewicz J. (1984) *Medical Microbiology, Vol. 2: Immunisation against bacterial disease*. Academic Press Inc.

Hahn H. & Kaufmann S.H.E. (1981) The role of cell-mediated immunity in bacterial infections. *Rev. Infect. Dis.* **3,** 1221.

Horwitz M.A. & Silverstein S.C. (1981) Activated human monocytes inhibit the intracellular multiplication of Legionnaires disease bacilli. *J. Exp. Med.* **154,** 1618.

Joiner K.A., Brown E.J. & Frank M.M. (1984) Complement and bacteria: Chemistry and biology in host defence. *Ann. Rev. Immunol.* **2,** 461.

Kaufmann S.H.E. & Hahn H. (1982) Biological function of T cell lines with specificity for the intracellular bacterium. *Listeria monocytogenes in vitro* and *in vivo. J. Exp. Med.* **155,** 1754.

Mims C.A. (1977) *The pathogenesis of infectious disease*. Academic Press.

Nahmias A.J. & O'Reilly, J. (eds.). (1981) *Comprehensive Immunology, Vol. 8. Immunology of human infection, Part 1: Bacteria, Mycoplasmae, Chlamydiae and Fungi*. Plenum Medical Book Company.

Nathan C.F., Murray H.W., Wiebe M.E. & Rubin B.Y. (1983) Identification of interferon-γ as the lymphokine that activates human macrophage oxidative metabolism and antimicrobial activity. *J. Exp. Med.* **158,** 670.

Rook G.A.W. (1983) The immunology of leprosy. *Tubercle* **64,** 297.

Segal A.W. (1980) The antimicrobial role of the neutrophil leukocyte. *Journal of Infection* **3,** 3.

Fungi

Calderon R.A. & Hay R.J. (1984) Cell-mediated immunity in experimental murine dermatophytosis. Adoptive transfer of immunity to dermatophyte infection by lymphoid cells from donors with acute or chronic infections. *Immunology* **53,** 465.

Cox R.A. (1979) Immunologic studies of patients with histoplasmosis. *Am. Rev. Resp. Dis.* **120,** 143.

Grayhill J.R. & Drutz D.J. (1979) Host defence in cryptococcosis in the nude mouse. *Cell. Immunol.* **40,** 263.

Nahmias A.J. & O'Reilly, J. (eds.). (1981) *Comprehensive Immunology, Vol. 8. Immunology of human infection, Part 1: Bacteria, Mycoplasmae, Chlamydiae and Fungi*. Plenum Medical Book Company.

Rogers T.J. & Balish E. (1980) Immunity to *Candida albicans*. *Microbiological Reviews* **44,** 660.

17 Immunity to Protozoa and Worms

Parasite infections typically stimulate more than one immunological defence mechanism, for example, both antibody and cell-mediated immunity, and the response that predominates depends upon the identity of the parasite. In order to illustrate the general principles of immunity to the diseases caused by parasites some of the more important infections of man are considered here, together with the main defence mechanisms that control the multiplication and spread of the parasites within the host. This discussion will therefore be devoted to the events that occur in nature, where a number of immunological effector mechanisms act simultaneously, rather than to the controlled experimental conditions associated with the laboratory investigation of these mechanisms, described previously.

Parasitic protozoa which infect man include amoebae which live in the gut, those protozoa which live in the blood, either free (eg. African trypanosomes) or in erythrocytes (*Plasmodium spp.*), and those which live in macrophages, either in the skin or lymphatics (Leishmania), or in the mononuclear phagocyte system of the liver, spleen and bone marrow (eg. *Trypanosoma cruzi* and *Leishmania spp.*). *T. cruzi* also lives in both smooth and striated muscle.

Parasitic worms which infect man include some Trematodes or flukes (eg. Schistosomes), some Cestodes (tapeworms) and some Nematodes or roundworms (eg. *Trichinella spiralis,* hookworms, Ascaris and the filarial worms).

Examples of these different parasites, their life cycles, their vectors, their geographical distribution and the diseases they cause are described in figures 17.26-17.31.

Parasites infect very large numbers of people and present a major medical problem, especially in tropical countries (Fig. 17.1). The diseases caused are diverse and the immune responses which are effective against the different parasites vary considerably. Parasitic infections do, however, share a number of common features.

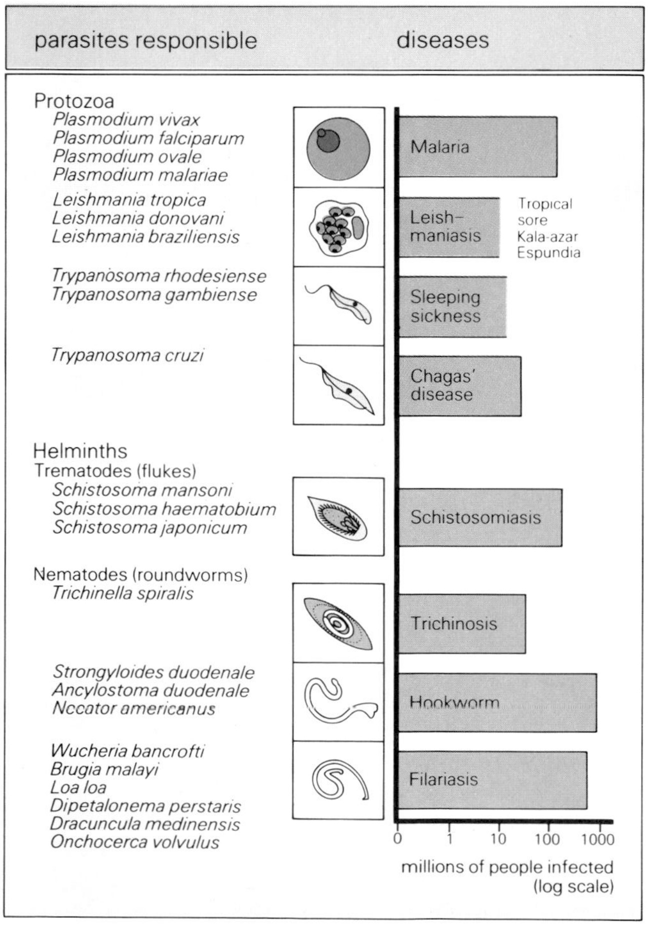

GENERAL FEATURES OF PARASITIC INFECTIONS

Protozoan parasites and worms are larger than other infectious agents such as bacteria and viruses (Fig. 17.2).

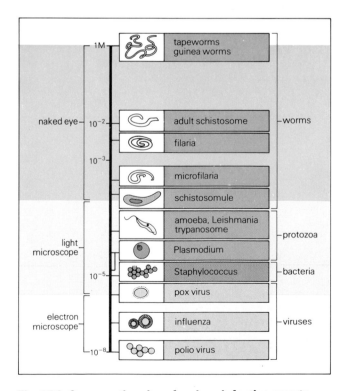

Fig. 17.1 The most important parasitic infections of man and the numbers of people infected. The precise figures for Leishmaniasis and sleeping sickness are not available.

Fig. 17.2 Comparative size of various infective agents.

These parasites often have complicated life cycles and additionally some depend upon a vector to transmit them from one host to another. Larger size entails the existence of more antigens, both in number and kind. In the case of parasites which display more complicated life histories, some of these antigens may be specific to a particular stage of development.

Parasitic infections are generally chronic. It is to the disadvantage of the parasite to kill its host and over millions of years of evolution the parasites that have survived are well adapted to their host and show marked host specificity. For example, the malarial parasite of birds, rodents or man can each multiply only in its own particular kind of host. There are some exceptions to this general rule, for example, the tapeworm of the pig is also able to infect man, but frequently the parasite cannot complete its life cycle in the incorrect host, indicating that host resistance is determined by particular genes.

Among the consequences of chronic infection are the presence of circulating antigens, persistent antigenic stimulation and the formation of immune complexes (Fig. 17.3). Characteristically levels of immunoglobulins are raised in some infections: IgM in trypanosomiasis and malaria; IgG in malaria and visceral leishmaniasis, and IgE in worm infections. Splenomegaly is pronounced in most parasitic infections, and there is evidence that parasite antigens can act directly as polyclonal mitogens for lymphocytes. Frequently, in addition to the immune responses directed against the parasite, immunosuppression and immunopathological effects are observed.

As a result of close adaptation of the parasite to its host, a balanced relationship has been set up. In the natural host no single immunological effector mechanism acts in isolation, there are always several, and in return parasites have evolved many different ways of evading the host's defences. In general terms however, cell-mediated responses are more effective against intracellular protozoa while antibody is more effective against extracellular parasites, in blood and tissue fluids. The following section considers the effector mechanisms by which cells and antibodies act.

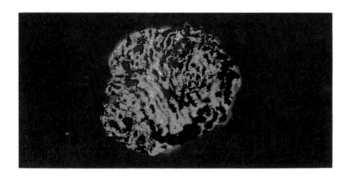

Fig. 17.3 Immune complex deposition in quartan malaria nephrotic syndrome – low power fluorescence micrograph of a renal glomerulus in a biopsy specimen from a Nigerian child with the syndrome. People infected with *Plasmodium malariae*, as in this case, may develop glomerulonephritis as a result of the deposition of immune complexes in the renal glomerulus. The section was stained with FITC conjugated anti-human IgG and shows granular deposition of immunoglobulin throughout the capillary loops of the glomerulus. Courtesy of Dr. V. Houba.

EFFECTOR MECHANISMS

In most parasite infections protection can be conferred on normal animals by the transfer of immune spleen cells. Normally T cells transferred from infected animals confer protective immunity, although in some cases (eg. *L tropica*) T cells can suppress the protective response, causing death of the recipients.

The T Cell Responses Important in the Control of Parasite Infections

1. Restraint of parasite proliferation and prolongation of host survival. This is demonstrable by the way in which nude (athymic) or T-deprived mice are unable to clear otherwise non-lethal infections of *T. cruzi* or rodent malaria (Fig. 17.4).

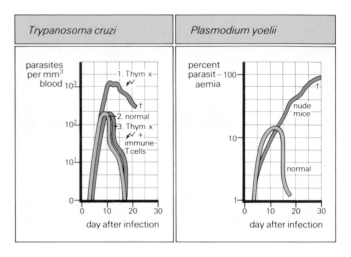

Fig. 17.4 Two examples of parasite infections in T-deprived mice that illustrate the importance of T cells in the control of acute infection. These graphs plot the increase in number of blood-borne parasites (parasitaemia) following infection of mice.
T. cruzi multiplies faster (and gives fatal parasitaemia) in mice that have been thymectomized (Thym x) and irradiated (⟿) to destroy T cells (1) than in normal mice, where parasites are cleared from the blood by 16 days (2). Reconstitution of T-deprived mice with T cells from immune mice (immune T) restores their ability to control the parasitaemia (3). In these experiments both experimental groups (1 and 3) were given foetal liver cells to restore vital haematopoietic function.
P. yoelii causes a self-limiting infection in normal mice and the parasites are cleared from the blood by day 20. In nude mice (which lack T cells congenitally) the parasites continue to multiply, killing the mice after about 30 days.

2. Cytotoxic T cells. Although it might be expected that cytotoxic T cells would play a role in reactions against intracellular parasites (as they do against other intracellular pathogens such as viruses), so far this has only been shown for *Theileria parvum*, which lives in the lymphocytes of cattle, and for *T. cruzi* infections, in which autoimmune destruction of parasitized heart cells and fibroblasts has been demonstrated.

3. Macrophage activation by lymphokines. Lymphokines are soluble factors released by certain kinds of sensitized T lymphocytes. They can activate macrophages by inducing the formation of more Fc and C3 receptors and by stimulating the production and secretion of various enzymes and other factors, including

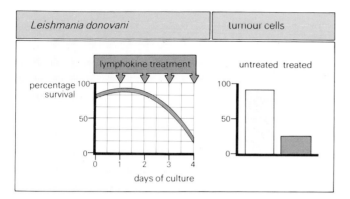

Fig. 17.5 The inhibition of parasite survival in macrophages treated with lymphokines. *Leishmania donovani* multiplies in normal macrophages *in vitro*. Daily treatment of the cultures with lymphokines from antigen activated spleen cells causes a progressive decrease in the number of Leishmania amastigotes compared with controls. Treated macrophages also become capable of killing tumour cells. Note that two other species of parasite which multiply in macrophages *in vitro, T. cruzi* and *Toxoplasma gondii,* are also unable to survive in macrophages that have been activated (whether *in vivo* as the result of infection or *in vitro* by treatment with lymphokines.)

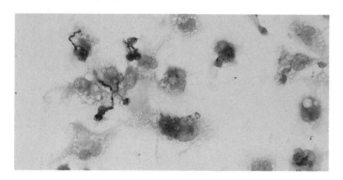

Fig. 17.6 The triggering of the respiratory burst of macrophages by *Leishmania donovani*. This picture shows a culture of resident peritoneal macrophages that have ingested promastigotes of *L. donovani* in the presence of nitroblue tetrazolium (NBT). The development of a black precipitate shows that the NBT has been reduced by products of the respiratory burst that was triggered by contact with the parasites, presumably by interaction with a specific receptor. More than 80% of promastigotes (the stages injected by the insect vector) are destroyed by normal macrophages but some escape from the phagolysosomes to become amastigotes. Amastigotes do not trigger the respiratory burst as well as do promastigotes and they survive well in normal macrophages. They can, however, be eradicated *in vitro* by incubation of the cells with lymphokines. Both stages are killed by H_2O_2 but not by the other O_2 metabolites. The promastigote is more sensitive to H_2O_2 than the amastigote. Courtesy of Dr. J. Blackwell.

oxygen metabolites, ultimately causing macrophages to become cytotoxic for tumour cells or parasites.

Activated macrophages are important, for example, in the control of infections caused by *T. cruzi, Leishmania* and *Plasmodium* spp. Figure 17.5 describes an experiment which shows that macrophages, activated by treatment with lymphokines to become tumoricidal, inhibit the multiplication of *L. donovani*. Perturbation of the membrane of macrophages, for instance during phagocytosis, can induce a respiratory burst, demonstrable by increased uptake of oxygen, activation of the hexose monophosphate shunt pathway and the production of oxygen metabolites that are cytotoxic for tumour cells and which kill bacteria and many parasites, including *T. cruzi, T. gondii, Leishmania*, malarial parasites, filarial worms and schistosomes (Fig. 17.6). Macrophages activated by lymphokines release more superoxide and hydrogen peroxide than resident macrophages.

4. Granulomata formation in liver and fibrous encapsulation. In some parasitic infections in which the immune system cannot completely eliminate the parasite, the body reduces damage by walling off the parasite behind a capsule of inflammatory cells. This reaction, which is T-dependent, is a chronic cell-mediated response to locally released antigen. Macrophages accumulate, release fibrogenic factors and stimulate the formation of granulomatous tissue and ultimately fibrosis. Granuloma formation around worm eggs is particularly marked in schistosome infections. Lack of T cells leads to lack of both granulomata formation and of the subsequent fibrous encapsulation (Fig. 17.7).

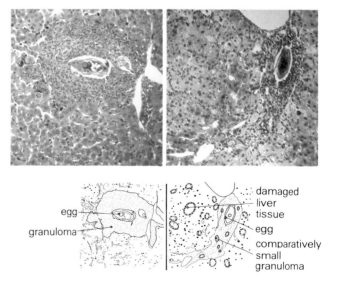

Fig. 17.7 T dependence of granuloma formation around schistosome eggs in the liver. Many of the eggs of schistosome worms are carried to the liver where they become insulated behind a capsule of inflammatory cells. In normal mice, the granulomata consist predominantly of eosinophils and are the result of a T-dependent reaction (left). In T cell deficient hosts, eggs of *S. mansoni* do not induce much granuloma formation and as a consequence of the lack of immune protection, toxic products of the eggs can diffuse out and cause damage to the surrounding liver tissue (right). Courtesy Dr. M. Doenhoff.

5. Eosinophils in worm infections. T cells recruit eosinophils into the gut mucosa in worm infections. The eosinophil appears to be a major effector cell against helminths and its recruitment is mediated by a specific factor, ESP (Eosinophil Stimulation Promoter) (Fig. 17.8).

6. Immunological responses of intestinal mucosa which cause expulsion of nematodes from the gut. T cells induce an increase in the number of inflammatory cells, mast cells and goblet cells and enhanced secretion of mediators and mucus (Fig. 17.9).

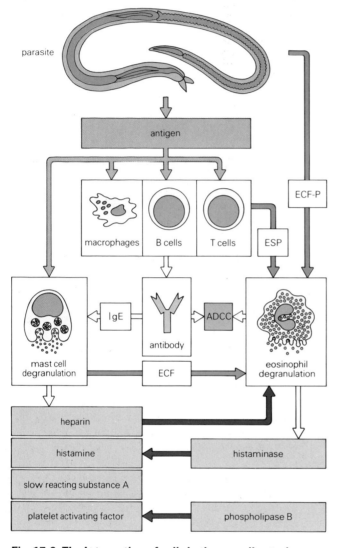

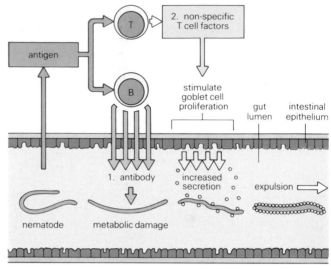

Fig. 17.9 Two-stage expulsion of nematodes from the gut. The expulsion of some intestinal nematodes occurs spontaneously a few weeks after a primary infection. It depends upon two sequential steps, following antigen sensitization of specific T cells and B cells:
1. the production of antibody (mainly IgG1) which damages the worms but is not itself sufficient to cause their elimination,
2. a T cell dependent secretory response. The T cells do not adhere directly to the worms but cause their expulsion through the release of non-specific factors acting on mucus secreting goblet cells in the intestinal epithelium. Although the T cell factors act non-specifically on the secreting cells, the initial triggering of the T cells is antigen specific.
The effector T cells are generated early in infection and the rate-limiting step is the onset of antibody damage. The numbers of goblet cells in the jejunal epithelium and the secretion of mucus increase in proportion to the worm burden. Mast cells also accumulate in the jejunal mucosa during infection, but worms can be eliminated quite normally by mice deficient in mast cells.

Fig. 17.8 The interaction of cells in the coordinated response to a worm infection. Antigens released by the parasite stimulate T cells and macrophages to interact with B cells to produce specific antibody. IgE-specific antibody sensitizes local mast cells so that they degranulate when they come into contact with antigen, releasing a variety of effector molecules (e.g. histamine). In addition, the mast cells also release eosinophil chemotactic factors (ECF). Eosinophils are attracted towards the worm by parasite-derived chemotactic factors (ECF-P) and are stimulated to proliferate by eosinophil stimulation promotor (ESP) derived from antigen-stimulated T cells. The eosinophils act in two main ways: (1) in association with specific antibody they kill the worm by antibody dependent cytotoxicity (ADCC), (2) enzymes released from the eosinophil granules exert a controlling effect on the substances released from the mast cells. The mast cell-derived factors are important in controlling the permeability of local blood vessels and inflammation at the site of infection. Heparin reduces eosinophil degranulation by feedback inhibition. (Note that green arrows indicate stimulation, and red arrows inhibition.)

In the presence of antibody, expulsion of worms enveloped in mucus is effected by the muscular activity that accompanies the increased secretions.

7. Production of specific antibody. T-helper cells cooperate in the production of specific antibody (including IgE) during parasite infections. T$_H$ cells cooperate specifically with B cells of each different class. In addition to the rise in specific antibodies many parasite infections provoke a non-specific hypergammaglobulinaemia. While T cells contribute to some of the generalized increase in immunoglobulin production, it is probable that much of the increase is due to antigens released from the parasite acting as polyclonal mitogens for B cells (ie. in a T-independent fashion). The effector functions of antibody are discussed in the following section.

Effector Functions of Antibodies

As previously stated, antibody is particularly important in the control of extracellular parasites. Thus, antibody is effective in preventing the reinvasion of cells by blood-borne parasites but is ineffective once the parasite has entered its host cell. The importance of antibody relative to cell-mediated immunity varies with the infection (Fig. 17.10). The mechanism by which specific antibody controls parasite infections and its effects are summarized in figure 17.11 and elaborated in figures 17.12-17.16.

parasite and habitat		antibody			cell-mediated immunity	
		importance	mechanism	means of evasion	importance	mechanism
T. brucei free in blood	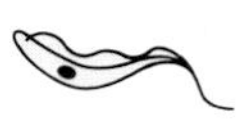	+ + + +	lysis with complement which opsonizes for phagocytosis	antigenic variation	–	
Plasmodium inside red cell	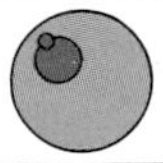	+ + +	blocks invasion opsonizes for phagocytosis	intracellular habitat	? +	macrophage activation
T. cruzi inside macrophage	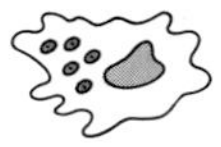	+ +	limits spread in acute infection	intracellular habitat	+ + + (chronic phase)	macrophage activation by lymphokines and killing by metabolites of O₂
Leishmania inside macrophage	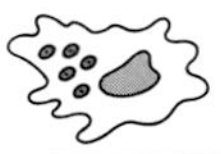	+	limits spread	intracellular habitat	+ + + +	

Fig. 17.10 Relative importance of antibody and cell-mediated responses in protozoal infections. This table summarizes the relative importance of the two immune responses, the mechanisms involved and, for antibody, the means by which the protozoan can evade damage by antibody. The mechanism by which the cell-mediated response is avoided is unknown. Antibody is the most important part of the immune response against those parasites that live in the bloodstream, such as African trypanosomes and malarial parasites, whereas cell-mediated immunity is active against those like *Leishmania* that live in the tissues. Antibody can damage parasites directly, enhance their clearance by phagocytosis, activate complement or block their entry into their host cell and so limit the spread of infection. Once inside, the parasite is safe from its effects. *T. cruzi* and *Leishmania* are both susceptible to the action of oxygen metabolites released by the respiratory burst of macrophages. Treatment of macrophages with lymphokines released by T cells enhances the release of these toxic products and diminishes both entry and survival of the parasites. Malarial parasites within the red cell may be destroyed by some products of activated macrophages, including hydrogen peroxide and other cytotoxic factors, but their importance in immunity to the disease is still under investigation. The means by which the organisms escape immunological control is discussed below.

parasite	Plasmodium sporozoite, intestinal worms, trypanosome	Plasmodium sporozoite, merozoite. T. cruzi Toxoplasma gondii	Plasmodium trypanosome	schistosomes T. spiralis filarial worms
mechanism	1 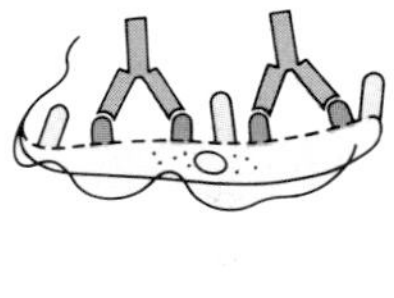	2 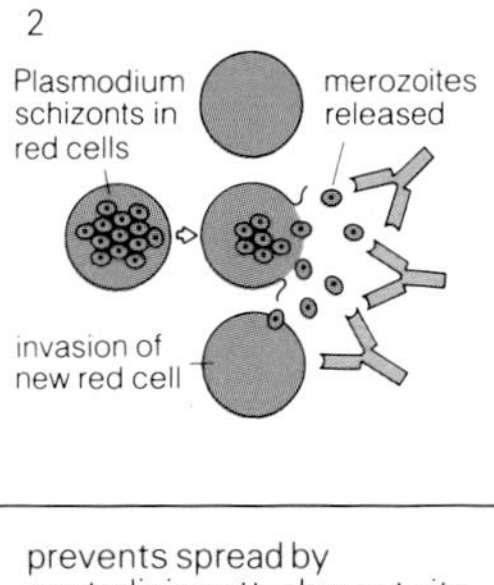 Plasmodium schizonts in red cells / merozoites released / invasion of new red cell	3 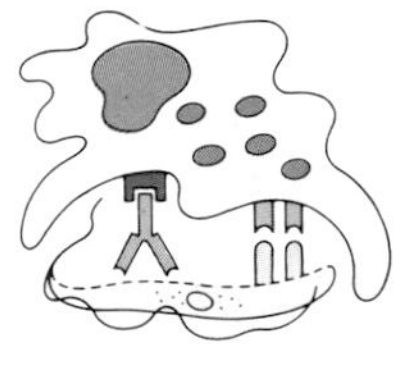	4 larval worm 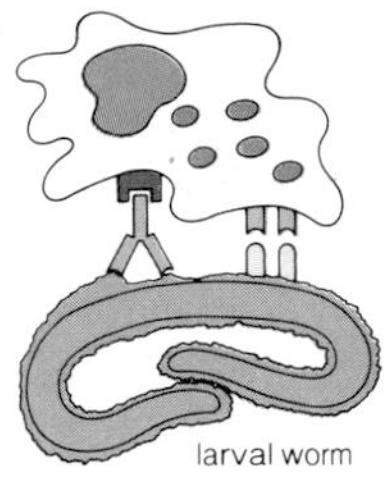
effect	direct damage or complement-mediated lysis	prevents spread by neutralising attachment site, prevents escape from lysosomal vacuole, prevents inhibition of lysosomal fusion	enhancement of phagocytosis	antibody dependent cytotoxicity (ADCC)

Fig. 17.11 Control of parasite infections by specific antibody: mechanisms and effects. 1) Direct damage caused by antibody activating the classical pathway of complement causes damage to the parasite membrane and increased susceptibility to other mediators. 2) Neutralization. For example, parasites such as *Plasmodium* spp. spread to new cells by specific receptor attachment: blocking the merozoite binding site with antibody prevents attachment to the receptors on the erythrocyte surface and hence further multiplication. 3) Enhancement of phagocytosis. Complement C3b deposited on parasite membrane opsonizes it for phagocytosis by cells with C3b receptors (eg. macrophages). Macrophages also have Fc receptors. 4) Eosinophils, neutrophils, platelets and macrophages may be cytotoxic for some parasites when they recognize the parasite via specific antibody (ADCC). The reaction is enhanced by complement.

1. Antibody can act directly on protozoa to damage them, either by itself or by interacting with the complement system (Fig. 17.12).

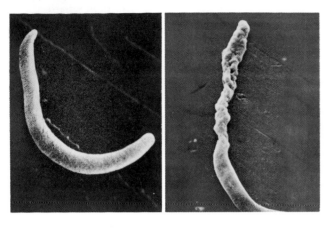

Fig. 17.12 Direct effect of specific antibody on sporozoites of malarial parasites. These scanning electron micrographs show a sporozoite of *P. berghei*, a parasite which causes malaria in rodents, before (left) and after incubation in immune serum (right). The surface of the parasite is damaged. Specific antibody protects against infection with *Plasmodium* spp. at several of the extracellular stages of the life cycle of the parasite and the antibody is stage specific in each case. It may act against sporozoites (the stage injected by the bite of a mosquito), against merozoites (the stage which penetrates the red blood cell) or against the gametocytes. Specific antibody perturbs the outer membrane of the sporozoite, causing leakage of fluid. Courtesy of Dr. R. Nussenzweig.

2. Antibody can neutralize a parasite directly by blocking its attachment to a new host cell. This effect can be observed in the case of *Plasmodium* spp.: the merozoites enter red blood cells through a special receptor and their entry is inhibited by specific antibody (Fig. 17.13). It may also act to prevent spread (eg. in the acute phase of infection with *T. cruzi*).

3. Antibody can enhance phagocytosis mediated by Fc receptors on macrophages. Phagocytosis (mediated by C3 receptors) of the parasites is increased even more by addition of complement. Both Fc and C3 receptors may themselves be increased in number as a result of macrophage activation. Phagocytosis plays a role in the control of infections with *Plasmodium* and *T. brucei*.

4. Antibody is also involved in antibody-dependent cytotoxicity, for example, in infections caused by *T. cruzi*, *T. spiralis*, *S. mansoni* and filarial worms. Cytotoxic cells such as macrophages, neutrophils and eosinophils in the presence of antibody adhere to worms by means of Fc and C3 receptors (Fig. 17.14). Damage to schistosomes is caused by the major basic protein (MBP) of the eosinophil crystalloid core (Fig. 17.15). Destructive effects are non-specific but the release of the MBP into a small space between the eosinophil and the schistosome surface localizes its action and minimizes damage to bystanding host cells (Fig. 17.16). The cells damage the tegument of the worms and kill them. Different kinds of cell and of antibody may act at different stages in the life cycle. For example, eosinophils are more effective at killing the newborn larvae of *T. spiralis* than other cells, macrophages are more effective against the microfilariae, and in each case antibody mediating the reaction is stage specific. IgG can mediate killing by eosinophils and IgE,

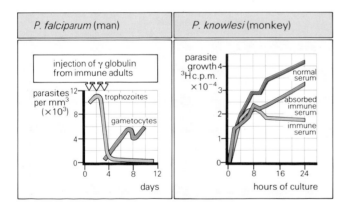

Fig. 17.13 Effect of antibody on malarial parasites.
P. falciparum. In man, transfer of γ-globulin from immune adults to a child infected with *P. falciparum* caused a sharp drop in parasitaemia. Specific antibody acts at the merozoite stage in the life of the parasite and prevents the initiation of further cycles of multiplication. The development of gametocytes from existing intracellular forms is unaffected.
P. knowlesi. In culture, the presence of immune serum blocks the continued increase in number of *P. knowlesi* (a malarial parasite of monkeys), as measured by incorporation of ³H-leucine. It stops multiplication at the stage after schizonts rupture, by preventing the released merozoites invading fresh red blood cells. The inhibitory activity of the immune serum can be removed by absorbing the specific antibody with free schizonts.

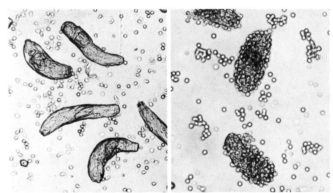

Fig. 17.14 Antibody-dependent cytotoxicity against schistosomes mediated by neutrophils. These photographs show a schistosomule of *S. mansoni* incubated with neutrophils in the presence of normal rat serum (left) and in the presence of fresh immune serum (contains active complement) (right). It demonstrates the adherence of neutrophils to the surface of the larva, mediated by antibody and complement, and is the first step in the killing of the parasite. The worm is probably killed by hydrogen peroxide and other oxygen metabolites released from the neutrophil during the respiratory burst that follows the membrane perturbation resulting from contact between parasite and neutrophil. Neutrophils from patients with chronic granulomatous disease that are incapable of generating hydrogen peroxide are markedly impaired in their ability to kill schistosomules. Courtesy of Dr. D. McLaren.

killing by macrophages. Killing of *S. mansoni* by eosinophils is enhanced by mast cell products (Fig. 17.8) and eosinophils from patients with schistosomiasis are more effective than those from normal subjects. The importance of these effector cells *in vivo* has been shown by experiments performed with antiserum against eosinophils, in which, for example, mice infected with *T. spiralis* and treated with the antiserum developed more cysts in their muscles than controls: with poorer protection by cells of the immune system the mice cannot eliminate the worms but encyst the parasites to minimize damage.

The role of the high levels of IgE that appear in nematode worm infections is unclear. It has been suggested that IgE sensitizes mast cells and basophils in the gut mucosa to induce the self-cure phenomenon seen in some of these infections. However, the phenomenon also occurs in animals deficient in mast cells and it appears therefore that the interaction of IgE and mast cells is not essential for expulsion of the worms.

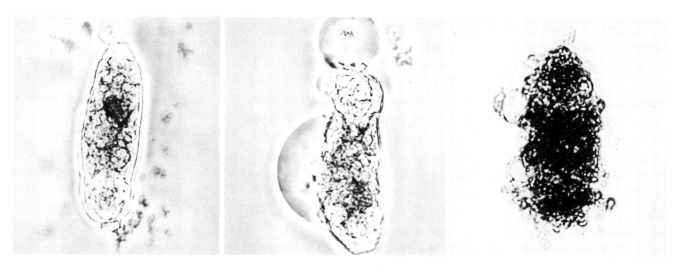

Fig. 17.15 Effect of basic protein of eosinophils on schistosomule larva. Killing of schistosomules by eosinophils can be associated with the major basic protein of the granules. These pictures show progressive surface damage and disruption of a larva caused by incubation in this cell product: intact worm (left), initial stage of damage to the tegument and worm surface (middle), total destruction of the worm (right). Courtesy of Dr. D. McLaren.

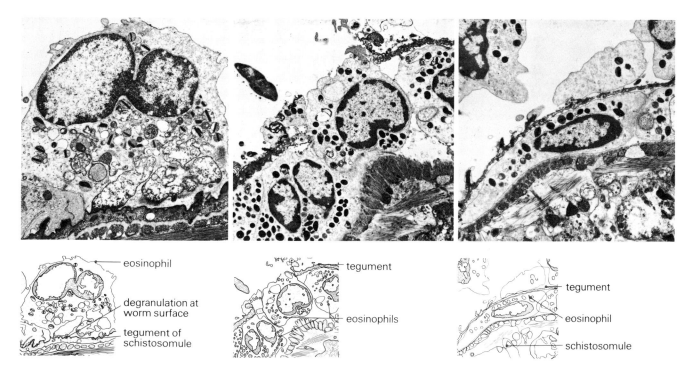

Fig. 17.16 Killing of schistosome larvae by eosinophils. Eosinophils can adhere to schistosomules and kill them. Damage is associated with degranulation of the eosinophils and release of the contents of the granules onto the surface of the worm. This series of views shows adherence of the eosinophil and degranulation onto the surface of the worm larva (left), and stages in the formation of lesions in the worm tegument and migration of eosinophils through the lesions (middle, right). Courtesy Dr. D. McLaren.

Non-Specific Effector Mechanisms

A variety of non-specific effector mechanisms act in parasitic infections. The blood phagocytes, both monocytes and granulocytes, and tissue macrophages all have some intrinsic anti-parasite activity although this is greatly enhanced by interaction with the different parts of the adaptive immune system, particularly antibody. It has also been postulated that NK cells may be active in some infections though this is still unproven.

Of the serum-soluble factors, complement has already been mentioned for its interaction with specific antibody via the classical pathway. Several parasites, including adult worms and infective larvae of *T. spiralis* and schistosomules of *S. mansoni,* activate the alternative pathway directly. This function is dependent on the nature of the molecules in their surface coats. The activation of the alternative pathway is dependent on both the species of host and the species of parasite.

ESCAPE MECHANISMS

It is a characteristic of all successful parasite infections that they can, in different ways, evade the full effects of the host's immune responses.

1. Location Many parasites are protected from the host's defences by their anatomical inaccessibility. For example, those that have an intracellular habitat avoid the effects of antibody (eg. *T. cruzi, Leishmania* spp. and the intracellular stages of *Plasmodium* spp.). Other parasites are protected by cysts (eg. *T. spiralis, E. histolytica*) or live in the gut (intestinal nematodes). Those that live inside macrophages have evolved different ways of avoiding killing by O_2 metabolites and lysosomal enzymes (Figs. 17.17 & 17.18).

Some parasites (eg. *T. gondii*) avoid triggering the oxidative burst while others break down its products. These escape mechanisms are of more limited efficiency in the immune host.

2. Avoidance of recognition Parasites that may be exposed to antibody have evolved different methods of evading its effects. African trypanosomes, by a process called antigenic variation, change the antigens of their surface coat (Fig. 17.19). Each variant possesses an antigenically distinct glycoprotein which forms its surface coat. The immunological uniqueness of these glycoproteins reflects diversity in amino acid sequence. Glycoproteins are identified on the organism by immunofluorescence or by radioimmunoassay of extracts. The surface coat presumably protects the underlying surface membrane from the host's defence mechanisms.

Some malarial parasites also show antigenic variation, but not, it seems, of antigens of the sporozoites or merozoites. Other parasites mask their presence by acquiring a surface layer of host antigens so that the host does not distinguish them from 'self' (eg. *Schistosome* spp., Fig. 17.20). Schistomules cultured *in vitro* in medium containing human serum and red blood cells can acquire surface molecules containing A, B and H specific blood group determinants. They can also acquire antigens of the major histocompatibility complex. The acquisition of

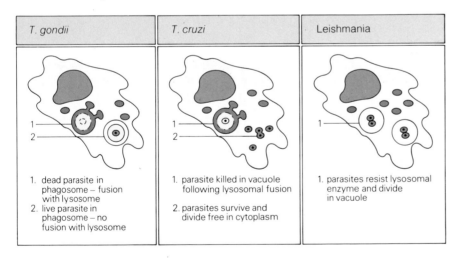

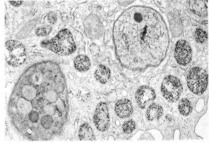

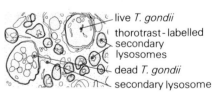
live *T. gondii*
thorotrast-labelled secondary lysosomes
dead *T. gondii*
secondary lysosome

Fig. 17.17 The different means by which protozoa that multiply within macrophages escape digestion by lysosomal enzymes.
Toxoplasma gondii Live parasites are not exposed to the enzymes because fusion of secondary lysosomes with the phagosomal vacuole within which the parasites live is inhibited. Dead parasites – or those coated with antibody – lose the capacity to block fusion and are destroyed.
Trypanosoma cruzi Survival of these parasites depends upon their stage of

development; trypomastigotes escape from the vacuole and divide in the cytoplasm whereas epimastigotes do not escape and are killed and digested. The proportion of parasites found in the cytoplasm is decreased if the macrophages are activated.
Leishmania spp. These parasites multiply in the phagocytic vacuole where they resist digestion. If the macrophages are first activated by treatment with lymphokines, the number of parasites entering the cell and the number that replicate diminish.

Fig. 17.18 Electron micrograph showing a macrophage infected with *T. gondii.* Following infection the macrophages are treated with thorotrast to make the contents of secondary lysosomes electron dense. The live parasite has inhibited fusion of the secondary lysosome with the phagosome. By contrast, a dead parasite lies in a vacuole that contains thorotrast and it can be seen that a lysosome has just fused with the vacuole and emptied its contents into it ×14,000. Courtesy Professor T. C. Jones.

host molecules may protect the parasite from damage by antibody while within that host. Schistosomules maintained in medium devoid of host molecules, however, also become refractory to attack by antibody and comple-

ment so that changes in the parasite tegument occur that are independent of the adsorption of host antigens. Thus, the importance of this antigen masking in protecting the worm from recognition is still controversial.

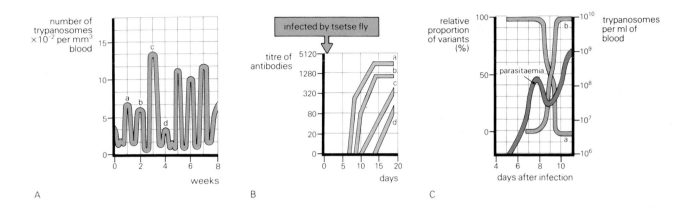

A

B

C

Fig. 17.19 Antigenic variation in African trypansomes.
Trypanosome infections, which can be initiated by a single parasite, may run for several months giving rise to successive waves of parasitaemia. Graph A shows a chart of the fluctuations in parasitaemia in a patient with sleeping sickness. Each wave is caused by an immunologically distinct population of parasites (a, b, c, d): protection is not afforded by antibody against preceding variants. There is a strong tendency for new variants to appear in the same order in different hosts. Variation does not occur in immunologically compromised animals (that is, treated in order to deprive the

animal of some aspect of its immune function). Graph B shows the time course of production of antibody against four variants in a rabbit bitten by a tsetse fly carrying *Trypanosoma brucei*. Antibody to successive variants appears shortly after the appearance of the variant and rises to a plateau. The appearance of antibody drives the parasite towards another variant type. Graph C shows the kinetics of one cycle of antigenic variation in a rat infected with a homogeneous population of one variant (a) of *T. brucei*. The new wave of parasitaemia develops as the new variant (variant b) emerges and predominates.

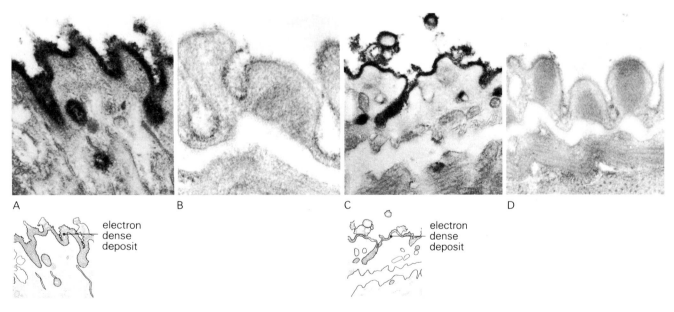

A

B

C

D

Fig. 17.20 Acquisition of host antigens by schistosomes.
These electron micrographs show sections of the surface of schistosomes that have been incubated with antibody (which has been labelled with horse radish peroxidase), directed against schistosome antigens or against mouse red blood cells. The presence of each particular antigen is shown by the layer of electron dense deposit of labelled antibody.
Young 3 hour schistosomules bind specific antibody *in vitro* (A) but fail to do so after 4 days in a mouse host (B). Antibody against mouse antigens binds to the 4 day old lung stage

parasite (C) but not to the newly transformed schistosomules (D). Thus, the older worms express the species specific antigens of their host but not the worm's own antigens. Lung stage worms are immune to attack by both complement and antibody-mediated effectors *in vitro*. Worms transferred from one species to another die within 24 hours. They are only susceptible to attack by specific antibody *in vitro* if they are not coated with protective antigens from their host, whereas antibody to host red cell antigens causes severe damage to the worm surface. Courtesy of Dr. D. McLaren.

3. Suppression of the host's immune responses. Parasites can cause disruption of lymphoid cells or tissue directly. For example, newborn larvae of *T. spiralis* release a soluble lymphocytotoxic factor. Similarly, schistosomes can cleave a peptide from IgG that inhibits many cellular immune responses. Soluble parasite antigens which can occur in enormous quantities may reduce the effectiveness of the host's response (Figs. 17.21 & 17.22). Non-specific immunosuppression is a universal feature of parasite infections and has been

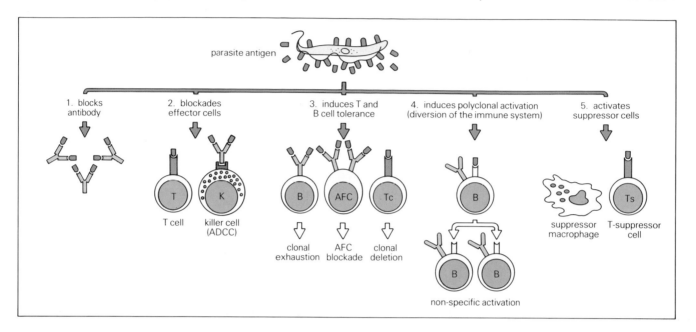

Fig. 17.21 Interference with host's immune response by antigens released from the parasite. The antigens interfere:
1. by combining with antibody and diverting it from the parasite.
2. by blockading effector cells, either directly or as immune complexes formed by combination with antibody. Circulating complexes for example, are able to inhibit the action of cytotoxic cells active against *S. mansoni*.
3. by inducing T or B cell tolerance, presumably by blockade of antibody-forming cells (AFC) or by depletion of the mature antigen-specific lymphocytes (ie. clonal exhaustion).

4. by polyclonal activation. Many parasite products are mitogenic to B lymphocytes, their action resembling that of bacterial lipopolysaccharide, and the high serum concentrations of non-specific IgM (and IgG) commonly found in parasitic infections probably result from this polyclonal stimulation. Its continuation is believed to lead to impairment of B cell function, the progressive depletion of antigen-reactive B lymphocytes and thus immunosuppression.
5. by activating suppressor cells, which may be T cells or macrophages or both.

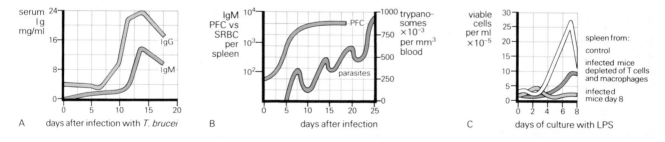

Fig. 17.22 Polyclonal activation by African trypanosomes. Graph A shows increasing concentrations of serum immunoglobulins observed in mice infected with *T. brucei*. These levels are only consistent with polyclonal activation and not specific antibody alone. Graph B shows the increase in number of IgM-secreting cells forming plaques with sheep red blood cells (SRBC) that occurs spontaneously during infection, that is, without injection of SRBC. The number increases with the parasitaemia to reach a plateau of 20-30 times normal. Cells secreting antibody against other antigens, including horse and donkey red cells, chicken gammaglobulin and TNP hapten, increase similarly. Soluble fractions derived from parasites have been shown to be mitogenic, their activity being enhanced by macrophages.

Trypanosomes – and other parasites – thus trigger and accelerate the proliferation of B lymphocytes and this may lead to the progressive depletion of antigen-reactive B cells. Graph C shows the failure of spleen lymphocytes taken from infected mice (at day 8) to proliferate in response to stimulation by lipopolysaccharide *in vitro*. Removal of T cells and macrophages from spleens taken soon after infection partly restores the response, but not later on when the B cell potential appears to become exhausted. Macrophages collected early in infection depress the ability of normal spleen cells to respond to LPS. Thus, the clonal exhaustion of B lymphocytes that have been stimulated directly to proliferate by parasites is partly mediated by the generation of suppressive macrophages and T cells.

demonstrated for both antibody (Fig. 17.23) and cell-mediated responses. Specific suppression may also occur, as has been demonstrated in Leishmaniasis (Fig. 17.24). In this case immunosuppression of T cell reactivity is harmful to the host because protection depends upon cell-mediated immunity. Experiments have demonstrated that elimination of the suppressor cells allows mice to recover from the infection. However, immunosuppression may be to the benefit of both host and parasite, as is seen in schistosomiasis. Many immune responses are depressed in this infection: the activity of T-helper cells is suppressed, as shown by decreased antibody responses to sheep red blood cells or to tetanus toxoid. Specific delayed hypersensitivity is suppressed, as shown by diminished foot pad responses to challenge by soluble worm egg antigen. Lymphocyte proliferation

in response to mitogens such as a phytohaemagglutinin or concanavalin A is depressed. A factor produced by the worm inhibits lymphocyte proliferation directly and the existence of both suppressor T cells and suppressive macrophages has been demonstrated. Liver granulomata caused by schistosome eggs diminish in size with time and it is thought that diminishing local production of lymphokines such as migration inhibition factor (MIF) and eosinophil stimulation promoter (ESP) may explain the decrease in size of the granulomata. This immunosuppression is to the benefit of both host and parasite because, although extensive granulomata formation damages the host's liver, some macrophage accumulation is helpful in protecting the tissue against the toxic secretions of the egg. Some of the escape mechanisms discussed above are summarized in figure 17.25.

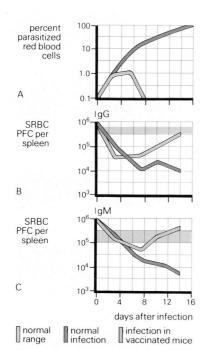

Fig. 17.23 Depression of non-specific antibody production in mice with malaria. Graph A shows the course of parasitaemia in unvaccinated and vaccinated mice infected with a lethal variant of the rodent parasite *Plasmodium yoelii*. Unvaccinated mice die about 16 days later: vaccinated mice survive and all parasites disappear from the blood by 8 days. The time course of parasitaemia correlates with the immunosuppression. Graphs B and C show numbers of IgM- and IgG- plaque forming cells (PFC) per spleen obtained 5 days after injection of sheep red blood cells into two groups of mice. Antibody producing cells decrease during infection: in vaccinated mice they return to normal as the mice recover. The depression of PFC, and thus antibody, appears to reflect parasite load. Its mechanism is unknown.

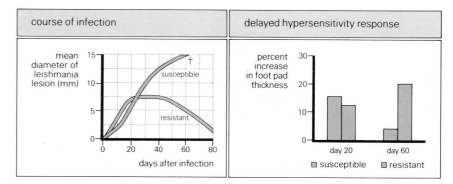

Fig. 17.24 Depression of specific delayed hypersensitivity in mice infected with Leishmania. The course of infection of *L. tropica*, as determined by the size of the lesion produced at the site of infection, is plotted for a susceptible strain and a resistant strain of mouse. Mice of the susceptible strain die about 70 days after infection. Delayed hypersensitivity to specific antigen injected into the footpad is

illustrated as the percentage increase in footpad thickness. In resistant mice the response increases as the mice recover, whereas it is significantly depressed in the susceptible mice. The depression is antigen specific and is mediated by a T-suppressor cell, which inhibits delayed hypersensitivity, but not antibody production. Recovery from this infection is associated with cell-mediated immunity.

parasite	habitat	effector	method of avoidance
African trypanosome	bloodstream	antibody + complement	antigenic variation
Plasmodium spp	blood (red cell)	antibody	intracellular habitat, antigenic variation
Toxoplasma gondii	macrophage	lysosomal enzymes and O_2 metabolites	inhibits fusion of lysosomes
Trypanosoma cruzi	macrophage	lysosomal enzymes and O_2 metabolites	escapes into cytoplasm
Leishmania	macrophage	O_2 metabolites	avoids digestion (mechanism unknown)
Trichinella spiralis	gut, blood, cysts in muscles	eosinophils etc. + antibody + complement	encystment
Schistosoma mansoni	gut, blood, lungs, portal vein	eosinophils etc. + antibody + complement	acquisition of host antigens, blockade by soluble antigen and immune complexes

Fig. 17.25 Examples of ways evolved by parasites to avoid host defences.

IMMUNOPATHOLOGICAL CONSEQUENCES OF PARASITE INFECTIONS

Apart from the directly destructive effects of some parasites and their products on host tissues, many immune responses themselves have pathological effects. The formation of immune complexes is common and apart from deposition in the kidneys, as in the nephrotic syndrome of quartan malaria, they may give rise to many other pathological changes. For example, tissue-bound immunoglobulins have been found in the muscles of mice with trypanosomiasis (cattle with this disease have a very wasted appearance) and in the choroid plexus of mice with malaria. Immune complexes have been postulated to cause cerebral malaria in man. Autoantibodies, probably arising as a result of polyclonal activation, have been detected against red blood cells, lymphocytes and DNA (eg. in trypanosomiasis and in malaria). Antibodies against the parasite may cross-react with host tissues. For example, the cardiomyopathy, enlarged oesophagus and megacolon that occur in Chagas' disease are thought to result from the autoimmune effects on nerve

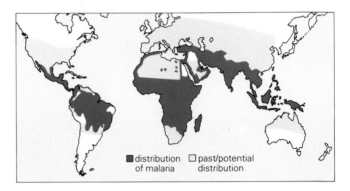

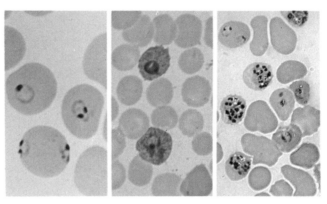

into schizonts and then merozoites which enter the blood. In red blood cells, parasites become first trophozoites (5) and then erythrocytic schizonts (6), from each of which 12-24 merozoites are released to invade further cells (7). Some merozoites become gametocytes (8) and are ingested by a mosquito in which they develop into microgametes and macrogametes (9) that fuse to form a zygote (11). This becomes a motile ookinete (12) which bores through the gut wall and forms an oocyst (13) from which large numbers of sporozoites are released (14). These invade the salivary glands from which they are injected into the human host when the mosquito feeds (1).

Bouts of fever are associated with the rupture of the schizonts (diagnostic stage) which occurs every 48 hours with *P. falciparum, P. vivax* and *P. ovale* (tertian fever) and every 72 hours with *P. malariae* (quartan fever). The liver and spleen are grossly enlarged and haemolytic anaemia may be severe. The three photographs illustrate blood films showing ring forms of *P. falciparum* (left) and trophozoites of *P. vivax* in human erythrocytes (middle) (both courtesy of Dept. of Protozoology, London School of Hygiene and Tropical Medicine) and placental blood showing schizonts of *P. falciparum* in erythrocytes (right, courtesy of Professor G. A. T. Targett).

Fig. 17.26 Life cycle of *Plasmodium vivax* and the geographical distribution of malaria.
1. The geographical distribution of malaria is shown for 1981.
2. The life cycle of *Plasmodium vivax* is associated with a relapsing form of human malaria. In man the infection begins when sporozoites are injected into the blood by a mosquito of the genus *Anopheles* (1) (infective stage). The sporozoites migrate to the liver where they enter hepatocytes (2) and develop into schizonts (3) which give rise to the invasive form, the merozoites (4), some of which enter red blood cells. Some sporozoites may remain dormant in the liver as hypnozoites. They may later, after an interval of several months, develop

ganglia of antibody or of cytotoxic T cells that cross-react with *T. cruzi*. The splenomegaly and hepatomegaly of malaria, sleeping sickness and visceral leishmaniasis are all associated with increases in the numbers and activity of macrophages and lymphocytes in the liver and spleen. The enlarged liver and its fibrosis in schistosomiasis are a consequence of granulomata formation around the worm eggs, resembling a delayed hypersensitivity reaction (Fig. 17.7). Lastly, the non-specific immunosuppression that is so universal, probably explains the fact that people with parasite infections are especially susceptible to bacterial infections and to viral infections (eg. measles) and it may account for the association of Burkitt's lymphoma with malaria.

EXAMPLES OF MAJOR HUMAN PARASITES

In the text above, a number of parasites infecting man are referred to. Their life cycles, geographical distributions and, in some cases, clinical and pathological presentation are illustrated in figures 17.26 – 17.31.

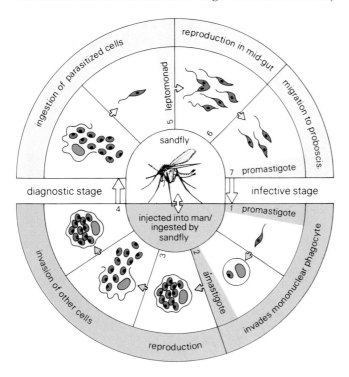

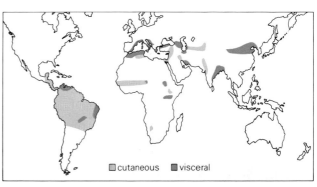

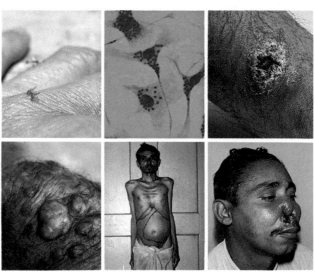

Fig. 17.27 Life cycle of *Leishmania* and the geographical distribution of Leishmaniasis.

The geographical distribution in 1981 of *Leishmania tropica* is shown, the parasite which causes cutaneous Leishmaniasis (involving skin), and *L. donovani,* which causes visceral Leishmaniasis (Kala-azar) (involving internal organs). Both the cutaneous and visceral forms are transmitted to man by certain species of Phlebotomines (sandflies). In India and some parts of E. Africa the parasite may be transmitted from man to man; in other areas dogs, rodents and some small mammals form a reservoir.

A generalized life cycle is shown. In man, infection begins when the promastigote is injected into the skin (1). It then enters mononuclear phagocytes (2) where it becomes an amastigote and multiplies (3). Further amastigotes are released which infect other cells (4). While in passage in the blood the infected cells may be picked up by the vector during feeding. After transformation into the leptomonad form (5), reproduction takes place in the mid-gut of the insect (6). From there the leptomonads migrate to the proboscis (7) to complete their maturation into promastigotes. *L. tropica* is restricted to macrophages of the skin, whereas *L. donovani* infects macrophages of the liver, spleen and bone marrow. *L. tropica* causes the self-healing ulcer of Oriental Sore, while *L. donovani* causes a systemic and often fatal disease.

A sandfly of the species *Lutzomyia longipalpis* photographed in Lapinha, Brazil (upper, left). Courtesy of Professor W. Peters. Resident peritoneal macrophages of a CBA/Ca strain mouse infected with amastigotes 72 hours previously (upper, middle). Giemsa stain. Courtesy of Dr. J. Blackwell. Tropical ulcer, caused by *Leishmania major,* on the arm of an individual in Saudi Arabia (upper, right). Courtesy of Professor W. Peters.

Diffuse cutaneous leishmaniasis, caused by *L. mexicana amazoniensis,* in the knee of an individual from Belem, in the Amazon region in Brazil (lower, left). The nodules indicate the spread of the disease that occurs in the absence of cell-mediated immunity. Courtesy of Professor W. Peters. Visceral leishmaniasis (Kala-azar), caused by *L. donovani* in a patient from Bilhar, India (lower, middle). Courtesy of Professor W. Peters. Mucocutaneous leishmaniasis (Espundia), caused by *L. brasiliensis brasiliensis,* showing severe destruction of nasopharyngeal tissues in a patient from Belo Horizonte, Brazil (lower, right). Courtesy of Professor W. Peters.

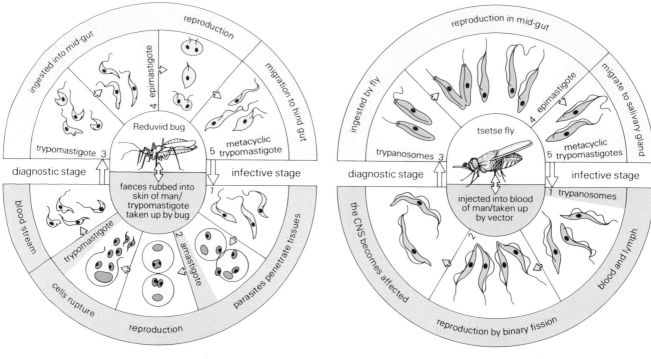

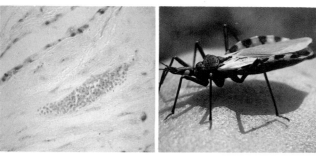

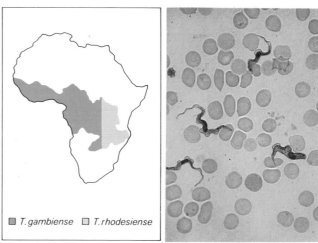

Fig. 17.28 Life cycle of *Trypanosoma cruzi.*

T. cruzi causes Chagas' disease which is widespread in S. America. The parasites exist in wild mammals such as armadillos and opossums as well as in domestic animals. They are transmitted to man by the bite of Reduviid bugs, called 'kissing' or 'assassin' bugs, particularly of the genera *Triatoma, Rhodnius* and *Panstrongylus.* The vectors live in cracks in the walls of mud huts and bite at night. They transmit *T. cruzi* while feeding, not by inoculation but by faecal contamination. They defaecate and the victim rubs the faeces into the skin when scratching. After an initial trypomastigote parasitaemia (1), associated with fever in the acute stage of the disease, the parasites penetrate the tissues, for example, cardiac muscle and smooth muscle of the gut, where they transform into amastigotes (2). There is a long chronic stage of infection, during which the heart may become enlarged and destruction of various ganglionic plexuses may occur, or various segments of the alimentary tract may become enlarged and denervated, causing such conditions as megacolon. Sudden death may result from heart block. The life cycle is completed when a feeding bug picks up blood trypomastigotes (3). The trypanosomes become epimastigotes (4) in the mid-gut, multiply and migrate to the hindgut where they become metacyclic trypomastigotes (5), the form which is the infective stage for man.
Morphological appearance of amastigotes of *T. cruzi* in heart muscle (left). Courtesy of the Wellcome Museum. The Reduviid bug (right). Courtesy of Dr. W. Petana.

Fig. 17.29 Life cycle and geographical distribution of the African trypanosomes.

African trypanosomiasis is confined to equatorial Africa. In man, disease (sleeping sickness) is caused by two species of trypanosome, *T. gambiense,* which is widespread in West and Central Africa and *T. rhodesiense,* which occurs in the East and east central areas. Trypanosomes are parasites of wild and domestic animals and are transmitted from host to host by the tsetse fly genus *Glossina.* Trypanosomiasis is a chronic and serious disease of domestic cattle, causing great economic loss. Trypanosomes at the metacyclic stage are injected from the salivary gland of the tsetse fly during feeding (1). The entire life cycle in man occurs in the blood and lymph. The parasites are extracellular and divide by binary fission (2). As the CNS becomes affected the patient becomes progressively more wasted and finally comatose. The parasites are picked up by the vector during feeding (3); they divide and mature in the mid-gut of the fly (epimastigote stage, 4), then return as a metacyclic trypanosome to the fly's salivary gland (5). Morphological appearance of the parasite in the blood. It is extracellular and motile, using its long free flagellum to propel itself (right). Courtesy of Professor W. Peters.

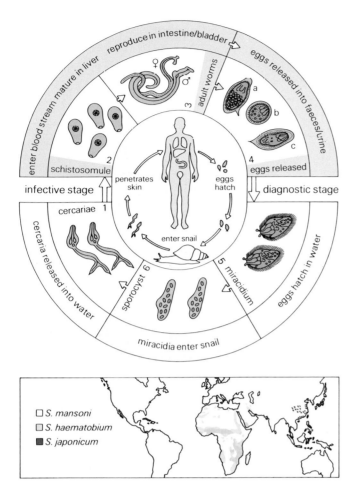

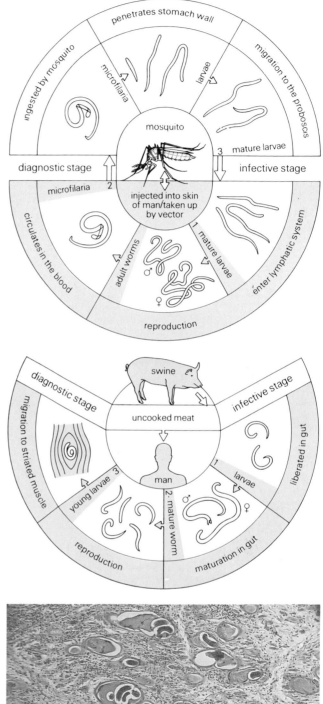

Fig. 17.30 Life cycle and geographical distributions of *Schistosoma mansoni*, *S. haematobium* and *S. japonicum*. Man becomes infected from water in which there are free swimming cercariae (larval form) which can penetrate the skin (1). The tail is shed and the worms (schistosomule stage) migrate through the circulation to the lungs and then to the liver, where they mature (2). They then enter the blood vessels of the gut or, in the case of *S. haematobium*, the bladder. The adult worms remain closely entwined in the portal vein (or blood vessels of the bladder) and the eggs released work their way out of the vessels into the tissues of the wall of the gut or bladder (3) and from there they escape into the faeces or urine (4). The three common species of Schistosome infecting man can be distinguished by their eggs. Some eggs are carried to the lungs or liver, where granulomata develop around them. In water, the eggs hatch to become ciliated miracidia (5) which must enter a snail of a suitable species within 24 hours or die (6).

Fig. 17.31 The life cycles of two representative nematodes (roundworms). One is spread by an insect vector (*Wucheria bancrofti*, upper right), and one (*Trichinella spiralis*, lower right) by direct transmission.
Trichinella spiralis develops through both adult and larval stages within a single mammalian host, which may be a carnivorous or omnivorous animal. The cycle in man is initiated by the ingestion of meat, usually undercooked pork, which contains encysted larvae. The larvae liberated in the gut (1) mature rapidly (2) and the fertilized females then deposit further young larvae (3) which migrate to the tissues (4) by way of the lymphatics and the blood. They usually develop only in striated muscle, where they become encysted. *Wuchereria bancrofti*, a typical filarial worm, lives in the lymphatic vessels of man (adult stage) (1) and produces a prelarval form, the microfilaria, which circulates in the blood (2). The parasite is transmitted by mosquitoes, in which the microfilariae pass through 3 stages of development to reach the infective stage (3). The arthropod host is necessary for cyclical development and microfilariae circulating in transfused blood are unable to cause infection.
The muscle biopsy of thigh muscle from a child in Kenya shows encysted larvae of *Trichinella spiralis*. Courtesy of Professor G. Nelson.

17.15

FURTHER READING

General

Capron A., Dessaint J. P., Haque A., Auriault C. & Joseph M. (1983) Macrophages as effector cells in helminth infections. *Trans. Roy. Soc. Trop. Med. & Hyg.* **77,** 631.

Cohen S. & Warren K. S. (eds) (1982) *Immunology of Parasitic Infections.* 2nd edition. Blackwell Scientific Publications, Oxford.

Evered D. C. & Collins G. M. (eds) (1983) *Cytopathology of Parasitic Disease.* Vol. 99 CIBA Foundation Symposium.

Jarrett E. E. & Miller H. R. P. (1982) Productions and activities of IgE in helminth infections. *Prog. Allergy.* **31,** 178.

Mitchell G. F. (1979) Effector cells, molecules and mechanisms in host-protective immunity to parasites. *Immunology.* **38,** 209.

Mitchell G. F. (1979) Responses to infection with metazoan and protozoan parasites in mice. *Adv. Immunol.* **28,** 451.

Nathan C. (1983) Mechanisms of macrophage antimicrobial activity. *Trans. Roy. Soc. Trop. Med. & Hyg.* **77,** 620.

Thorne K. J. & Blackwell J. M. (1983) Cell-mediated killing of protozoa. *Adv. Parasitol.* **22,** 44.

Wakelin D. (1984) *Immunity to parasites: how animals control parasite infections.* E. J. Arnold, London.

Malaria

Brown K. N. (1983) Host resistance to malaria. *Critical Reviews in Tropical Medicine.* **1,** 171.

Deans J. A. & Cohen S. (1983) Immunology of malaria. *Ann. Rev. Microbiol.* **37,** 25.

Trypanosoma cruzi

Brener Z. (1980) Immunity to *Trypanosoma cruzi. Adv. Parasitol.* **18,** 247.

Wood J. N., Hudson L., Jessel T. M. & Yamamoto M. (1982) A monoclonal antibody defining antigenic determinants on subpopulations of mammalian neurones and *Trypanosoma cruzi* parasites. *Nature.* **296,** 34.

African trypanosomes

Cross G. A. M. (1979) Immunological aspects of antigenic variation in trypanosomes. The Third Fleming Lecture. *J. Gen. Microbiol.* **113,** 1.
Turner M. J. (1982) Biochemistry of the variant surface glycoproteins of salivarian trypanosomes. *Adv. Parasitol.* **21,** 70.

Schistosomes

Butterworth A. E., Taylor D. W., Veith M. C., et al. (1982) Studies on the mechanisms of immunity in schistosomasis. *Immunol. Rev.* **61,** 5.

McLaren D. J. & Terry R. J. (1982) The protective role of acquired host antigens during schistosome maturation. *Parasite Immunol.* **4,** 129.

Simpson A. J. G., Singer D., McCutchan T. F., Sacks D. L. & Sher A. (1983) Evidence that schistosome MHC antigens are not synthesized by the parasite but are acquired from the host as intact glycoproteins. *J. Immunol.* **131,** 962.

Other helminths

Bell R. G., Adams L. S. & Ogden R. W. (1984) Intestinal mucus trapping in the rapid expulsion of *Trichinella spiralis* by rats: induction and expression analyzed by quantitative worm recovery. *Inf. Immun.* **45,** 267.

Bell R. G., McGregor D. D. & Adams L. S. (1982) Studies on the inhibition of rapid expulsion of *Trichinella spiralis* in rats. *Int. Arch. Allergy. Appl. Immunol.* **69,** 73.

Ha T. Y., Reed N. D. & Crowle P. K. (1983) Delayed expulsion of adult *Trichinella spiralis* by mast cell-deficient W/W mice. *Inf. Imm.* **41,** 445.

18 Immunity to Tumours

A ROLE FOR THE IMMUNE SYSTEM?

Solid human tumours removed at surgery are sometimes characterized by a marked mononuclear cell infiltrate, unrelated to tissue necrosis, which is suggestive of host resistance of an immunological nature (Fig.18.1). Modern enzyme immunohistochemical techniques reveal that such infiltrates are heterogeneous and frequently comprise mononuclear phagocytes, lymphocytes of different subtypes as well as minority populations of other cells (such as plasma cells and mast cells). In man, the opportunity to monitor the *in situ* immune responses usually arises only once (at surgery for removal of the primary lesion): this reflects the situation at an isolated, often very late point in the pathogenesis of the tumour. Although for some rare neoplasms mononuclear cell infiltration is a good indicator of prognosis (for example, in medullary carcinoma of the breast) and may even contribute to conventional anti-cancer therapy (for example, in seminoma of the testis), there is no simple relationship between infiltration and prognosis and/or survival. The view that mononuclear cell infiltration has a defensive connotation is therefore an assumption. Infiltration may vary from the florid example in figure 18.1 to none at all, and with the exception of the specific neoplasms mentioned above, it rarely follows a consistent or predictable pattern. Although the *in situ* function of these cells is not

determined their presence does suggest an involvement of cells of the immune system with established cancers which could have important implications for the host response to the disease at earlier stages.

Many experimentally induced neoplasms are characterized by mononuclear cell infiltrates. For some, for example, Moloney virus-induced sarcomas, host cell infiltration is clearly associated with the frequent spontaneous regression of this tumour. This neoplasm is probably unique in this respect and its biological behaviour has little relevance for human neoplasia. For the majority of tumours – clinical and experimental – the relationship is much more complex.

EXTENT OF POSSIBLE IMMUNE RESPONSES TO TUMOURS

Malignant transformation may be accompanied by phenotypic changes in the involved cells including the loss of normal cell surface antigenic components, gain of neoantigens (antigens not detectable in the corresponding normal tissue) and other membrane changes which influence cell:cell interactions in the host. Whether 'public' (that is, expressed on cells other than the tumour) or 'private' (that is, expressed exclusively by the tumour), some of these neoantigens are capable of evoking an adaptive immune response (Fig.18.2).

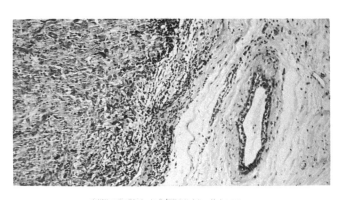

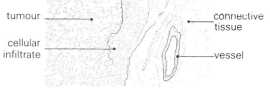

Fig.18.1 Immunological reaction to a mammary carcinoma. The section shows a mammary carcinoma heavily infiltrated with mononuclear cells, suggesting that carcinomas may be recognized by cells of the immune system which are *potentially* active in limiting or eliminating the tumour cells. H&E stain, ×50.

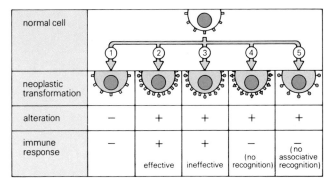

Fig.18.2 Host recognition of tumours and adaptive immune responses. Cells which undergo neoplastic transformation do not necessarily change their surface phenotype, in which case no adaptive immune response can result (1). If the neoplastic cells do change their surface phenotype, immune responses may develop and are either effective (2) or ineffective (3), a condition referred to as 'immunological escape'. Some changed neoplastic cells do not induce immune responses, either because there is a failure to recognize the new antigens (4) or because other surface antigens (such as MHC products) are changed and there is no associative recognition of the neoplastic cell with its new antigens (5).

In some systems, the immune response to these antigens may be as strong as an allogeneic reaction. At the other end of the spectrum, tumours which show minimal antigenic changes might be expected to elicit little or no adaptive immune response. (Spontaneous tumours of experimental animals are the major group in this category.) Between these two extremes lie the theoretical possibilities that tumours express neoantigens which evoke no response at all, or generate a response which is successfully evaded, a condition referred to as 'immunological escape' (discussed below). While neoantigens appear to be a stable, heritable property of some selected experimental tumours, the majority of cancers should probably be regarded as heterogeneous, genetically unstable and subject to phenotypic change.

In addition to changes in the antigenic phenotype of malignant cells, tumour cell membranes apparently acquire new 'structures' which render them susceptible to natural effector cells. The relationship of these structures, which are present in a wide variety of tumour cells, to the well-defined cell surface antigens is presently unknown.

CELL-MEDIATED IMMUNITY TO TUMOURS – T CELL RESPONSES

The adaptive immunity induced to tumour antigens is essentially similar to that evoked against T cell dependent transplantation and other cell surface glycoprotein antigens (Fig. 18.3). T cell activation includes the generation of helper (T_H) and suppressor (T_S) subsets as well as cytolytic T lymphocytes (T_C). Amplification of these

responses requires an optimal supply of interleukins. Cytotoxic T cells recognize tumour antigen in association with MHC products. Activation also gives rise to the production of lymphokines by T_H cells which are important for the recruitment and activation of macrophages and natural killer (NK) cells (Fig. 18.4).

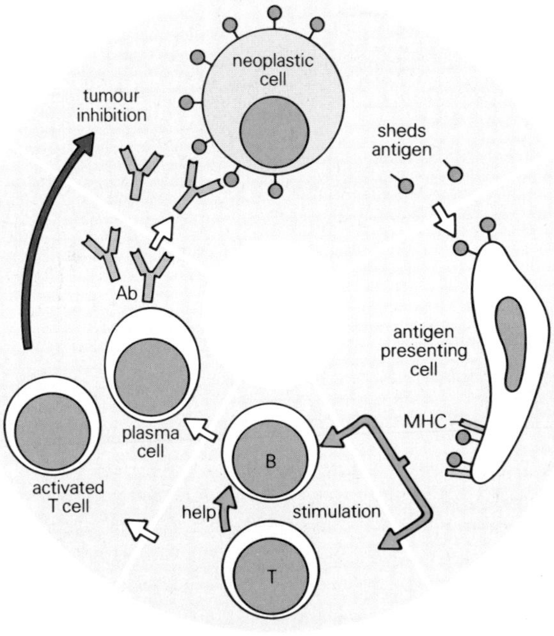

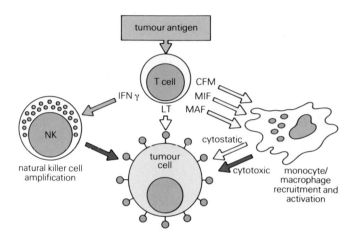

Fig. 18.4 The role of Lymphokines in tumour killing. T cells activated by tumour antigen: (1) release interferon (IFNγ) to amplify the lytic action of natural killer (NK) cells, (2) release lymphotoxin (LT) which acts directly and, (3) release chemotactic factors (CFM), migration inhibition factor (MIF) and macrophage activating factor (MAF) all of which attract and activate macrophages. Macrophages have a cytotoxic effect on the tumour and prevent multiplication. Other lymphokines, including IL−2, amplify antigen-specific immune reactions by B cells and other T cells.

The important lymphokines are:
1. Migration inhibition factor (MIF) increases the level of intracellular cyclic AMP, resulting in increased polymerization of microtubules and decreased cell migration. Its function is probably to arrest macrophages at the (antigenic) tumour site.
2. Macrophage activating factor (MAF), has similar properties to MIF and is probably identical to IFNγ (see below). Macrophages cultured with this factor develop some of the properties of 'activated' macrophages.
3. Chemotactic factor for macrophages (CFM), is distinguishable from MIF and is the molecule responsible for recruitment of phagocytes to the tumour site.
4. Lymphotoxin (LT), is a protein also distinct from MIF that can lyse some tumours *in vitro* but of unknown *in vivo* significance.
5. Transfer factor (TF) is a lymphocyte product found, to date, only in man, with the ability to enhance resistance to fungal infection *in vivo* and found to be therapeutically beneficial in some patients.
6. Interferons (IFNs) were first described as antiviral proteins which exert many effects on the immune response. The type of IFN generated in the immune response is IFNγ (formerly Type II IFN). This is a more probable candidate for an immunoregulatory molecule than the virus-induced IFNs (Type I; IFNα, IFNβ), the *primary* function of which is probably direct inhibition of virus replication. To date, the antiviral and immunomodulatory properties of the two major classes of IFN largely

Fig. 18.3 Adaptive immunity to tumours. Antigens shed from neoplastic cells bind to antigen-presenting cells and in association with MHC class II antigens stimulate specific T and B cells. The activated lymphocytes cooperate in the production of tumour specific antibody and activated T cells may also have cytostatic or cytolytic activity. (Memory cells are generated during the response.)

overlap though quantitative differences and even qualitative differences exist. Depending upon the conditions, IFNs may suppress or enhance immune responses, and their possible immunomodulatory roles include the regulation of antibody production, various T cell functions, expression of cell surface antigens, regulation of natural killer activity and macrophage functions.

7. Mitogenic factors (MF) comprise a family of molecules generated by antigen, or lectin stimulation of T cells. The most important factor in this context is interleukin-2 (IL–2) which is an antigen non-specific, soluble factor, the production of which is dependent upon the presence of both macrophages and T_H cells.

Detection of T Cell-Mediated Immunity

The methodology for the detection of tumour antigens on both human and experimental neoplasms which evoke adaptive immune responses relies upon T cell activation and the concomitant elaboration of lymphokines following exposure of T cells to tumour (target) cells. Tests have direct implications for the tumour-host relationship only if conducted (for animal tumours) in strictly syngeneic systems (targets and effector T cells derived from members of the same inbred strain) or (for human tumours) in autologous combinations (targets and T cells from same donor). Otherwise irrelevant allogeneic interactions may intrude. The tests fall into 3 major categories. Assays may be made of: 1. T cell proliferation, 2. lymphokine production and 3. effector function (Fig. 18.5).

1. Specific T cell proliferation is measured by incorporation of ³H–thymidine into autologous (or syngeneic) responder lymphocytes after 6 days cocultivation with 'inactivated' tumour cells (MLTI) (Fig. 18.6). Proliferating T cells may be of cytotoxic, helper or suppressor subsets. Cytotoxic T cells (Tc) may be assayed by cytotoxicity assays as described below, helper T cells (T_H) by their capacity to undergo restimulation with the appropriate antigen (primed lymphocyte test, PLT) and suppressor T cells (Ts) by their capacity to inhibit primary lymphocyte transformation by lectins.

2. Lymphokine production is assayed by inhibition of leucocyte migration (LMI) (Fig. 18.7) or adherence (LAI).

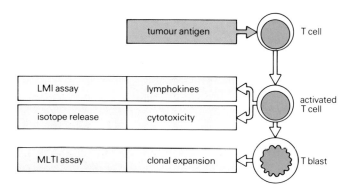

Fig.18.5 Demonstration of T cell-mediated immunity to tumours _in vitro_. Cell-mediated immunity is measured in 3 assays. Following antigenic stimulation of specific T cells, the cells release lymphokines and develop anti-tumour cytotoxic activity measured in the leucocyte migration inhibition assay (LMI) and isotope release assays respectively. Clonal expansion and proliferation of the cells is measured in the mixed lymphocyte/target cell interaction assay (MLTI).

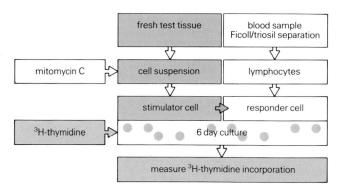

Fig.18.6 Mixed lymphocyte/target cell interaction (MLTI) test. A cell suspension (target cells) is prepared from normal or tumour tissue. The cells are then treated with mitomycin C which prevents them from dividing but does not alter their antigenicity. Meanwhile lymphocytes are prepared on a Ficoll/triosil gradient from a fresh heparinized blood sample and the lymphocytes and target cells cocultivated for 6 days. Any antigen-specific lymphocytes are stimulated to divide as measured by pulsing the culture with tritiated thymidine and measuring the amount incorporated into the responder cells.

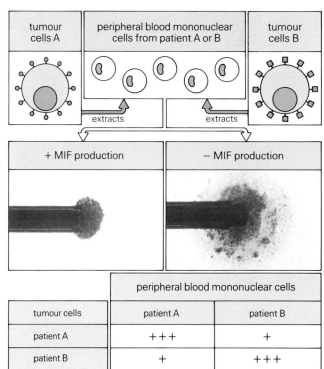

tumour cells	peripheral blood mononuclear cells	
	patient A	patient B
patient A	+++	+
patient B	+	+++

Fig. 18.7 Leucocyte migration inhibition assay (LMI). Peripheral blood mononuclear cells from patients with different tumours (A or B) are mixed separately with extracts derived from the patient's tumour. The cells are spun down into capillary tubes and the tubes are incubated on the surface of an agar plate. Under normal circumstances the adherent cells (chiefly macrophages) in the mixture will migrate out of the tube. However if the T cells in the mixture react to the tumour antigen they release macrophage Migration Inhibition Factor (MIF) and migration is reduced. MIF production is greatest to the autologous extract although there is also some non-specific release. This assay can also be used to detect responses to tumours of different histogenic type. Note that in all cases the assay detects primed T cells, not T cell priming.

3. Tc effector function is commonly monitored in short-term cytotoxicity assays such as release of ^{51}Cr from pre-labelled tumour targets (Fig.18.8). Since unfractionated or only partially-purified T cells are generally used in such assays, it is important to distinguish T cell effector function from that of Natural Killer (NK) cells (see below) by using appropriate specificity controls.

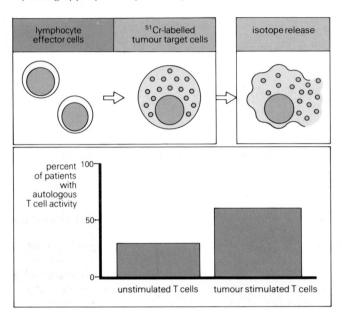

Fig.18.8 Isotope release assay. Autologous T cell cytotoxicity (ATC) can be measured in an isotope release assay. Lymphocytes from peripheral blood or lymph node are incubated with autologous radiolabelled tumour cells (above). The lytic action of these effectors is measured by assaying released isotope. Approximately 30% of patients operated on to remove tumours display ATC against the tumour. If their lymphocytes are stimulated in an MLTI assay for 6 days prior to the isotope release assay up to 60% now display ATC implying that antigen specific lymphocytes are present in the majority of patients but they may need stimulation, as in MLTI, to become actively cytotoxic for the tumour (below).

Approximately one-third of all cancer patients who undergo surgery exhibit peripheral blood (or lymph node) lymphocyte cytotoxicity which is directed against fresh autologous tumour cells. If the effector lymphocytes are first pre-incubated *in vitro* with inactivated tumour targets (as in the MLTI assay) and subsequently (day 6) assayed against cryopreserved autologous targets the incidence of cytotoxicity increases to approximately two-thirds. This suggests that the frequency of Tc activity in the majority of operable patients is too low for detection without clonal amplification. Increased cytotoxicity can also be achieved if effector lymphocytes are cultured for short periods in exogenous IL–2, or under conditions in which IL–2 is generated endogenously. In patients in whom autologous lymphocyte cytotoxicity is demonstrable in peripheral blood or draining lymph nodes, the activity of tumour-infiltrating lymphocytes recovered by disaggregation of the tumour mass, is significantly depressed (see below). This observation suggests *in situ* modulation of T cell function by tumour-related products or accumulation of suppressor cells.

NATURAL IMMUNITY

Natural immunity is effected by cells capable of lysing tumours spontaneously, that is, without prior sensitization. Strictly speaking, the effectors of *natural immunity* include mononuclear phagocytes and polymorphonuclear leucocytes as well as NK cells, a term usually, though not invariably, used for cells of lymphocyte lineage (Fig.18.9). This is based upon their apparent predilection for tumour cells adapted to tissue culture, against which cytotoxicity can be readily monitored in isotope release assays. Even so, NK cells and macrophages, the most studied of the trio call for separate discussion. Unlike cytotoxic T cells, NK cells appear to lack both immunological memory and MHC restriction and are characterized by an ability to lyse a wide variety of targets including those which are syngeneic, allogeneic and xenogeneic to the NK cell donor. Virus-infected targets are also highly sensitive as are certain normal cells of thymic and bone marrow origin. This has led to the hypothesis that the capacity to regulate tumours is an extension of the normal regulatory role of NK cells which is to combat virus-infected cells and regulate cellular differentiation in the thymus and bone marrow.

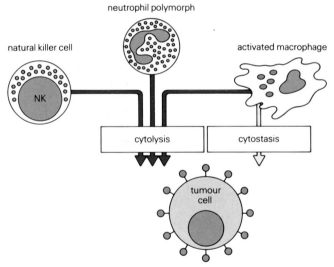

Fig.18.9 Natural immunity to tumours. Natural immunity to tumours is mediated by activated macrophages, neutrophils and NK cells. Their action may be cytolytic, causing tumour cell lysis or cytostatic, inhibiting growth. This type of immunity does not require antibody and displays no antigen specificity – the cells attack all tumour cells of a particular type, the origin of the cell donor being irrelevant.

NK Cells

In man, the principal NK cell is the large granular lymphocyte (LGL), so called because of its intracytoplasmic azurophilic granules and high cytoplasmic:nuclear ratio. These cells comprise 2–5% of peripheral blood lymphocytes. However, cytolysis experiments performed at the single cell level indicate that not all LGLs are lytic and not all lytic cells are LGLs. LGLs display a number of phenotypic and functional markers but studies on NK clones indicate marked heterogeneity within this population, not only in respect of cell surface phenotype (as determined by reactivity with monoclonal antibodies against lymphoid and monocytoid determinants) but also the target cell which they recognize (Fig.18.10). In addition to peripheral blood, NK activity is demonstrable in the spleen, but to a much lesser extent in lymph nodes, bone marrow, thoracic duct and thymus. Certain extravascular NK cells (eg. in the tonsils) are different in some functional and morphological respects from peripheral NK cells such as their capacity to respond to interferon and the absence of intracytoplasmic granules. Whether this is a reflection of a different maturational status of the same cell type as that detectable in peripheral blood, or of intrinsically different NK populations (eg. of different lineage) has not been resolved.

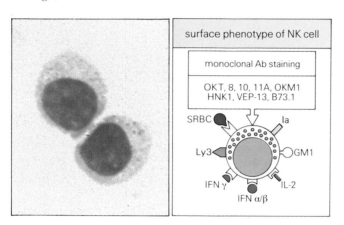

Fig. 18.10 The NK cell. The NK cells are a heterogeneous group of cells, but a major proportion of them are large granular lymphocytes seen here stained with Jenner-Giemsa (left). The surface phenotype has been delineated with the monoclonal antibodies listed right. They also carry the Ly3, Ia and GM1 antigens, and have receptors for Fc (with which B73.1 is reactive), interferons (IFN), interleukin 2 (IL-2) and sheep red blood cells (SRBC). Not all NK cells carry all surface markers. In addition to target structures recognized by NK cells, the lytic process probably involves release of soluble cytotoxic factors for which the susceptible target cell has additional receptors.

The target cell structure(s) recognized by NK cells have yet to be defined. They do not correlate with any of the well-characterized cell surface antigens such as MHC products. Some evidence suggests that the transferrin receptor (trf) present on all dividing cells may be implicated, though this is probably not the whole story. Indeed, it appears from experiments using human NK clones that some determinants recognized by NK cells are ubiquitous while others have a more restricted distribution. The determinants recognized by NK cells are more prevalent on tumours adapted to tissue culture. Susceptibility of a target to lysis by the NK cell also depends on the differentiation status of the target and its capacity to repair membrane damage.

There is virtually total overlap of the NK population in peripheral blood with that population (K cells) which mediates antibody-dependent cellular cytotoxicity (ADCC). The Fc receptor of the NK cell is, however, not involved in the lytic process. There are also other mechanistic differences and K cell activity is less consistently augmented by interferon and other immunomodulators.

NK activity is subject to both positive and negative regulation, both *in vivo* and *in vitro* (Fig.18.11). Pretreatment with various types of IFN markedly augments lysis of sensitive targets and may induce lysis of resistant ones.

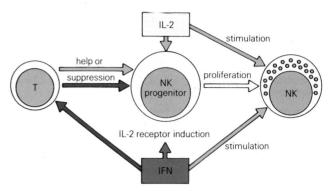

Fig.18.11 Schematic representation of IL–2 (TCGF), IFN and T cell regulatory mechanisms influencing NK cell activity. The proliferation of NK cells is under T cell control. IL-2 may also induce proliferation and stimulate the NK activity of proliferating NK cells. Interferon (IFN) induces expression of IL–2 receptors on the NK progenitor, enhancing proliferation, however, IFN also feeds back on T cells to reduce their activity.

The action of IFN in this context is two-fold: (i) to transform non-cytolytic NK precursors into a lytic state and (ii) to enhance the cytolytic capacity of already active cells. NK cells themselves produce IFN (detectable by anti-IFNα antibody) on binding to their targets: this most likely acts as a positive feedback mechanism regulating their lytic potential (Fig. 18.12).

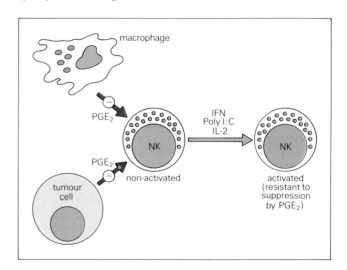

Fig.18.12 Involvement of IFN and PGE$_2$ in the regulation of NK activity. Major sources of PGE$_2$ are macrophages and certain tumour cells. Suppressor macrophages and tumour cells produce PGE$_2$ which suppresses NK activity. However, if NK cells are activated by IFN poly I: C (poly Inosinic: Cytidylic acid, a synthetic nucleotide) or IL–2, they become partially resistant to suppression by PGE$_2$.

The biological role of NK cells is uncertain. There is circumstantial evidence from experimental systems that they participate in the rejection of transplanted tumour cells, in the prevention of metastases and in bone marrow graft rejection. However they have no impact on established cancers where their numbers are few and their functional ability greatly depressed. Anti-tumour effects are likely to be in the nature of a 'first line of defence' against a tumour nidus before the development of adaptive immune responses. Peripheral blood NK activity tends to wane with progressive disease and is undetectable in some malignant lymphoproliferative disorders (Fig.18.13).

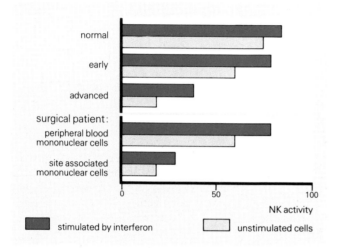

Fig.18.13 **NK activity in disease.** The activity of NK cells (defined as the percentage of maximum possible lysis of target cells) declines as the tumour progresses (upper chart). Activity is slightly reduced in the mononuclear cell population of early cancer patients but is much reduced in advanced patients. NK activity can be enhanced in all groups by interferon (red) by comparison with unstimulated cells (grey). Mononuclear cells derived from the tumours of early surgical patients have less NK activity than their peripheral blood mononuclear cells (lower chart).

Macrophages

In common with NK cells, macrophages can properly be regarded as effectors of natural immunity, though this represents only one of their several central roles in cellular immunity. As effectors, macrophages generally express little cytotoxicity unless 'activated' by lymphokines (see Fig.18.4) or by substances (eg. endotoxin, double stranded RNA, polyanionic IFN inducers) acting on them directly. 'Activation' is characterized by several other morphological, biochemical and functional changes. Activated macrophages are frequently nonspecifically cytotoxic for tumour cell lines *in vitro* which lack contact inhibition. The nature of the tumour cell 'receptor' to which macrophages bind and discriminate from normal cells which exhibit contact inhibition is unknown (Fig.18.14). The cytotoxic process involves a sequence of events and includes both cytolytic and cytostatic components. Tumour destruction results predominantly from a non-phagocytic, contact-mediated event and a later step in the process involves secretion of

effector substances from the activated macrophages. Macrophages may also function as effectors in ADCC reactions against tumours. Macrophages derived from tumour infiltrates recovered by disaggregation and adherence frequently possess the characteristics of activated macrophages.

Macrophages can also mediate negative or inhibitory effects on various immune functions. This suppressive activity does not represent an abnormal state but a normal regulatory mechanism that may be intensified by the presence of a tumour or by certain treatments. Suppressor macrophages inhibit lymphoproliferative responses to allo- and tumour-associated antigens, which is partially reversible by indomethacin which inhibits PGE_2 synthesis. The fact that this reversal is rarely complete suggests that macrophages may be able to suppress via mechanisms not involving PGE_2. The primary effect of suppressor macrophages is not necessarily confined to the proliferation of lymphocytes, since some cellular responses independent of lymphocyte proliferation are also inhibited. For example, suppressor macrophages interfere with the production of MIF, MAF and other lymphokines, which is not dependent on lymphocyte proliferation. Like NK cells, macrophages themselves may be involved in the regulation of their own activity. A hypothetical scheme, based on data derived from *in vitro* studies, for the interaction of natural and adaptive immunity *in vivo* is shown in figure 18.15.

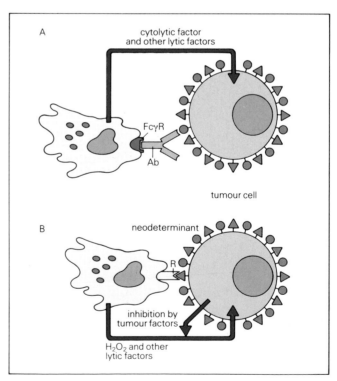

Fig.18.14 **Macrophage action against tumours.**
Macrophages act against tumours in two ways. The tumours are recognized by antibody binding to target cell antigen and to the macrophage's Fc gamma receptor (FcγR) (A). Some tumour cells which lose the normal cell property of contact inhibition display a new surface determinant for which macrophages have a receptor (R) (B). Macrophage action is by cytotoxic factor, a cytolytic proteinase, H_2O_2 and/or other oxygen reduction intermediates.

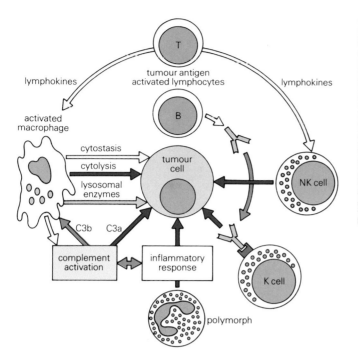

Fig.18.15 **Summary of the interactions between natural and adaptive immunity.** Lymphokines activate macrophages and NK cells. Activated macrophages produce complement components locally which are involved in the development of the inflammatory response. C3a is cytolytic and chemotactic for neutrophils while C3b induces macrophage enzyme release. K cells are armed by antibody from tumour specific B cells. This scheme should be interpreted in the awareness that amplifying mechanisms only are shown. Negative interactions are discussed below

IN SITU CELLULAR RESPONSES

The study of the *in situ* host immune response was alluded to above where a mammary carcinoma infiltrated by mononuclear cells was presented (see Fig. 18.1). With the advent of monoclonal antibodies to leucocytes and their subpopulations, the cellular nature of inflammatory infiltrates can now be more definitively analysed. Ideally the immunohistological examination of tumours should be accompanied by functional analysis of the recovered, purified cell populations. In man, however, this combined approach frequently presents insurmountable logistical problems. Monoclonal antibodies to T cell subsets, monocytes/macrophages and NK cells can determine the preponderance of a given subpopulation at the tumour site and its microanatomical distribution. The efficacy of this technique is exemplified in figure 18.16 for carcinoma of the breast. Much additional information can be obtained with monoclonal antibodies to MHC Class 1/Class 2 antigens. On the one hand, some tumours fail to express Class 1 antigens (Fig. 18.17) while others express Class 2 (DR) antigens. Expression of Class 1 antigens has implications for effector T cell function because tumour antigens are recognized in association with these MHC products. Expression of Class 2 antigens, may determine the capacity of tumours to stimulate lymphocytes, as in the MLTI assay.

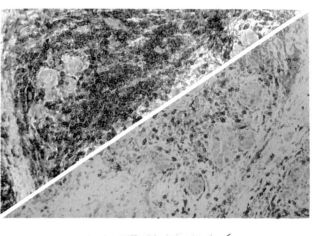

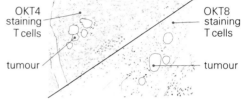

Fig.18.16 **Helper/inducer (OKT4⁺) and cytotoxic/suppressor (OKT8⁺) T lymphocyte subsets in carcinoma of the breast.** Numerous dark staining OKT4⁺ cells are present throughout the tumour, whereas the fewer OKT8⁺ cells tend to cluster round the periphery. Indirect immunoperoxidase technique, counterstained with Haematoxylin.

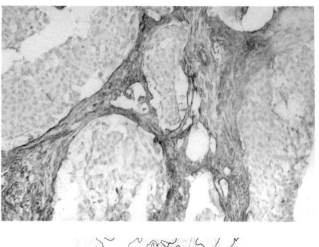

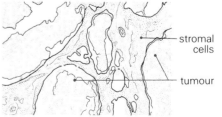

Fig. 18.17 **Breast cancer tissue reactive with monoclonal antibody (2A1) to the monomorphic determinant of HLA Class I antigens.** Only the stromal cells are stained indicating that malignant epithelial cells fail to express MHC Class 1 antigens. Some 50% of primary human breast cancers fall into this category. Indirect immunoperoxidase technique, counterstained with Haematoxylin.

B CELL RESPONSES

That antibodies are produced against antigen expressed on the tumour cells may be demonstrated by a variety of techniques (Fig.18.18).

Although cell-mediated reactions are probably of greatest significance, antibodies against tumour antigens which are detectable in autologous sera, may have important implications for host resistance. Such antibodies may be directly lytic for tumour cells or recruit cells carrying Fc receptors (eg. K cells and macrophages). Alternatively, antibodies forming soluble immune complexes with tumour antigen may subvert cellular immune responses (see below). Monoclonal antibodies and conventional polyclonal antibodies have been used to determine the complicated antigenic profile expressed by different tumours.

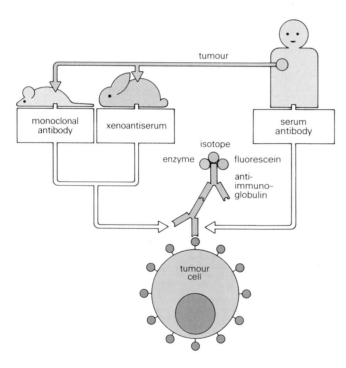

Fig.18.18 Detection of tumour antigens by particular antibodies. The antibodies may occur in the patient's serum or they may be raised in experimental animals by immunization with the tumour. If this is done in mice monoclonal antibodies can be produced. Binding of the antibody to the tumour is detected by a second layer of antibody specific for the first antibody and conjugated to an enzyme, or an isotope or a fluorochrome.

TUMOUR SPECIFIC ANTIGENS

There are inherent difficulties in defining 'tumour-specific' antigens regardless of the type of antibodies used for their analysis. First, a tumour may anomalously express cell surface antigens, not found on the normal cell from whence it is derived, but which are produced by other normal cell types. This might result from the ability of tumours to make products inappropriate to their normal state of differentiation. Second, because most tumours result from the clonal expansion of single cells they frequently express differentiation antigens (antigens normally only seen at particular phases of differentiation of a cell type) which would normally only be expressed by a minority of cells of that type. This is exemplified by the four major phenotypes of human acute leukaemias which can be distinguished by membrane and enzyme markers. The antigenic profile of the leukaemic cells is qualitatively similar to the characteristics of the corresponding normal haemopoietic cells. Clonally-expanded normal antigens (or simply 'clonal antigens') may masquerade as tumour-specific especially if the target normal cell which undergoes transformation is present only as a small proportion of the normal cells of the tissue from which the tumour arises. For example, another type of antigen appears when tumours inappropriately express particular alloantigens such as blood group determinants. Some blood group antigens are determined by carbohydrate chains present on the cell surface. The loss or gain of these chains is a common occurrence in foetal erythrocytes. In isolated cases 'illegitimate blood' group antigens appear, that is, normal blood group antigens different from those present on the normal tissues of the host.

Antigens associated with solid tumours are classified serologically as follows:–

Class 1 antigens (not to be confused with MHC Class 1 antigens) show an absolute restriction to a single tumour and are not found on any other normal or malignant cells. Class 2 antigens (not to be confused with MHC Class 2 antigens) are shared tumour antigens and are found on tumour cells in different individuals. (Recent data have shown that Class 2 antigens are also found on a restricted range of normal cells and therefore should be classified as *autoantigenic differentiation antigens*.) Class 3 antigens are pervasive and expressed on a wide variety of normal and malignant cells of animal and human origin. In the experimentally observed immune response to a patient's or animal's own tumour (autologous tumour typing) Class 3 antigens are encountered more frequently than Class 1 or 2 antigens. In order to identify autologous reactions against the different classes it is necessary to absorb out reactivity against other classes using appropriate normal or tumour tissues.

Retrogenetic Antigens

Certain tumours express antigens or synthesize proteins normally expressed only by foetal and not by adult tissue, a phenomenon known as '*retrogenetic expression*'. Most of these oncofoetal antigens (OFA) are not strictly tumour-associated and with the use of sensitive assays they have also been detected in small amounts in non-malignant adult cells. The two most important and best studied are α foetoprotein (αFP) and carcinoembryonic antigen (CEA). αFP is a serum protein associated with normal foetal and neonatal development and with the growth of hepatocellular carcinoma. However, it is also produced during liver regeneration and low serum αFP levels have been found in the normal adult. CEA is a foetal colon cell surface glycoprotein that is produced by tumours of ectodermal origin – intestinal, pulmonary, pancreatic, gastric and mammary adenocarcinomas. Elevated CEA levels are associated with smoking and with inflammatory diseases of the bowel, lung and pancreas.

Both αFP and CEA have a limited utility in the monitoring of patients with certain types of neoplasm following primary tumour removal (Fig.18.19) and in the *in vivo* localization of metastatic disease, with radiolabelled antibody (Fig.18.20).

Numerous other oncofoetal antigens have been described in association with particular experimental and human neoplasms.

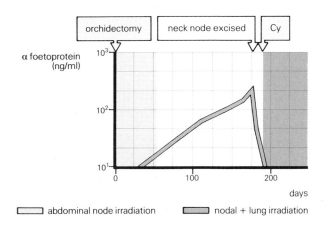

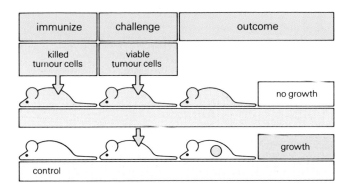

Fig.18.21 Demonstration of tumour-associated transplantation antigens (TATA). The presence of TATA on transplantable tumours can be demonstrated by taking tumour cells from an animal and inactivating them chemically (eg. with mitomycin C) or by irradiation. Animals which have been innoculated with inactivated tumour fail to produce a tumour when injected with viable tumour cells, whereas control, uninnoculated animals permit tumour growth.

Fig. 18.19 Relationship of serum α foetoprotein levels to clinical course in a patient with teratoma of the testes. The progressive rise in the αFP precedes relapse in the neck and lungs by about 150 days. After further therapy and treatment with cyclophosophamide (Cy) and irradiation the αFP level returns to normal. Courtesy of Prof. T. J. McElwain.

of these antigens is a feature of many though not all, experimental neoplasms. The term TATA (or tumour rejection antigen, TRA) is purely functional and several different types of cell surface antigen (eg. embryonic, viral, differentiation, altered histocompatibility etc.) could theoretically possess this capability.

Where detectable, the major TATA of chemically-induced experimental neoplasms are unique ('private') for each tumour (Fig.18.22).

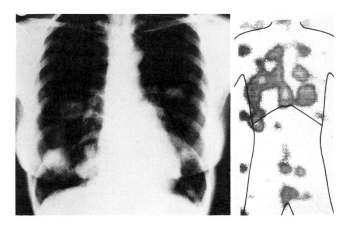

Fig.18.20 Chest radiograph and immunoscintigraphy scan of a colon carcinoma patient with lung and liver metastases. The monoclonal antibody YPC2/12.1, raised against human colorectal cancer, binds to CEA and reacts with a glycoprotein of Mol.Wt. 180 Kdaltons. The antibody was radiolabelled with ^{131}I, administered intravenously and scintigrams obtained at 48 hours. The image is that obtained after a subtraction procedure to eliminate background blood borne antibody. Courtesy of Dr. K. Sikora.

Tumour Associated Transplantation Antigens

An important class of cell surface antigens are the tumour-associated transplantation antigens (TATA) so called because they evoke the rejection of tumour cells in pre-immunized syngeneic hosts (Fig.18.21). Expression

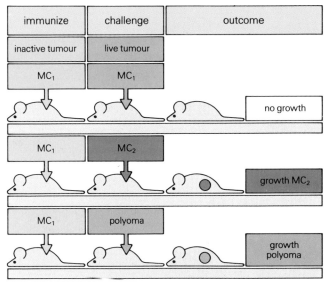

Fig.18.22 Absence of common antigens on chemically induced tumours. Three groups of animals were immunized to a methyl cholanthrene-induced sarcoma (MC_1) by repeated implantation of inactivated tumour.
(Methylcholanthrene is a chemical carcinogen.) Subsequently the groups were challenged with MC_1 or another methylcholanthrene induced tumour (MC_2) or a virally-induced tumour (polyoma). Immunization was effective only for the specific tumour, MC_1 indicating that tumours induced by the same chemical do not share antigens nor do they share antigens with virally induced tumours.

Moreover, sarcomas which are morphologically indistinguishable from each other are antigenically different even if they are different clonotypes from a single host. The reason for this degree of polymorphism among TATA is presently obscure but probably reflects the multiplicity of genomal changes coding for cell surface antigens induced by carcinogen/DNA interaction.

TATAs induced by the same virus cross-react regardless of the cell type from which the tumours are derived but do not cross-react with tumours induced by other viruses (Fig. 18.23).

In the case of the DNA viruses (for example, polyoma and SV40), the TATA is coded by the viral DNA integrated into the cellular genome. The TATA is thus a *cellular* antigen which reflects the specificity of the inducing virus. Other antigens (for example, nuclear T antigen) are also expressed concomitantly but by virtue of their cellular location have no role in transplantation resistance. In the case of RNA tumour viruses the cellular antigens are distinguishable serologically from the structural components of the virus including the envelope glycoproteins which enter the cell membrane as part of the budding process.

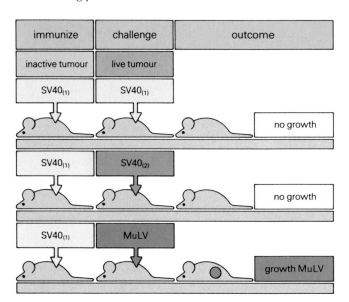

Fig.18.23 Common antigens on virally induced tumours. Three groups of animals were immunized to an SV40 virus induced tumour (SV40$_{(1)}$) by repeated implantation of inactivated tumour. Subsequently the groups were challenged with live SV40$_{(1)}$ tumour or another similarly induced tumour, SV40$_{(2)}$, or with a tumour induced by murine leukaemia virus, MuLV. Immunization to SV40$_{(1)}$ protected against SV40$_{(1)}$ and SV40$_{(2)}$ but not against MuLV induced tumours indicating that tumours induced by the same virus may have common antigens.

Malignant transformation in laboratory animals is sometimes accompanied by activation of latent oncogenic RNA viruses. For example, the antigens expressed by radiation-induced murine leukaemias are those of the MuLV (Murine Leukaemia Virus) complex. Similar concomitant expression of virus-induced tumour antigens can occur during chemical carcinogenesis. 'Spontaneous' animal tumours, where the aetiological agent is

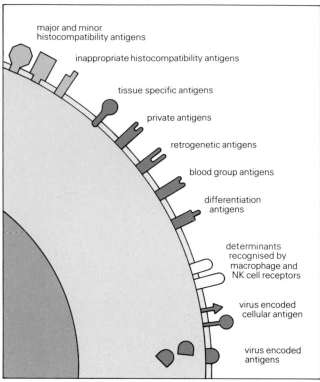

Fig.18.24 Tumour antigens and other cell surface antigens. Tumour cells may display one or several of the antigen types listed here. Private neoantigens are unique to a particular tumour; retrogenetic antigens, also referred to as oncofoetal antigens are antigens which appear normally on tissue at an early stage of differentiation but are inappropriate on differentiated normal tissue.

unknown, possess very weak TATA. A composite scheme of tumour cell surface antigens based on *in vivo* studies and serology is given in figure 18.24. While not all of these may be immunogenic in the original host, they may still be of practical interest in immunodiagnosis and immunotherapy (see below).

IMMUNE COMPLEXES

The body fluids of cancer patients frequently contain immune complexes. To this extent they differ little as a group from the sera of patients with non-malignant inflammatory or degenerative conditions of the same tissue or organs (lung, intestinal tract, etc.). Theoretically, circulating immune complexes detectable in the sera of cancer patients and those with other pathological disorders may consist of several disparate antigens, including in the case of cancer patients some which are tumour-associated. In some malignant diseases, for example, breast carcinoma, levels of circulating immune complexes have a tendency to rise in patients who suffer relapse and to fall in patients who remain free of the disease. However, the nature of the complexes detected in the sera of cancer patients is largely unknown and precise immunochemical characterization using monoclonal antibodies is awaited (Fig. 18.25).

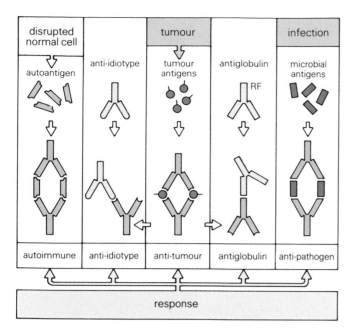

Fig. 18.25 Possible origin of circulating immune complexes in neoplasia. Immune complexes are detected in the body fluids of many tumour-bearers. They may be due to antibodies reacting with autoantigens of damaged tissue or with microbial antigens. Intercurrent infections are seen more frequently in cancer patients who may be immunosuppressed by the action of the tumour or by cytotoxic drug therapy. They may also be due to anti-tumour antibodies. Anti-tumour antibodies could form complexes with tumour antigens, antiglobulin rheumatoid factor (RF) or with specific anti-idiotypes.

IMMUNOSURVEILLANCE

Immunosurveillance could conceivably occur during oncogenesis, or after cancer has developed. There is evidence that both forms may actually occur, depending at least in experimental systems on the tumour type and the inducing agent. It is important to stress that *immuno-surveillance* is only one form of host surveillance which might limit tumour development. Other local and systemic mechanisms are concerned with the orderly maintenance of cells within tissues and the constant anatomical relationship between tissues of different kinds in controlling growth and development and in repair and regeneration after injury. Furthermore, immuno-surveillance may be mediated by more than one component of the cellular immune respones (eg. T cells and natural killer cells). Surveillance of all categories of neoplasm by a single mechanism (eg. T cells) is highly unlikely. The most convincing evidence for T cell-mediated immunosurveillance during oncogenesis is provided by tumours induced by the murine oncogenic DNA viruses (eg. polyoma and SV40) (Fig. 18.26). Here, the frequency of neoplasms in T cell deficient mice is unequivocally greater than that in normal immuno-competent siblings. For other onocogenic agents (oncor-naviruses, carcinogens), the frequency of neoplasms in T cell deficient hosts is broadly comparable with that in their normal counterparts. In these circumstances T cell

surveillance does not occur to any measurable extent and the fact that many of the emergent tumours express strong TATA is not necessarily at variance with this (see "Im-munological Escape" below).

cause	incidence of tumour		anti-tumour immune mechanisms
	nude	control	
spontaneous tumours	+	+	
chemical carcinogens	+	+	NK cells natural antibodies
oncornaviruses (RNA tumour virus)	+	+	
DNA tumour viruses	++	+	NK cells T cells antibodies

Fig. 18.26 Evidence for and against the role of T cells in immunosurveillance. The incidence of tumours (+) caused by different agents or spontaneously occurring in T cell deficient (nude) and control (littermate heterozygote) mice is given. Only tumours caused by DNA viruses have a higher incidence in nudes than controls. This implies that if immunosurveillance is important for most types of tumour the function is performed by NK cells and other natural immune mechanisms. Only in the case of DNA virus induced tumours is there evidence for T cell mediated surveillance.

Spontaneous tumours occur in approximately 10% of genetically T cell deficient patients (DiGeorge syndrome, ataxia telangiectasia), with cancer of the lymphoreticular system being particularly prevalent (Fig. 18.27).

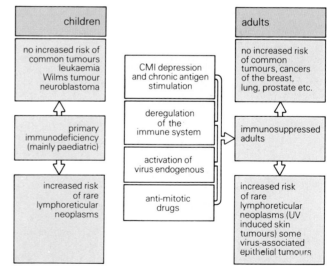

Fig. 18.27 A diagrammatic scheme relating to immunosurveillance in humans. Certain groups of tumours in children and adults can be related to impaired immune functions. It would be anticipated if immunosurveillance is operative that defects in the immune system would result in increased tumour incidence. In fact there is *no* increase in common tumours in primarily immunodeficient children or in immunosuppressed adults (usually transplant recipients), but there is an increase in the rarer tumours listed.

A consequence of immunodepression in these patients may be the release of ubiquitous viruses with oncogenic potential from immunological control. Several human viruses are oncogenic and their evasion of control may result from abrogation of the T cell response to virus-infected and transformed cells. Alternatively, the tumours might arise from an immunoregulatory abnormality in an already pathologically disturbed immune system. This avoidance of the regulatory action of the immune system is termed 'immunological escape'.

Recent examples of the failure of immunosurveillance in human populations could be the unusual occurrence of Burkitt-like lymphoma (of Epstein-Barr virus association) and Kaposi's sarcoma (of CMV association) in homosexual males with AIDS (acquired immuno-deficiency syndrome).

Provisional evidence of a role for NK cells in immunosurveillance derives from the 'beige' mouse, the mutant gene of which confers some impairment of *in vitro* NK function, but which is neither selective nor absolute. However, in comparison with normal heterozygous littermates, these mice are marginally more susceptible to tumour transplantation and primary tumour development by chemical carcinogens.

Immunological escape does not necessarily invalidate immunosurveillance, since many tumours may be eliminated before their presence is detected. The relative ineffectiveness of immunotherapy to date neither disproves surveillance nor excludes the possibility that it may be made more effective. If immunosurveillance exists its effectiveness is likely to depend on a balance between mechanisms minimizing tumour viability, immunological escape or immunodepression.

IMMUNOLOGICAL ESCAPE

Mechanisms of immunological escape address the central paradox of tumour immunology which is why neoplasms which are demonstrably immunogenic elude the effector arm of the immune response. Immunological escape occurs when the balance between factors favouring tumour growth and destruction is tilted in favour of the tumour. Some escape mechanisms are so potent that they could circumvent immunological therapy as well as the normal autologous response.

The factors that may contribute to immunological escape include:

1. Tumour kinetics ('sneaking through') – In immunized animals, tumour cells administered in sufficiently low doses (see above) develop into cancers where greater doses are rejected, that is, under conditions theoretically optimized for rejection, tumour cells may 'sneak through' and not be recognized until growth is established and beyond recall. This mechanism could account for many failures of immunosurveillance in both clinical and experimental situations.

2. Antigenic modulation – In the presence of antibody some antigens are *modulated off* the cell surface – this involves antigen shedding, endocytosis and redistribution within the cell membrane without a complete loss of

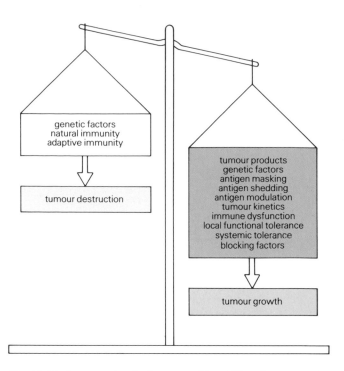

Fig.18.28 Immunological escape. The ability of a tumour to escape from immunological control may depend on a balance between the effectiveness of the immune system and a variety of factors promoting escape.

the determinant from the cell surface – it is a process distinct from capping. This facilitates escape by removing the target antigens that the immune system's effector cells would recognize.

3. Antigen masking – Facilitation of tumour escape from effector cells may occur because certain molecules such as sialomucin, which are frequently bound to the surfaces of tumour cells, mask tumour antigens and prevent adhesion of attacking lymphocytes. Masking can be overcome by treatment which degrades sialomucin (eg. *Vibrio cholera* neuraminidase).

4. Antigen shedding – Circulating, soluble tumour antigens have been demonstrated in the sera of tumour-bearing animals and patients, where they have the capability to compromise the expression of T cell-mediated immunity by saturation of antigen-binding sites, particularly in the tumour microenvironment where the concentration of shed antigen is likely to be highest. A similar paralysis of the local effector response can be produced by antigen-antibody complexes.

5. Tolerance – Specific inhibition of the normal immune response to tumour antigens is exemplified by another murine tumour-host system, the mammary tumour virus (MTV). The virus is transmitted through the milk. Fostered mice are not infected and do not develop tumours.

Transplantation experiments show that mammary tumours are far more antigenic in mice that lack the virus than in those that acquired it at birth. Those mice which are infected congenitally become immunologically tolerant to certain antigens common to the virus and the resulting tumours. Suppressor cells may also appear which inhibit murine T and B cell responses to tumour antigens causing accelerated tumour growth. Antisera against the I-J subregion determinants which are expressed on suppressor T cells retard tumour growth.

6. Lymphocyte trapping – It is possible that tumour escape may be facilitated *in vivo* by trapping of tumour specific lymphocytes in lymph nodes draining the tumour. In these lymph nodes the level of tumour antigen could tolerize the local lymphocytes, while the reactivity of lymphocytes at distant sites is normal. It is noted, however, that appreciable numbers of cytotoxic effector cells can be demonstrated in the circulation of patients even with advanced disease.

7. Genetic factors – Failure to induce an effector T cell response to a tumour could be a function of the MHC haplotype of the host in an analogous fashion to the T cell responses seen to virally infected cells (see 'MHC'). It has been shown with several viruses in mice and with influenza virus in humans, that hosts with certain MHC haplotypes are poor inducers of a cytotoxic T cell response, probably on account of the inability of the MHC products to form a suitable associated complex with the foreign antigen. Indeed, some neoplasms fail to express MHC Class I antigens altogether. Genetically-determined unresponsiveness to tumour antigens need not deter immunological approaches to tumour therapy because it may be overcome by appropriate modification or presentation of the relevant antigen.

8. Blocking factors – When tumour cell antigens are shed they may form complexes with the host's specific antibody. These complexes could block the cytotoxicity of host T lymphocytes in two ways:
1. by binding directly to the T_C cells and so preventing them engaging the tumour cells,
2. by binding to T_H cells and preventing them from recognizing the tumour and delivering help to T_C cells.

Additionally, if the antibody induced by the shed antigens is ineffective, it could bind the antigen on tumour cells and prevent T_C and T_H from engaging the tumour. Even if the antibodies can fix complement and are potentially able to kill the tumour, they may still be rendered ineffective by shed antigens which bind to the anti-tumour antibody before it reaches its target.

The major action of blocking factors may be local rather than systemic, otherwise it is difficult to explain the phenomenon of 'concomitant immunity' where small inocula of tumour cells can be rejected at a site distal from a progressively growing tumour in the same animal.

9. Tumour products – The subversion of immune responses by products of tumours other than antigens can also be envisaged. Prostaglandins which negatively regulate NK and K cell functions constitute one such example. Similarly, other humoral factors act non-specifically to impair inflammatory responses, chemotaxis, the complement cascade or to augment the formation of a blood supply within solid tumours.

10. Growth factors – Amplification of T cell responses is critically dependent on the availability of interleukins. Any perturbation in production of IL–1 by macrophages

or in the degree of cooperation between the T cell subsets or in the availability of IL–2 could conceivably limit the overall response to a tumour. All of these factors in immunological escape are listed in figure 18.28.

POTENTIAL FOR THERAPY

It is important to stress that in no cancerous state is the efficiency of immunotherapy presently greater than that of conventional treatments. At best immunotherapy may facilitate the removal of tumour foci inaccessible to conventional treatment or may be exploited to enhance specific or non-specific anti-tumour activity (Fig.18.29).

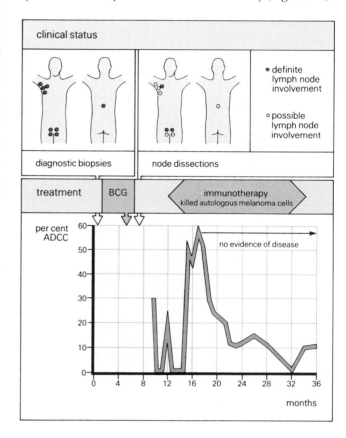

Fig.18.29 Potential for immunotherapy of cancer. A patient with malignant melanoma was immunized with BCG (the key component of complete Freunds adjuvant) and separately with killed autologous melanoma cells and tested for the incidence of ADCC (K cell activity) to the melanoma expressed as percentage killing of the melanoma target cells. The patient's lymph nodes were examined for metastasis during the treatment. The clinical incidence of the tumour was inversely related to the activity of the effector cells. Data from Dr. L. J. Old and colleagues.

The complexity of the immune response to tumours necessitates a multilateral approach to the problem of immunotherapy. Ideally this should attempt to enhance specific and non-specific host resistance at the same time as minimizing the prospects of escape from immunological control by the induction of other potentially deleterious changes in immune regulation.

In practice, this may be approached either by active manipulation of the immune response in the patient, adoptive immunotherapy, passive administration of serological reagents of predefined activity and specificity (eg. monoclonal or polyclonal antibodies), or depletive immunotherapy.

Active intervention means vaccination, and this seeks either to enhance specific, or non-specific mechanisms of host resistance, or both. In animals this form of therapy has been successful only in exceptional circumstances. It has been found possible to induce resistance in experimental animals in advance of tumour challenge. However, the same control of tumour cell growth is not produced when tumour cells are inoculated simultaneously with immunization. Modified cancer vaccines may offer a means whereby the immunogenicity of the tumour cells may be artificially enhanced for use in active immunization protocols (Fig.18.30). These comprise (1) infection with certain viruses; (2) chemical attachment of foreign determinants; (3) introduction of foreign determinants by somatic cell hybridization and (4) isolation and purificiation of the relevant tumour specific antigens.
1. Studies in mice have shown that homogenates prepared from virus-infected tumours (viral oncolysates) are more effective immunogens than comparable preparations of non-infected tumour cells for the induction of transplantation immunity. In mice the myxoviruses are the viruses of choice and vesicular stomatitis virus (VSV) – infected melanoma cells are under study in man.
2. Augmentation of the immunogenicity of tumour cells by chemical, enzymatic (eg. haptenization or antigenic modification) has been achieved with chemically-induced murine sarcomas. PPD (purified protein derivative of BCG) bound to tumour cell surfaces provides

effective 'help' if the host is preimmune to BCG. The widespread use of BCG in clinical immunotherapy suggests that this approach could have advantages in man.
3. Cell hybridization offers another means of introducing foreign helper determinants on the tumour cell surface.
4. Vaccines containing complex microorganisms such as pneumococci, meningococci or influenza bacilli are considerably less effective than vaccines prepared from isolated capsular polysaccharides of these bacteria. By analogy, this suggests that immunization with purified tumour antigens may be more effective than using whole killed tumour cells.

Non-specific active immunization employs a diversity of reagents which affect the immune response and are called biological response modifiers (BRM). The prototypes are BCG and *C. parvum* (Fig. 18.31). Both agents affect several components of the immune response, modify the activity of several cell types and may induce positive (stimulatory) or negative (inhibitory) effects depending on the system and how they are used. However, their limited anti-tumour effects are thought to be mainly mediated through macrophage activation.

Agents which restore normal T cell activity to cancer patients who otherwise manifest abnormalities in both T cell number and function (as a consequence rather than a cause of the disease) include thymic hormones and related factors.

Adoptive immunotherapy involving the transfer (xenogeneic, allogeneic or syngeneic) of immunocompetence or tumour immunity from one individual to another via leucocytes, transfer factor or immune RNA has met with virtually no therapeutic success. The most likely prospect for adoptive immunotherapy depends upon the

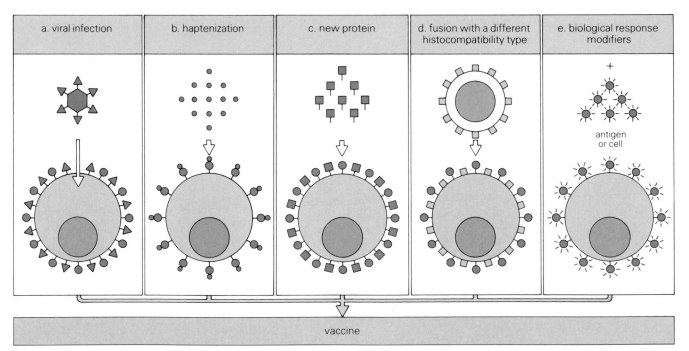

a. viral infection	b. haptenization	c. new protein	d. fusion with a different histocompatibility type	e. biological response modifiers

antigen or cell

vaccine

Fig.18.30 Augmentation of host response. Vaccination against tumours is aimed at increasing the host response to tumour by a) infecting the tumour with virus, b) coupling haptens to the tumour surface antigens, c) coupling protein antigens to the tumour surface, d) fusing the tumour with cells of a different histocompatibility type, e) increasing the immune response with adjuvants and other biological response modifiers.

type	examples	major effect
bacterial products	BCG, *C. parvum* muramyl dipeptide trehalase dimycolate	macrophage and NK activation
synthetic molecules	pyran copolymer MVE, poly I:C pyrimidines	interferon induction
cytokines	IFNα, IFNβ IL-2	macrophage and NK activation
hormones	thymosin, thymulin thymopoetin	modulate T cell function

Fig.18.31 Examples of biological response modifiers.
Biological response modifiers are used to enhance immune responses and they fall into four major groups. Broadly speaking, bacterial products have adjuvant effects on macrophages; a variety of synthetic polymers, nucleotides and polynucleotides induce interferon production and release; the cytokines administered directly act on macrophages and NK cells, and a variety of hormones including the thymic hormones, can be used to enhance T cell function. (MVE = maleic anhydride divinyl ether.)

successful preparation of T cell clones with tumour-directed cytotoxic or helper/inducer activity. Clones of autologous lymphocytes with cytotoxic or helper properties could be repeatedly administered for therapeutic benefit, an objective already achieved to a limited extent in animal models, such as the MSV system and antigenic chemically-induced sarcomas. In combination with chemotherapy, the approach is particularly effective against experimental leukaemias.

Passive immunotherapy entails the transfer of anti-tumour antibody to cancer patients in order to cause tumour regression or prevent tumour recurrence. Occasional therapeutic effects have been reported in leukaemias, lymphomas (including Burkitts lymphoma), malignant melanoma and kidney carcinoma. Currently, there is considerable interest in using partially-purified xenogeneic antibody to deliver drug or radioactive isotopes to the tumour. Antibodies coupled to chlorambucil have some activity against malignant melanomas and antiferritin antibody linked to ^{131}I against hepatomas. Monoclonal antibodies coupled to adriamycin have a limited effectiveness against very weakly immunogenic tumours such as spontaneous rat mammary carcinomas. There is currently much interest in the possible exploitation of antibody/toxin conjugates. Substances such as diphtheria toxin A, abrin and ricin require only a few molecules to kill a cell. The specificity of antibodies used to target such highly toxic agents is clearly crucial. A promising area of development is that of anti-idiotype antibodies against B cell tumours where the tumour population is relatively homogenous and accessible.

Success against other tumours is likely to depend on a multiplicity of factors including antibody avidity, affinity, class, subclass, retention of specificity after coupling to the toxic agent and resistance to *in vivo* cleavage etc. The therapeutic efficacy of monoclonal antibodies against human tumours growing as xenografts in experimental animals has been shown to be antibody subclass dependent, reflecting a capacity to recruit host macrophages (via FcR) into the attack.

Immunodepletive therapy involves the reduction of certain circulating serum factors produced by, or related to tumours which are immunosuppressive and inhibit the optimal expression of tumour immunity. These comprise prostaglandins, blocking antibodies and complexes and suppressor cell-activating factors.

The potential for immunological intervention is summarized in figure 18.32. There is potential for cancer therapy using immunological methods, based on the observation that leucocytes expressing anti-tumour reactivity are found in cancer patients. However, since their activity is insufficient to control developed tumours it is necessary to enhance the activity of tumour reactive leucocytes. This in turn requires the identification of antigens or other structures on the tumour surface which can stimulate the immune system and through which the immunological attack can be directed. It is not certain that these target antigens exist for every tumour, but if immunological surveillance does occur those tumours which arise in immunocompromized patients may be potentially immunogenic and thus susceptible to immunological destruction. On the other hand, those tumours which arise in normals may be insufficiently immunogenic. Thus, there is sufficient evidence to offer hope of useful immunological intervention in some tumours. Even if immunology does not offer therapeutic solutions to the problems of cancer it is still useful in cancer diagnosis and monitoring.

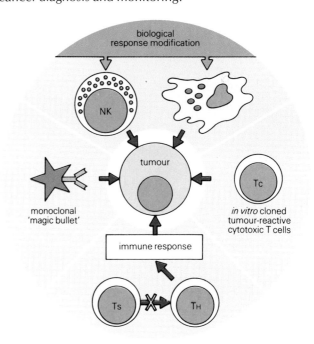

Fig. 18.32 The prospects for immunological intervention.
Biological response modifiers could be used to activate NK cells and macrophages. Monoclonal antibodies directed to tumour antigens and coupled to cytotoxic drugs provide a possible 'magic bullet' against the tumour. Cloning of cytotoxic (Tc) and helper (TH) T cells of appropriate specificities could also be effective, particularly if they were resistant to the action of host T-suppressor cells (Ts).

FURTHER READING

Fefer A. & Goldstein A.L. (eds) (1982) The Potential Role of T Cells in Cancer Therapy. *Progress in Cancer Research and Therapy* **22.**

Fishman W. H. (ed) (1983) *Oncodevelopmental markers: biologic, diagnostic and monitoring aspects.* Academic Press, New York & London.

Haskill S. (ed) (1982) Tumour Immunity in Prognosis: the role of mononuclear cell Infiltration. *Immunology Series* 18. Marcel Dekker, Inc. New York & Basel.

Herberman R. B. (ed) (1982) *NK cells and other natural effector cells.* Academic Press, New York & London.

Herberman R. B. (ed) (1983) *Basic and Clinical Tumour Immunology.* Martinus Nijhoff, Boston.

19 Hypersensitivity–Type I

TYPES OF HYPERSENSITIVITY

When an adaptive immune response occurs in an exaggerated or inappropriate form, causing tissue damage, the term hypersensitivity is applied. Hypersensitivity is a characteristic of the individual and is manifested on second contact with a particular antigen. Coombs and Gell have described four types of hypersensitivity reaction (Type I, II, III and IV) but in practice, these types do not necessarily occur in isolation from each other. It should be stressed that these reactions are no more than expressions of the beneficial immune responses already described, acting inappropriately, and sometimes causing inflammatory reactions and tissue damage. The first three types are antibody mediated, and the fourth mediated primarily by T cells and macrophages.

Type I, or immediate hypersensitivity occurs when an IgE response is directed against innocuous antigens, such as pollen, and the resulting release of pharmacological mediators, such as histamine, by IgE-sensitized mast cells produces an acute inflammatory reaction with symptoms such as asthma or rhinitis. Type II, or antibody-dependent cytotoxic hypersensitivity, occurs when antibody binds to antigen on cells leading to phagocytosis, killer cell activity or complement-mediated lysis. Type III, or immune complex mediated hypersensitivity develops when complexes are formed in large quantities, or cannot be cleared adequately by the reticuloendothelial system, leading to serum sickness type reactions.

Finally, Type IV or delayed type hypersensitivity (DTH) is most seriously manifested when antigen, for example tubercle bacilli, trapped in a macrophage, cannot be cleared. T lymphocytes are then stimulated to elaborate lymphokines which mediate a range of inflammatory responses. Other aspects of DTH reactions are seen in graft rejection and allergic contact dermatitis. These four types of hypersensitivity reaction are summarized diagrammatically in figure 19.1.

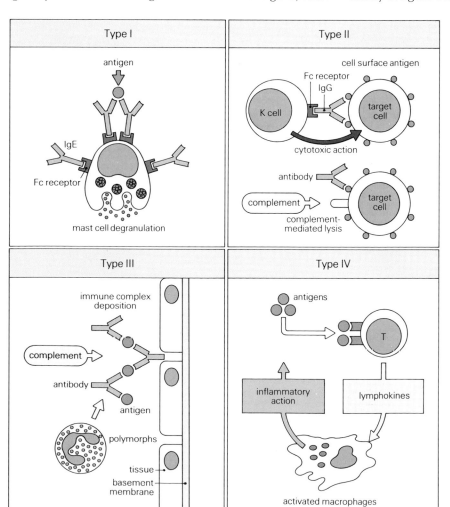

Fig.19.1 Summary diagram of the four types of hypersensitivity reactions.

Type I Mast cells bind IgE via their Fc receptors. On encountering antigen the IgE becomes crosslinked, inducing degranulation and release of mediators.

Type II Antibody is directed against antigens on an individual's own cells (target cell). This may lead to cytotoxic action by K cells or complement-mediated lysis.

Type III Immune complexes are deposited in the tissue. Complement is activated and polymorphs are attracted to the site of deposition, causing local damage.

Type IV Antigen-sensitized T cells release lymphokines following a secondary contact with the same antigen. Lymphokines induce inflammatory reactions and activate and attract macrophages which release mediators.

19.1

TYPE I – IMMEDIATE HYPERSENSITIVITY

Definition

Type I hypersensitivity is characterized by allergic reactions immediately following contact with the antigen (allergen) (Fig.19.2). The term 'allergy' was originally coined in 1906 by von Pirquet meaning 'changed reactivity' of the host when meeting an 'agent' on a second or subsequent occasion. He made no strictures as to the type of immunological response made by the host and it is only in recent years that 'allergy' has become synonymous with Type I hypersensitivity. The reactions are dependent on the specific triggering of IgE-sensitized mast cells by antigen resulting in the release of pharmacological mediators of inflammation (Fig.19.3).

Atopy

Originally described by Coca and Cooke (1923), the term atopy describes the clinical features of Type I hypersensitivity, which include asthma, eczema, hayfever and urticaria, in subjects with a family history of similar complaints and showing positive immediate wheal and flare skin reactions to common inhalent allergens.

It had already been suggested that anaphylaxis in animals, discovered by Portier and Richet (1902) was related to hay fever or asthma in humans, but whereas 90% of animals developed precipitating antibodies to injected heterologous proteins or toxins, only 5-10% of the human population exposed to an airborne allergen became sensitized to it. Furthermore, human allergy shows strong hereditary linkages which were not then appreciated in the animal model. For these reasons, Coca and Cooke felt that human allergic disease was fundamentally different from animal anaphylaxis and called them 'atopic diseases'. There is still some advantage in keeping the term atopy as it is a convenient umbrella term for a number of diseases, which share some common features – asthma, eczema, and hay fever.

The first description of the mechanism of the allergic reaction was by Prausnitz and Kustner (1921), who showed that a serum factor (termed reagin) could mediate the reaction on passive transfer to the skin of a normal subject. Some 45 years later Ishizaka and colleagues showed that this 'atopic reagin' was a new class of immunoglobulin – ImmunoGlobulin-E: IgE.

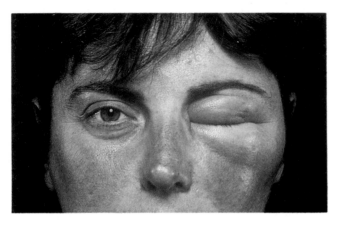

Fig.19.2 The anaphylactic response to bee venom. This patient has been stung on her face by a bee. The immediate hypersensitivity to bee venom is a clear cut example of Type I hypersensitivity, due to the release of pharmacological mediators, including histamine, from mast cells. The reaction can produce generalized anaphylaxis and even death since the allergen is injected into the patient rather than being inhaled. The reaction can be aggravated by mellitin in the venom which can trigger mast cells non-immunologically.

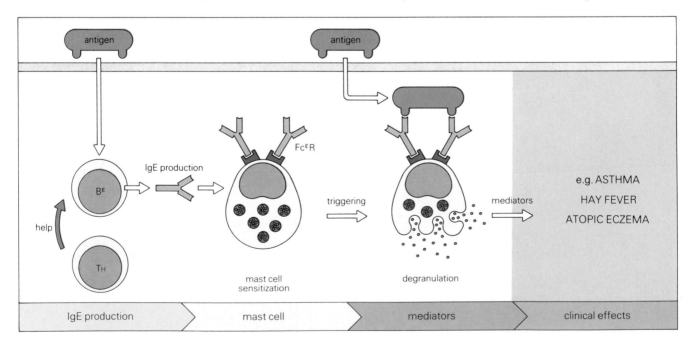

Fig.19.3 Overall scheme for Type I hypersensitivity.
Antigen stimulates B$^\varepsilon$ cells to produce specific IgE with T cell help. This antigen-specific IgE binds to mast cells via Fc$^\varepsilon$ receptors (Fc$^\varepsilon$R) thus sensitizing them. When antigen subsequently reaches the sensitized mast cell, it crosslinks surface bound IgE and the cell degranulates, releasing mediators which cause the symptoms associated with Type I hypersensitivity.

IMMUNOGLOBULIN E

Following the initial contact of allergen with the mucosa there is a complex series of events before IgE is produced and before allergic symptoms result after a second contact with the same allergen. The IgE response is a local event occurring at the site of the allergen's entry into the body, that is, at mucosal surfaces and/or at local lymph nodes. IgE production by B cells involves antigen presentation via antigen-presenting cells, T cell help and the stimulation of B cells to produce IgE. Locally produced IgE will first sensitize local mast cells and 'spill-over' IgE enters the circulation and binds to receptors on both circulating basophils and tissue-fixed mast cells throughout the body.

The structure of immunoglobulin E is compared with that of IgG in figure 19.4. As with other immunoglobulins, IgE is comprised of two heavy and two light chains but the IgE heavy chain has five domains.

The major characteristics of IgE include its heat lability and its ability to bind to mast cells and basophils. It is notable that although the serum half-life of IgE is only two and a half days, mast cells may remain sensitized for up to 12 weeks following passive sensitization with atopic serum containing IgE. As has been mentioned, the original description of passive transfer of allergy by a serum component was by Prausnitz and Kustner. Kustner was allergic to fish and his serum injected into the skin of

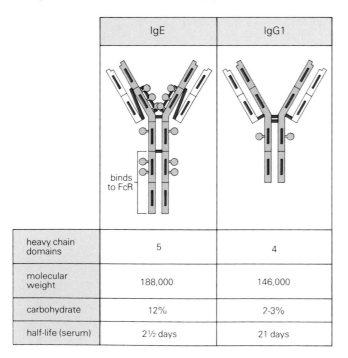

	IgE	IgG1
heavy chain domains	5	4
molecular weight	188,000	146,000
carbohydrate	12%	2-3%
half-life (serum)	2½ days	21 days

Fig.19.4 IgE structure compared with IgG1. IgE is a trace protein in serum (< 0.001% of total serum immunoglobulin). It has five domains in the heavy chain and varies from the basic IgG structure as indicated. A part of the Fc region of IgE (C_H3 and C_H4) is involved in binding to Fc^ε receptors (FcR) on mast cells and basophils. This Fc binding is heat labile and activity is destroyed by heating at 56°C for 30 min, whilst antigen binding to the Fab portion is not heat labile. IgE serum levels are raised in parasitic infections and atopy.

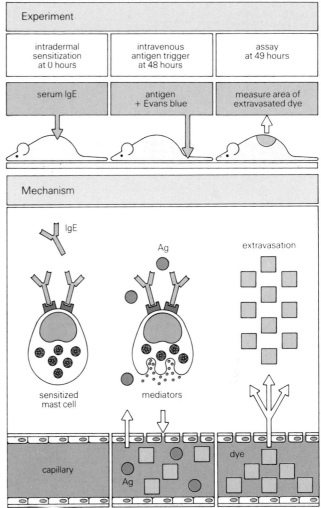

Fig.19.5 Passive cutaneous anaphylaxis (PCA). Antigen-specific IgE is classically measured by passive cutaneous anaphylaxis (PCA). A rat is injected intradermally with test serum and the IgE in this serum binds to mast cells and sensitizes them. 48 hours later the antigen and a dye, Evans blue, are injected intravenously. The antigen triggers degranulation and mediator release at the site of the first injection causing locally increased vascular permeability and extravasation of the dye. The skin of the animal is then examined: the area of dye in the dermis is a measure of the amount of antigen-specific IgE present in the original injection. IgE can also be measured by specific radioimmunoassay (see 'Immunological Tests').

Prausnitz (allergic to pollen) led to an immediate wheal and flare reaction when fish antigen was subsequently injected into the sensitized site. This test is similar to the passive cutaneous anaphylaxis test which is used for the assay of IgE production in experimental animals (Fig.19.5). The skin-sensitizing capacity of IgE resides in the Fc portion of the molecule and by heating the immunoglobulin at 56°C for half an hour the skin sensitizing capacity is destroyed: the antigen-binding capacity, which resides in the Fab portion, is preserved. Thus, a test to distinguish IgE from other antibodies which may sensitize mast cells (eg. IgG1 in the guinea pig) is to perform PCA tests before and after heating the serum.

IgE Levels in Disease

IgE levels are often raised in allergic disease and grossly elevated in parasitic infestations. When assessing children or adults for the presence of atopic disease, a raised level of IgE aids the diagnosis although it must be emphasized that a normal IgE level does not exclude atopy (Fig.19.6.). The determination of IgE alone will not predict an allergic state as there are genetic and environmental factors which play an important part in the production of clinical symptoms. When skin tests are performed on a large number of subjects, many more give positive skin tests than complain of symptoms. A recent survey has shown that up to 30% of a random group of 5000 subjects tested had a positive wheal and flare reaction to one or more common allergens. Thus, these subjects can produce specific IgE but they lack some factor (factor 'X': see Fig.19.35), which precipitates the symptoms of atopy.

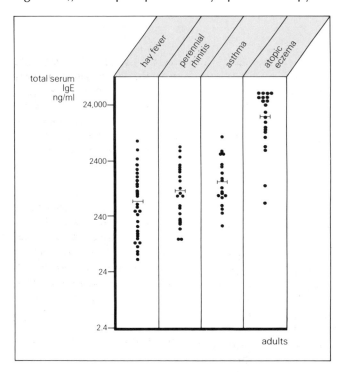

Fig.19.6 IgE levels in allergic patients. Each point in this chart represents the serum IgE level of a patient. IgE levels vary over a wide range, but the levels in atopic patients are generally elevated above the levels in normal subjects of the same age. For many atopic individuals with less severe disease, the serum IgE level falls within the normal range. IgE titres are usually expressed in international units per ml, by reference to standard sera, where 1IU = 2.4 ng. The normal range of IgE in non-atopic subjects is shaded yellow.

Control of IgE Production

The early studies by Tada using rats clearly demonstrated the T cell control of IgE production. Animals immunized with the antigen DNP-Ascaris, with *B. pertussis* as adjuvant, showed a rise in IgE titres peaking between five and ten days returning to normal over the next six weeks. If these animals were thymectomized or irradiated as adults, the IgE response was enhanced and prolonged. If during this phase of enhanced IgE production the animal was passively given thymocytes or spleen cells from

Ascaris-primed animals, IgE production was suppressed (Fig.19.7). Since there was no reduction in IgM or IgG responses in the treated animals this suggests that the enhanced IgE production was not due to defective negative feedback regulation by serum IgG antibodies but was due to decreased T-suppressor cell activity. However, neonatal thymectomy completely abolishes the capacity to produce IgE to DNP–Ascaris showing the need for T-helper cells in the IgE response. In several clinical conditions there is an association between low T-suppressor cell numbers and high levels of IgE, thus supporting the hypothesis for T cell control of IgE production.

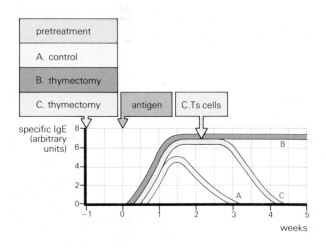

Fig.19.7 T cell control of the IgE response. The IgE response is under both T-helper and T-suppressor cell control. This experiment uses three groups of rats – a control group (A) receiving no pre-treatment one week before antigen challenge, and two groups which are first thymectomized (B, C). Following antigen challenge the IgE response is measured regularly. On immunization with antigen there is a transient rise in antigen-specific IgE (A. control). Thymectomy (or irradiation) causes a prolonged response (B) which can be curtailed by the addition of antigen-stimulated spleen cells containing Ts cells (C). (If neonatally thymectomized rats are immunized no IgE response is seen indicating the requirement for T-helper cells in the IgE response.)

The finding that different strains of animal vary in their ability to produce IgE suggests that the production of IgE is under direct genetic control. Low responder strains of mice such as SJL do not produce high titres of IgE even when subjected to an optimum injection schedule for its production. In these studies, both the dose of antigen and the mode of its administration is critical (Fig.19.8). It must be emphasised that although many animal model systems are available for studying IgE production, these are not models of allergy; there are no strains of laboratory mouse that develop hayfever spontaneously, although some dogs do. However, clinically, man is sensitized with multiple low dose exposures to allergen such as pollen during the summer and the route of sensitization is by mucosal surfaces and not by intraperitoneal injection! The production of IgE in response to allergen, which is under genetic control, is just one factor in the development of atopy as discussed below.

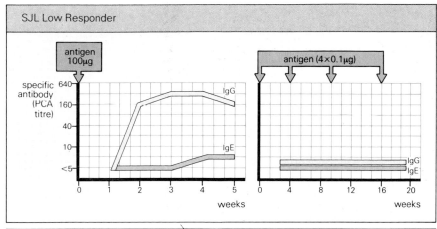

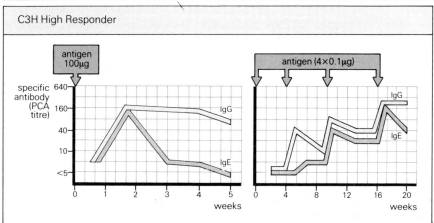

SJL Low Responder

Fig. 19.8 Dependence of the IgE response on the antigen dose and the genetic constitution of the animal. A 'low responder' SJL mouse (top) makes predominantly IgG to a single large dose (100 µg) of antigen (left), but makes little or no specific IgG or IgE in response to repeated small doses (0.1 µg). By contrast a C3H 'high responder' mouse (bottom) makes a transient large IgE response to a single high antigen dose which decays over 3-4 weeks, whilst repeated low dose antigen stimulation produces rising titres of both IgE and IgG with each injection.

GENETICS OF THE ALLERGIC RESPONSE

Early studies in the 1920s showed that allergic parents tended to have a higher proportion of allergic children than parents who were not allergic. When large numbers of families were examined the figures showed that with two allergic parents there is a 50% chance of the children having allergy. Even with one allergic parent the chances are still almost 30%. Thus, both genetic background and elevated serum IgE levels are risk factors (Fig. 19.9). It has been calculated that the annual challenge of individuals by airborne pollens is in the order of 1 microgram, which is clearly a low-dose challenge. It is perhaps surprising that some 15% of the population respond to this exceptionally low dose challenge. A variety of non-genetic factors also play an important role, such as the quantity of the exposure, nutritional status of the individual and the presence of either chronic underlying infections or acute viral illnesses (see Fig. 19.36). There are three main genetic mechanisms regulating the allergic response:

1. Total IgE levels. Studies of families in which at least one member has high IgE levels have confirmed the hypothesis that a low IgE level is associated with a dominant gene.

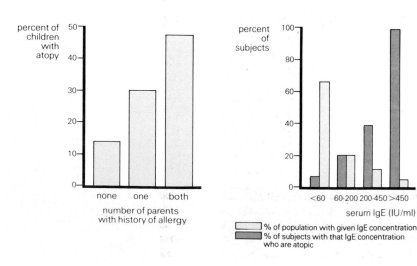

% of population with given IgE concentration
% of subjects with that IgE concentration who are atopic

Fig. 19.9 Risk of allergy: family and IgE levels. The left hand bar diagram shows the percentage of atopic children born to parents where either none, one or both of the parents have a history of allergy. The greater the parental or family history of allergy, the greater is the risk of atopy in the child. The right hand diagram shows that the majority of the population has low levels of IgE. However, the higher the level of total serum IgE, the greater the likelihood of atopy.

2. HLA-linked Ir response. In general, HLA-linked genetic responsiveness to airborne allergens can only be shown when a pure antigen isolated from a crude extract is used and these antigens may be minor determinants of the allergen. For example, only one in six of ragweed-allergic patients respond to Ra 3, a minor determinant. Of the Ra3$^+$ patients with low total IgE levels, 9 out of 10 subjects carry HLA-A2 (Fig.19.10). With increasing total IgE levels the number of determinants recognized is less restricted and the HLA association disappears. A weak association of ragweed Ra5 antigen responsiveness with HLA–A3, B7 has been shown by skin tests and RAST. An even greater association is shown with the D locus antigen, Dw2 where more than 90% of Ra5$^+$ subjects have Dw2 compared to 20% of Ra5$^-$. Following hyposensitization to ragweed it is only the HLA–Dw2, Ra5$^+$ subjects who make a good IgG response to the Ra5 antigen showing that the immune response to Ra5 is not restricted to IgE but includes other immunoglobulin classes.

3. General hyperresponsiveness. The concept of hyperresponsiveness to a broad range of antigens has been tested in patients attending an allergy clinic who were divided solely on the basis of having positive or negative skin tests (Fig.19.11). The results show that HLA–B8 and HLA–Dw3, but not HLA–A1, are present at a significantly higher frequency in the allergic group. This hyperresponsiveness can also be seen in those already making anti-ragweed IgE antibodies, where those with HLA–B8 have higher titres of antibody and also high levels of total IgE.

| HLA | skin test | | p |
	positive (%)	negative (%)	
A1	28.7	24.1	0.4
B8	22.3	11.5	0.01
Dw3	25.2	11.7	0.002

Fig.19.11 IgE response: genetic association. In atopic subjects skin test positive to a number of common environmental allergens (eg. pollens, housedust mite), there is a significant association between HLA-B8 and HLA-Dw3 and skin test positivity compared with skin test negative non-allergic controls. The IgE response to antigens is clearly genetically linked, both in terms of the ability to respond to a given antigen and the general 'atopic ability' to produce an IgE antibody response to any antigen.

HLA–B8 is also strongly associated with other forms of immune 'hyperactivity', such as autoimmune diseases, raising the possibility that it is linked to T-suppressor cell control of immune responses, since depressed T-suppressor activity is thought to be involved in the development of both autoimmune and IgE responses. The three genetically controlled parameters predisposing to allergy are summarized below.

1. Basal IgE levels   ANTIGEN NON-SPECIFIC
Dominant for low levels
Not HLA linked
IgE class specific

2. HLA linked antigen-   ANTIGEN SPECIFIC
specific response
HLA-linked Ir genes
Not IgE class specific

3. General   ANTIGEN NON-SPECIFIC
hyperresponsiveness
HLA-linked
Not IgE class specific

There is also a fourth possible mechanism, HLA-linked, associated with immune-suppressive genes.

MAST CELLS

It has long been recognized that there is a species difference in mast cell morphology. Morphological differences may be seen in staining properties of the cells, the outer structure of their granules and in the detailed mechanism of the degranulation process. This last point is clearly seen in man where the membranes surrounding the mast cell granules fuse before exocytosis compared to rats where the granules are expelled singly (Figs. 19.12 & 19.13). In addition to morphological differences there are also functional differences between species and between the mast cells derived from different sites within the same

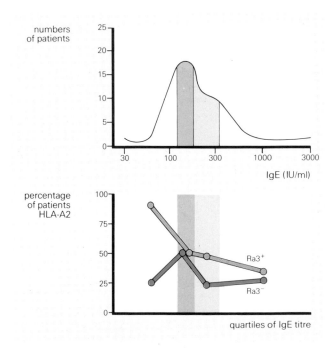

Fig.19.10 Atopy: IgE levels and tissue type. The upper chart shows the numbers of ragweed allergic patients (Ra3$^+$) with given levels of total IgE as a frequency distribution. The quartiles of the range are indicated in different shades. The lower chart shows the percentage of patients in these four quartiles possessing the HLA antigen A2 for both Ra3$^+$ and Ra3$^-$ individuals. It appears that a person is more likely to be sensitive to Ra3 if they possess HLA-A2. This genetic association is most marked where the IgE level is low (first quartile). HLA-A2 is present in 47% of the population.

animal. The functional differences are seen in response to secretagogues (histamine liberators) and to drugs which block or enhance histamine release.

It used to be thought that mast cells comprised a homogeneous population of cells, the morphology being similar to that which is now recognized as the connective tissue mast cell (CTMC). The staining technique used to demonstrate CTMCs involves formalin fixation of sections and toluidine blue staining. It is now realized that these stains do not adequately show up the mucosal mast cell (MMC) which is only shown with special fixatives and stains (Figs. 19.14 & 19.15).

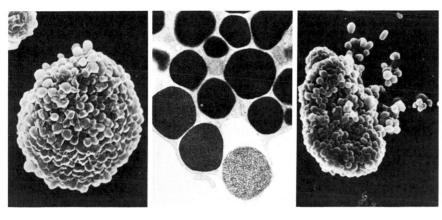

Fig.19.12 Electron micrograph study of mast cells I. These micrographs of rat peritoneal mast cells show an undegranulated cell (left, scanning EM, × 1,500); granule in the process of exocytosis (middle, transmission EM, × 15,000), and exocytosis of granules following incubation with anti-IgE at 37°C for 30 seconds (right, scanning EM, × 1,500). Courtesy of Dr. T. S. C. Orr.

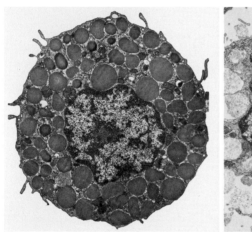
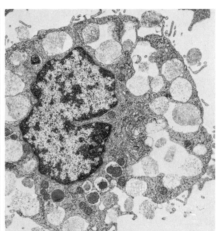

Fig.19.13 Electron micrograph study of mast cells II. These transmission EMs of rat peritoneal mast cells show electron-dense granules (left) and following incubation with anti-IgE (right) – vacuolation with exocytosis of the granule contents has occurred. × 2,700. Courtesy of Dr. D. Lawson.

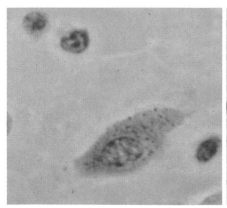
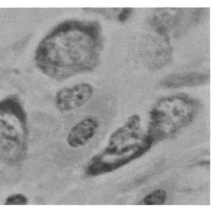

Fig.19.14 Histological appearance of human gut mast cells. Connective tissue mast cell showing dark blue cytoplasm with brownish granules (left) and a mucosal mast cell with light blue-staining cytoplasm and blue granules (right). There is marked heterogeneity of mast cell morphology, these appearances being relatively clear-cut examples from each end of the spectrum. The sections were fixed in Carnoys and stained with Alcian blue and Safranin, ×400. Courtesy of Drs. T. S. C. Orr and B. Greenwood.

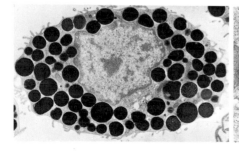
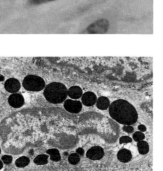

Fig.19.15 Electron micrographs showing a rat peritoneal CTMC and intestinal MMC. The CTMC (left) has multiple electron-dense granules and the nuclear size is small compared with the total cytoplasmic mass. In the MMC from the core of a rat intestinal villus (right) the granules are more sparse and the nucleus is large. ×4,000. Courtesy of Dr. T. S. C. Orr.

	mucosal mast cell (MMC)	connective tissue mast cell (CTMC)
location *in vivo*	gut and lung	ubiquitous
life span	<40 days (?)	>40 days (?)
T cell dependent	+	–
number of Fc$^\varepsilon$ receptors	2×10^5	3×10^4
histamine content	+	+ +
cytoplasmic IgE	+	–
major AA metabolite LTC$_4$:PGD$_2$ ratio	25:1	1:40
DSCG/theophyline inhibits histamine release	–	+
major proteoglycan	chondroitin sulphate	heparin

Fig.19.16 Differences between mast cell populations.
There are at least two sub-populations of mast cells, the MMC
and the CTMC. The differences in their morphology and
pharmacology suggest different functional roles *in vivo*.
MMCs are associated with parasitic worm infections and
possibly allergic reations. In contrast to the CTMC the MMC is
smaller, shorter lived, T cell dependent, has more surface Fc
receptors and contains intracytoplasmic IgE. Both cells
contain histamine and serotonin in their granules; the higher
histamine content of the CTMC may be accounted for by the
greater number of granules. Major arachidonic acid
metabolites, prostaglandins and leukotrienes, are produced
by both mast cell types but in different amounts. For example,
the ratios of production of the leukotriene LTC4 to the
prostaglandin PGD$_2$ is 25:1 in the MMC and 1:40 in the
CTMC. The effect of drugs on degranulation is different
between the two cell types. Sodium cromoglycate (DSGC)
and theophylline both inhibit histamine release from the
CTMC but not the MMC and this may have important
implications in the treatment of asthma. Much of the data
comes from rodent studies and may not apply to man.

Distribution of Mast Cells
CTMCs are found around blood vessels in most tissues.
Although CTMCs from different sites may have similar
properties, the gross morphology of CTMCs from the peri-
toneum and the skin for example, may be quite different
in terms of the number and size of the granules, the density of staining and their pharmacological properties.
MMCs show a distribution different to that of the CTMC,
in man the highest concentration being found in the mucosa of the midgut and the lung. During parasitic infections there is a marked increase in MMCs in the gut. This
increase is also seen in Crohn's disease and ulcerative
colitis.

Difference Between MMCs and CTMCs
T cell dependence of mast cells In rats infected with *Nip-
postrongylus brasiliensis* there is an increase in lymphoblasts in the gut mucosa. It has been suggested that these
lymphoblasts (of T cell origin) arise in the mesenteric
lymph nodes which drain the gut and then migrate via the
thoracic duct back to the intestine. It is clear that MMC
proliferation after such infection is T cell dependent since
it does not occur in nude mice. However, it is still unclear
whether MMCs are T-lymphoblast derived rather than
merely T cell dependent as regards maturation and proliferation. By contrast, CTMC clones arise in culture from
fibroblast layers, independent of T cells or T cell factors,
and are found in normal numbers in nude mice.

Effect of drugs Crucial from the functional and clinical
points of view is the effect of drugs on mast cell degranulation. Sodium cromoglycate and theophylline both
inhibit histamine release from rat CTMCs but not from
MMCs. Because of mast cell heterogeneity and species
differences, the development of 'pure' human mast cell
lines may be of great use in the development of drugs for
the management of the allergic patient. MMCs and
CTMCs are compared in figure 19.16.

Other Fc$^\varepsilon$ Receptor-bearing Cells
In addition to mast cells and basophils, a number of other
cells have Fc receptors for IgE (Fc$^\varepsilon$) (Fig.19.17). It is notable that Fc$^\varepsilon$ receptor positive T cells and IgE levels rise
during the pollen season. Monocytes possessing Fc$^\varepsilon$ receptors are increased in the circulation in some atopics
and especially so in those with severe atopic eczema.

cell type	comment
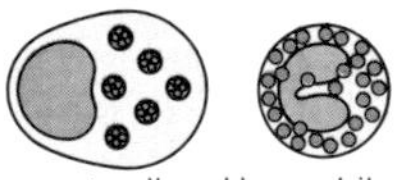 mast cell and basophil	main effectors of IgE-mediated reactions
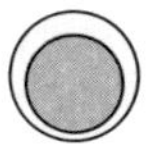 T cell and B cell	T cells: about 1% Fc$^\varepsilon$R positive, increase in atopics during pollen season. B cells: about 30% Fc$^\varepsilon$R positive increasing as above
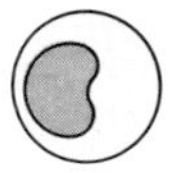 monocyte	about 2% Fc$^\varepsilon$R positive increasing up to 20% in some allergic disorders
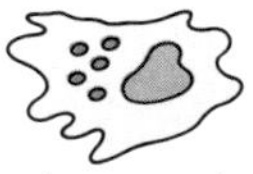 alveolar macrophage	receptors demonstrated by IgE-mediated enzyme release
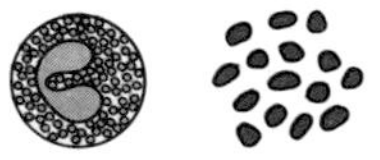 eosinophil and platelets	effectors of IgE-mediated damage to schistosomes

Fig.19.17 Fc$^\varepsilon$ receptor-bearing cells. Mast cells and
basophils express high affinity (Kd$\approx 10^{10}$) Fc receptors. The Fc
receptors on other cells are of much lower affinity (Kd$\approx 10^6$)
and their function on T and B lymphocytes and monocytes is
not yet clear. IgE bound to alveolar macrophage Fc$^\varepsilon$ receptors
when reacted with antigen can stimulate lysosomal enzyme
release and production of leukotrienes, which may be
important in asthmatic reactions. Fc$^\varepsilon$ receptor-bearing
eosinophils and platelets have been shown to mediate killing
of IgE sensitized schistosomes.

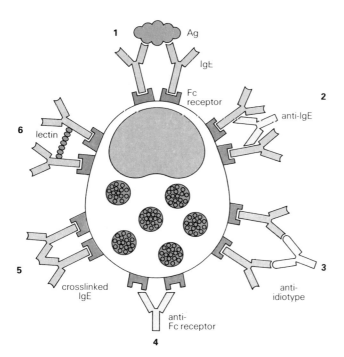

alpha and two beta chains and antibodies have been made against these components. These antibodies can crosslink the receptors thereby leading to degranulation of basophils without the need for the presence of IgE. Lectins, including PHA and Concanavalin A can also crosslink IgE by binding to carbohydrate residues on the Fc region thus causing degranulation. This might explain the urticaria induced in some individuals by strawberries which contain large amounts of lectin.

As well as the methods of bridging the Fc^ε receptors described in figure 19.18 there are other compounds that are extremely active in degranulating mast cells. Probably the most important of these *in vivo* are the breakdown products of complement activation, that is, the anaphylatoxins C3a and C5a. The anaphylatoxins also affect a variety of other cells including neutrophils, platelets and macrophages, so the mast cell is only one of many cells to be affected by them. There are a number of compounds that directly activate mast cells such as calcium ionophore, mellitin and compound 48/80 as well as some drugs such as synthetic ACTH, codeine and morphine (Fig. 19.19). All these compounds activate the mast cell by causing an influx of calcium ions.

Fig.19.18 Fc^ε receptor-mediated mast cell triggering.
Mast cells are triggered when their Fc^ε receptors are crosslinked. This may occur when 1) surface bound antigen-specific IgE binds antigens (Ag); 2) by divalent antibody to the Fc region of IgE or (3) by anti-idiotypic antibodies to the idiotopes of that IgE. The receptors may be crosslinked by direct binding of anti-receptor antibody (4). Experimentally, covalently crosslinked IgE dimers can bridge the receptors (5) or lectins (carbohydrate binding glycoproteins) can link sugar residues on IgE and thus cause degranulation (6). It is the perturbation of the mast cell membrane caused by crosslinking of the Fc^ε receptors that is the first stage in mast cell activation. Thus, monovalent antigen or antibody will not cause mast cell activation, since crosslinking is not achieved.

These cells when armed with IgE may have a local cytotoxic potential. Alveolar macrophages may also be sensitized with IgE and release enzymes when challenged by allergen. This could play an important role in allergen-induced lung disease.

Both eosinophils and platelets have been shown to bear Fc^ε receptors and when these cells are sensitized with IgE they are found to have a greatly enhanced capacity for cytotoxicity against some parasites including schistosomes. It may be that these cells perform important functions in allergic patients when sensitized by circulating immune complexes containing IgE, since they both contain a variety of active pharmacological mediators capable of accentuating (platelets) or controlling (eosinophils) allergic reactions.

Mast Cell Triggering

Once IgE binds to the Fc^ε receptors on the mast cells and basophils, degranulation may be triggered by crosslinking the IgE thereby crosslinking the Fc^ε receptors. Degranulation may also be effected by manoeuvres which directly crosslink the receptors (Fig.19.18).

Using a rat basophil leukaemic cell line, the receptor for IgE has been isolated. It has a four chain structure; two

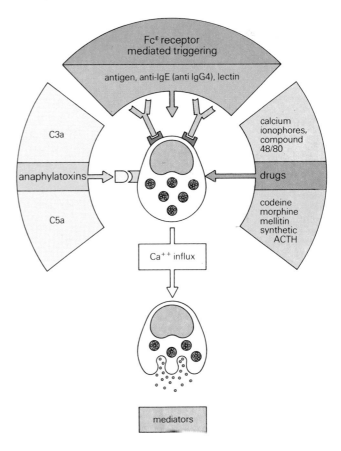

Fig.19.19 Mast cell activation-1. Mast cell activation can be produced by immunological stimuli which crosslink Fc^ε receptors and by other stimuli such as anaphylatoxins and secretagogues (eg. compound 48/80, mellitin and calcium ionophore A23187). Some other drugs such as codeine, morphine and synthetic ACTH have also been found capable of activating the mast cell directly. The common feature in each case is the influx of Ca^{++} ions into the mast cell which initiates the biochemical processes leading to mast cell degranulation and mediator release.

T Cells and Mast Cell Triggering

The mucosal mast cell needs T cells for maturation but there also seems to be a more direct relationship between these cells in the induction of mediator release. Lymphokines from stimulated human lymphocytes can release histamine from basophils and this release is additional to that due to IgE and antigen. This histamine releasing factor (HRF) may be involved in non-specifically amplifying delayed hypersensitivity and also modulating Type I hypersensitivity reactions. In addition to this non-specific factor, an antigen-specific T cell factor (TCF) can also arm mast cells to release mediators following contact with antigen. This factor sensitizes mast cells for a few hours only, by comparison with IgE, which sensitizes them for days. Thus, T cells are linked to mast cells not only by growth factors but by the release of specific factors (TCF) and non-specific histamine releasing factor (HRF).

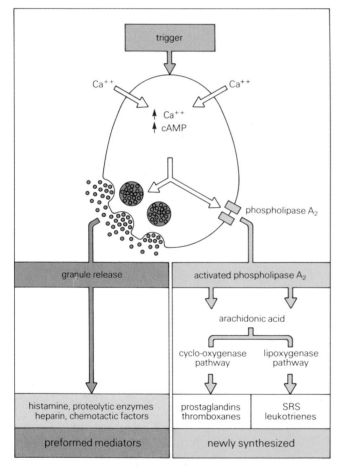

Fig.19.20 Mast cell activation-2. Immunological triggers (eg. antigen or anti-IgE) perturb the mast cell membrane, leading to calcium ion influx which is crucial for degranulation. Microtubule formation and movement of granules to the cell membrane leads to fusion of granule and plasma membrane and release of granule-associated mediators into the intercellular space. Changes in the plasma membrane associated with activation allows phospholipase A_2 to release arachidonic acid which can then be metabolized by lipoxygenase or cyclo-oxygenase enzymes, depending on the mast cell type. The newly synthesized products include prostaglandin A_2 and thromboxane A_2 (cyclo-oxygenase pathway), and SRS (which is leukotriene $LTC_4 + LTD_4$) and chemotactic LTB_4 (lipoxygenase pathway).

granule-associated preformed mediators		
histamine	Mol.Wt. = III	vasodilation, increased capillary permeability chemokinesis bronchoconstriction
heparin	Mol.Wt. = 60,000	anticoagulant
enzymes	tryptase (Mol.Wt. = 130,000) β-glucosaminidase (Mol.Wt. = 150,000)	proteolytic C3 convertase cleaves glucosamine residues
chemotactic and activating factors	ECF-A (Mol.Wt. = 380/2000) NCF (Mol.Wt. >750,000) PAF (Mol.Wt. = 600)	chemotaxis of eosinophils, neutrophils platelet activation

newly formed mediators		
SRS ($LTC_4 + LTD_4$) chemotactic leukotrienes (LTB_4)	lipoxygenase pathway products	vasoactive, bronchoconstriction, chemotactic and/or chemokinetic
prostaglandins thromboxanes	cyclooxygenase products	bronchial muscle contraction, platelet aggregation, vasodilation

Fig.19.21 Human mast cell derived mediators. In man the major vasoactive amine is histamine, which leads to immediate inflammatory effects and is stored in the granule in association with heparin. Granule-associated proteases, such as tryptase and chemotactic factors may lead to the inflammation associated with late phase reactions. Of the newly formed mediators, SRS ($LTC_4 + LTD_4$) is associated with early inflammation, although later than that induced by histamine. Prostaglandins, thromboxane and chemotactic factors such as ECF-A, NCF and LTB_4 may be involved in initiating the late phase reaction and inducing the cellular infiltrate which includes neutrophils, eosinophils, basophils and mononuclear cells.

Mediator Release

The calcium ion influx has two main results. Firstly, there is an exocytosis of granule contents with the release of *preformed mediators*, the major one being histamine. Secondly, there is the induction of synthesis of *newly formed* mediators from arachidonic acid leading to the production of prostaglandins and leukotrienes (Figs.19.20 & 19.21). These mediators have a direct effect on the local tissues and in the lung cause immediate bronchoconstriction, mucosal oedema and hypersecretion leading to asthma (Fig. 19.22).

It is becoming clear that different newly-formed mediators arise from the different populations of mast cells as indicated previously (Fig.19.16), thus the different clinical effects in different organs may be related to the varying population of mast cells in each. An overall scheme of the allergic reaction is shown in figure 19.23.

Drugs may block the release of mediators in two ways; firstly by increasing the intracellular levels of cAMP by stimulation of β-receptors with drugs such as isoprenaline, or secondly by drugs which prevent breakdown of cAMP by phosphodiesterase, for example, theophylline. The mode of action of sodium cromoglycate in preventing histamine release is not clear.

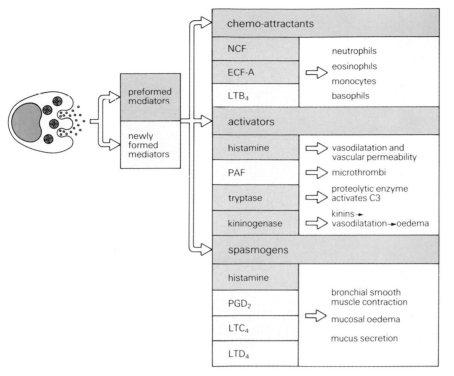

chemo-attractants		
NCF		neutrophils
ECF-A	⟹	eosinophils
		monocytes
LTB₄		basophils

activators		
histamine	⟹	vasodilatation and vascular permeability
PAF	⟹	microthrombi
tryptase	⟹	proteolytic enzyme activates C3
kininogenase	⟹	kinins → vasodilatation → oedema

spasmogens		
histamine		
PGD₂	⟹	bronchial smooth muscle contraction
LTC₄		mucosal oedema
LTD₄		mucus secretion

Fig.19.22 Physiological effects of mast cell derived mediators. Both the preformed granule-associated and the newly formed mediators have three main areas of action.

As *chemotactic agents*: a variety of cells can be attracted to the site of mast cell activation, in particular eosinophils, neutrophils and mononuclear cells including lymphocytes.

Inflammatory *activators* can lead to vasodilatation, oedema and, via PAF, to microthrombi – leading to local damage. Tryptase, the major protein of human lung mast cells can activate C3 directly, this function being inhibited by heparin. Kininogenases are also released and these affect small blood vessels by generating kinins from tissue kininogens, again leading to inflammation.

The *spasmogens* have a direct effect on bronchial smooth muscle but can also increase mucus secretion leading to bronchial plugging.

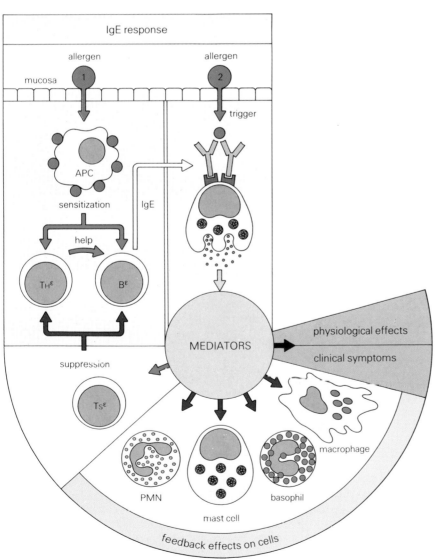

Fig.19.23 Activation and control of the allergic response. Initial exposure to allergen (1) stimulates an IgE response in atopic subjects, involving the interaction of antigen-presenting cells (APC) and antigen-specific T-helper cells with Bᵋ cells at the mucosal site of antigen entry and/or in the local lymph nodes. Locally produced IgE sensitizes local mast cells which will degranulate on future exposure to allergen (2). This can also boost the IgE response. The mediators produce the clinical symptoms of allergy but there are negative feedback effects of these mediators (particularly histamine) on other cells of the immune system. For example, histamine has been shown to suppress PMN lysosomal enzyme release, mast cell and basophil degranulation and monocyte production of complement components. In addition, histamine can activate antigen non-specific T-suppressor cells, which may have a feedback effect on the IgE response. Some data suggest that these feedback mechanisms are defective in atopics and this may represent another factor in the development of atopic allergy in susceptible subjects. The mediators exert a variety of physiological effects and produce the clinical symptoms of allergy.

CLINICAL TESTS FOR ALLERGY

The classical skin test in atopy is the Type I wheal and flare reaction in which antigen is introduced into the skin leading to the release of preformed mediators, increased vascular permeability, local oedema and itching (Figs.19.24 & 19.25). A positive skin test usually correlates with a positive RAST (a test for antigen-specific IgE) and the relevant provocation test, for example, nasal or bronchial provocation with the allergen.

The late response following skin testing is not often seen because is it rarely looked for and when it does occur it has the appearance of a lump in the skin which is painful rather than itchy. Endpoint titration of skin testing is a useful clinical method of determining a rough approximation of the patient's sensitivity to the allergen. There is a small group of patients who give a clear-cut history of, for example, allergic rhinitis, but in whom skin tests and RAST are negative. These patients, however, do make a local mucosal antibody response as can be shown by a positive nasal provocation test and by the presence of the relevant specific IgE in the nasal secretion.

Patients with a variety of atopic disorders show the classical immediate wheal and flare response following skin prick tests demonstrating that IgE is bound to skin mast cells. If the lymphocytes of these patients are stimulated with allergen, lymphocyte transformation and lymphokine production result, indicating T cell reactivity to the allergen. This does not necessarily imply that delayed hypersensitivity is contributing directly to the disease process but indicates that T cells specific for allergen are present in these patients and may be providing 'help' in the IgE response.

In patients with atopic eczema (Fig.19.26) who have IgE antibodies to the house dust mite, it has been shown that when mite allergen is applied to abraded non-affected skin, a positive patch test results (Fig.19.27).

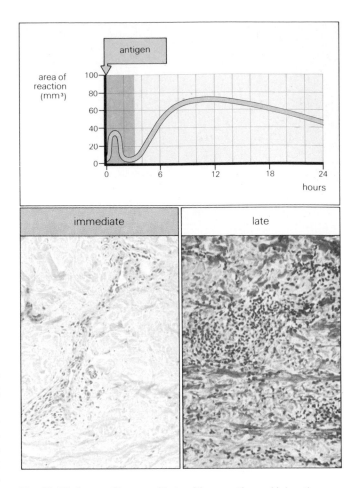

Fig.19.25 Immediate and late skin reactions. Using the skin prick or intradermal method of skin testing, an immediate wheal and flare reaction is often followed by a late phase reaction. This phase may last 24 hours and the reaction is larger and generally more oedematous than the immediate response. The immediate type of reaction (here exemplified by a biopsy of chronic urticaria) has a sparse cellular infiltrate around the dermal vessels consisting primarily of neutrophils, whereas the late reaction has a dense infiltrate, with many basophils. The late phase reaction can be seen following challenge of the skin, nasal mucosa and bronchi and may be particularly important in the development of chronic asthma. Courtesy of Dr. A. K. Black (left) and Dr. G. Boyd (right).

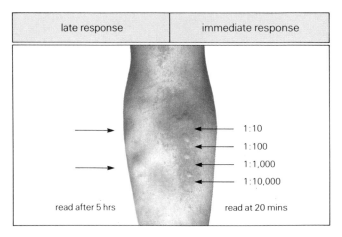

Fig.19.24 Skin prick tests with grass pollen allergen in a patient with typical summer hay fever. Skin tests were performed 5 hours (left) and 20 minutes (right) before the photograph was taken. The tests on the right show a typical end point titration of a Type I immediate wheal and flare reaction. The late phase skin reaction (left) can be clearly seen at 5 hours, especially where a large immediate response has preceded it. Figures for allergen dilution are given.

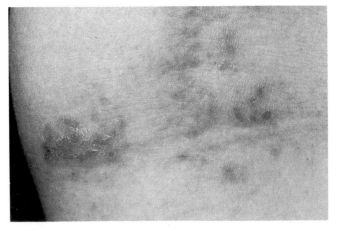

Fig.19.26 The appearance of atopic eczema on the back of a knee in a child allergic to rice and eggs.

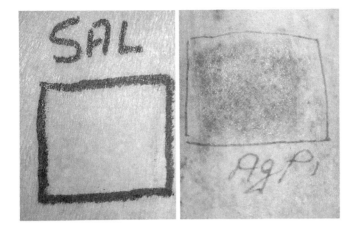

Fig.19.27 Skin patch tests in a patient with atopic eczema using purified house dust mite (Dermatophagoides pteronyssinus) antigen. The surface keratin of an unaffected area is removed by gentle abrasion (left) and the extract is placed on the skin and occluded for 48 hours at which time the site is examined (right). The lesions are macroscopically eczematous and microscopically contain infiltrates of eosinophils and basophils. Courtesy of Dr. E. B. Mitchell.

It is interesting that a proportion of patients with allergic rhinitis due to the house dust mite (Fig.19.28) also show positive patch tests with basophil infiltration, suggesting that the infiltration is an immune response to house dust mite antigen and is not specific for atopic eczema. The recruited basophils may be sensitized to many different allergens and could degranulate in response to allergens other than the one used to induce the lesion.

When the late phase skin reaction was originally described it was thought that the mechanism might have been a Type 3 reaction (immune complex mediated) due to a precipitating IgG antibody, as is seen in bronchopulmonary aspergillosis. However, precipitating anti-

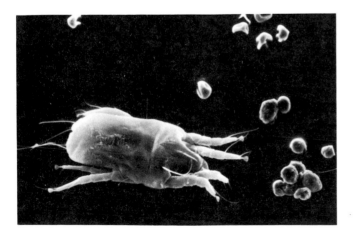

Fig.19.28 House dust mite – a major allergen. Electron micrograph showing the house dust mite, *Dermatophagoides pteryonyssinus*, and faecal pellets (bottom right) which represent the major source of allergen. Biconcave pollen grains (top right) are shown for comparison of size showing that the faecal pellet and not the mite itself can become airborne and reach the lungs. Courtesy of Dr. E. Tovey.

bodies have not been found associated with this late reaction and further research has confirmed that the late response is an IgE-dependent sequel to the immediate response.

Bronchial reactions to allergens also show an immediate and late phase response (Fig.19.29). Sodium cromoglycate is a very effective treatment in allergic asthma and it prevents both the immediate and late phase responses following bronchial provocation with allergen. This implies that the development of a late reaction in the lung is dependent on an initial allergen/IgE/mast cell interaction; preventing degranulation with sodium cromoglycate prevents all subsequent events. If patients are pretreated with corticosteroids or prostaglandin synthetase inhibitors, late reactions alone are abolished leaving the immediate response unchanged. This indicates a role for mast cell-derived arachidonic acid metabolites such as prostaglandins and leukotrienes in the late response (see Figs.19.20 & 19.22).

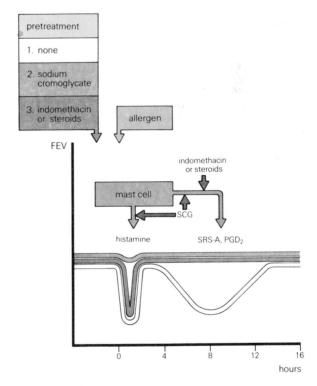

Fig.19.29 Immediate and late phase bronchial reactions. This graph plots the forced expiratory volume (FEV) in three groups of individuals prior to and several hours after bronchial provocation with an allergen. Each group is pretreated differently. As can be seen from the control group (1) there is a biphasic (initial and late) bronchial constriction. The initial reaction lasts for 1 hour and is followed by a late reaction lasting several hours. Histamine released from degranulating mast cells is thought to cause the immediate reaction. Pretreatment with sodium cromoglycate (SCG) inhibits mast cell degranulation thus preventing both early and late reactions (2). Pretreatment with indomethacin and corticosteroids, which block arachidonic acid metabolic pathways, inhibit the late phase reaction but not the immediate (3) thus implicating SRS-A and PGD_2 in the development of the late reaction.

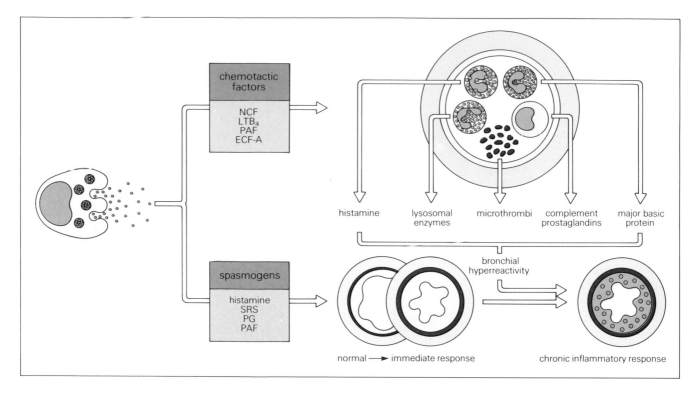

Fig. 19.30 The inflammatory response in the asthmatic lung. Mast cell mediators may be divided into chemotactic and direct acting (spasmogenic) factors. The chemotactic factors lead to active cell accumulation, the production of a further set of inflammatory molecules by these cells and the late phase response. The spasmogenic mediators produce the immediate response on bronchial provocation and also lead to increased small vessel permeability, oedema and cell emigration. All these factors, including hypersecretion of mucus, smooth muscle hypertrophy and cell infiltration with associated bronchial hyperreactivity lead to subacute or chronic inflammation.

Most asthmatics with reversible airway obstruction benefit from treatment with corticosteroids, although these drugs have little or no effect on the immediate IgE-mediated reaction. The fact that it is the late reaction which is abolished by corticosteroids suggests that in chronic asthma the late reaction is of major clinical importance. The beneficial effect of corticosteroids in chronic asthma may be related to the reduction of cell infiltration in the bronchii (Fig. 19.30).

Associated with asthma is hyperreactivity of the bronchi to histamine and non-specific stimuli such as cold air and water vapour. Normal subjects become asthmatic following inhalation of 10ng of histamine whereas asthmatics respond to amounts at least 20 fold less.

The fact that this hyperreactivity is a response to chronic antigen challenge is strongly supported by the data of Platts-Mills who removed asthmatics from their allergenic environment (house dust mite) for up to 3 months and showed that at the end of that time their sensitivity to histamine was greatly reduced and in some cases had completely returned to normal.

THE CAUSES OF ALLERGY

1. T Cell Deficiency

There is substantial evidence for a role for T cells in the IgE response (see Fig. 19.7). This has led to the suggestion that a defect in T cells and in particular, suppressor T cells, may be involved in the aetiology of atopy. Reduced numbers of E-rosette forming cells and suppressor T cells are seen in severe atopic eczema patients but not so clearly in patients with rhinitis and asthma (Fig. 19.31).

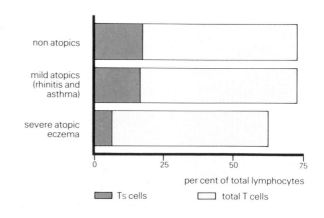

Fig. 19.31 Suppressor T cells in atopy. The total number of T cells was estimated by E-rosetting, and T-suppressor cells by staining with an anti-T-suppressor monoclonal antibody (OKT8). Patients with severe atopic eczema, but not patients with rhinitis or asthma, have a reduced total number of T cells, which is almost wholly accounted for by fewer OKT8 staining, T-suppressor cells. Decreased numbers of circulating T-suppressor cells are associated with the often grossly elevated serum IgE levels seen in atopic eczema.

In addition, T cell mitogen responses are reduced in the severe atopics (those with eczema) (Fig.19.32) and these reduced T cell responses *in vitro*, correlate with reduced cell-mediated immunity seen *in vivo* as depressed delayed hypersensitivity skin responses.

Until recently it has not been clear whether this T cell defect is a cause or a consequence of the atopic disease. Interestingly, recent studies have provided some evidence for a causal relationship between the T cell defect in atopy and the type of feeding in infancy. Studies by Soothill and colleagues have shown that the incidence of eczema in children is reduced if they are breast fed and work by other groups has shown a relationship between bottle feeding in infancy, IgE level and T cell numbers (Fig.19.33). The implication is that bottle feeding in infancy associated with reduced numbers of some subsets of regulatory T cells causes increased IgE levels, although it is not certain whether the bottle feeding itself affects T cell numbers.

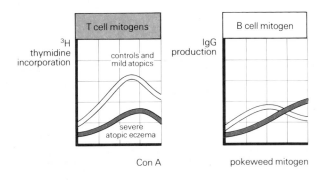

Fig.19.32 Mitogen responses in atopy. *In vitro* studies show that the response of purified peripheral blood lymphocytes (PBLs) to the two mitogens, Con A and pokeweed mitogen, can be used as a measure of T cell and B cell activity respectively. Mitogens react with cell surface glycoproteins, stimulating cell transformation and proliferation, measured by ^{3}H-thymidine incorporation into cellular DNA. PBLs from mild atopics — those with rhinitis or asthma — and non-atopics respond similarly to the T cell mitogen (Con A), whilst the response of PBLs from patients with severe atopic eczema is generally depressed. In contrast, the response of atopic and non-atopic subjects to a B cell mitogen (pokeweed) is very similar when measured by either ^{3}H-thymidine incorporation or IgG antibody production.

2. Abnormal Mediator Feedback

Histamine is one of the major mediators of Type I hypersensitivity reactions and it has been shown to inhibit T cell responses to mitogens such as Con A and PHA. The histamine suppression of T cell proliferation is greater in atopics than non-atopics and can be reduced in atopics, but not in normals, by the addition of indomethacin, a drug which inhibits prostaglandin production by monocytes present in the cell preparations (Fig.19.34). This finding suggests that histamine can stimulate monocytes from atopics (but not from normal subjects) to produce prostaglandins which can both suppress T cell responses *in vitro* and may contribute to the inflammatory reactions *in vivo*.

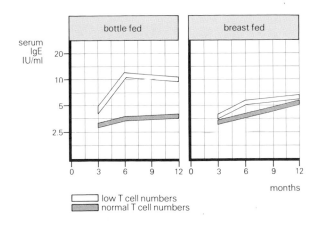

Fig.19.33 Effect of early bottle feeding and T cell deficiency on serum IgE levels. In infants with low numbers of circulating T cells, IgE levels in the serum were found to be elevated when those children were bottle fed early in life. Other infants with low T cells, but breast fed, had similar IgE levels to those infants with normal levels of T cells who were breast or bottle fed. These data show that the type of feeding and T cell numbers affect IgE levels and suggest that a T cell defect in association with an environmental factor (feeding) may influence development of the atopic state.

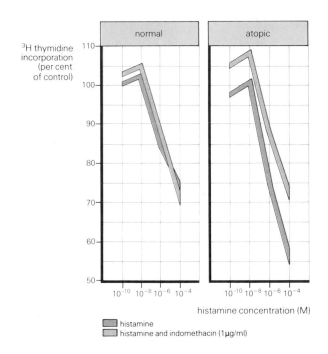

Fig.19.34 Graphs showing the effect of histamine on lymphocyte transformation and proliferation (determined by ^{3}H-thymidine incorporation) in normal and atopic subjects. Increasing concentrations of histamine initially enhance and then suppress the T cell response to the mitogen Con A. The histamine suppression is greater in atopics than in normals and can be reduced to levels seen in normals by indomethacin, which inhibits prostaglandin production. This suggests that atopic monocytes can produce suppressive prostaglandins in response to histamine. This mechanism may be involved in the late reaction *in vivo*.

3. Environmental Factors: The Concept of Allergic Breakthrough

It is evident that a number of factors must contribute to allergy and this has led to the hypothesis of allergic break-through, where clinical symptoms of allergy are only seen when an arbitrary level of immunological activity (allergic breakthrough) is exceeded (Fig.19.35). This will depend on a number of conditions, including exposure to allergen, genetic predisposition of the patient, the tendency to make IgE, and other factors, such as the presence of upper respiratory tract viral infections, decreased suppressor activity or transient IgA deficiency. Viral infections may exacerbate allergic symptoms and this may be due to the fact that some viruses (eg. *Herpes simplex*) enhance basophil histamine release (Fig.19.36). Both live and UV light-inactivated viruses can enhance histamine release, and interferon has been shown to be the mediator of this effect. Additionally, viruses can also enhance allergen entry through damaged epithelial surfaces and the responsiveness of target organs to histamine. Thus the role of viruses in the development of allergy is an area of particular interest.

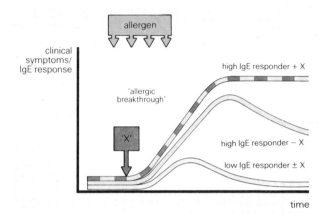

Fig.19.35 Allergic breakthrough in man: hypothesis. On exposure to allergen an IgE response may develop transiently in low IgE responders before being controlled by normal T-suppressor cell activity. In high responders, the IgE response to allergen is much greater than in low responders, but the overt expression of clinical symptoms is only seen when allergic breakthrough is exceeded. This may depend on the presence of concomitant factors ('X') such as viral infections of the upper respiratory tract, transient IgA deficiency or decreased T-suppressor cell activity, which will allow unrestrained IgE responses and clinical symptoms to develop. In the absence of factor 'X', the high responder subject may not show clinical symptoms after a short period of allergen exposure alone, but may be induced to express clinical symptoms of allergy by future exposure to allergen and factor 'X'.

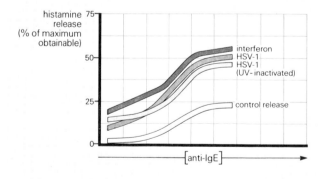

Fig.19.36 Virus enhancement of IgE-mediated histamine release. Basophils can be induced to release histamine by anti-IgE which crosslinks the Fc receptors (control). Histamine release is enhanced in the presence of live *Herpes simplex* virus (HSV-1) or UV-inactivated HSV. Interferon is thought to be responsible for this enhancement because it mimics the virus effect. This might explain the exacerbation of asthma seen in atopics following upper respiratory tract virus infections.

HYPOSENSITIZATION

Hyposensitization therapy involves the injection of increasing doses of allergen and although clinical benefit is

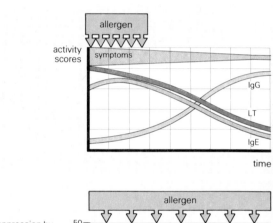

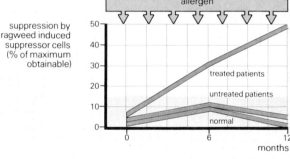

Fig.19.37 Hyposensitization: a prospect for allergy treatment. Hyposensitization treatment involves repeated injection of increasing doses of allergen. There is an increase in antigen-specific IgG (upper graph) accompanied by a fall in antigen-specific IgE. This fall is thought to be due to an increase in activity of T-suppressor cells, which is reflected in reduced antigen-induced lymphocyte transformation (LT) *in vitro*. The lower graph shows evidence to support this concept. Following successful hyposensitization of ragweed-sensitive patients over 6 or 12 months there is an increase in antigen-specific T-suppressor activity by comparison with untreated patients or controls. This is measured by co-cultivating the patient's lymphocytes with autologous antigen-generated T-suppressor cells, and then measuring proliferation of the lymphocytes in response to allergen. The background level of suppression (brown) seen with an irrelevant antigen (SKSD) is the same in all groups.

often obtained, the exact mechanism by which it occurs is unknown. Following treatment there is an increase in serum levels of allergen-specific IgG and suppressor T cell activity whilst specific IgE levels tend to fall (Fig. 19.37, upper graph). However, in most cases, there is no clear-cut correlation between any of these findings and clinical improvement in the patient. One exception is in the case of people allergic to bee venom where IgG produced by hyposensitization protects by neutralizing the injected venom antigen. In these cases there is an excellent correlation between specific IgG antibodies and clinical protection. In addition it has been shown that allergen-specific suppressor T cells develop in successfully hyposensitized ragweed allergic patients and this may have a number of effects such as suppression of the IgE response and may also lead to suppression of T cell dependent mast cell recruitment (Fig. 19.37, lower graph).

It is now realized that IgE isotype suppression may be as important a factor in the control of IgE responses as antigen-specific T-suppressor cell activity. Katz and colleagues have demonstrated the presence of an IgE, antigen non-specific factor called suppressor factor of allergy (SFA). This molecule, demonstrated in human lymphocyte culture is claimed to supress IgE, but not IgG, synthesis. Future treatment of allergy may be centered around such specific inhibition of IgE synthesis by molecules such as SFA. Another possible mode of treatment could

be to use antibodies to receptor on T-helper cells (an anti-idiotype) to block binding of T cells to the allergen and thus block T-B lymphocyte cooperation.

THE BENEFICIAL ROLE OF IgE

With so many disadvantages inherent in producing an IgE response to an allergen the question arises as to what useful function IgE actually has. If IgA does not stop the penetration of the gut mucosa by an organism or worm, contact with IgE-sensitized mast cells will lead to release of mediators which recruit serum factors (IgG and complement) whilst chemotactic factors will attract eosinophils and neutrophils needed for local defence. It is significant that IgA deficiency has been implicated in the aetiology of atopy thus drawing a parallel between the induction of an immune response to infectious agents and airborne allergens. It has long been considered that IgE plays a major role in the defence against parasitic worms and the mechanisms involved are indicated in figure 19.38. It is worth noting that since approximately one-third of the world's population has parasitic worm infections this may have represented the evolutionary pressure which initiated development of the IgE class, allergies being an unfortunate by-product of this evolutionary step.

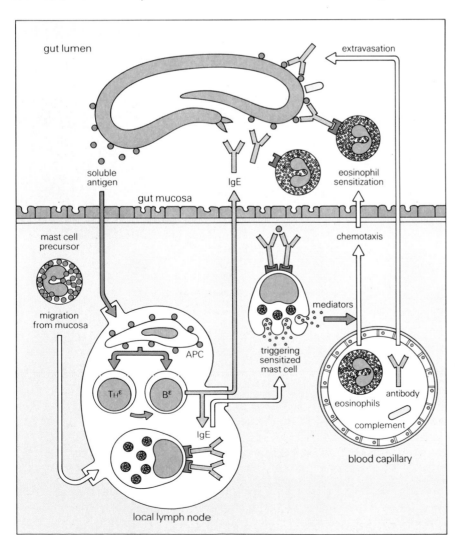

Fig. 19.38 The beneficial role of IgE in parasitic worm infections. During a parasitic worm infection soluble worm antigens diffuse across the gut mucosa into the body and are transported to the local lymph node where an IgE response occurs. Mast cell precursors migrate from the gut mucosa to the same local lymph nodes where they mature, and acquire worm-specific IgE on their surface and then migrate back to the gut mucosa via the thoracic duct and bloodstream. These mast cells degranulate following contact with worm antigen releasing mediators, which increase vascular permeability and attract inflammatory cells, including eosinophils, to the area. IgE from the lymph node also sensitizes the worm to attack by eosinophils which bear Fc receptors for IgE. Complement and worm-specific IgG also enter the site due to increased vascular permeability caused by mediators such as histamine. All of these mechanisms lead to worm damage and expulsion.

FURTHER READING

Brostoff J. & Challacombe S. (1982) Food Allergy. *Clinics in Immunology and Allergy* 2.1 W.B. Saunders.

Cooke R.A. & Vander-Veer A. (1916) Human sensitization. *J. Immunol.* **1,** 201.

Gleich G.J. (1982) The late phase of the immunoglobulin E-mediated reaction: a link between anaphylaxis and common allergic disease. *J. Allergy Clin. Immunol.* **70,** 160.

Ishizaka K., Ishizaka T. & Hornbrook M.M. (1966) Physicochemical properties of human reaginic antibody. IV Presence of a unique immunoglobulin as a carrier of reaginic activity. *J. Immunol.* **97,** 75.

Ishizaka K. (ed.) (1982) Regulation of the IgE antibody response. *Progress in Allergy* **32.** Karger, Basle.

Ishizaka K. (ed.) (1984) Mast cell activation and mediator release. *Progress in Allergy* **34.** Karger, Basle.

Joseph M., Tonnel A.B., Capron A. & Voisin C. (1980) Enzyme release and superoxide anion production by human alveolar macrophages stimulated with immunoglobulin E. *Clin. Exp. Immunol.* **40,** 416.

Juto P. (1980) Elevated serum immunoglobulin E in T cell deficient infants fed cows milk. *J. Allergy Clin. Immunol.* **66,** 402.

Katz D.H. (1978) The allergic phenotype: manifestation of 'allergic breakthrough' and imbalance in normal damping of IgE antibody production. *Immunol. Rev.* **41,** 77.

Marsh D.G. & Bias W.B. (1978) The genetics of atopic allergy. *Immunogenetics* **6,** 248.

Muller G. (ed.) (1978) Immunoglobulin E. *Immunological Reviews* **41.** Munksgaard, Copenhagen.

Rocklin R.E. (1983) Clinical and immunologic aspects of allergen specific immunotherapy in patients with seasonal allergic rhinitis and/or allergic asthma. *J. Allergy Clin. Immunol.* **72,** 323.

Stanworth D.R. (1973) *Immediate hypersensitivity.* North Holland Publications. Amsterdam.

Wide L., Bennich H. & Johansson S.G.O. (1967) Diagnosis of allergy by an *in vitro* test for allergen antibodies. *Lancet* **ii** 1105.

20 Hypersensitivity–Type II

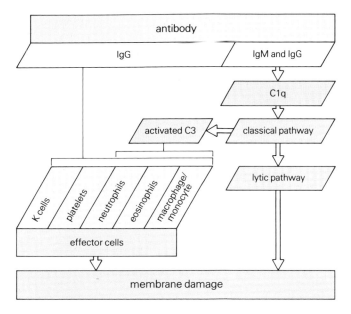

In this form of hypersensitivity antibody, directed against cell surface or tissue antigens, interacts with molecules of the complement pathways and a variety of effector cells to bring about damage to those cells and surrounding tissues (Fig.20.1). The antibodies interact with complement (Clq) and the effector cells via their Fc regions, and thus the antibody acts as a bridge between antigen and the effectors. The damage mechanisms are a reflection of the normal physiological processes involved in dealing with pathogenic microorganisms.

DAMAGE MECHANISMS

The complement system has a dual function. Acting alone it can cause lysis of the membranes of antibody-sensitized cells. Complement activation takes place via the classical pathway and results in the formation of a C5b6789 membrane attack complex. Additionally, binding of activated C3 to target cells and antigens opsonizes the target for effector cells carrying receptors for activated C3 (Fig.20.2).

C3b binds to targets by a short-lived highly reactive site exposed following activation of C3 by C3 convertases. Bound C3b is broken down by the actions of factors I and H (β_1H) and other serum proteases to produce successively C3bi and C3d which remain attached to the target. Receptors for C3b and C3d are separate structures. Both are present on macrophages and some neutrophils. Neutrophils appear to lose C3d receptors as they age.

Fig.20.1 Antibody dependent cytotoxicity. The action of antibody occurs through Fc receptors. Platelets, neutrophils, eosinophils and cells of the mononuclear phagocyte series all have receptors for Fc, by which they can engage target tissues. K cells are functionally defined Fc receptor⁺ cytotoxic cells. Clq is a soluble Fc receptor and the first molecule of the complement classical pathway. Activation of complement C3 can generate complement-mediated lytic damage to target cells directly, and also allows phagocytic cells with receptors for activated C3 to bind to the target.

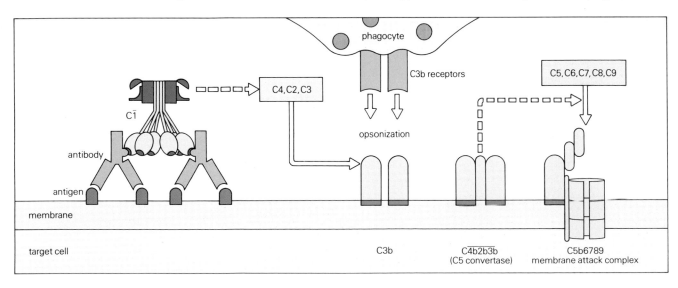

Fig.20.2 The action of complement in mediating Type II hypersensitivity reactions. Antibody binds to antigens on the target cell membranes and activates the first component of the complement pathway, C1. This activates the classical pathway depositing C3b and C4b2b3b on the target cell. C3b (and C3d) act as opsonins for cells with appropriate receptors. The deposition of C3b may be amplified by the amplification loop (alternative pathway). C5 convertases can activate the lytic pathway causing membrane damage by the C5-9 membrane attack complex.

The different antibody subclasses vary in their ability to interact with different effector cells in an analogous way to their varied ability to bind C1q and activate the complement classical pathway (Fig.20.3). This is related to the different types of Fc receptors found on macrophages, neutrophils and K cells.

Figure 20.4 shows a neutrophil interacting with a basement membrane which has been opsonized by antibody.

Chemotactic stimuli attract effector cells to sites of type II hypersensitivity reactions in the same way as they attract them to inflammatory foci caused by microbial damage. Particularly important in this respect is C5a, split by C5 convertases off C5. It is a short range signalling peptide, inactivated by carboxypeptidase B (normally present in serum), and capable of attracting both neutrophils and macrophages (Fig.20.5).

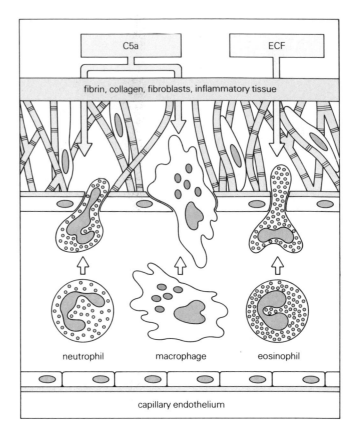

Fc receptor of effector system	IgG subclass				IgG fragment		
	IgG1	IgG2	IgG3	IgG4	Cγ2	Cγ3	Fc
macrophages	+	−	+	−	−	+	+
neutrophils	+	+	+	some	−	+	+
K cells	+	+	+	some	−	−	+
C1q	+	±	+	−	+	−	+

Fig.20.3 Human IgG subclass domains activating different effector systems. The ability to interact with Fc receptors on cells and Clq varies with the different IgG subclasses. Additionally the site recognized on the Fc region varies for the different cell types. For example, neutrophils bind to a site in Cγ3 whereas K cells bind a site which requires the whole Fc region (Cγ2 and Cγ3).

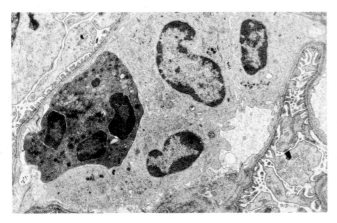

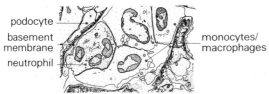

Fig.20.4 Phagocytes attacking a basement membrane. This electron micrograph shows a neutrophil and three monocytes binding to the capillary basement membrane in the kidney of a rabbit containing anti-basement membrane antibody. ×3500. Courtesy of Professor G. A. Andres.

Fig.20.5 The chemotactic stimuli acting on effector cells of hypersensitivity reactions. C5a acts on neutrophils and macrophages to induce movement out of blood vessels and into inflammatory foci. (C5b67 may also be chemotactic. C3a was thought to act similarly to C5a in this respect but this is now questionable.) Eosinophil chemotactic factor (ECF) attracts eosinophils. The fibrils of inflammatory tissue act as guideways for the arriving cells and thus facilitate their migration into the tissue. Other peptides from the inflammatory tissue, including fibrin products, have chemokinetic and chemotactic actions.

neutrophil function	activator					
	IgG	C3	IgG+C3	C5a	C5b67	IgA
adherence	+	+++	+++	+	−	+
oxygen metabolism	+	±	++++	+++	++	+
lysosomal enzyme release	+	+	++++	+++	++	+
chemotaxis	+	−	+	+++	++	?
phagocytosis	+	±	++++	−	−	?

Fig.20.6 Neutrophil activation. Neutrophils are activated by complexed IgG and activated complement components. Each mediator has a particular spectrum of activity. Note how activated C3 (including C3b, C3bi and C3d, depending on the maturity of the cells involved) and activation via IgG Fc receptors potentiate each other and present a particularly powerful signal to the cells when both are present.

The complement components also perform an important function in potentiating the effects of antigen-complexed IgG. This includes enhancing its phagocytic and bactericidal functions (Fig.20.6).

The mechanisms by which phagocytes damage cells in type II hypersensitivity reactions reflects their normal physiological functions in dealing with infectious pathogens (Fig.20.7). Most pathogens, unless they are resistant to phagocyte mediated attack are killed inside the phagolysosome by a combination of oxygen metabolites, radicals, ions, enzymes and other factors interfering with their metabolism. Phagocytes cannot adequately phagocytose large targets and so granule and lysosome contents are released in apposition to the sensitized target, damaging host tissue (Fig. 20.8). This is referred to as exocytosis. In some reactions, such as the eosinophil reactions against schistosomes the function is beneficial, but if the host tissue has been sensitized by antibody it will activate similar effector mechanisms and damage, rather than benefit occurs.

The susceptibility of different target cells to the actions of different effector cells varies (Fig.20.9). This is due to such factors as the amounts of particular antigens and target structures expressed on the cell's surface, and secondly on the inherent ability of the target cell to withstand damage. For example a red cell may be lysed by a single active C5 convertase site, whereas it takes many such sites to destroy most nucleated cells.

The remainder of the chapter examines some of the instances where antibody dependent cytotoxicity is thought to be of prime importance in causing cell destruction or pathological damage.

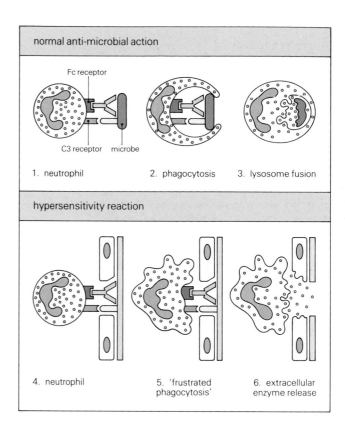

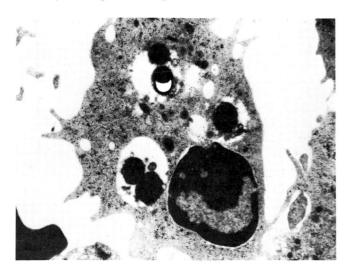

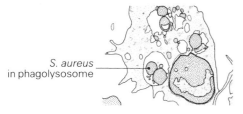

S. aureus
in phagolysosome

Fig.20.7 Neutrophil phagocytosis. This electron micrograph shows *Staphylococcus aureus* in phagolysosomes in a human neutrophil. The *S. aureus* was phagocytosed by the neutrophil following opsonization with human serum. ×5000.

Fig.20.8 Damage mechanisms. Neutrophil-mediated damage is a reflection of normal anti-bacterial action. Neutrophils engage microbes with their Fc and C3 receptors (1). The microbe is then phagocytosed (2) and destroyed as lysosomes fuse to form the phagolysosome (3). In hypersensitivity reactions host cells coated with antibody are similarly phagocytosed, but where the target is large, for example a basement membrane (4), the neutrophils are frustrated in their attempt at phagocytosis (5) and release their lysosomes to the outside causing damage to cells in the vicinity (6).

effector	target			
	nucleated mammalian cells	group A human erythrocytes	pyogenic micro-organisms	parasites
K cells	+++	−	±	?
mononuclear phagocytes	++	+++	+++	?
neutrophils	±	+++	++++	?
eosinophils	?	?	?	++
platelets	±	?	?	?

Fig.20.9 The susceptibility of different targets to damage by effector cells. Susceptibility differs with the cell type. For example, K cells are inactive against pyogenic bacteria. The standard cell on which to test K cells is the chicken red blood cell – a nucleated red cell, particularly susceptible to damage. Note that cytotoxic T cells and K cells both require extracellular Mg^{++} and Ca^{++} for optimum killing – neutrophil and macrophage activation by aggregated IgG does not.

TRANSFUSION REACTIONS

At least fifteen different blood group systems have been recognized in man, each system consisting of a gene locus specifying antigens appearing on the erythrocyte surface. An individual with a particular blood group can recognize red cells carrying different blood group antigens and produce antibodies to them. Antibodies may be produced naturally, without immunization with the foreign red cells as is the case with the ABO system (Fig.20.10). Here it is thought that the subject becomes immunized to the non-self ABO antigens by reacting to identical antigenic determinants which are expressed coincidentally on a variety of microorganisms. In most cases however, an individual only acquires antibodies to non-self blood group antigens following exposure to those antigens on some foreign tissue, a graft or an incompatible blood transfusion. Since antibodies to the ABO system antigens occur naturally, it is particularly important to match donor blood to the recipient for this system.

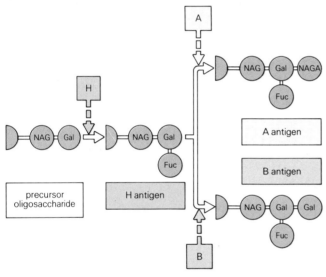

blood group (phenotype)	genotypes	antigens	antibodies to ABO in serum
A	AA, AO	A	anti-B
B	BB, BO	B	anti-A
AB	AB	A and B	none
O	OO	H	anti-A and anti-B

Fig.20.10 ABO blood group reactivities. The diagram presents a simple account of the way the ABO blood groups are constructed. The enzyme produced by the H gene attaches a fucose residue (Fuc) to the terminal galactose (Gal) of the precursor oligosaccharide. Individuals possessing the A gene now attach N-acetyl galactosamine (NAGA) to this galactose residue while those with the B gene attach another galactose producing A and B antigens respectively. People with both genes make some of each. The table indicates the genotypes and antigens of the ABO system. Most people naturally make antibodies to the antigens they lack.

system	gene loci	antigens	phenotype frequencies	
ABO	1	A, B or O	A B AB O	42% 8% 3% 47%
Rhesus	3 closely linked loci: major antigen=RhD	C or c D or d E or e	RhD$^+$ RhD$^-$	85% 15%
Kell	1	K or k	K k	9% 91%
Duffy	1	Fy^a, Fy^b or Fy	Fy^{a}Fy^b Fy^a Fy^b Fy	46% 20% 34% 0.1%
MN	1	M or N	MM NN MN	28% 50% 22%

Fig.20.11 Five major blood group systems involved in transfusion reactions. Not all are equally antigenic in transfusion reactions. Thus RhD evokes a stronger reaction in an incompatible recipient than the other Rhesus antigens and Fy^a is stronger than Fy^b. Frequencies stated are for caucasian populations – other races have different gene frequencies.

Figure 20.11 lists five of the more important blood groups involved in transfusion reactions.

Transfusion of blood into a recipient who has antibodies to those red cells produces an immediate transfusion reaction (Fig.20.12). The severity of the reaction depends on the class and amounts of the antibodies involved. Antibodies to the ABO system antigens are usually of the IgM class, they cause agglutination, complement activation and intravascular haemolysis. Other blood groups induce IgG antibodies, and although these agglutinate the cells less well than IgM antibodies they activate Type II hypersensitivity mechanisms and cause red cell destruction. The cell destruction may cause circulatory shock, and the released contents of the red cells can produce acute tubular necrosis of the kidneys. Transfusion reactions to incompatible blood may also develop over days or weeks in previously unsensitized individuals as antibodies to the foreign cells are produced, resulting in anaemia and jaundice.

Transfusion reactions to other components of blood, including leucocytes and platelets may also occur, though their consequences are not usually as severe as reactions to erythrocytes.

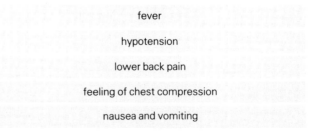

Fig.20.12 Clinical indications of transfusion reactions.

HAEMOLYTIC DISEASE OF THE NEWBORN (HDNB)

This condition appears in newborn infants where the mother has been sensitized to the blood group antigens on the infant's erythrocytes and makes IgG antibodies to these antigens. These cross the placenta and react with the foetal red cells causing their destruction. Rhesus D (RhD) is the most commonly involved antigen. A risk arises when a Rh⁻ mother carries a Rh⁺ infant. Sensitization of the Rh⁻ mother to the Rh⁺ red cells usually occurs during birth, when some foetal red cells leak back across the placenta into the maternal circulation to be recognized by the maternal immune system. For this reason the first incompatible child is usually unaffected but the second and later children have an increasing risk of being affected as the mother is repeatedly immunized with successive pregnancies (Figs. 20.13 & 20.14). Reactions to other blood groups may cause HDNB, the second most common being the Kell system K antigen. This is much less frequent than reactions due to Rhesus D due to the relative infrequency of the K antigen (9%) and its weaker antigenicity.

It was noticed that in cases where haemolytic disease of the newborn due to Rhesus incompatibility was expected, there was a lower incidence of the condition if the father was also of a different ABO group to the mother. This led to the idea that Rh⁺ foetal cells would be destroyed in a Rh⁻ mother by the mother's natural antibodies if they were also ABO incompatible. Consequently they would not be available to sensitize the maternal immune system to the Rhesus D antigen. This observation formed the basis of Rhesus prophylaxis, in which anti-RhD antibodies were given to Rhesus negative mothers immediately after delivery of Rhesus positive infants. This has led to a fall in the incidence of the condition due to Rhesus incompatibility (Fig.20.15). Although it is not certain that the prevention of sensitization is due to destruction of foetal red cells, this is assumed to be so.

Fig.20.13 Haemolytic disease of the newborn I. Erythrocytes from a Rhesus⁺ (RhD⁺) foetus leak into the maternal circulation during a first incompatible pregnancy. This stimulates the production of anti-rhesus antibody of the IgG class *post partum* which, during subsequent pregnancies, is transferred across the placenta into the foetal circulation (IgM antibodies cannot cross the placenta). If the foetus is again incompatible these antibodies will cause red cell destruction.

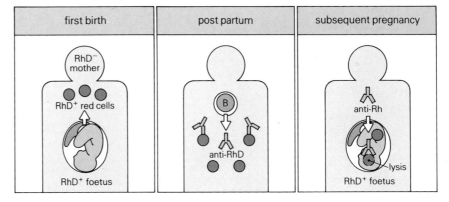

Fig.20.14 Haemolytic disease of the newborn II. The child is suffering from HDNB. There is considerable enlargement of the liver and spleen associated with red cell destruction caused by maternal anti-red cell antibody in the foetal circulation. The child had elevated bilirubin (breakdown product of haemoglobin) and the facial petechial haemorrhaging was due to impaired platelet function (courtesy of Dr. K. Sloper). The most commonly involved antigen is RhD. The table indicates the phenotype of children from parents with different RhD

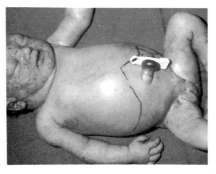 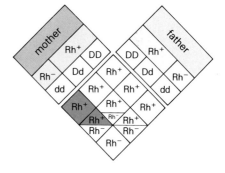

phenotypes. The Rh⁺ individuals may be homozygous (DD) or heterozygous (Dd). Rh⁻ individuals are always homozygous (dd). The danger of HDNB arises in Rh⁻ mothers carrying Rh⁺ children (red).

Fig.20.15 Rhesus prophylaxis. Without prophylaxis Rh⁺ red cells leak into the circulation of a Rh⁻ mother and sensitize her to the Rh antigen(s) (A). If anti-Rh antibody (anti-D) is injected *post partum* it eliminates the Rh⁺ red cells and this prevents sensitization (B). The incidence of deaths due to haemolytic disease of the newborn was falling over the period 1950–1966 with improved patient care, but the decline in the disease accelerated with the general advent of rhesus prophylaxis in 1969.

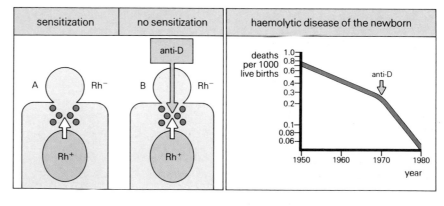

AUTOIMMUNE HAEMOLYTIC ANAEMIAS

Reactions to blood group antigens also occur in the autoimmune haemolytic anaemias, in which patients produce antibodies to their own red cells. A diagnosis of autoimmune haemolytic anaemia would be suspected if a patient gave a positive Coomb's test (Fig.20.16). This test identifies antibodies present on the patient's red cells, and is usually indicative of either a) antibodies directed towards erythrocyte antigens or b) immune complexes adsorbed onto the red cells' surface. The Coomb's test is also used to detect antibodies on red cells caused by mismatched transfusions and in haemolytic disease of the newborn. Autoimmune haemolytic anaemias can be divided into three types depending upon whether they are due to:

1. warm-reactive autoantibodies which react with the antigen at 37°C,
2. cold-reactive autoantibodies which only react with antigen below 37°C,
3. antibodies provoked by allergic reactions to drugs.

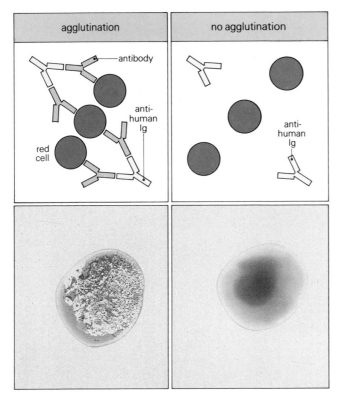

Fig.20.16 Indirect Coomb's test. This test, also called the direct antiglobulin test is used to detect antibody on a patient's erythrocytes. If antibody is present the erythrocytes can be agglutinated by anti-human immunoglobulin, as shown below. If no antibody is present on the red cells they will not be agglutinated by the anti-human Ig.

Warm-Reactive Autoantibodies
Warm-reactive autoantibodies are frequently found against Rhesus system antigens, including determinants of the Rh C and Rh E loci as well as Rh D. The type of reactivity displayed by these autoantibodies is, however, not typical of the antibodies which develop in transfusion reactions to these antigens in the sense that they appear to react with different epitopes on the Rh antigens than otherwise occurs. Occasionally autoantibodies to other blood group antigens are found. . The cause of the majority of warm antibody haemolytic anaemias is unknown but some are associated with other autoimmune diseases. The anaemia seen in these patients appears to be more often caused by accelerated clearance of the sensitized red cells by spleen macrophages than by complement mediated lysis.

Cold-Reactive Autoantibodies
Cold-reactive autoantibodies are often present in higher titres than the warm-reactive autoantibodies. The majority react against the I blood group system (not described above) and fix complement. The reaction of the antibody with the red cells takes place in the peripheral circulation (particularly in winter) where the temperature in the capillary loops of exposed skin may fall below 30°C. This can cause peripheral necrosis in severe cases. Since organs such as the spleen and liver are at 37°C, and the antibodies do not bind at this temperature, anaemia is apparently not caused by Fc-mediated removal of sensitized red cells in the centre of the body but by complement mediated destruction in the periphery. The severity of the anaemia is related to the complement fixing ability of the patient's serum.

Most cold antibody autoimmune haemolytic anaemias occur in older people, their cause is unknown, but it is notable that the autoantibodies produced are usually of very limited clonality. Other cases may follow infection with *Mycoplasma pneumoniae*. This is usually an acute onset disease of short duration and with polyclonal autoantibodies. The reason for its occurrence is thought to be due to cross-reacting antigens on the bacteria and the red cells producing bypass of normal tolerance mechanisms as described in 'Autoimmunity and Autoimmune Disease'.

DRUG INDUCED REACTIONS TO COMPONENTS OF BLOOD

Drugs can provoke allergic and autoallergic reactions against blood cells including erythrocytes and platelets. This can occur in three different ways (Fig.20.17). Usually the reaction occurs to the drug or drug metabolites, in which case it is necessary for both the drug and the antibody to be present to produce the reaction. The first observation of this type was made by Ackroyd who observed thrombocytopoenic purpura (destruction of platelets) following administration of the drug Sedormid. Haemolytic anaemias have been reported following administration of a wide variety of drugs, including penicillin, quinine and sulphonamides. All these conditions are rare.

Occasionally drugs may induce allergic reactions where autoantibodies directed against the red cell antigens are produced, as is the case with 0.3% of patients given α-methyl dopa. The antibodies produced are similar to those in patients with warm-reactive antibody, but unlike those diseases, the condition remits shortly after the cessation of drug treatment.

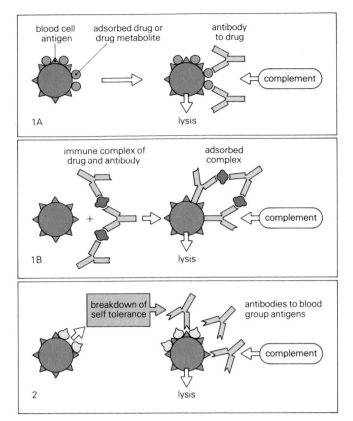

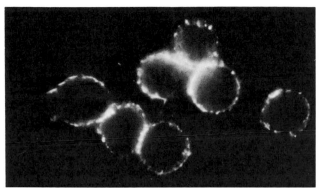

Fig.20.18 Immunofluorescence of normal neutrophils incubated with SLE serum and goat anti-human F(ab')$_2$FITC. Antibodies to neutrophils occur in SLE demonstrated by immunofluorescence of normal neutrophils. Acute transfusion reactions to neutrophils may cause pyrexia, presumably due to pyrogens released from the damaged neutrophils. This indicates that anti-neutrophil antibodies can damage neutrophils, although their role in the pathogenesis of SLE is uncertain. Reproduced from the Journal of Clinical Investigation, *64*, 1979, p 902–912.

HYPERACUTE GRAFT REJECTION

This reaction occurs when a transplant recipient has pre-formed antibodies directed against the graft. The reaction occurs between a few minutes and forty eight hours following completion of the transplantation; the recipient's antibodies react immediately against antigens exposed on the graft cells. The reaction is only seen in grafts which are revascularized directly after transplantation, such as kidney grafts. Within one hour of revascularization there is an extensive infiltration of neutrophils and this is followed by major damage to the glomerular capillaries and haemorrhage. Thrombi deposit in the arterioles and the graft is irreversibly destroyed (Fig.20.19).

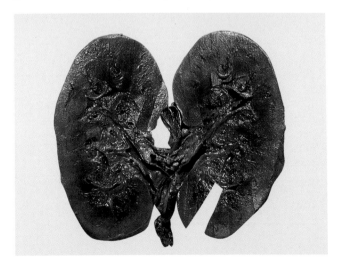

Fig.20.19 Hyperacute graft rejection. This human kidney removed 18 hours after transplantation is thrombosed and haemorrhagic. The whole tissue is dark and necrotic. Courtesy of Dr. K. Welsh.

Fig.20.17 Drug induced reactions to blood cells: three ways in which damage can occur to elements of blood, induced by drug treatment.

1A. Drugs (or metabolites) adsorb to cell membranes. If the patient makes antibodies to them they will bind to the cell and complement-mediated lysis occurs.

1B. Immune complexes of drugs and antibody become adsorbed to the red cell. This appears to be mediated by the immune adherence (C3b) receptor and/or the immunoglobulin Fc region. It is uncertain whether Fc dependent binding is specific. Damage occurs by complement-mediated lysis.

2. Drugs, preumably adsorbed onto cell membranes induce a breakdown of self tolerance possibly by stimulating T$_H$ cells. This leads to formation of antibodies to other blood group antigens on the cell surface. Note that in 1A and 1B the antibody is to the drug while in 2 it is to normal cell surface antigens, therefore in 2 the antibody can destroy cells whether they carry adsorbed drug or not.

REACTIONS TO LEUCOCYTES

Autoantibodies to neutrophils and lymphocytes are sometimes reported. The autoantibodies to neutrophils are true tissue specific antibodies unlike antibodies to ABO system antigens. (ABO antigens are found on many tissues, for example, red cells, kidney, salivary gland etc. – the neutrophil-specific antigens are found only on the PMNs). Antibodies to both neutrophils and lymphocytes are observed in SLE (Fig.20.18) but their contribution to the pathogenesis of the disease appears to be relatively small, possibly because these cells modulate bound antibodies off their surface quite rapidly.

The major effectors are the neutrophils and platelets, interacting with the sensitized cells, via their Fc, C3b and C3d receptors. The antibodies directing the effectors may be of the ABO system, since many tissues as well as red cells carry the ABO antigens. Alternatively the antibody may be directed against MHC class 1 antigens, if the recipient has been previously sensitized with an incompatible graft.

SENSITIVITY TO GLOMERULAR BASEMENT MEMBRANE

A number of patients with nephritis are found to have antibodies to a glycoprotein (not collagen) of the glomerular basement membrane (Fig.20.20). The antibody is usually IgG and in at least 50% of patients appears to fix complement. The condition usually results in severe necrosis of the glomerulus with fibrin deposition. Presumably complement and neutrophils are again the main effectors. The association of this kind of nephritis with lung haemorrhage was noticed by Goodpasture (Goodpasture's syndrome). It is now apparent that lung basement membrane crossreacts with glomerular basement membrane, explaining this association. Although other causes may also produce the syndrome as originally described, anti-glomerular basement membrane antibody nephritis is now synonymous with Goodpasture's syndrome. The appearance of this type of nephritis is compared with that produced by immune complex deposition in 'Hypersensitivity – Type III' (Fig.21.3).

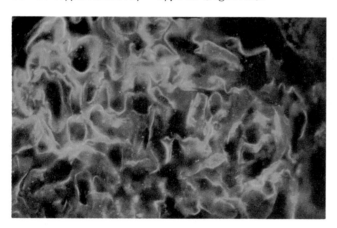

Fig.20.20 Immune complex formation in Goodpasture's syndrome. Antibody to a basement membrane antigen forms an evenly bound layer on the basement membrane. This is visualized with fluorescent anti-IgG. Courtesy of Dr. F. Hay.

MYASTHENIA GRAVIS

It has recently been recognized that the disease myasthenia gravis, a condition in which there is extreme muscular weakness, is associated with antibodies to the acetylcholine receptor present on the surface of muscle membranes. The acetylcholine receptors are located at the motor end plate where the neuron contacts the muscle.

Transmission of impulses from the nerve to the muscle takes place by the release of acetylcholine from the nerve terminal which diffuses across the gap to the muscle fibre.

It was noticed that immunization of experimental animals with purified acetylcholine receptors produced a condition of muscular weakness, closely resembling myasthenia in humans. This suggested a role for antibody to the acetylcholine receptor in the human disease. Analysis of the lesion in myasthenic muscles indicated that the disease was not due to an inability to synthesize acetylcholine nor was there any problem in secreting it, in response to a nerve impulse. It appeared that the released acetylcholine was less effective at triggering depolarization of the muscle (Fig.20.21).

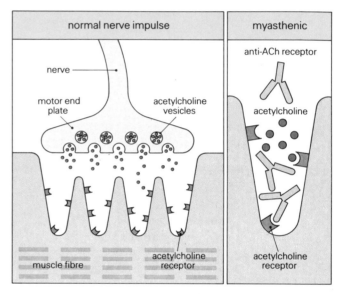

Fig.20.21 Myasthenia gravis. Normally a nerve impulse passing down a neuron which arrives at a motor end plate causes fusion of acetylcholine-containing vesicles with the cell membrane and release of the acetylcholine (ACh). This diffuses across the neuromuscular junction and combines with ACh receptors on the muscle causing opening of ion channels in the muscle membrane. In myasthenia gravis antibodies to the receptor block binding of the ACh transmitter and so the effect of each released vesicle is reduced. This is probably only one of the factors operating in the disease.

Examination of neuromuscular end plates by immunochemical techniques has demonstrated IgG, C3 and C9 deposited on the post-synaptic folds of the muscle (Fig. 20.22). The IgG and complement is thought to act in two ways. Firstly there is an increased rate of turnover of the acetylcholine receptors and secondly there may be some blockage of acetylcholine binding with reduced ability to depolarize the muscle. It was noted that myasthenic serum injected into experimental animals reduces the size of the MEPPS (the amount of depolarization caused by a single vesicle quantum of acetylcholine). Cellular infiltration of myasthenic end plates is rarely seen, so it is assumed that damage does not involve effector cells. The transient muscle weakness in babies born to myasthenic mothers is further evidence for a pathogenetic role for IgG antibody, which can cross the placenta.

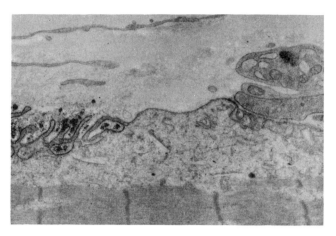

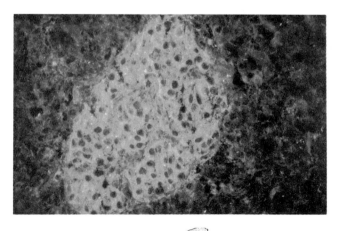

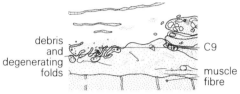

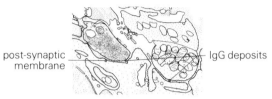

post-synaptic membrane — IgG deposits

debris and degenerating folds — C9 — muscle fibre

Fig.20.22 Electron micrographs showing IgG autoantibody (left) and complement C9 (right) localized at the motor end plate in myasthenia gravis. The micrograph on the left shows IgG deposits in discrete patches on the post-synaptic membrane (×13000).

The micrograph illustrating C9 shows the post-synaptic region denuded of its nerve terminal: it consists of debris and degenerating folds. There is a strong reaction for C9 on this debris. ×9000. Courtesy of Dr. A. G. Engel.

SENSITIVITY TO TISSUE ANTIGENS

Although a great number of autoantibodies react with tissue antigens, their significance in causing tissue damage and pathology *in vivo* is uncertain. For example, it is possible to demonstrate an *in vitro* cytotoxicity to thyroid cells using sera containing antibodies to the thyroid microsomes (Fig.20.23) and cytotoxicity to pancreatic islet cells using sera of diabetic patients (Fig.20.24). This does not necessarily mean that the antibodies have caused the tissue damage however, they may be formed as a consequence of the disease process.

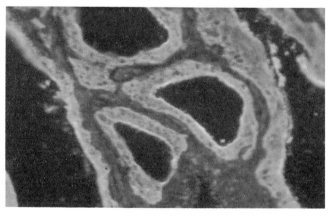

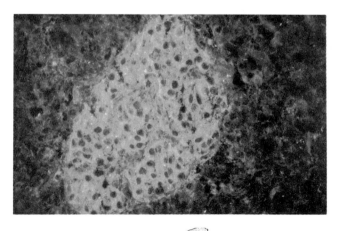

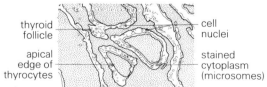

thyroid follicle — cell nuclei
apical edge of thyrocytes — stained cytoplasm (microsomes)

acinar cells of exocrine pancreas — islet of Langerhans
unstained nuclei — stained cytoplasm

Fig.20.23 Antibodies to thyroid microsomes demonstrated by indirect immunofluorescence. This shows antibody binding to microsomes in human thyroid follicular cells. These antibodies are cytotoxic for thyroid cells *in vitro*. Courtesy of Dr. B. Dean.

Fig.20.24 Islet cell autoantibodies. Autoantibodies to the pancreas in diabetics may be demonstrated by immunofluorescence. They are cytotoxic for islet cells *in vitro*, indicating a pathological role in disease. Courtesy of Dr. B. Dean.

FURTHER READING

Fearon D. T. (1984) Cellular receptors for fragments of the third component of complement. *Immunol. Today* **5,** 105.

Horwitz D. A. & Bakke A. C. (1984) An Fc receptor bearing third population of human mononuclear cells with cytotoxic and regulatory function. *Immunol. Today* **5,** 148.

Hughes-Jones N. S., Clarke C. A. (1982) Haemolytic disease of the newborn. In *Clinical Aspects of Immunology* 4th Edition. Lachmann P. J. & Peters D. K. (eds.) Blackwell Scientific Publications, Oxford.

Lalezari P. (1983) Autoimmune hemolytic disease. In *Recent Advances in Clinical Immunology 3*. Thompson R. A. & Rose N. R. (eds.) Churchill Livingstone, Edinburgh.

McCluskey R. T. & Colvin R. B. (1978) Immunological aspects of renal tubular and interstitial disease. *Annu. Rev. Med.* **29,** 191.

Newsom-Davis J. (1981) Myasthenia gravis: immune mechanisms and implications. *Clin. Exp. Neurol.* **18,** 14.

Sturgeon P. (1983) Erythrocyte antigens and antibodies. In *Hematology*. Williams W. J., Bentler E., Erslev A. & Rundles W. (eds.) McGraw Hill, New York.

21 Hypersensitivity–Type III

TYPES OF IMMUNE COMPLEX DISEASE

Immune complexes are formed every time antibody meets antigen and generally they are removed effectively by cells of the reticuloendothelial system, but occasionally their formation can lead to a hypersensitivity reaction. Diseases resulting from immune complex formation can be placed broadly into three groups (Fig.21.1).

cause	antigen	sites of complex deposition
persistent infection	microbial antigen	infected organ(s), kidney
autoimmunity	self antigen	kidney, joint, arteries, skin
extrinsic	environmental antigen	lung

Fig.21.1 Three categories of immune complex disease.
This table indicates the source of the antigen and the organs most frequently affected.

First, where there is persistent infection such as the α–haemolytic viridans streptococci or staphylococcal infective endocarditis, or with a parasite such as *Plasmodium vivax*, or in viral hepatitis, the combined effects of a low grade persistent infection together with a weak antibody response leads to chronic immune complex formation with the eventual deposition of complexes in the tissues (Fig.21.2).

Second, immune complex disease is a frequent complication of autoimmune disease where the continued production of autoantibody to a self-antigen leads to prolonged immune complex formation, overload of the mononuclear phagocyte system (which is responsible for the removal of complexes) and tissue deposition of complexes, as in the disease systemic lupus erythematosus (SLE) (Fig.21.3).

Third, immune complexes may be formed at body surfaces, for example in the lungs, following repeated inhalation of antigenic materials from moulds, plants or animals. This is exemplified in Farmer's lung disease and Pigeon Fancier's disease (which are examples of extrinsic allergic alveolitis) where there are circulating antibodies to actinomycete fungi following repeated exposure to mouldy hay or pigeon antigens. The antibodies induced by these antigens are primarily IgG, rather than IgE, which are produced in an immediate (Type 1) hypersensitivity reaction.

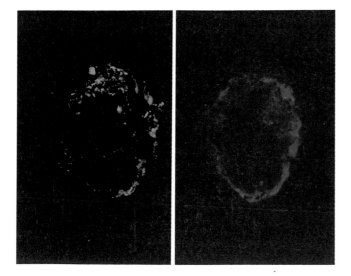

Fig.21.2 Immunofluorescence study of immune complexes in infectious disease. These two serial sections of the renal artery of a patient with chronic hepatitis B infection are stained with fluoresceinated anti-hepatitis B antigen (left) and rhodaminated anti-IgM (right). The presence of both antigen and antibody in the intima and media of the arterial wall indicate the deposition of the complexes at this site. IgG and C3 deposits are also detectable with the same distribution. Courtesy of Dr. A. Nowoslawski.

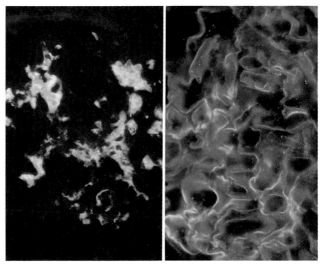

Fig. 21.3 Immunofluorescence study of immune complexes in autoimmune disease. In these renal sections from patients with SLE and Goodpastures syndrome the antibody is detected with fluorescent anti-IgG. Complexes deposited in the kidney form characteristic 'lumpy bumpy' deposits (left). The anti-basement membrane antibody in Goodpastures syndrome (lung and kidney) in this Type II reaction (right) forms an even layer on the basement membrane.

When antigen enters the body again by inhalation of fungal spores, local immune complexes are formed in the alveoli leading to inflammation (Fig.21.4).

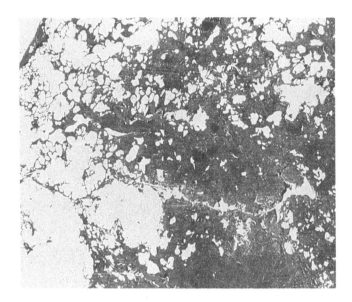

Fig.21.4 Histological appearance of the lung in extrinsic allergic alveolitis (Pigeon Fancier's disease). There is considerable destruction of the alveoli with consolidated areas of (darkly stained) inflammation and fibrosis. H & E stain, ×150. Courtesy of Dr. G. Boyd.

Precipitating antibodies to the inhaled antigens are found in the sera of 90% of patients with Farmer's lung, but since they are also found in some people with no disease and are absent from some sufferers, it seems that other factors are also involved, including Type IV hypersensitivity reactions. Diseases in which immune complexes are important are summarized in figure 21.5.

INFLAMMATORY MECHANISMS IN TYPE III HYPERSENSITIVITY

Immune complexes trigger a variety of inflammatory processes. They can interact with the complement system leading to the generation of C3a and C5a, which have anaphylatoxic and chemotactic properties. They cause the release of vasoactive amines from mast cells and basophils, thus increasing vascular permeability and attracting polymorphs. Immune complexes can also interact with platelets through their Fc receptors leading to aggregation and microthrombus formation and hence a further increase in vascular permeability due to the release of vasoactive amines (Fig.21.6).

The attracted polymorphs will attempt to phagocytose the complexes but in the case of tissue-trapped complexes this is difficult and the phagocytes are more likely to release their lysosomal enzymes to the exterior, causing tissue damage (Fig. 21.7). Simply released into the blood or tissue fluids these lysosomal enzymes are unlikely to cause much inflammation as they will soon be neutralized by serum enzyme inhibitors, but if the phagocyte applies itself closely to the tissue-trapped complexes serum inhibitors will be excluded and the enzymes will then damage the underlying tissue.

EXPERIMENTAL MODELS OF IMMUNE COMPLEX DISEASE

Experimental models are available for each of the three main types of disease described above: serum sickness representing the presence of a persistent infection, the NZB/NZW mouse for autoimmunity and the Arthus reaction for local damage by extrinsic antigen.

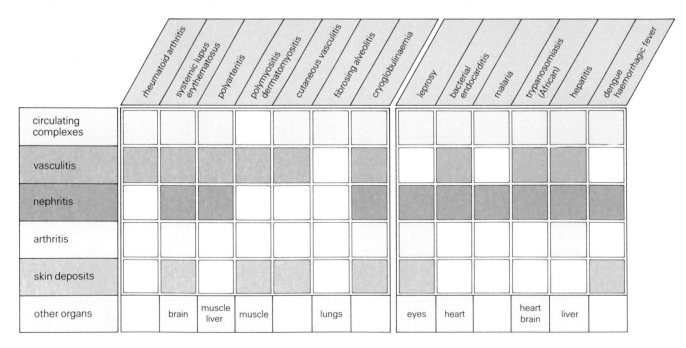

	rheumatoid arthritis	systemic lupus erythematosus	polyarteritis	polymyositis dermatomyositis	cutaneous vasculitis	fibrosing alveolitis	cryoglobulinaemia	leprosy	bacterial endocarditis	malaria	trypanosomiasis (African)	hepatitis	dengue haemorrhagic fever
circulating complexes													
vasculitis													
nephritis													
arthritis													
skin deposits													
other organs		brain	muscle liver	muscle		lungs		eyes	heart		heart brain	liver	

Fig.21.5 Some of the main diseases in which immune complexes are implicated, indicating sites of deposition. Those diseases on the left of the table are primarily autoimmune, those on the right are due to microbial antigens.

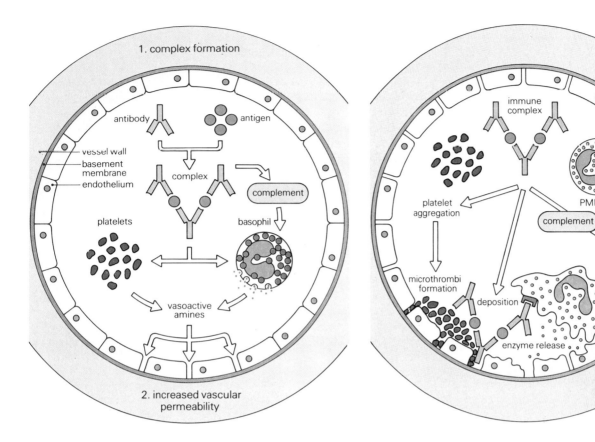

Fig.21.6 Deposition of immune complexes in blood vessel walls I. Antibody and antigen combine to form immune complexes (1). The complexes act on complement (to release C3a and C5a), which in turn acts on basophils to release vasoactive amines. The complexes also act directly on basophils and platelets (in humans) to produce amine release. The amines released include histamine and 5–hydroxytryptamine, which cause endothelial cell retraction and thus increased vascular permeability (2).

Fig.21.7 Deposition of immune complexes in blood vessel walls II. With increased vascular permeability, complexes become deposited in the vessel wall. The complexes induce platelet aggregation and complement activation. The platelets aggregate to form microthrombi on the exposed collagen of the basement membrane of the endothelium. Polymorphs (PMN) attracted to the site by chemotactic complement peptides cannot phagocytose the complexes and so release their lysosomal enzymes to the exterior of the cell causing damage to the vessel wall.

Serum Sickness

In serum sickness circulating immune complexes deposit in the tissues when vascular permeability is increased, thus leading to inflammatory diseases such as glomerulonephritis and arthritis. In the pre-antibiotic era serum sickness was a complication of serum therapy with massive doses of antibody for diseases such as diphtheria – horse anti-diphtheria serum was usually used and some individuals made antibodies against this foreign protein. Serum sickness is now commonly studied in rabbits. Animals are given an intravenous injection of a foreign soluble protein such as bovine serum albumin. After about one week antibodies are formed which enter the circulation and complex with antigen in antigen excess (Fig.21.8). These small complexes are only removed slowly by the mononuclear phagocyte system and persist in the circulation. With the formation of complexes there is an abrupt fall in total haemolytic complement and the clinical signs of serum sickness develop as granular deposits of antigen-antibody and C3 form along the glomerular basement membrane and in small vessels elsewhere. As the complexes are cleared the animals recover but the disease may be made chronic by the continued daily administration of antigen.

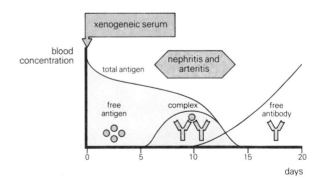

Fig.21.8 Time course of experimental serum sickness. Following an injection of xenogeneic serum there is a lag period of approximately 5 days in which free antigen is detectable in serum. After this period, antibodies are produced to the foreign proteins and complexes are formed in serum. During this period the symptoms of nephritis and arteritis appear. As antibody titres rise the complexes are cleared and the syndrome resolves.

Autoimmune Immune Complex Disease

This is demonstrated using the F_1 hybrid NZB/NZW mouse which simulates various features of human systemic lupus erythematosus. These mice make a range of autoantibodies including anti-red cell, anti-nuclear, anti-DNA and anti-SM. The animals are born clinically normal but within 2–3 months show signs of haemolytic anaemia, positive Coombs' tests (for anti-red cell antibody), anti-nuclear antibodies, positive lupus cell tests, circulating immune complexes together with deposits in glomeruli and the choroid plexus. The disease is much more marked in the females and these die within a few months of developing symptoms (Fig.21.9).

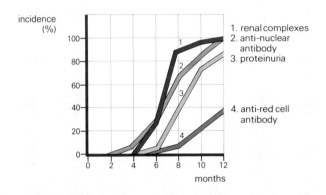

Fig.21.9 Autoimmune disease in NZB/NZW mice. The graph shows the onset of autoimmune disease in female NZB/NZW mice with advancing age. Incidence refers to the number of mice with the features identified. Immune complexes were detected by immunofluorescent staining of kidney sections. Anti-nuclear antibodies were detected in serum by indirect immunofluorescence. Proteinuria reflects kidney damage. Autoantibodies to red cells develop later in the disease and are therefore less likely to relate to kidney pathology. The onset of autoimmune disease is delayed in male mice by approximately 3 months.

The Arthus Reaction

The Arthus reaction takes place at a local site in and around the walls of small blood vessels; it is most frequently demonstrated in the skin. Animals are immunized repeatedly until they have appreciable levels of precipitating, mainly IgG, antibody. On injecting antigen subcutaneously or intradermally a reaction develops which reaches peak intensity in 4 to 10 hours (Fig.21.10).

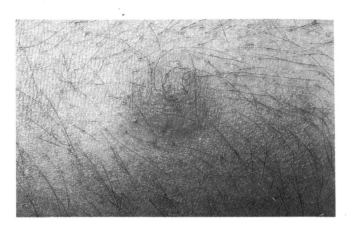

Fig.21.10 The gross appearance of the Arthus reaction. The area consists of a reddened area of inflammation which is maximal 5–6 hours after injection of antigen.

Depending on the amount of antigen injected, marked oedema and haemorrhage develop at the site of injection. The reaction then wanes and is usually markedly decreased by 48 hours. Immunofluorescent studies have shown that initially antigen, antibody and complement are deposited in the vessel wall followed by a polymorphonuclear neutrophil infiltration and the intravascular clumping of platelets (Fig.21.11). This platelet reaction can lead to vascular occlusion and necrosis in severe cases. After 24–48 hours the polymorphs are replaced by mononuclear cells and eventually some plasma cells

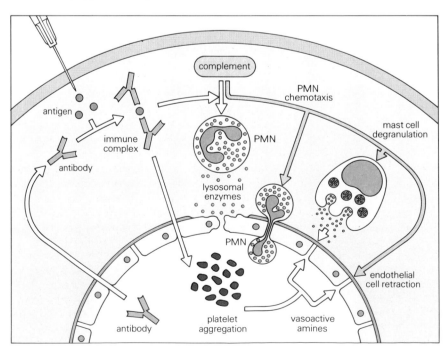

Fig.21.11 The Arthus reaction. Antigen injected intradermally combines with specific antibody from the blood to form immune complexes. The complexes activate complement and act on platelets, which release vasoactive amines. Complement C3a and C5a fragments cause endothelial cell retraction, mast cell degranulation and polymorph chemotaxis into the tissues. Mast cell products, including histamine and leukotrienes, induce increased blood flow and capillary permeability. The inflammatory reaction is potentiated by lysosomal enzymes released from the polymorphs. Furthermore, C3b deposited on the complexes opsonizes them for phagocytes.

appear. Complement activation via either the classical or alternative pathways is essential for the Arthus reaction to develop and only a mild oedema will occur in the absence of the polymorphs. The ratio of antibody to antigen is important for producing maximum reactivity. Generally, complexes formed in either antigen or antibody excess are much less toxic than those formed at equivalence.

WHY DO COMPLEXES PERSIST?

Normally immune complexes are removed by the mononuclear phagocyte system particularly in the liver, spleen and lungs. Size is important – in general larger complexes are rapidly removed by the liver within a few minutes, while smaller complexes circulate for longer periods (Fig.21.12). The major factor governing removal of large complexes appears to be liver blood flow. Factors which affect the size of the complexes are therefore likely to influence their clearance. It has been suggested that a genetic defect leading to the enhanced production of low affinity antibody could well lead to the formation of smaller complexes and so, immune complex disease. Generally, when an individual forms antibodies to self-antigens, only a few epitopes on the antigen are recognized and this will favour the formation of small complexes since the formation of a cross-linked complex is restricted.

There is controversy over the need for complement activation for the removal of immune complexes. It appears to depend on whether the complexes are particulate or soluble. *In vivo* the main site for immune complex removal is the liver where Kupffer cells are responsible for phagocytosing the complexes. Both complement (C3) and IgG appear to be necessary for the removal of particulate immune complexes, for example, red cells coated with antibody and complement first adhere to receptors on the Kupffer cells through C3 and are then phagocytosed through recognition of IgG Fc. If red cells coated solely with C3 are used, these are found to adhere in the liver but are then released again intact, probably through the action of C3 inactivator. Red cells coated only with antibody are not removed by the liver but, instead are slowly taken up in the spleen. With soluble complexes, however, complement does not seem to be involved; in animals depleted of complement (by cobra venom factor) the clearance of complexes is virtually unaffected, but the possible involvement of locally manufactured complement cannot be ruled out (Fig.21.13).

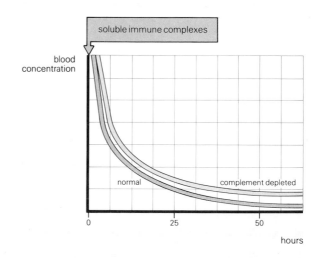

Fig.21.13 Complex clearance by the reticuloendothelial system II. Soluble complexes were injected into a normal and a complement-depleted animal and their persistence measured during the following hours. The graph shows that the clearance rate of these complexes (principally 14S–22S) is little affected by the presence or absence of complement, even though they are large enough to fix complement.

In contrast, the *in vitro* uptake of complexes by phagocytic cells is markedly enhanced by the addition of complement. When large amounts of complex are present the mononuclear phagocyte system may become overloaded. Certainly in experimental animals it is possible to block the mononuclear phagocyte system which then leads to prolonged circulation of immune complexes with some complex deposition in the glomerulus. There is some evidence for a defective mononuclear phagocyte system in human immune complex disease but this may well be the result of overload rather than a primary defect.

Recently the carbohydrate groups on immunoglobulin molecules have been shown to be important for removal of immune complexes by Kupffer cells in the liver and there may be abnormalities of the immunoglobulin carbohydrates in certain immune complex diseases, particularly in rheumatoid arthritis and SLE. It is not certain, however, whether the abnormalities of carbohydrate are primary or are themselves caused by the disease.

Although complexes may persist in the circulation for prolonged periods simple persistence is not usually harmful in itself, problems start to occur when they deposit in the tissues.

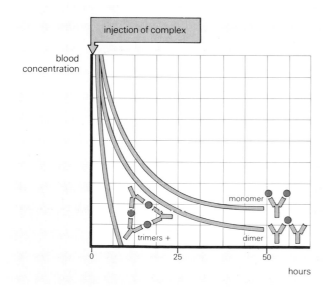

Fig.21.12 Complex clearance by the reticuloendothelial system I. Large complexes are cleared most quickly because they present an IgG-Fc lattice to reticuloendothelial cells with Fc receptors, permitting higher avidity binding to these cells. They also fix complement (C1q) better than small complexes.

WHY DO COMPLEXES DEPOSIT IN TISSUES?

Two questions are relevant to tissue deposition: why do complexes deposit, and why in different diseases do the complexes show affinity for particular tissues?

Increase in Vascular Permeability
The most important trigger for tissue deposition is probably an increase in vascular permeability. This can be initiated by a range of mechanisms which may vary in importance in various diseases and in different species. This makes interpretation of some of the animal models difficult. Complement, mast cells, basophils and platelets must all be considered as potential contributors to the release of vasoactive amines. Inert substances (eg. colloidal carbon) can be made to deposit in vessel walls if animals are given vasoactive substances such as histamine or serotonin. Similarly, circulating immune complexes may be made to deposit by the infusion of agents which cause liberation of mast cell vasoactive amines. Pretreatment with antihistamines blocks this effect. In studies of experimental immune complex disease, long-term administration of vasoactive amine antagonists, such as chlorpheniramine or methysergide, considerably reduced complex deposition (Fig. 21.14). More importantly, young NZB/NZW mice treated with methysergide showed less renal pathology than controls (Fig. 21.15).

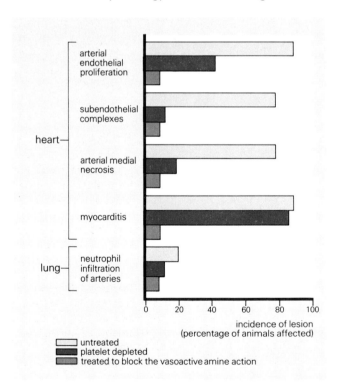

Fig.21.14 **Effect of vasoactive amine antagonists on immune complex disease.** Serum sickness was induced in rabbits with a single injection of bovine serum albumin. Animals were either untreated (pink), platelet depleted (red) or treated with drugs to block vasoactive amine action (purple). The incidence of serum sickness lesions in the heart and lung was scored. Drug treatment considerably reduces the signs of disease by minimizing complex deposition.

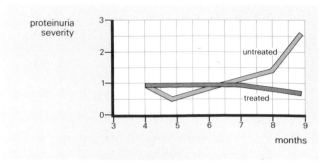

Fig.21.15 **Effect of the vasoactive amine antagonist methysergide on kidney damage.** Kidney damage, assessed by proteinuria, was measured in NZB/NZW mice over a period of months. Untreated animals developed severe proteinuria, while methysergide-treated animals did not. Methysergide blocks formation of the vasoactive amine, 5 HT and thus platelets are depleted of this.

Haemodynamic Processes
Immune complex deposition is more probable in sites where there is high blood pressure and turbulence (Fig.21.16). In the glomerular capillaries the blood pressure is about four times that of most other capillaries — many macromolecules favour a glomerular localization. If the pressure is reduced by partially constricting the renal artery, or ligating the ureter, complex deposition is reduced; experimentally induced hypertension enhances the development of the symptoms of acute serum sickness in the rabbit. Similarly at other sites, such as the walls of arteries, the most severe lesions occur either at sites of turbulence, such as vessel bifurcations, or in filters such as the choroid plexus or the ciliary body of the eye.

Antigen Tissue Binding
Local high blood pressure, while explaining a general tendency for certain organs to be particular sites for complex deposition does not explain why complexes in various diseases home in on different organs. For example, in SLE the kidney is a particular target whereas in rheumatoid arthritis, although circulating complexes are present, the kidney is usually spared and the joints are the principal target. It is possible that the antigen in the complex provides the organ specificity. It has been shown that DNA has a strong affinity for collagen in the basement membrane of the glomerulus and this could lead to the deposition of DNA:anti-DNA antibody complexes in the kidney in SLE where these antibodies are such a marked feature. A convincing model has been established where mice are given endotoxin, which causes cell damage and the release of DNA, which binds to the glomerular basement membrane. Anti-DNA is then produced by polyclonal activation of B cells and is bound by the fixed DNA leading to local immune complex formation (Fig.21.17). It is possible that in other diseases further antigens will be identified with affinity for other organs. In certain diseases the antibodies and antigens are both produced within the target organ. The extreme of this is reached in rheumatoid arthritis where the anti-human IgG is produced by plasma cells within the synovium: the antibodies combine with each other and self-associate so setting up an inflammatory reaction.

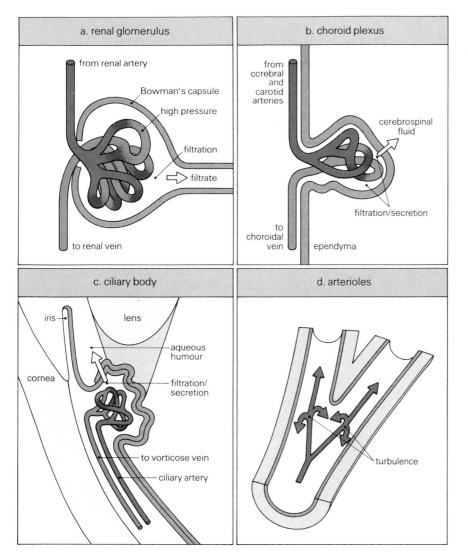

Fig. 21.16 Haemodynamic factors affecting complex deposition. Factors include filtration, which occurs in the formation of the glomerular ultrafiltrate (a), the formation of the cerebrospinal fluid by the choroid plexus, which lies along the ventricles of the brain (b), and in the formation of the aqueous humour by the epithelium of the ciliary body in the eye (c). High pressure in the renal glomerulus also favours deposition as does turbulence such as occurs at curves or bifurcations of arteries (d).

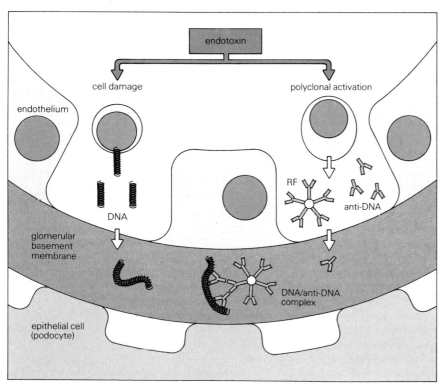

Fig. 21.17 A model for the formation and deposition of immune complexes in the kidney. Endotoxin induces cell damage with release of DNA which becomes deposited on the collagen of the glomerular basement membrane. Endotoxin also induces a polyclonal stimulation of B cells, some of which produce anti-DNA antibodies and auto-anti-IgG antibodies – these are termed rheumatoid factors (RF). Anti-DNA binds to the deposited DNA, and rheumatoid factors, which have low affinity for monomeric IgG bind to the assembled DNA/anti-DNA complex. Thus immune complex formation occurs *in situ*.

Size of Immune Complexes

The exact localization of immune complexes is partly dependent on the size of the complex. This is shown in the kidney where small immune complexes are able to pass through the glomerular basement membrane so ending up on the epithelial side of the membrane, while large complexes are unable to cross the membrane and largely accumulate between the endothelium and the basement membrane or in the mesangium (Fig.21.18). The size of immune complexes depends on the valency of the antigen and the titre and affinity of the antibody.

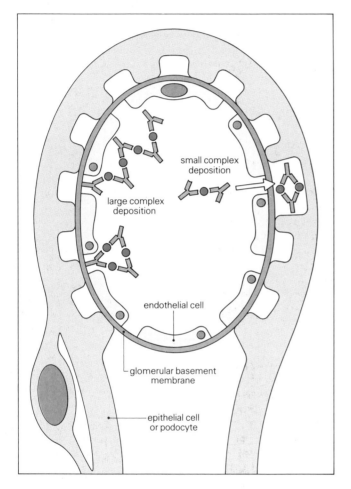

Fig.21.18 The site of complex deposition in the kidney is dependent on the size of the complexes in the circulation. Large complexes become deposited on the glomerular basement membrane, while small complexes pass through the basement membrane and are seen on the epithelial side of the glomerulus.

Immunoglobulin Class

The class of immunoglobulin can influence the deposition of immune complexes. With anti-DNA antibodies in SLE there are marked age and sex-related variations in the class and subclass distribution. As the NZB/NZW mice age there is a class switch of these antibodies from predominantly IgM to IgG2a. This occurs earlier in females than in males and coincides with the onset of renal disease preceding the time at which death occurred by 2–3 months, indicating the importance of antibody class in the tissue deposition of complexes (Fig.21.19).

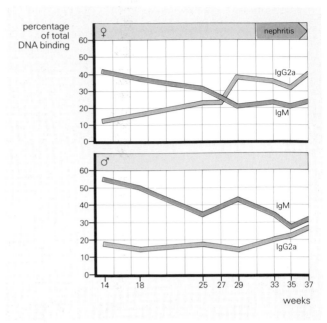

Fig.21.19 Antibody classes in immune complex disease. Immune complex disease in the NZB/NZW mouse follows a class switch from IgM to IgG2a. The graphs show the titres of anti-DNA antibodies (IgM and IgG2a) in females (top) and males (bottom). The class switch and fatal renal disease occurs earlier in female mice of this strain.

COMPLEMENT SOLUBILIZATION OF IMMUNE COMPLEXES

Once complexes have deposited in the tissues a mechanism, complement, exists for making them soluble again.

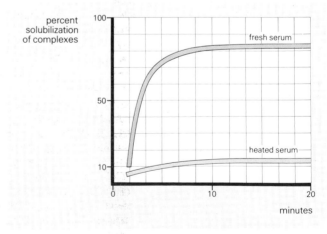

Fig.21.20 Solubilization of immune complexes by complement. Complement can solubilize precipitable complexes *in vitro*. Addition of fresh serum containing active complement to insoluble complexes induces solubilization over about 15 minutes at 37°C. Some of the complexes resist resolubilization. Heated serum (56° for 30min) lacking active complement cannot resolubilize the complexes. It appears that intercalation of complement components C3b and C3d, into the complex causes their solubilization.

Complement can rapidly resolubilize precipitated complexes (Fig. 21.20). The solubilization appears to occur by the insertion of complement C3b and C3d fragments into the complex. It may be that complexes are continually being deposited in normal individuals, but are removed by solubilization. If this is the case, the process would be inadequate in hypocomplementaemic patients, leading to prolonged complex deposition. Solubilization defects have been observed in sera from patients with systemic immune complex disease, but whether the defect is primary or secondary is not known.

DETECTION OF IMMUNE COMPLEXES

There are many techniques for detecting and quantitating immune complexes. The ideal place to look for the complexes is in the affected organ. Tissue samples may be examined by immunofluorescence for the presence of

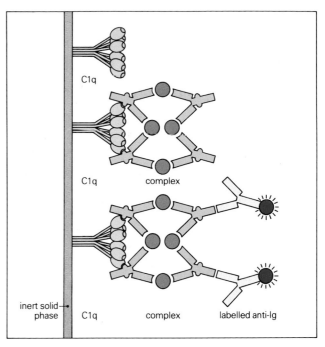

Fig. 21.22 A three layer radioimmunoassay for immune complexes based on the use of C1q.
1. C1q is linked to an inert solid phase support, usually a polystyrene tube or plate.
2. Serum containing complexes is added and the complexes bind to the solid phase C1q via the array of Fc regions presented to the C1q.
3. The amount of complex bound to the C1q is detected using a radiolabelled antibody to IgG and the radioactivity measured in a gamma counter.

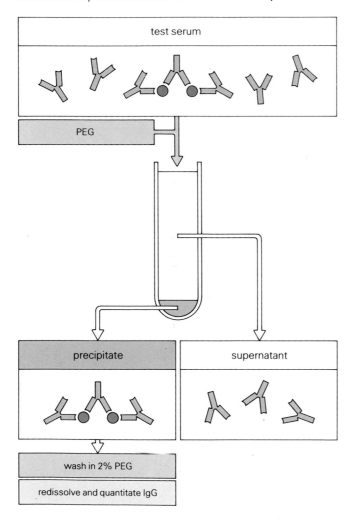

Fig.21.21 An assay for complexes based on polyethylene glycol (PEG). PEG is added to test serum containing complexes of IgG and IgG monomer, to produce a final concentration of 2% PEG. At 2% PEG, complexes are selectively precipitated and the supernatant contains free antibody. After washing the precipitate it is redissolved and complexed IgG can be quantitated (eg. by single radial immunodiffusion, nephelometry, or radioimmunoassay).

immunoglobulin and complement. The composition, pattern and particular area of tissue affected all provide useful information on the severity and prognosis of the disease. For example, one can contrast the poor prognosis for the patient with continuous, granular, subepithelial deposits of IgG found in membranous glomerulonephritis with the relatively good prognosis where the complexes are localized in the mesangium. Not all tissue-bound complexes give rise to an inflammatory response; for example in SLE, complexes are frequently found in skin biopsies from unaffected, as well as inflamed areas. Complexes may also be found in the circulation where they may be detected physically as high molecular weight immunoglobulin.

Precipitation of the immune complex with polyethylene glycol and estimation of the precipitated IgG is frequently used to identify high molecular weight IgG and forms the basis for one of the commercial assays (Fig. 21.21). Circulating complexes are often identified by their affinity for complement, C1q, utilizing either radiolabelled C1q or C1q linked to a solid support (solid phase C1q) (Fig. 21.22). Other receptors may be used such as the C3 receptor on RAJI cells or the Fc receptor on platelets. Even more care than that exercized over the interpretation of tissue complexes must be given to the evaluation of the importance of circulating complexes since many circulating complexes will not in themselves be harmful unless they deposit in the tissue.

FURTHER READING

Agnello V. (1983) Immune complex assays in rheumatic diseases. *Hum. Pathol.* **14,** 343.

Inman R. D. (1982) Immune complexes in SLE. *Clin. Rheum. Dis.* **8,** 49.

Sedlacek H. H. & Seiler F. R. (eds.) (1979) Immune Complexes. *Behring Inst. Mitt.* **64.**

Theofilopoulos A. N. & Dixon F. J. (1979) The biology and detection of immune complexes. *Adv. Immunol.* **28,** 89.

Williams R. C. (1980) *Immune complexes in clinical and experimental medicine.* Harvard University Press, Cambridge, Massachusetts.

World Health Organisation Scientific Group (1977) Technical Report 606. *The Role of Immune Complexes in Disease.* W.H.O., Geneva.

22 Hypersensitivity – Type IV

In the classification of hypersensitivity suggested by Coombs and Gell in 1963 delayed hypersensitivity (cell-mediated hypersensitivity or Type IV) was used as a general category to describe all those hypersensitivity reactions which took more than 12 hours to develop. At that time the mechanisms underlying the phenomena were not known, and they are still not well understood. It has become evident, however, that several different types of immune reaction can produce delayed hypersensitivity.

Unlike other forms of hypersensitivity it cannot be transferred from one animal to another by serum, but can be transferred by T lymphocytes bearing a variety of surface phenotypes eg. in the mouse, Ly1 or Ly1,2,3. It is obviously associated with T cell protective immunity but does not necessarily run parallel with it. The T cells necessary for producing the delayed response, T-delayed hypersensitivity or T_D cells, are cells which have become sensitized to the particular antigen by a previous encounter. But although sensitized T cells are instrumental in producing delayed hypersensitivity reactions, they frequently act by recruiting other cell types to the site of the reaction.

REACTIONS OF DELAYED HYPERSENSITIVITY

Four types of delayed hypersensitivity reaction are recognized and of these the first three – the Jones-Mote reaction, contact hypersensitivity and tuberculin-type hypersensitivity – all occur within 72 hours of antigen challenge. By contrast, the fourth type, granulomatous reactions, develop over a period of weeks. The position is complicated because these different types of reaction may overlap to some extent, or occur sequentially following a single antigenic challenge; therefore many of the hypersensitivity reactions seen in practice do not correspond to one category alone.

The four different types of delayed hypersensitivity were originally distinguished according to the reaction they produced when antigen was applied directly to the skin or injected intradermally. The degree of the reaction is assessed in animals by measuring thickening of the skin, which occurs at the site of antigen application and is accompanied by a variety of immune reactions.

The first type of reaction to appear is the Jones-Mote, which is maximal at 24 hours. Contact and tuberculin-type hypersensitivities both peak at 48-72 hours after antigen challenge. These may be followed by an even more delayed response characterized histologically by the aggregation and proliferation of macrophages which form granulomas which may persist for weeks. The granulomatous hypersensitivity reaction is, in terms of its clinical consequences, by far the most serious type of delayed response.

The four types of reaction and times taken to produce maximal skin swelling, are listed in figure 22.1. In addition to the difference in timing and degree of skin swelling the four types of delayed hypersensitivity are characterized in other ways which will now be described.

delayed reaction	maximal reaction time
Jones-Mote	24 hours
contact	48-72 hours
tuberculin	48-72 hours
granulomatous	at least 14 days

Fig. 22.1 The four types of delayed hypersensitivity. The Jones-Mote response is maximal at 24 hours. Contact and tuberculin-type hypersensitivities, which have a similar time course, are maximal at between 48-72 hours. In certain circumstances, tuberculin-type reactions may develop at 21-28 days into a granulomatous hypersensitivity reaction which may continue for several weeks (eg. skin testing in leprosy).

JONES-MOTE HYPERSENSITIVITY

Jones-Mote hypersensitivity is characterized by infiltration of the area immediately under the epidermis by basophils, and is frequently called cutaneous basophil hypersensitivity when induced in experimental animals such as the guinea pig. It is induced by soluble antigen, is maximal seven to ten days after induction and tends to disappear when antibody appears. The skin swelling is maximal 24 hours after antigen challenge. A reaction with a similar time course may be induced in the guinea pig by an intradermal injection of the antigen ovalbumin in Freund's Incomplete Adjuvant (FIA), a mild antigenic stimulus. If, however, a powerful antigenic stimulus is applied by injecting ovalbumin with Freund's Complete Adjuvant (adjuvant containing tubercle bacilli), a tuberculin-type response is seen. In the Jones-Mote reaction studies of the cellular infiltrate reveal numerous basophils, but less basophils may be seen in guinea pig tuberculin reactions. Interestingly, if ovalbumin in FIA is combined with cyclophosphamide pre-treatment, a skin response with a longer time course is seen which superficially resembles the tuberculin response but may not be identical.

It is concluded that the Jones-Mote response is strongly regulated by cyclophosphamide-sensitive lymphocytes (suppressor lymphocytes). (Fig. 22.2).

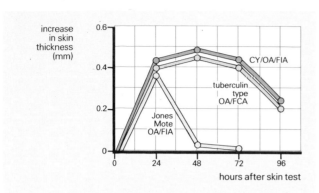

Fig. 22.2 The induction of Jones-Mote and tuberculin-type reactions in the guinea pig using ovalbumin (OA) and Freund's Adjuvant. This graph plots the skin swelling induced when guinea pigs are injected with different combinations of ovalbumin, Freund's Adjuvant and cyclophosphamide. Intradermal injection of OA with Freund's Incomplete Adjuvant (FIA) induces skin swelling which is maximal at 24 hours – the Jones-Mote response. If OA and Freund's Complete Adjuvant (FCA) are injected a swelling is induced, which is maximal at 48 hours – the tuberculin-type response (which may also show a basophil leucocyte infiltration). When the animal is pretreated with cyclophosphamide (Cy) before injection of OA and FIA, a reaction is obtained which has a similar time course to the tuberculin-type reaction. However, B cells from Jones-Mote animals are able to suppress the skin response of Jones-Mote animals treated with cyclophosphamide but not the skin responses of animals immunized with FCA. This provides some evidence to suggest that the tuberculin-response and the skin test of Jones-Mote animals treated with cyclophosphamide – although of similar time course – have different immunological effector mechanisms.

CONTACT HYPERSENSITIVITY

Contact hypersensitivity, characterized clinically in humans by eczema of the skin at the site of contact with the allergen, is usually maximal at 48 hours both in sensitized humans and experimental animals. In Europe the most common antigens are haptens such as nickel, acrylates and chemicals found in rubber, whereas in the USA, poison ivy and poison oak are the most important antigens (Fig. 22.3).

The small haptens which induce contact hypersensitivity would not normally be antigenic, however, it appears that these low molecular weight compounds can traverse the skin and then become conjugated, either covalently or non-covalently to normal body proteins. For example, it has been shown that following skin sensitization with the hapten dinitrochlorobenzene (DNCB) about 85% of the compound binds to the epidermal cell proteins (by their lysine $-NH_2$ residues). The conjugate then serves to sensitize the animal. T cell recognition of the conjugate is specific for the hapten/carrier conjugate and is not dependent on conventional hapten recognition plus carrier recognition, which occurs in antibody formation.

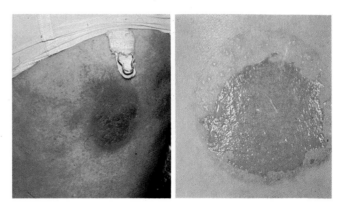

Fig. 22.3 Clinical and patch test appearances of contact hypersensitivity. The eczematous area is due to sensitivity to the rubber component of this individual's undergarment (left). The suspected allergen may be confirmed by applying it, in a weak, non-irritant concentration to a patch of skin (patch test). An eczematous reaction (right) induced between 48 and 72 hours, confirms the allergen.

Contact hypersensitivity is predominantly an epidermal reaction (as distinct from tuberculin-type hypersensitivity, which is a dermal reaction). The antigen-presenting cell for contact sensitization is the Langerhans cell (Fig. 22.4).

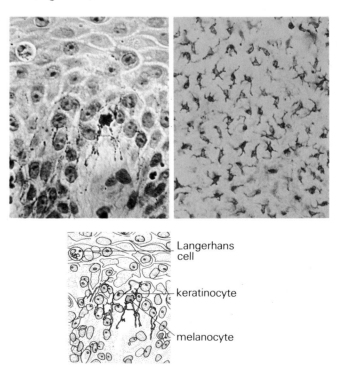

Fig. 22.4 The Langerhans cells seen in a skin section. These cells constitute only a small percentage of the cells in the epidermis, but when visualized by a specific stain (ATPase in a trypsinized section) they are seen to form a continuous network within the skin: DOPA reaction counterstained with toluidine blue, ×300 (left); ATPase stain ×110 (right).

The Langerhans cell is characterized in electron microscopy by the presence of 'Birbeck granules', which are unique to this cell (Fig. 22.5).

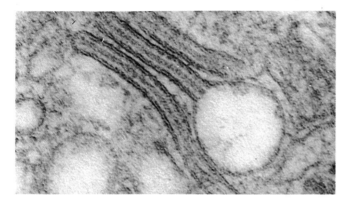

Fig. 22.5 The Langerhans cell under electron microscopy showing the characteristic 'Birbeck granule'. This is a racket-shaped organelle containing an array of particles delineated by a membrane. × 132,000.

The function of these granules is not known with certainty but it is probable that they are involved in antigen presentation. The Langerhans cell is a dendritic antigen-presenting cell carrying Ia antigens and it has been shown to recirculate, carrying antigen to the lymph nodes draining the skin. The lesion of a contact hypersensitivity reaction shows a mononuclear cell infiltrate first appearing at 6-8 hours and peaking at 12-15 hours. The

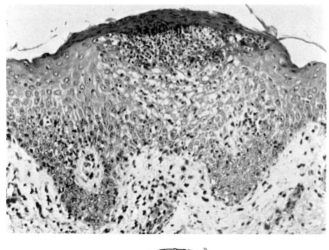

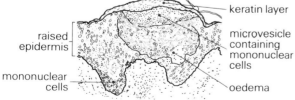

Fig. 22.6 Histological appearance of the lesion in contact hypersensitivity. There is infiltration of the epidermis (which is pushed outwards) by mononuclear cells, and microvesicle formation with oedema of the epidermis. The dermis is typically infiltrated by an increased number of leucocytes. H&E stain, × 130.

infiltration is accompanied by oedema of the epidermis with microvesicle formation (Fig. 22.6). A contact hypersensitivity reaction is distinguished from the inflammatory reaction following skin penetration by pyogenic bacteria, by the absence of neutrophil polymorphs. Increased numbers of leucocytes are characteristically seen in the dermal infiltrate.

TUBERCULIN-TYPE HYPERSENSITIVITY

This form of hypersensitivity was originally described by Koch, who observed that patients with tuberculosis reacted with fever and generalized sickness following a subcutaneous injection of tuberculin, a lipoprotein antigen derived from the tubercle bacillus.

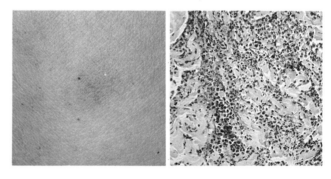

Fig. 22.7 Clinical and histological appearances of tuberculin-type sensitivity. Shown here is the dermal reaction to antigens of the leprosy bacillus in a sensitive individual (Fernandez reaction). The response is characterized clinically by red induration of the skin maximal at 48-72 hours after challenge (left) and histologically (right) by a dense dermal infiltrate of lymphocytes and macrophages. H&E stain, × 80.

This reaction was accompanied by an area of induration and swelling at the site of injection. Soluble antigens from a number of organisms, including *Mycobacterium tuberculosis*, *Mycobacterium leprae* and *Leishmania tropica*, induce similar reactions in sensitive people. The skin reaction is frequently used as the basis of a test for sensitivity to the organisms following previous exposure (Fig. 22.7). It has also been shown that this form of hypersensitivity may be induced by non-microbial antigens.

Twenty-four hours after exposure to the antigen the site of reaction shows an intense infiltration by mononuclear cells of which about 50% are lymphocytes and the remainder monocytes. In man polymorphs are very uncommon in this reaction. By 48 hours there is an extensive infiltration of lymphocytes around the blood vessels extending outwards and disrupting the organization of the collagen bundles in the dermis. The percentage of macrophages falls somewhat over the following 48 hours as the reaction becomes maximal. As the lesion develops it may become a granulomatous reaction. The progression from tuberculin-like to granulomatous reaction appears to depend on the persistence of the antigen in the tissues. Subepidermal infiltration with basophils is not a characteristic of this reaction.

22.3

GRANULOMATOUS HYPERSENSITIVITY

Granulomatous hypersensitivity is clinically the most important form of delayed hypersensitivity, causing many of the pathological effects in diseases which involve T cell-mediated immunity. It results from the presence of a persistent agent within macrophages, usually micro-organisms, which the cell is unable to destroy. On occasion it may also be caused by the continued presence of immune complexes, for example in allergic alveolitis. The process results in epithelioid cell granuloma formation. The histological appearance of the granuloma reaction is quite different from the tuberculin-type reaction, which is usually a self-limiting response to antigen while the former is due to the persistence of antigen. Nevertheless they often result from sensitization to similar microbial antigens, for example, *M. tuberculosis* and *M. leprae* (Fig. 22.8).

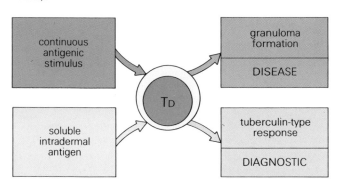

Fig. 22.8 Unifying role of T_D cells in tuberculin and granulomatous reactions. Both tuberculin-type and granulomatous hypersensitivity reactions are dependent on T_D cells which have been sensitized to particular antigens. Where there is a continuous antigenic stimulation either due to persistent or recurrent infection, or where macrophages and lymphocytes are incapable of destroying the antigen, granuloma formation will occur. The presence of sensitized T_D cells may be detected by the tuberculin reaction to the antigen in question.

As with the infectious agents, immunological granuloma formation also occurs in zirconium sensitivity and in sarcoidosis. Granulomas are also produced by certain non-antigenic stimuli, such as talc. In this case the macrophages are unable to digest the inorganic matter. These non-immunological granulomas may be distinguished by the absence of lymphocytes in the lesion. Examples of granulomatous hypersensitivity in various diseases will be discussed later.

The characteristic cell of granulomatous hypersensitivity is the epithelioid cell which on electron microscopic examination appears as a large flattened cell with increased endoplasmic reticulum (Fig. 22.9). The nature of the cell is poorly understood; it has been suggested that epithelioid cells are derived from activated macrophages but examination reveals that whereas activated macrophages have many phagosomes this is not true of epithelioid cells. Also seen in this type of reaction are multinucleate giant cells which are also

referred to as Langhans giant cells (not to be confused with the Langerhans cell discussed earlier). Giant cells have several nuclei distributed about the periphery leaving the central area of the cytoplasm free. The cytoplasm contains membrane-lined vesicles and

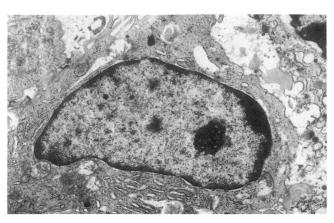

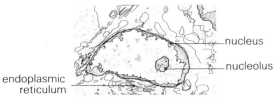

Fig. 22.9 Electron micrograph of an epithelioid cell. This is the characteristic cell of granulomatous hypersensitivity. Note the increased endoplasmic reticulum compared with a monocyte/macrophage. × 4,800.

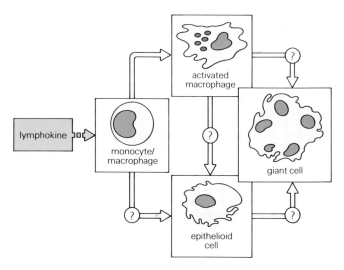

Fig. 22.10 A proposed scheme for the terminal differentiation of cells of the monocyte/macrophage system. These developments represent the pathological changes resulting from the inability of the macrophage to deal effectively with the pathogen. Lymphokines from active T cells induce monocytes and macrophages to become activated macrophages. Where prolonged antigenic stimulation exists it is hypothesized that the activated macrophages may differentiate further into epithelioid cells and then into giant cells. This process occurs only *in vivo*, in granulomatous tissue. It is believed that the multinucleate giant cell is derived from fusion of several epithelioid cells, although the functional significance of this fusion is obscure.

intracellular particles. The giant cell has little endoplasmic reticulum, and its mitochondria and lysosomes appear to be undergoing degeneration. For this reason it is thought that the cell may be a terminal differentiation stage of the monocyte/macrophage line (Fig. 22.10). The typical immunologically-induced granulomatous lesion has a core of epithelioid cells and macrophages, sometimes with giant cells. In some diseases, such as tuberculosis, this central area may have a zone of necrosis (cell death), with complete destruction of all cellular architecture. The macrophage/epithelioid core is surrounded by a cuff of lymphocytes, and there may also be considerable fibrosis (deposition of collagen fibres) caused by proliferation of fibroblasts and increased collagen synthesis. An example of a granulomatous reaction can be seen in the Mitsuda reaction to leprosy antigens or in the Kveim test, where patients suffering from sarcoidosis (a disease of unknown aetiology) react to splenic antigens derived from other sarcoid patients. The Mitsuda reaction is illustrated in figure 22.11.

The four types of delayed hypersensitivity reaction are summarized in figure 22.12.

type	Jones-Mote	contact	tuberculin	granulomatous
reaction time	24 hours	48 hours	48 hours	4 weeks
clinical appearance	skin swelling	eczema	local induration and swelling ± fever	skin induration
histological appearance	basophils, lymphocytes, mononuclear cells	mononuclear cells, oedema, raised epidermis	mononuclear cells, lymphocytes and monocytes, reduced macrophages	epithelioid cell granuloma, giant cells, macrophages, fibrosis, ± necrosis
antigen	intradermal antigen eg. ovalbumin	epidermal: eg. nickel, rubber, poison ivy etc.	dermal: tuberculin, mycobacterial and leishmanial antigens	persistent Ag or Ag/Ab complexes in macrophages or 'non immunological' eg. talcum powder

Fig. 22.12 Summary of the important characteristics of the four types of delayed hypersensitivity reaction.

CELLULAR REACTIONS IN DELAYED HYPERSENSITIVITY

Delayed hypersensitivity reactions are initiated by cells rather then antibody. It was shown by Simon and Rackeman in 1934 that there was no association between the tuberculin-type reaction and the incidence of serum antibodies to the sensitizing antigen. Moreover, in 1942 Landsteiner and Chase showed that the reactivity may only be transferred to a non-sensitive individual by cell suspensions containing lymphocytes. By eliminating T lymphocytes in the transfer it is relatively easy to show that these cells are the effectors in tuberculin-type hypersensitivity (Fig. 22.13).

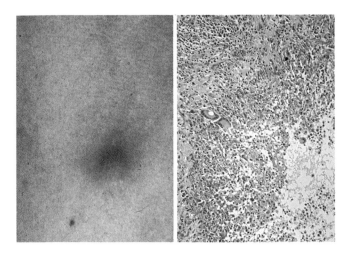

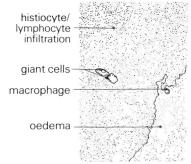

histiocyte/ lymphocyte infiltration

giant cells

macrophage

oedema

Fig. 22.11 Clinical and histological appearances of the Mitsuda reaction in leprosy seen at 28 days. The resultant skin swelling (which may be ulcerated) is much more indurated, and is better defined than at 48 hours (left). Histology demonstrates a typical epithelioid cell granuloma. Giant cells are also visible in the centre of the lesion which is surrounded by a cuff of lymphocytes (right, H & E stain, ×60). This response is more akin to the pathological processes in delayed hypersensitivity diseases than the self-resolving tuberculin-type reaction, the reaction is due to the continued presence of antigen.

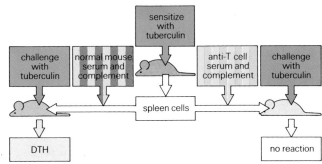

Fig. 22.13 Demonstration of the role of T lymphocytes in the tuberculin response. A mouse is sensitized to tuberculin by intradermal injection. Its spleen cells are later removed and treated with either (1) normal serum and complement or (2) anti-T lymphocyte serum and complement. The treated cells are injected into recipient mice which are challenged with tuberculin. The mouse with spleen cells treated with normal serum develops a tuberculin-type reaction, whereas the mouse donated anti-T cell-treated spleen cells fails to respond. It is concluded that sensitized T cells are responsible for producing the response to tuberculin.

Similarly, T lymphocytes are responsible for initiating the other delayed reactions. The lymphocytes interact with macrophages by releasing soluble factors, termed lymphokines.

Lymphokines have several functions but their main purpose is to activate macrophages and attract them to the site of antigen challenge and amplify the local response (Fig. 22.14). The biochemistry of lymphokines is not well established, they are usually defined by their biological activities, and it is likely that many lymphokines have more than one effect (Fig. 22.15).

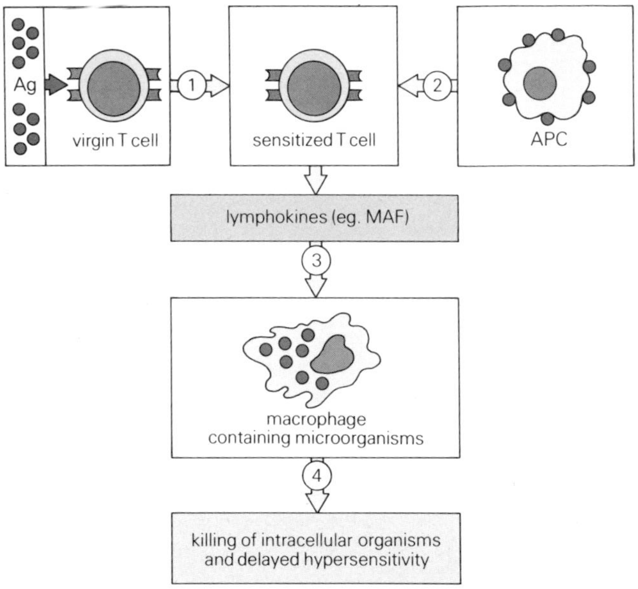

One of the tests for T cell reactivity to antigens measures production of one lymphokine, by the macrophage migration inhibition factor (MIF) test. In the presence of antigen, sensitized lymphocytes produce a lymphokine (MIF) which inhibits the normal migration of macrophages (Fig. 22.16).

Fig. 22.14 The production and role of lymphokines in delayed hypersensitivity. During infection. T cells recognize the microorganism's antigens and proliferate, giving rise to a population of sensitized T cells (1). When these cells are presented with antigen by the antigen-presenting cell (2), they release lymphokines. The lymphokine Macrophage Activating Factor (MAF) activates the macrophages (3), stimulating them to kill any microorganisms they may contain. These macrophages may participate in a delayed hypersensitivity response (4).

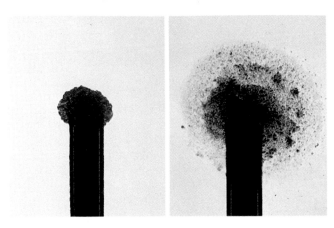

Fig. 22.16 Macrophage Migration Inhibition Test. Macrophages are packed into capillary tubes with either test lymphocytes (suspected as being sensitive to an antigen) together with antigen (left) or control lymphocytes and the antigen (right), and set up in short term tissue culture. Where migration is inhibited (left) it is concluded that the lymphocytes are sensitive to the antigen and produce the lymphokine, Migration Inhibition Factor, which inhibits the normal migration of macrophages.

Another useful *in vitro* test in the diagnosis of delayed hypersensitivity is the lymphocyte transformation test (LTT). When sensitized lymphocytes are cultured in the presence of the appropriate antigen they respond by undergoing transformation into blast cells (lymphoblasts) which divide (Fig. 22.17).

lymphokine	effect
Macrophage Activating Factor (MAF)	killing of intracellular organisms
Mononuclear Phagocyte Chemotactic Factor, Migration Inhibition Factor	localization of macrophages
Interleukin II (TCGF)	promotes T cell clone proliferation
Interferon (IFNγ)	Inhibition of viral multiplication
Mitogenic Factor	T helper function
Lymphocyte Inhibitory Factor (LIF)	T suppressor function
Lymphotoxin	? tumour inhibition
Skin Reactive Factor	? facilitation of cell recruitment from circulation

Fig. 22.15 Effects of different lymphokines. This table lists some of the lymphokines released by T cells. They are usually defined by their effect on other cells.

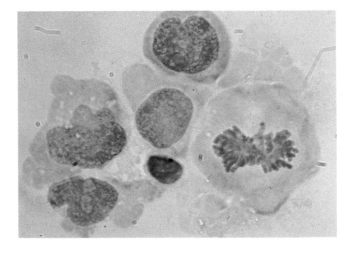

Fig. 22.17 Transformed lymphocytes. Following stimulation with appropriate antigen, T cells undergo lymphoblastoid transformation prior to cell division. Blast cells with expanded nuclei and cytoplasm (as well as one lymphocyte in the metaphase of cell division) are shown.

The transformation is accompanied by DNA synthesis, and this is measured by assaying the uptake of tritiated thymidine into the cells. (Thymidine is a nucleotide used by the cells for DNA synthesis.) The lymphocyte transformation test is described in figure 22.18. It is important to stress that the LTT is a test for T cell memory and this does not necessarily imply the presence of protective immunity in the host, that is, the strength of the effective immune response against an invading organism.

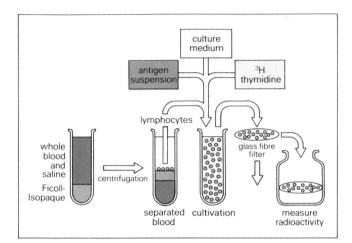

Fig. 22.18 The Lymphocyte Transformation Test. Whole blood in saline solution is layered on Ficoll-Isopaque (which has a density between, and therefore separates, white cells and red cells) and centrifuged (400×G). This separates the lymphocytes from the other cell and serum constituents. The cells are washed (to remove contaminants such as antigen) and then put into test tubes with a suspension of antigen and culture medium (cells from lymphoid tissues may also be used). Tritiated thymidine (³H-thymidine) is added sixteen hours before the cells are harvested. The cells are harvested on a glass fibre filter disc and their radioactivity is measured by placing the disc in a liquid scintillation counter. A high count indicates that the lymphocytes have undergone transformation and confirms their sensitivity to the antigen.

DISEASES MANIFESTING DELAYED HYPERSENSITIVITY

There are a considerable number of chronic diseases in man which manifest delayed hypersensitivity, and most are due to infectious agents such as mycobacteria, protozoa, and fungi. Important diseases in this respect include:
1. Tuberculosis
2. Leprosy
3. Leishmaniasis
4. Listeriosis
5. Deep fungal infections (eg. blastomycosis)
6. Helminthic infections (eg. schistosomiasis)
These diseases are caused by pathogens which present a persistent chronic antigenic stimulus. The threat they pose is met by lymphocytes and macrophages. Although these diseases are liable to induce protective immunity, as previously stated, protective immunity and delayed hypersensitivity are not always coincident.

Leprosy
A dramatic example of delayed hypersensitivity occurs in the borderline leprosy reaction. Leprosy is a disease where protective immunity depends on cell-mediated immunity and where humoral immunity apparently plays no protective role.

There is a spectrum of disease dependent on the competence of the host's immune response; those with good responsiveness to the organism are 'tuberculoid', and those with no response, 'lepromatous'. In between these two extremes lies borderline leprosy, and these patients tend to develop characteristic reactions to the leprosy bacillus.

Borderline reactions occur either naturally or following drug treatment. In this case the hypopigmented skin lesions become swollen and inflamed (Fig. 22.19, left) with the histological appearance becoming more tuberculoid.

The same process may occur in peripheral nerves, and this is the most important cause of nerve destruction in this disease. The lesion in leprosy patients who have borderline reactivity is typical of granulomatous hypersensitivity (Fig. 22.19, right).

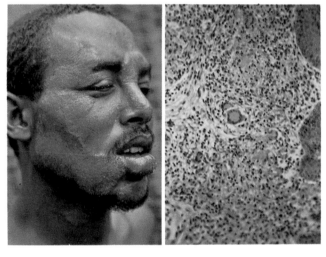

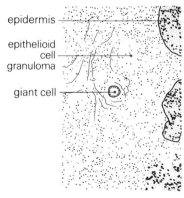

epidermis

epithelioid cell granuloma

giant cell

Fig. 22.19 A borderline leprosy reaction. The previously hypopigmented skin lesions have become swollen and inflamed following sensitization to antigens of *Mycobacterium leprae* (left). The histological appearance of the borderline leprosy reaction (right) is typical of granulomatous hypersensitivity. Note the giant cell and infiltration by monocytes and lymphocytes. H&E stain, ×140.

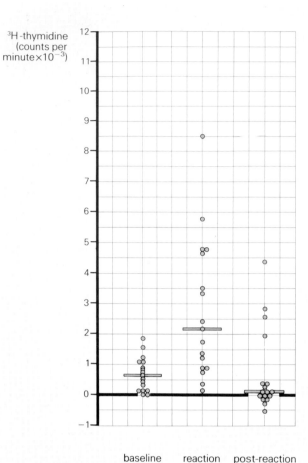

Fig. 22.20 Results of a LTT in a borderline leprosy reaction. During a borderline leprosy reaction, the lymphocyte transformation response to *M. leprae* rises, and there is a fall in response when the reaction is treated successfully. The lymphocyte transformation responses (uptake of ^{3}H-thymidine) to sonicated *M. leprae* are shown for 17 patients who developed such reactions:
(a) before starting steroid treatment (baseline) (b) during the reaction, and (c) on cessation of steroids. Medians are indicated by horizontal bars.

When a patient develops immunity associated with tuberculoid-type hypersensitivity T cell sensitization may be assessed *in vitro* by the lymphocyte transformation test using either whole or sonicated *Mycobacterium leprae* as the source of antigen (Fig. 22.20).

Tuberculosis

In tuberculosis there is granuloma formation in the lung and other infected organs. Lung damage caused by the granulomatous reaction leads to cavitation and spread of bacteria.

The reactions are frequently accompanied by extensive fibrosis and the lesions may be seen in the chest radiographs of affected patients (Fig. 22.21).

The histological appearance of the lesion is typical of a granulomatous reaction, with central caseous (cheesy) necrosis (Fig. 22.22).

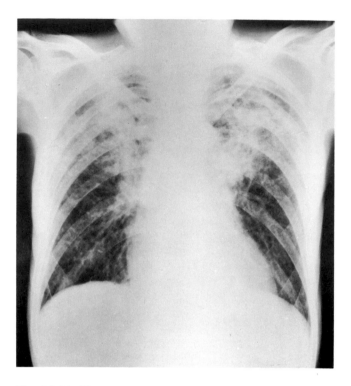

Fig. 22.21 Chest radiograph of a patient with pulmonary tuberculosis. This shows marked tuberculous infiltration of both lungs.

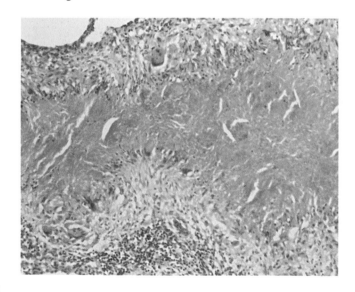

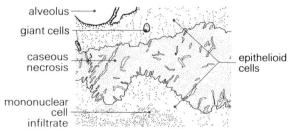

Fig. 22.22 Histological appearance of a tuberculous section of lung. This demonstrates epithelioid cell granuloma and giant cells typical of a granulomatous reaction. There is also marked caseation and necrosis within the area of the granulomatous reaction. Part of an alveolus is visible at the top left of the section. H&E stain, × 75

Sarcoidosis

Sarcoidosis is a disease of unknown aetiology, although it has been postulated that it might be due to an infectious agent such as mycobacterium, since the condition produces all the features of immunological granuloma formation frequently accompanied by fibrosis typical of mycobacterial infection (Fig. 22.23).

There may also be manifestations of Type III hypersensitivity such as cutaneous vasculitis or uveitis. The disease particularly affects lymphoid tissue and lymphadenopathy may be detected in chest radiographs of affected patients (Fig. 22.24).

One of the paradoxes of clinical immunology is that this disease is usually associated with the depression of delayed hypersensitivity both *in vivo* and *in vitro*. These patients are anergic on testing with tuberculin but when cortisone is injected with the tuberculin antigen, skin tests become positive. This suggests that cortisone-sensitive suppressor T cells are responsible for the anergy. Cortisone itself would normally suppress these responses.

Schistosomiasis

Another disease which exemplifies granulomatous hypersensitivity is schistosomiasis caused by parasitic trematode worms called schistosomes. The host becomes sensitized to the ova of the worms leading to a typical granulomatous reaction in the parasitized tissue (Fig. 22.25).

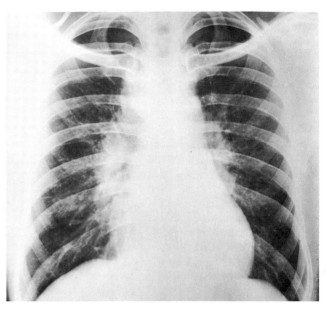

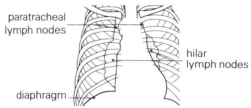

Fig. 22.24 The chest radiograph of a patient with sarcoidosis. There is bilateral hilar and paratracheal lymphadenopathy with diffuse pulmonary infiltration characteristic of the disease.

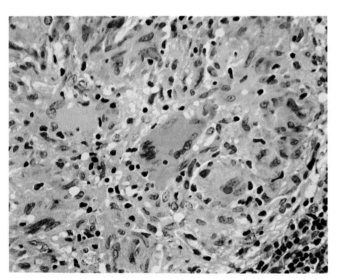

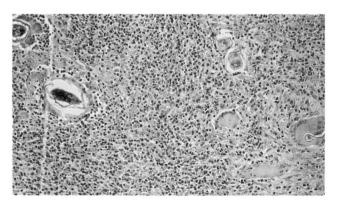

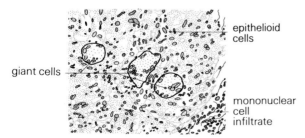

Fig. 22.23 Histological appearance of sarcoid lymph node tissue. This appearance is typical of epithelioid cell granuloma without necrosis. H&E stain, × 240.

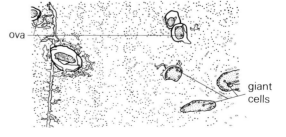

Fig. 22.25 Histological appearance of the liver in schistosomiasis. The epithelioid cell granuloma is surrounding ova of schistosomes. Note also the giant cells. H&E stain, ×100.

FURTHER READING

Bjune G., Barnetson R. StC., Ridley D.S. & Kronvall G. (1976) Lymphocyte transformation test in leprosy: correlation of the response with inflammation of lesions. *Clinical and Experimental Immunology* **25**, 85.

Turk J.L. (1980) *Delayed Hypersensitivity, 3rd edition.* Research Monographs in Immunology **1**. Elsevier/North Holland, Amsterdam.

Wolff K. & Stingl G. (1983) The Langerhans Cell. *Journal of Investigative Dermatology* **80**, supplement, 175.

23 Autoimmunity and Autoimmune Disease

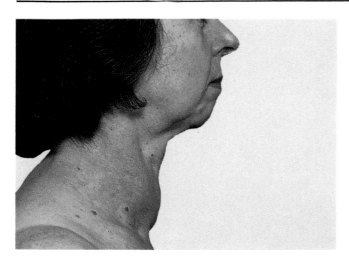

Fig.23.1 Enlarged thyroid in Hashimoto's thyroiditis.

The immune system has tremendous diversity and the repertoire of specificities expressed by the B and T cell populations are bound to include many which are directed to self-components. In earlier chapters, we have discussed the complicated mechanisms which the body must establish to distinguish between self and non-self determinants so as to avoid the embarrassment of auto-reactivity. However in the nature of things, all mechanisms have a risk of breakdown and the self-recognition mechanisms are no exception. So it is that a number of diseases have been identified in which there is copious production of autoantibodies and autoreactive T cells.

One of the earliest examples in which the production of autoantibodies associated with disease in a given organ was recognized was Hashimoto's thyroiditis. This is a disease of the thyroid which is more common in middle-aged women and often leads to formation of a goitre and to hypothyroidism. The gland is infiltrated, sometimes to an extraordinary extent, with inflammatory lymphoid cells (Fig.23.1). These are predominantly mononuclear cells of the lymphocytic and phagocytic series, and plasma cells: *secondary lymphoid follicles* are frequent features (Fig.23.2). The gland in Hashimoto's disease often shows regenerating follicles but this is not a feature of the thyroid in a related condition, primary myxoedema, in which comparable immunological features are seen but the gland undergoes almost complete destruction and shrinks (Fig.23.3).

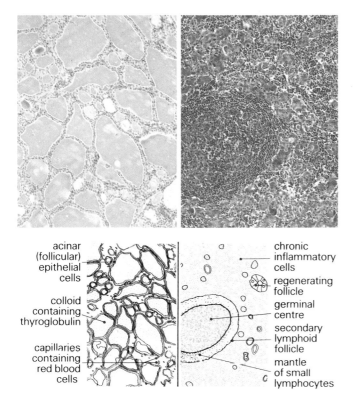

Fig. 23.2 Histological changes in Hashimoto's thyroiditis.
A normal thyroid showing the follicular cells lining the colloid space into which they secrete thyroglobulin, which is broken down on demand to provide thyroid hormones (left). A Hashimoto gland (right). The normal architecture is virtually destroyed and replaced by the invading cells which consist essentially of lymphocytes, macrophages and plasma cells. A secondary lymphoid follicle with a germinal centre and a small regenerating thyroid follicle are present. H & E stain, ×80.

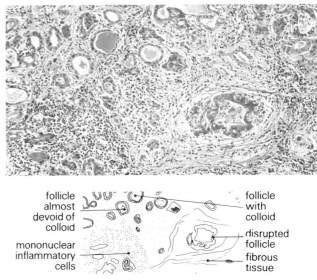

Fig. 23.3 Histological appearance of a primary myxoedema gland. There is destruction of the gland by chronic inflammatory cells associated with fibrosis. Isolated thyroid follicles, some in the process of breakdown, are seen. Unlike the appearance in Hashimoto's disease there is no tendency for follicular regeneration, and the gland shrinks instead of becoming a goitre. H & E stain, ×100.

The serum of patients with Hashimoto's disease usually contains antibodies to thyroglobulin, the major iodine-containing protein in the follicular fluid of the thyroid acinae, which acts as a depot for the thyroid hormone. These antibodies are demonstrable by immunofluorescence and also, when present in high titre, by precipitin reactions (Fig. 23.4). The immunofluorescence method led to the finding of antibodies directed against a cytoplasmic or microsomal antigen (Fig. 23.5).

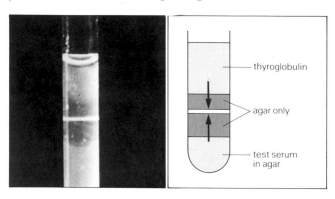

Fig.23.4 Thyroglobulin autoantibodies in the sera of Hashimoto patients demonstrated by precipitation in agar (Oudin's method). Test serum is incorporated into agar in the bottom of the tube; the layer above that contains agar only while the autoantigen, thyroglobulin, is present in the top layer. As serum antibody and thyroglobulin diffuse towards each other, they form a zone of opaque precipitate in the middle layer. The control serum is negative.

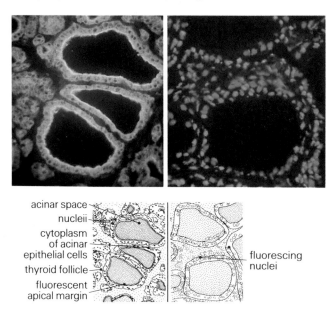

Fig.23.5 Autoantibodies to thyroid demonstrated with double layer immunofluorescence. An unfixed human thyroid section is treated successively with a patient's serum and then a fluoresceinated rabbit anti-human immunoglobulin. The acinar epithelial cells are stained by antibody in Hashimoto serum which reacts with cytoplasm (left). Note the unstained nuclei. The colloid is lost from the unfixed section so thyroglobulin staining is not seen. In contrast, serum from a patient with systemic lupus erythematosus contains antibodies which react with the nucleus but leave the cytoplasm unstained (right).

THE SPECTRUM OF AUTOIMMUNE DISEASES

The antibodies which we have just described react only with the thyroid, not any other tissues in the body. In contrast, the serum from patients with diseases such as systemic lupus erythematosus (SLE) reacts with many if not all the tissues in the body; in the particular case of SLE, one of the dominant antibodies is directed against the cell nucleus (see Fig.23.5). Diseases associated with autoimmune phenomena in fact tend to distribute themselves within a spectrum in which at one pole, typified by Hashimoto's thyroiditis, the antibodies and the invasive destructive lesion are directed against just one organ in the body whereas at the other end of the spectrum, typified by SLE, the antibodies are directed to antigens widespread throughout the body and the lesions characteristic of the disease are also widely disseminated. We speak of organ specific and non-organ specific diseases and in figure 23.6 the diseases are classified so that they lie within such a spectrum.

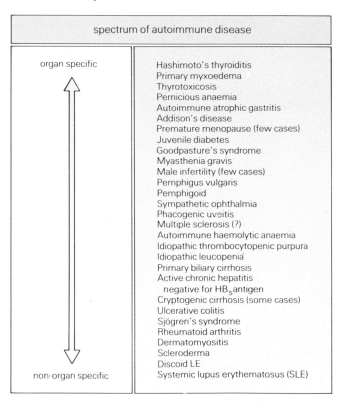

Fig.23.6 The spectrum of autoimmune diseases.

Common target organs affected in organ specific disease include thyroid, adrenal, stomach and pancreas, whereas the non-organ specific diseases, which include the so-called rheumatological disorders, involve skin, kidney, joints and muscle (Fig.23.7).

Interestingly, there are remarkable overlaps at each end of the spectrum. For example, thyroid antibodies occur with a high frequency in patients with pernicious anaemia who have stomach autoimmunity; furthermore, these patients even have a higher incidence of thyroid autoimmune disease than the normal population.

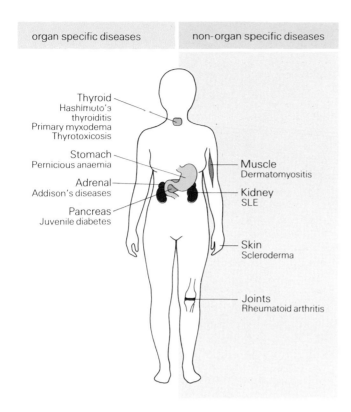

| organ specific diseases | non-organ specific diseases |

Thyroid
Hashimoto's
thyroiditis
Primary myxodema
Thyrotoxicosis

Stomach
Pernicious anaemia

Adrenal
Addison's diseases

Pancreas
Juvenile diabetes

Muscle
Dermatomyositis

Kidney
SLE

Skin
Scleroderma

Joints
Rheumatoid arthritis

Fig.23.7 Two types of autoimmune diseases – organ specific and non-organ specific. Examples are given of each. Although the organ non-specific diseases produce symptoms in different organs, particular diseases affect particular organs more markedly, eg. the kidney in SLE, the joint in rheumatoid arthritis etc.

In the same way, patients with thyroid autoimmunity have an abnormally high incidence of stomach autoantibodies and to a lesser extent, the clinical disease itself, pernicious anaemia. The cluster of rheumatological disorders at the non-organ specific end of the spectrum

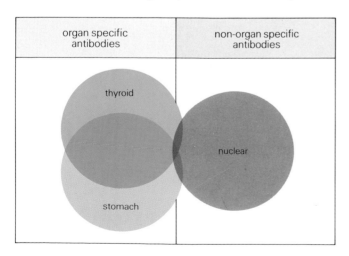

| organ specific antibodies | non-organ specific antibodies |

thyroid

nuclear

stomach

Fig. 23.8 Overlap of autoantibodies. The organ specific autoantibodies directed against thyroid and stomach often occur together in the same individual but there is little overlap with non-organ specific antibodies such as those with reactivity for nuclear components such as DNA and nucleoproteins.

shows considerable overlap amongst themselves and features of rheumatoid arthritis for example, are frequently associated with the clinical picture of SLE. In organ non-specific disease, complexes formed with the antigens involved deposit systemically, particularly in kidney, joints and skin so giving rise to the more disseminated features of the disease (Fig.23.8). In contrast, the overlap between diseases at the two ends of the spectrum is relatively rare, and cases in which thyroiditis and SLE occur together are extremely unusual; those reported are likely to be highly selective because they are so unusual. In the case of organ specific diseases, the lesions are restricted because the antigen in the organ acts as a target for immunological attack. Organ specific and non-organ specific disorders are compared in figure 23.9.

	organ specific	non-organ specific
antigen	essentially localized to given organ	widespread throughout the body
lesions	antigen in organ is target for immunological attack	complexes deposit systemically particularly in kidneys, joints and skin
overlap	with other organ-specific antibodies and diseases	with other non-organ specific antibodies and diseases

Fig.23.9 Comparison of organ specific and non-organ specific disorders.

GENETICS

There is an undoubted familial incidence of autoimmunity, a remarkable example of which is shown in figure 23.10.

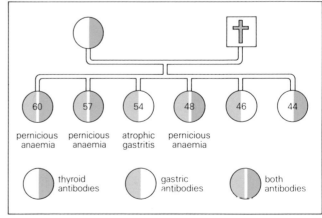

| 60 | 57 | 54 | 48 | 46 | 44 |

pernicious anaemia   pernicious anaemia   atrophic gastritis   pernicious anaemia

thyroid antibodies   gastric antibodies   both antibodies

Fig. 23.10 Autoimmunity in a family. The family chart shows the incidence of organic-specific abnormalities affecting the thyroid and stomach. Although the siblings present with gastric autoimmune disease (green), unlike the mother, who has primary myxoedema, there is a striking overlap with thyroid autoimmunity (blue) at the serological level, although the subjects lack clinical symptoms of thyroid disease. Autoantibodies are more prevalent with increasing age (ages are given at which autoantibodies were detected).

This familial incidence is almost certainly largely genetic rather than environmental, as may be seen from studies of identical and non-identical twins and from the association of, say, thyroid autoantibodies with abnormalities of the X-chromosome.

Just as there is an overlap between organ specific disorders in given individuals, so the tendency to develop autoimmunity within families tends to show a bias towards organ specific autoimmunity (Fig.23.11). In addition to this predisposition to develop organ specific antibodies, it is clear that other genetically controlled factors tend to select the organ which will be largely affected. It is interesting to note that although relatives of Hasimoto patients have a higher than expected incidence and titre of thyroid autoantibodies and that the same is seen in pernicious anaemia relatives, the latter are distinguished by having a far higher frequency of gastric autoantibodies indicating that the stomach as an organ is being differentially selected within the pernicious anaemia relative group.

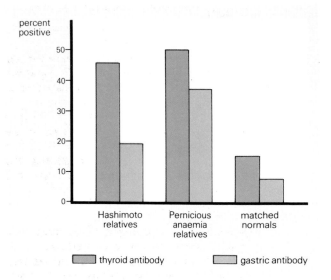

Fig.23.11 **Thyroid and stomach antibodies in first degree relatives of patients with Hashimoto's disease or pernicious anaemia.** A remarkably high proportion of the first degree relatives of Hashimoto patients have thyroid autoantibodies and to a lesser degree parietal cell (gastric) autoantibodies. The pernicious anaemia relatives also have a very high incidence of thyroid autoimmunity, indicative of a predisposition to develop organ specific autoantibodies; the percentage with gastric autoantibodies is also high even when compared with the Hashimoto relatives, suggesting an inherent bias of the immune system for reactivity against particular organs.

Further evidence for the operation of genetic factors in autoimmune diseases comes from the realization that in general they tend to show associations with particular HLA specificities (Fig.23.12). The haplotype B8,DR3 occurs with particular frequency in the organ specific diseases, although Hashimoto's disease tends to be associated more with DR5. Rheumatoid arthritis, which originally showed no HLA associations when only the specificities at the A and B loci were studied has now

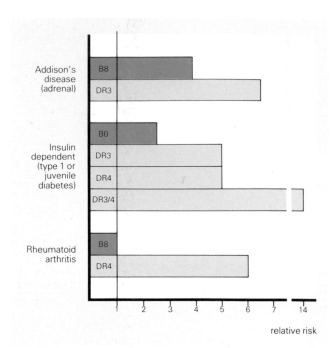

Fig.23.12 **HLA associations in autoimmune disease.** The relative risk is a measure of the increased chance of contracting the disease for individuals bearing the antigen relative to those lacking it. Virtually all autoimmune diseases studied show an association with some HLA specificity. The greater relative risk for Addison's disease associated with DR3 as compared with B8 suggests that DR3 is closer to, if not identical with, the 'disease susceptibility gene'. In this case B8 has a relative risk greater than 1 because it is known to occur together with DR3 more often than expected by chance in the population, a phenomenon termed linkage disequilibrium. Both DR3 and DR4 are associated with type 1 diabetes but strikingly, the DR3/4 heterozygote shows a greatly increased relative risk supporting the concept of multiple genetic factors. Rheumatoid arthritis is linked to HLA-DR4 but not to any HLA-A or B specificities.

been shown to be associated with HLA-Dw4 and DR4: individuals with this tissue type have a higher chance of developing the disease. Of note is the finding that in the organ specific disease, insulin-dependent or Type 1 diabetes, heterozygotes for DR3 and DR4 have a greatly increased relative risk. This supports the concept of several genetic factors being involved in the development of autoimmune diseases and these must include factors predisposing individuals to develop autoimmunity, either of the organ specific or non-organ specific kind, and others which determine the particular antigen or antigens to be implicated.

PATHOGENESIS

If autoantibodies are found in association with a particular disease there are logically three possible implications. Either:
1. the autoimmunity is responsible for producing the lesions characteristic of the disease,

2. there is a separate disease process which, through the production of tissue damage, leads secondarily to the development of autoantibodies,

3. it is possible that some quite separate factor directly produces both the lesions and the autoimmunity (Fig. 23.13).

Autoantibodies secondary to a lesion have been found in some circumstances as, for example, the cardiac auto-antibodies which may follow myocardial infarction. However, in many other cases, the autoantibodies are rarely induced following release of the autoantigens in question by simple trauma. The first proposition, namely that a number of diseases are caused by the autoimmune process is an attractive hypothesis and evidence will be adduced which is consistent with this view.

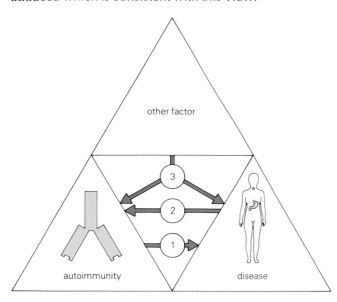

Fig. 23.13 Implications of an association of disease with autoimmunity. Three explanations for an association are possible: 1. autoimmunity may produce the disease, 2. the disease is responsible for the generation of autoimmunity, or 3. a third factor may lead to both.

The most direct test of the hypothesis is to say that if autoimmunity is responsible for the lesions of a given disease, then deliberate induction of autoimmunity in an experimental animal should lead to the production of those lesions. In fact, it is possible to provoke certain organ specific diseases in experimental animals by injecting the antigen in question with Complete Freund's Adjuvant. Figure 23.14 gives examples in which thyroglobulin can induce an inflammatory disease of the thyroid while myelin basic protein can bring about the production of encephalomyelitis in animals so autoimmunized. Strict organ specificity may be seen since the lesions are confined in both cases to those organs or organ systems in which the antigen used for immunization is located. In the case of the thyroglobulin-injected animals, not only are thyroid autoantibodies produced but the gland becomes infiltrated with mononuclear cells and the acinar architecture crumbles under their influence (Fig. 23.15). Although not identical in every respect with Hashimoto's disease, the thyroiditis produced bears a remarkable overall similarity to the human condition.

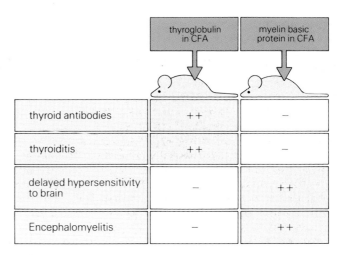

	thyroglobulin in CFA	myelin basic protein in CFA
thyroid antibodies	+ +	−
thyroiditis	+ +	−
delayed hypersensitivity to brain	−	+ +
Encephalomyelitis	−	+ +

Fig. 23.14 Deliberate induction of autoimmunity to produce diseases in the organ containing the autoantigen. Injection of an aqueous solution of thyroglobulin in Complete Freund's Adjuvant (CFA) produces thyroid antibodies and a destructive inflammatory lesion in the thyroid reminiscent of that seen in Hashimoto's thyroiditis. Immunization with the basic protein from myelin in CFA induces T cell activity, demonstrable as delayed hypersensitivity, which leads to paralysis due to demyelination associated with lymphoid infiltration (encephalomyelitis).

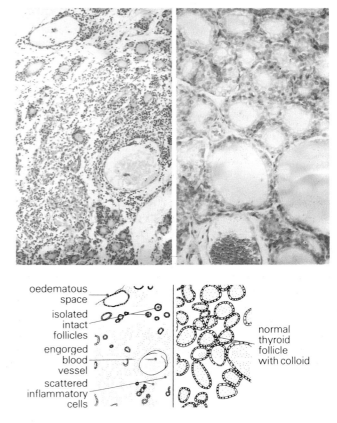

Fig. 23.15 The histological appearance of experimental autoallergic thyroiditis. In the section from a thyroglobulin-injected animal (left, ×200) there is gross destruction of the follicular architecture with extensive invasion by mononuclear inflammatory cells, associated with distended blood vessels, oedema and fibrosis. A control section is shown (right, ×110). H & E stain.

There is much to learn from spontaneous examples of autoimmune disease in animals. One well-established example is the Obese strain chicken in which thyroid autoantibodies occur spontaneously and the thyroid undergoes progressive destruction associated with a chronic inflammatory lesion (Fig.23.16).

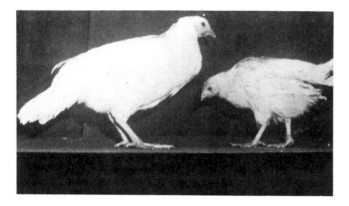

Fig.23.16   The Obese strain (OS) chicken: an example of spontaneously occurring autoimmune thyroid disease in animals. The birds grow poorly and look dishevelled because of the thyroxine deficiency which results from thyroid destruction.

If one examines the sera of these animals, not only do they show thyroglobulin autoantibodies, but approximately 15% react with the proventriculus (stomach) of the normal chicken giving a pattern similar to that obtained if the test is carried out with the sera from patients with pernicious anaemia who have parietal cell autoantibodies (Fig. 23.17).

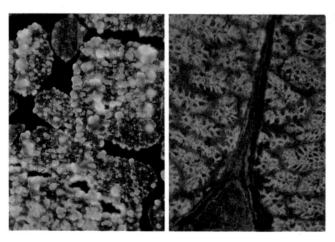

Fig.23.17   Autoantibodies in OS chickens. Fluorescent staining of a fixed thyroid section showing reaction in colloid (left). Approximately 15% of the birds have serum antibodies which stain the chicken stomach (proventriculus) giving the characteristic pattern shown (right) which is also seen if human sera containing parietal cell antibodies are tested against this organ.

This parallels spontaneous human autoimmune thyroid disease both in terms of the lesion in the gland, the production of antibodies to different components in the

thyroid, and lastly the overlap with gastric autoimmunity. When the immunological status of these animals is altered, quite dramatic effects on the outcome of the disease are seen. For example, if the bursa of Fabricius is removed soon after hatching, the severity of the thyroiditis is greatly diminished, indicating a role for antibody in the pathogenesis of the disease (Fig.23.18). Paradoxically, removal of the thymus at birth appears to exacerbate the lesion suggesting that the thymus in some way is exerting a controlling effect on the outcome of the disease. Clearly, the severity of the disease process is significantly influenced by the state of the immune system and this would be consistent with an important role for immunological processes in the causation of the disease.

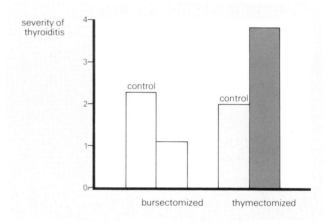

Fig.23.18   Modification of thyroiditis in Obese strain chickens by neonatal bursectomy and thymectomy. Neonatal bursectomy reduces the spontaneous development of thyroiditis suggesting an important role for antibody in the pathogenesis of the lesions. Paradoxically, removal of the thymus at birth exacerbates the disease indicating a controlling effect of T-suppressor cells. The severity of thyroiditis is assessed by lymphocyte infiltration.

With human autoimmunity it is of course more difficult to carry out direct experiments because of ethical limitations but there is a great deal of evidence which favours the view that the autoantibodies are of importance in pathogenesis. A number of diseases have been recognized in which autoantibodies to hormone receptors are present which may actually mimic the function of the normal hormone concerned (Fig.23.19). Thyrotoxicosis was perhaps the first disorder in which anti-receptor antibodies were clearly recognized and the phenomenon of neonatal thyrotoxicosis provides us with a 'natural' passive transfer study in which the IgG antibodies from the mother, can cross the placenta and if they are capable of acting *in vivo*, should stimulate the thyroid of the baby. Indeed, many examples of babies born to thyrotoxic mothers showing thyroid hyperactivity have been reported (Fig.23.20). As might be expected, as the maternally derived thyroid stimulating IgG is catabolized in the baby over several weeks, so the overactivity of the thyroid spontaneously resolves. A similar phenomenon has been observed in neonatal myasthenia gravis, where antibodies to acetyl choline receptors cross the placenta into the foetus and cause transient muscle weakness.

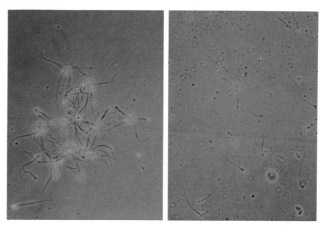

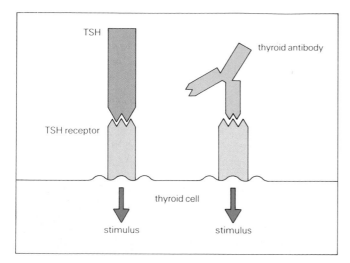

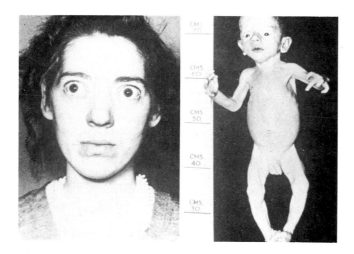

Fig.23.19 Autoimmunity to cell surface receptors. The thyroid cell is stimulated when its receptors for thyroid stimulating hormone (TSH, from the pituitary) bind the hormone (left). Antibody to the TSH receptor present in the serum of a patient with thyrotoxicosis (Graves' or Basedow's disease) combines with the receptor in a similar fashion to pituitary TSH thereby delivering a comparable stimulus to the thyroid cell (right).

Fig.23.20 Neonatal thyrotoxicosis. The TSH-receptor autoantibodies are IgG and therefore cross the placenta. If they act *in vivo* the baby should show evidence of thyroid stimulation. The appearance of both mother and child is characteristic of thyrotoxicosis.

Yet another example of autoimmune disease is seen in rare cases of male infertility where antibodies to spermatozoa lead to the clumping of spermatozoa either by their heads or their tails in the semen (Fig.23.21). It is surely difficult to imagine that spermatozoa in this stage of aggregation would be capable of the hard swim required to fertilize the ovum. A small proportion of cases of male infertility have been attributed to this cause.

In the disease pernicious anaemia, an autoantibody interferes with the normal uptake of oral vitamin B_{12}. B_{12} is not absorbed directly but must first associate with a protein called intrinsic factor, the complex then being transported across the intestinal mucosa. Early studies of

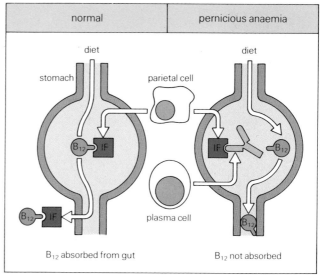

Fig.23.21 Sperm agglutination. The presence of sperm autoagglutinins produces either head to head (left) or tail to tail (right) agglutination.

pernicious anaemia demonstrated that the intrinsic factor-mediated uptake of oral vitamin B_{12} could be inhibited if the intrinsic factor: B_{12} complex was fed together with serum from the patient. Evidently there is a factor (antibody) in the serum of pernicious anaemia patients which blocks the uptake of the B_{12}: intrinsic factor complex. It is known that plasma cells in the gastric mucosa of patients with this disease secrete antibodies directed against intrinsic factor into the lumen of the stomach and it would therefore seem probable, based on the results of these experiments, to consider that such antibodies mixed with intrinsic factor derived from parietal cells would block the physiological action of this protein in transporting dietary vitamin B_{12} into the body (Fig.23.22).

normal	pernicious anaemia

diet   diet

stomach   parietal cell

B_{12} IF   IF B_{12}

plasma cell

B_{12} IF B_{12}

B_{12} absorbed from gut B_{12} not absorbed

Fig.23.22 Failure of vitamin B_{12} absorption in pernicious anaemia. Normally, dietary B_{12} is transported across the small intestine into the body as a complex with intrinsic factor synthesized by the parietal cells in the gastric mucosa. In pernicious anaemia, locally synthesized intrinsic-factor specific autoantibodies occur in the gastric juice and combine with intrinsic factor to inhibit its role as a carrier for B_{12} which now cannot be absorbed.

An excellent study bearing on the point in question, was carried out in Goodpasture's syndrome in which antibodies to the glomerular capillary basement membrane are bound to the kidney *in vivo* (Fig.23.23, left). These antibodies were eluted from the kidney of a patient who died with this disease and transferred to a primate whose antigens were sufficiently similar to those of the human for the injected antibodies to localize on the glomerular basement membrane of the kidney. The injected monkeys subsequently died with glomerulonephritis, the disease which proved fatal for the original patient.

In contrast to the linear staining seen in Goodpasture's syndrome kidney biopsies from patients with SLE show punctate staining of irregular deposits using fluorescent anti-human IgG (Fig. 23.23, right). Since a fluorescent anti-C3 gives a similar staining pattern, it has been assumed that what is revealed are complexes deposited in the kidney. In other words, the lesion in the kidney is associated with the deposition of complexes. The production of chronic immune complex disease by repeated injection of high doses of antigen also leads to the deposition of complexes in the kidney associated with glomerulonephritis and proteinurea. Turning to experimental animals, the hybrid of the New Zealand black and white strains provides a spontaneous model of murine SLE in which immune complex glomerulonephritis and anti-DNA antibodies are major features (Fig.23.24). What is particularly relevant to our argument, is that measures which suppress the immune response in these animals (eg. the drug cyclophosphamide), likewise suppress the development of disease and prolong the survival of these mice.

Taken together, all these studies provide powerful evidence that in many circumstances the autoimmune process appears to play a dominant role in the causation of disease.

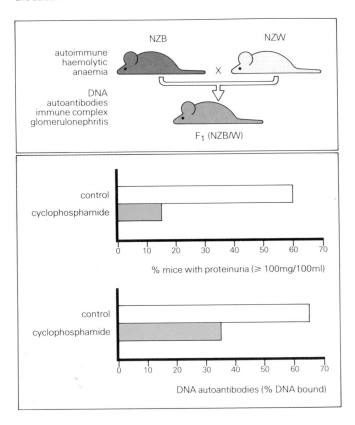

Fig.23.24 Suppression of autoimmune disease in NZB/W hybrids. The New Zealand Black spontaneously develops autoimmune haemolytic anaemia and when crossed with the New Zealand White strain, the F_1 develops DNA autoantibodies and immune complex glomerulonephritis like patients with SLE. Immunosuppression with cyclophosphamide (an anti-mitotic agent) considerably reduces the severity of the glomerulonephritis and the DNA autoantibodies showing the relevance of the immune processes to the generation of the disease.

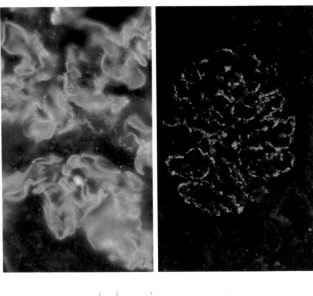

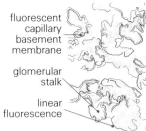

Fig.23.23 Immunofluorescent studies in Goodpasture's syndrome (left) and SLE (right). The presence of antibodies bound to the glomerular capillary basement membrane are revealed by immunofluorescent staining with fluoresceinated anti-human antibody. Note the linear staining pattern. The same antibody also binds to basement membrane in the lung. By contrast the irregular deposits of complexes in the SLE kidney produce a 'punctate' pattern.

AETIOLOGY

It is generally accepted that self-reactive lymphocytes exist in the body and some of the evidence for this is listed in figure 23.25. In addition, the autoantigens with which they can react, even proteins such as thyroglobulin which was previously thought to be secluded within the thyroid, are now known to be available to the recirculating lymphocyte pool. We therefore have a situation in which both self-reactive lymphocytes and autoantigen can make contact in the normal individual and therefore there

Evidence for self-reactive lymphocytes

1. thyroglobulin in CFA and other adjuvants (eg. lipopolysaccharide, poly A:U) induces autoimmunity in normal animals

2. small percentage of normal B cells bind self-thyroglobulin to surface

3. brain specific T cell line from normal rat induces encephalomyelitis

4. lymphocytes cultured with syngeneic testes or thyroid become autosensitized

Fig.23.25 Evidence for self-reactive lymphocytes.

must be controlling mechanisms which operate in normal circumstances to inhibit the triggering of the autoimmune reaction. It seems most likely that the operation of suppressor cells will be demonstrated as an important component in the containment of this autoreactivity. Figure 23.26 outlines a possible scheme by which the normal controls on autoreactivity may be by-passed. These controls include different types of suppressor T cells which go to make up a complex of T-suppressor activity. For a fuller discussion of this subject see 'Immunological Tolerance'. It has been postulated that defects in perhaps more than one type of T-suppressor may be important for the development of an autoimmune response.

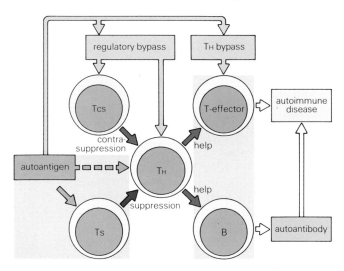

Fig.23.26 Autoimmune disease resulting from evasion of the controls on autoreactivity. Self-reactive B cells, T effector cells and autoantigens are all normally present (indicated in this and later figures by blue backshading) but T-helper cells capable of inducing an autoimmune response are functionally absent, either due to clonal abortion or the action of T-suppressor cells (antigen-, idiotype-, or non-specific). Thus the self-reactive T cells and B cells are not activated. (Idiotype-specific Ts cells may also act directly on B cells.) Autoimmunity may arise by a regulatory bypass which either causes direct activation of the TH cell or by activating another cell, the T-contrasuppressor (Tcs), which renders the TH cell resistant to suppression. The existence of contrasuppressors is still equivocal. Autoantigen could also bypass the TH cell to directly stimulate T-effectors and B cells.

It is interesting to note that studies on the clinically unaffected relatives of patients with SLE share with the patients themselves a defect in the generation of non-specific T-suppressors, suggesting first that the defect is not a consequence of the disease, and secondly that it is unable by itself to cause SLE. This is consistent with the previous discussion indicating several factors in the causation of autoimmune disease and it may be necessary to postulate further abnormalities in either antigen-specific or idiotype-specific regulatory T cells.

Some cell surface receptor molecules might be immunologically 'silent' because the cell membrane does not express MHC class 2 molecules; recent work showing that thyroid cells can be induced to make HLA-D molecules on stimulation with the plant lectin, phytohaemagglutinin has provoked the intriguing suggestion that inappropriate expression of such class 2 molecules may enable a surface receptor to stimulate autoreactive cells. In effect the tissue cell now acts as an antigen-presenting cell (Fig. 23.27).

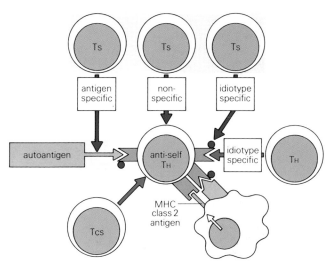

Fig.23.27 Induction of autoimmunity through bypass of regulatory mechanisms. The anti-self T-helper cell may be triggered through defects in antigen specific Ts, non-specific Ts or idiotype specific Ts, which would counteract the action of idiotype specific TH. (There is evidence that the various types of Ts may induce the activity of the others via soluble factors.) Stimulation of contrasuppressors (Tcs) can render the anti-self TH cells insusceptible to suppression, while the inappropriate cellular expression of MHC class 2 antigens on a cell carrying an autoantigen could convert that cell into an antigen-presenting cell to the autoreactive TH cell. In this scheme an idiotype specific TH cell is shown acting via the idiotype on the anti-self TH cell.

These are not the only possibilities however, and other not necessarily exclusive factors could operate. Particular interest was aroused by the suggestions of Allison and Weigle that a T cell bypass mechanism might operate. It was argued that since the unresponsiveness of the final effector T and B cells could be a consequence of suppression or tolerization of the autoantigen specific T-helper cells (inducer T cells) any circumstances leading to the circumvention of these tolerant T cells would lead directly to the triggering of effector lymphocytes.

A number of different ways in which this could be achieved are outlined in figures 23.28 – 23.30. A novel idea presented in figure 23.30 is that the idiotype network could be involved through triggering of a self-reactive T or B cell carrying a public idiotype cross-reacting with the idiotype on an antibody stimulated by microbial agents or with a structure on the microbe itself. Even in this case, it seems unlikely that the autoimmune response would be maintained unless there was some defect in the anti-idiotypic T-suppressor cell and this re-emphasizes the considerable importance of multiple factors in the establishment of prolonged autoimmunity.

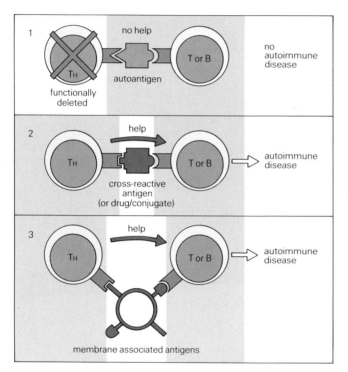

Fig.23.28 Induction of autoimmunity by T cell bypass-1. Normally autoimmune disease does not occur since T cells reacting with autoantigen are functionally deleted or suppressed (1). In the presence of a cross-reacting antigen a new population of T$_H$ cells reacting with a foreign carrier determinant can supply help (2). The binding of a drug to self-antigen may act as the determinant recognized by the T$_H$ cells, that is, a carrier determinant. The new carrier determinant can either be on a molecule which also bears the autoantigenic determinant (as in 2) or it can be on a different molecule associated with the autoantigen on a cell membrane (3).

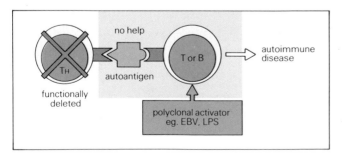

Fig.23.29 Induction of autoimmunity by T cell bypass-2. Self-reactive cells can be stimulated directly by polyclonal activators eg. Epstein Barr virus or bacterial lipopolysaccharides.

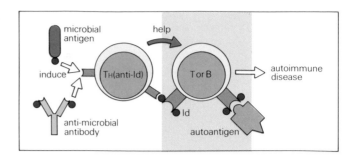

Fig.23.30 Induction of autoimmunity by stimulation via idiotype. Autoimmunity could arise if self-reactive T or B cells carry a public idiotype (Id) which cross-reacts with the idiotype on antibody stimulated by a microbial agent or even with a structure on the microbe itself.

DIAGNOSTIC AND PROGNOSTIC ASPECTS

Whatever the relationship of autoantibodies to the disease process, it is undeniable that they provide valuable markers which can be exploited for diagnostic purposes and indeed in the clinical immunology laboratory of today, tests for a wide range of different autoantibodies are carried out with this end in view. A particularly good example is the test for mitochondrial antibodies for distinguishing primary biliary cirrhosis (Fig.23.31). This differential diagnosis avoids the need for exploratory laparotomy which was previously necessary, and was often hazardous because of the age and condition of the patients concerned.

The autoantibodies may have a predictive value. For example, figure 23.32 shows a case in which a child related to siblings with insulin-dependent diabetes shared an HLA haplotype with them and developed complement fixing antibodies to the islet cells of the pancreas. Within 3 years after the study had begun, the sibling became frankly diabetic, showing the predictive value of these antibodies and the relatively long period of time before the disease becomes overt.

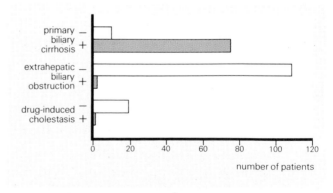

Fig.23.31 Diagnostic value of anti-mitochondrial antibodies. Mitochondrial antibody tests using indirect immunofluorescence together with percutaneous liver biopsy can be used to assist in differential diagnosis of the diseases listed above. A large proportion of primary biliary cirrhosis patients have anti-mitochondrial antibodies but this is rare in the other diseases.

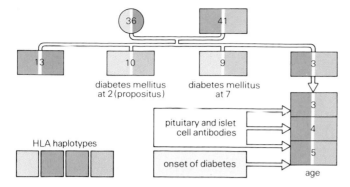

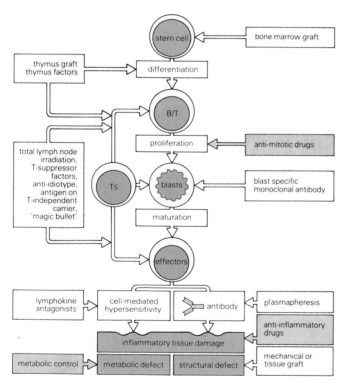

Fig.23.32 Prospective study of a family with insulin dependent diabetes. The sibling sharing a haplotype with the propositus and having complement fixing islet cell antibodies became diabetic 3 years after the study had begun.

TREATMENT

Conventionally, in organ specific disorders, the lesion can very often be corrected by metabolic control. For

Fig.23.33 The treatment of autoimmune disease. Current treatments for arresting the pathological developments are shown in dark grey, those that may become feasible, in light grey. For example, anti-mitotic drugs are given in serious cases of SLE or chronic active hepatitis. Anti-inflammatory drugs are widely prescribed in rheumatoid arthritis. Organ specific disorders such as primary myxoedema or pernicious anaemia which lead to a metabolic defect can usually be treated by supplying the defective component, in the examples cited, thyroid hormone and depot vitamin B₁₂. Where a live graft becomes necessary, the immunosuppressive therapy used may protect the tissue from autoimmune damage.

example, in hypothyroidism the lack of thyroid hormone can be controlled by administration of thyroxine while in thyrotoxicosis, anti-thyroid drugs are normally prescribed. In pernicious anaemia, metabolic correction is achieved by injection of depot vitamin B_{12} and in myasthenia gravis by administration of cholinesterase inhibitors. Where function is completely lost and cannot be substituted for by hormones, as may happen in lupus nephritis or chronic rheumatoid arthritis, mechanical or tissue grafts may be appropriate but in the latter case protection from the immunological processes which originally necessitated the transplant may be required.

Conventional immunosuppressive therapy with anti-mitotic drugs may be employed to damp down the immune response but because of the dangers involved, this tends to be used only in life-threatening disorders such as SLE and dermatomyositis. Anti-inflammatory drugs are, of course, prescribed for rheumatoid disease.

As we understand more about the precise defects in different autoimmune diseases and learn how to manipulate the immunological status of the patient, a number of the less well established approaches may become practical (Fig.23.33). In particular, the exploitation of the idiotype network to inhibit the idiotypes on T-inducer and effector cells could provide a promising approach.

POSITIVE INDUCTION OF AUTOIMMUNITY

There are areas in which the deliberate induction of an autoimmune response would be desirable (Fig.23.34). Although these represent academically feasible enterprises, the major (but not the only) problems in man concern the identification of the correct autoreactive epitopes which do not cross-react with other autoantigens, the attachment to an effective carrier, and the identification of an acceptable adjuvant.

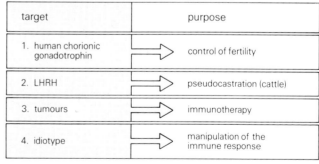

target	purpose
1. human chorionic gonadotrophin	control of fertility
2. LHRH	pseudocastration (cattle)
3. tumours	immunotherapy
4. idiotype	manipulation of the immune response

Fig.23.34 Positive induction of autoimmunity.
1. HCG is necessary for the maintenance of the implanted ovum at an early stage in pregnancy. Autoimmunization to the unique determinants on HCG (not shared with pituitary hormones such as LH) by coupling to carrier such as tetanus toxoid provides a basis for a possible contraceptive vaccine.
2. Neutralization of the releasing hormone for LH by autoimmunization can produce pseudo-castration in cattle.
3. The destruction of tumours through identification and exploration of tumour specific antigens has for long been a 'holy grail' for cancer immunologists.
4. Monoclonal anti-idiotypes may well have a potential for either boosting or damping down immune responses.

23.11

FURTHER READING

Cunningham A. J. (1975) Active suppressor mechanisms maintaining tolerance to some self components. *Nature* **254,** 143.

Davies, T. F. (ed) (1983) *Autoimmune Endocrine Disease.* John Wiley & Sons, New York.

Lachmann P. J. & Peters D. K. (eds) (1982) *Clinical Aspects of Immunology,* 4th edn. Blackwell Scientific Publications, Oxford.

Marchalonis J. J. & Cohen N. (eds) (1980) *Self/Non-self Discrimination.* Contemporary Topics in Immunobiology, Vol. 9. Plenum Press, New York.

Sites D. P., Stubo J. D., Fudenberg H. H. & Wells J. V. (1984) *Basic and Clinical Immunology,* 5th edn. Lange Medical Publications, Los Altos, California.

Yamamura T. & Tada T. (eds) (1984) *Progress in Immunology V.* Academic Press, Tokyo.

24 Transplantation and Rejection

Tissue transplantation is the third area (after hypersensitivity and autoimmunity) in which the immune system acts detrimentally. The phenomenon of graft rejection between unrelated individuals has been recognized for a long time but it is only since the 1950s that this has been shown to be due to the adaptive immune system. Graft rejection displays the two key features of adaptive immunity namely, memory and specificity. These characteristics can be demonstrated by grafting skin from one animal to another. Memory is demonstrated when a second allogeneic skin graft from one donor is rejected by the recipient more quickly than the first graft from that donor. This accelerated rejection is specific for the one donor – it is observed that grafts from other individuals applied at the same time do not suffer faster rejection (Fig. 24.1). These two types of rejection reaction are referred to as 'first set' and 'second set' reactions.

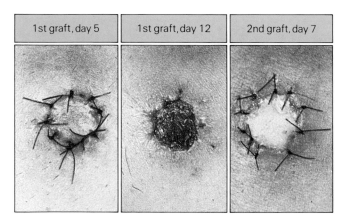

| 1st graft, day 5 | 1st graft, day 12 | 2nd graft, day 7 |

Fig. 24.1 Graft rejection displays immunological memory. A human skin allograft at day 5 (left) is fully vascularized and the cells are dividing, but by day 12 it is totally destroyed (middle). A second graft from the same donor (right) shown here on day 7 does not become vascularized and is destroyed rapidly. This indicates that sensitization to the first graft produces immunological memory.

Only sites in the recipient which are accessible to the immune system are susceptible to the graft rejection phenomenon. There are certain 'privileged' sites in the body where allogeneic grafts can survive indefinitely. It is also found that the ability to reject grafts can be transferred with previously sensitized lymphocytes. These, and many other observations, confirm the responsibility of the immune system for graft rejection. In view of the unphysiological nature of tissue transplantation it may seem surprising that the immune system has thrown such a formidable barrier in the path of transplantation surgery but it appears that this is an unfortunate side effect of a system which has evolved to recognize and destroy virally-altered cells.

GENETICS OF TRANSPLANTATION

In 1914 Little proposed that successful transplantation would depend on the donor and recipient sharing a number of independently segregating alleles, in effect histocompatibility genes. This hypothesis has been confirmed in all mammalian species studied, a process which was greatly facilitated by the development of haplotype identical inbred strains of mice (see 'MHC'). Grafting between such isogeneic mouse strains showed that animals could reject any graft carrying allogeneic histocompatibility determinants and would accept any graft that did not have allogeneic determinants (Fig. 24.2). These observations also confirm that histocompatibility genes are co-dominantly expressed in the F_1 animals.

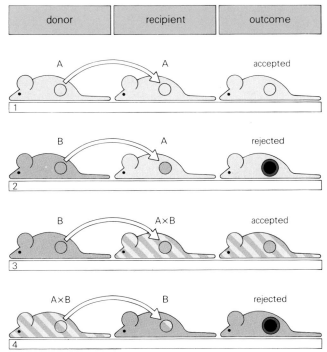

| donor | recipient | outcome |

Fig. 24.2 The laws of transplantation. Grafts between genetically identical animals are accepted. Grafts between genetically non-identical animals are rejected with a speed which is dependent on where the genetic differences lie. For example, syngeneic animals which are identical at the MHC locus, accept grafts from each other (1). Animals which differ at the MHC locus reject grafts from each other (2). The ability to accept a graft is dependent on the recipient sharing all the donor's histocompatibility genes. This is illustrated by grafting between parental and F_1 (A × B) animals (3 and 4). Animals which differ at loci other than the MHC reject grafts from each other, but much more slowly. Exceptions to these rules are discussed below.

In special circumstances there are exceptions to these simple rules. The first exception is seen where animals have been tolerized to the donor tissue either by having encountered the donor tissue antigens during neonatal life, or through immunopharmacological manipulation as described in 'Immunological Tolerance'. Indeed, the ability to accept grafts between allogeneic individuals is viewed as the most stringent criterion of immunological tolerance to allogeneic tissue. The second exception can be seen when immunocompetent cells are transferred from a donor to an allogeneic recipient which is incapable of reacting against them. In this case the donor cells react to the recipient's tissues, particularly those of the skin, gut epithelia and the liver and may destroy them. This is known as graft versus host disease (Fig. 24.3). The precise mechanism by which the recipient's cells are damaged is uncertain since many of the cells seen at the sites of damage are of recipient origin. Nevertheless, the condition is frequently fatal and graft versus host disease is a problem which is particularly associated with bone marrow transplantation.

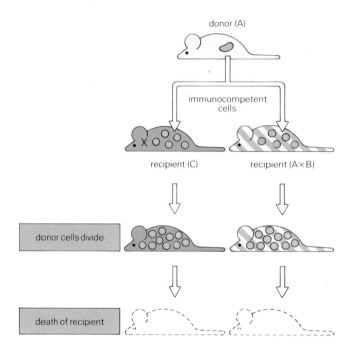

Fig.24.3 Graft versus host disease. Immunocompetent cells from a donor of type 'A' are injected into an immunosuppressed (X-irradiated) host of type 'C' or a normal F_1 (A × B) recipient. The immunosuppressed individual is unable to reject the cells and the F_1 animal is fully tolerant to parental type 'A' cells. In both cases the donor cells recognize the foreign tissue types 'B' and 'C' of the recipient. They divide and react against the recipient tissue cells and recruit large numbers of host cells to inflammatory sites. Very often the process leads to the death of the recipient.

Another exception to the basic scheme of figure 24.2 is noted where female mice reject skin grafts from autosomally isogeneic males. This is a function of a histocompatibility gene (H-Y) located on the Y chromosome which the female mice lack and therefore react against (Fig. 24.4). Unlike many other histocompatibility antigens H-Y appears to be monomorphic in different strains.

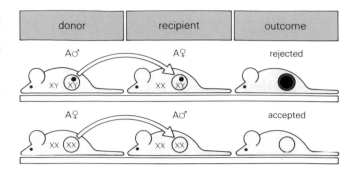

Fig.24.4 The H-Y antigen. Female mice will reject a graft from male mice of the same strain while the reciprocal graft (ie. female to male) is accepted. The rejection is due to the recognition of an antigen (H-Y) encoded by the Y chromosome and which is therefore, only present on male cells.

HISTOCOMPATIBILITY GENES

Genetic studies on the segregation of histocompatibility genes have demonstrated a large number of independently segregating loci in all species. As many as thirty different loci have been identified in mice designated H1, H2, etc. However, in all species there is one locus, the major histocompatibility complex, which elicits stronger allogeneic reactions than the others. With the discovery of the importance of the MHC in many other immune reactions (as described in previous sections), the minor histocompatibility loci have been less well studied. Nevertheless, second set allogeneic rejection reactions to minor locus antigens, or to minor locus differences may be as fast as to an MHC allogeneic graft (Fig. 24.5). In man it is found that approximately 50% of kidney grafts between HLA-matched siblings are rejected after five years suggesting that in man also, minor loci differences are sufficient to cause rejection. In spite of this, the major obstacle to successful transplantation is the MHC, since rejection arising from allogeneic differences of minor loci can usually be overcome by immunosuppressive therapy provided the recipient has not been previously sensitized to the minor locus antigens.

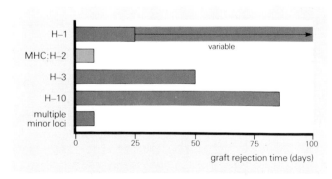

Fig.24.5 Histocompatibility antigens and graft survival. This chart gives the rejection time for skin grafts between individuals differing at the minor histocompatibility loci (red) or at the MHC locus (H-2) (turquoise) listed. Grafts which differ at multiple minor loci are rejected as quickly as those that differ at H-2. Data from Graff & Bailey.

THE ROLE OF T CELLS

Evidence has accumulated which indicates that the T cell is mainly responsible for rejection of solid grafts. First, nude mice do not reject foreign skin grafts. It is even possible to give nudes xenogeneic grafts (ie. from a different species) which would still be accepted. Furthermore, it appears that the T cells alone are sufficient to cause graft rejection since neonatally bursectomized chickens, which totally lack B cells, are still able to reject allogeneic grafts. This does not mean that antibody has no role in graft rejection: as indicated below, antibody can cause rapid graft rejection but it usually plays a lesser role than cell-mediated immunity except in some cases where the recipient has been previously sensitized to particular donor antigens, or in reactions to haemopoietic cells.

Histological examination of an allogeneic skin graft during the process of rejection shows the dermis becoming infiltrated by mononuclear cells, many of which are small lymphocytes (Fig.24.6). The accumulation of lymphocytes precedes the destruction of the graft by several days. It is assumed that these cells are responsible for graft rejection and for some time it was thought that graft destruction was effected by cytotoxic T cells. However, in some reactions this is not the case, for example, in H-Y mediated allograft rejection in syngeneic mice. Here, the destruction of the grafts in the female mice of different strains is not correlated with the ability of those mice to develop cytotoxic T cells to the H-Y antigen and other studies have shown that helper cells are effectors in rejection reactions elicited by MHC gene differences. These observations have led to the idea that graft rejection may be a specialized form of response related to delayed hypersensitivity reactions, in which case the ultimate effector of graft destruction would be monocytes and macrophages which may be recruited to the site. It is debatable however, whether the macrophages seen in grafts are effectors of graft destruction or arrive consequent to inflammatory processes and cell damage. These two different hypotheses are summarized in figure 24.7.

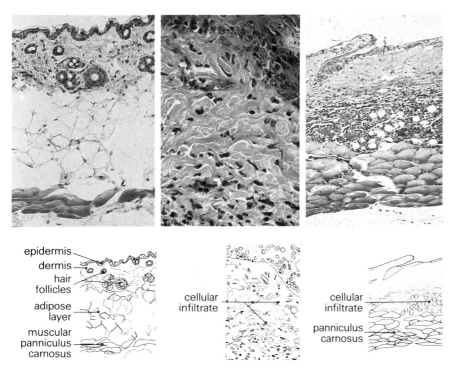

Fig.24.6 Sections of strain A mouse skin showing the normal appearance (left) and the allograft 5 days (middle) and 12 days (right) after transplantation to a CBA host. At 5 days there is a substantial infiltration by host mononuclear cells. At 12 days the epithelium has been totally destroyed and is lifting off the dermis, which is now free of cells; the infiltrating host cells have been destroyed by anoxia but there is still a brisk cellular traffic in the graft bed between the dermis and the panniculus carnosus. Courtesy of Professor L. Brent.

epidermis
dermis
hair follicles
adipose layer
muscular panniculus carnosus

cellular infiltrate

cellular infiltrate
panniculus carnosus

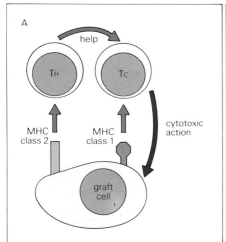
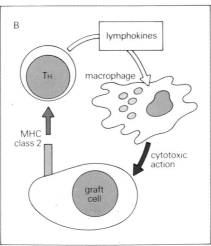

A
help
T_H T_C
MHC class 2   MHC class 1   cytotoxic action
graft cell

B
lymphokines
T_H macrophage
MHC class 2
cytotoxic action
graft cell

Fig.24.7 Graft cell destruction. Two ways in which T cells may mediate graft cell destruction are illustrated.
A. Foreign MHC class 2 antigens on the graft stimulate host T_H cells to help T_C cells destroy the target graft cell. T_C cells recognize the graft via the foreign MHC class 1 antigens.
B. T_H cells reacting to the graft release lymphokines, which stimulate macrophages to enter the graft and destroy it.

24.3

ALLOGENEIC RECOGNITION

In view of this debate on the relative importance of cyto-toxic T cells in graft destruction it is worth examining which classes of MHC antigens are primarily responsible for allograft rejection. Studies in which donor kidneys from cadavers were matched either for A and B (class 1) antigens or DR (class 2) antigens with the recipient, indicate that DR matching is most valuable in producing graft survival (Fig.24.8). Although there are technical differ-ences between the two studies the figures indicate that matching class 2 antigens is more valuable and this equates with the central role of the class 2 restricted T cells illustrated in figure 24.7. With the recent discovery of additional class 2 gene loci in the human HLA-D locus (DC and SB) it is possible that further improvement in acceptance rates could result from matching these loci. The mixed lymphocyte reaction (MLR) is most commonly used to determine D region differences between recipient and donor and it is notable that even with DR region matching there is still some variability in the degree of MLR between different stimulator cells acting on the same responder cells. This is presumably due to non-DR class 2 gene loci. It is found that donor/recipient pairs with the lowest MLR reactivity in these circumstances have a better graft survival. Cross-matching for MHC class 1 and D loci is usually performed by using antisera to the specific antigen (see 'MHC').
Allogeneic MHC antigens are highly immunogenic. For

example, they do not need to be recognized in associa-tion with self MHC molecules in order to stimulate T cells. They appear to be able by themselves to provide the dual recognition signal of self MHC plus antigen. In nor-mal, unprimed mice the proportion of T cells which can recognize allogeneic MHC is high. Up to 10% of the T cells can react to particular alloantigens, many times greater than the proportion which can recognize any other type of antigen. This implies that T cells recognizing MHC alloantigens also recognize other antigens, a hypothesis confirmed by the identification of T cell clones expressing specificity for an MHC alloantigen as well as to the antigen to which they were raised. These observations suggest that allogeneic MHC appears to the recipient's T cells as antigen-altered self MHC.

ANTIGEN PRESENTATION

Since allogeneic MHC antigens are capable of stimulat-ing recipient T cells without the necessity to associate with host MHC antigens the graft cells themselves are capable of eliciting rejection reactions. Allogeneic MHC is most immunogenic when presented on viable cells; purified MHC antigens or membrane fragments contain-ing the antigens are no more immunogenic than other non-MHC antigens. Thus, the presence of antigen-presenting cells in the graft tissues is particularly likely to elicit graft rejection. The most common of these cells are leucocytes which have entered the graft through the donor's circulation. Such antigen-presenting cells are re-ferred to as passenger cells (Fig.24.9). In human trans-plantation a problem may arise from immunogenic

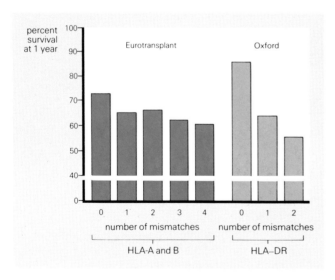

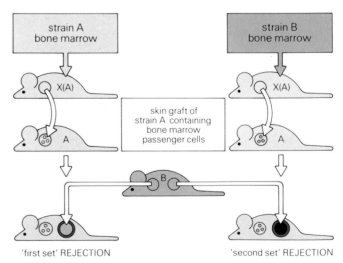

Fig.24.8 Kidney graft survival and HLA matching. The bar chart shows the percentage survival of cadaver kidney grafts at 12 months in humans, in two separate studies. In the first study (Eurotransplant) donors were matched as far as possible for the HLA-A and B antigens (class 1). In the second study (Oxford) the donors were matched for HLA-DR antigens (class 2). Note that the fewer mismatches present, the greater is the number of grafts surviving in both studies, but that DR matching has a greater effect on survival; the best results were obtained where there were no DR mismatches. The detrimental effects of HLA class 1 mismatches (but not class 2) is abrogated if patients are given blood transfusions prior to transplantation.

Fig. 24.9 The role of passenger cells in graft destruction. Strain A mice were irradiated (X) and reconstituted with bone marrow cells of either strain A or strain B. Skin grafts from these mice were transplanted to strain A recipients and are accepted. The recipients subsequently received skin grafts from strain B animals. Animals whose first graft came from an animal reconstituted with strain A cells reject the strain B graft more slowly than animals whose first graft came from a mouse reconstituted with strain B bone marrow. This implies that strain B bone marrow cells carried as passengers in the first graft primed the recipient to the strain B alloantigen.

Immunogenicity of different tissues
bone marrow
skin
islets of Langerhans
heart
kidney
liver

type	time of damage	effector mechanism	cause
hyperacute rejection	within minutes	Ab	preformed cytotoxic antibodies to donor antigens
accelerated rejection	2-5 days	CMI ± Ab	previous sensitization to donor antigens
acute rejection	7-21 days	CMI (± Ab)	development of allogeneic reaction to donor antigens
chronic rejection	later than 3 months	CMI (± Ab)	disturbance of host/graft tolerance
immuno-pathological	later than 3 months	immunopathological events related to those which necessitated the transplant damage the new organ	

Fig. 24.10 Immunogenicity of different tissues. This table orders different tissues according to their capacity to induce allogeneic reactions. Bone marrow is most immunogenic.

Fig. 24.11 Immune destruction of kidney grafts. This table lists the ways in which kidney grafts may be rejected. Acute rejection is equivalent to a first set allograft in experimental animals and accelerated rejection is equivalent to a second set allograft; both are primarily mediated by cells. Immunopathological changes include the presence of immune complex deposition and other hypersensitivity reactions already present in the recipient.

passenger cells leaving the graft after transplantation and entering the draining lymphatic system where they are particularly effective in sensitizing the host. Various manoeuvres have been performed to circumvent this problem including infusion of donor kidney with cytotoxic drugs before transplantation and u.v. irradiation of donor skin grafts, which induces emigration of Langerhans cells. Organs vary with respect to their susceptibility to rejection (Fig. 24.10). This is probably due to two factors:
1. the expression of class 2 MHC antigens by the graft varies for different tissues. For example, some strains of pig are able to accept liver grafts from other strains without immunosuppression but cannot accept kidney grafts from the same animals: swine liver parenchymal cells lack MHC class 2 antigens but tolerance in this system may also be due to a second factor.
2. the lack of suitable antigen-presenting cells in some tissues. It is noted that the most immunogenic tissues, bone marrow and skin, contain dendritic cells (or Langerhans cells which develop into dendritic cells) which are powerful stimulators of T_H cells in the MLR.

EFFECTS OF ANTIBODY

While cell-mediated immunity is the major effector in graft rejection, antibodies can also be involved. This is particularly true if the individual is already sensitized to donor antigens, and antibodies are either present before grafting or develop concomitantly with the cell-mediated immunity. The effects of antibody are most frequently seen in grafts which are connected directly to the host's blood supply for example, the kidney. Rejection of kidney grafts can be subdivided according to the time of occurrence and the effector mechanisms involved (Fig. 24.11). Hyperacute graft rejection is caused entirely by cytotoxic antibodies, usually those to A1 or B blood group substances or to class 1 MHC antigens (see

'Hypersensitivity – Type II'). The ABO blood group antigens are present on kidney grafts and naturally-occurring antibodies are present in mismatched recipients. However, those to the A2 blood group do not induce hyperacute graft rejection. Hyperacute graft rejection causes irreversible kidney damage within 48 hours due to polymorph infiltration, with thrombosis of the small arterioles and glomerular capillaries (Fig. 24.12).

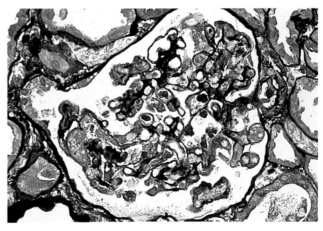

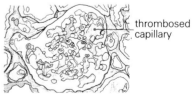

thrombosed capillary

Fig. 24.12 Renal histology showing hyperacute graft rejection. There is extensive necrosis of the glomerular capillary associated with massive interstitial haemorrhage. This extensive necrosis is preceded by an intense polymorphonuclear infiltration which occurs within the first hour of the graft's revascularization. The changes shown here occur 24-48 hours after this. H&E stain, × 200.

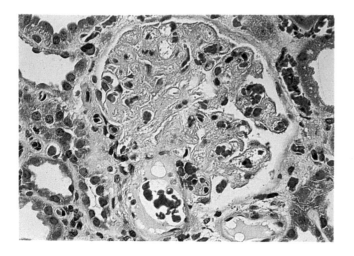

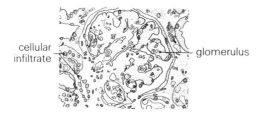

Fig. 24.13 Renal histology showing acute graft rejection
I. Small lymphocytes and other cells are accumulating in the interstitium of the graft. Such infiltration is characteristic of acute rejection and occurs before the appearance of any clinical signs. H&E stain, × 200.

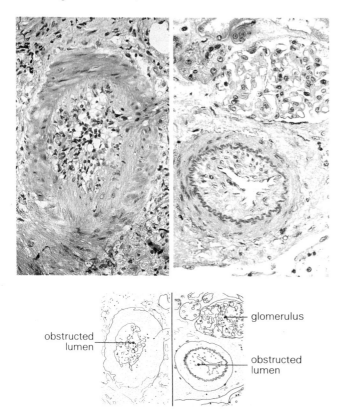

Fig. 24.14 Renal histology showing acute graft rejection
II. The section shown on the left (H&E stain) shows vascular obstruction and that on the right (Van Giesen stain) shows the end stage of this process. × 140.

The occurrence of this type of rejection is now rare since red cell and white cell crossmatching is carried out prior to all renal allografting. There is, so far, no evidence for hyperacute rejection occurring in transplanted livers.

With accelerated and acute graft rejection the importance of antibodies depends on circumstances. Acute graft rejection is more usually mediated by T cell immunity although antibodies may develop concomitantly. The second set accelerated rejection is more likely to involve antibody-mediated damage since secondary antibody responses develop early after implantation. The histological appearance of an acutely rejecting kidney is illustrated in figures 24.13 and 24.14.

GRAFT FACTORS AFFECTING REJECTION

As mentioned above, different tissues vary considerably in their immunogenicity but in addition the site of implantation also affects the eventual outcome. These two special conditions are referred to as 'privileged tissues' and 'privileged sites'. Privileged sites for transplantation include the brain, cornea and specially prepared skin flaps; these sites normally lack a lymphatic drainage. With corneal transplantation the rate of rejection is dependent upon whether the cornea becomes vascularized, and so whether it becomes accessible to the recipient's immune system (Fig.24.15). It is only within vascularized corneal transplants that HLA incompatibility increases the likelihood of rejection.

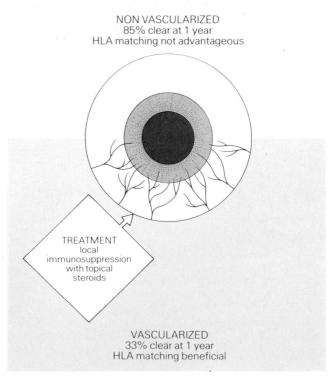

Fig. 24.15 Corneal transplantation. The success of corneal transplantation depends on whether the graft becomes vascularized. Grafts which do become vascularized are treatable with topical steroids to produce local immunosuppression.

CLINICAL TISSUE TRANSPLANTATION

The most frequent types of transplantation in humans are listed in figure 24.16. In practical terms the frequency with which transplants are performed depends upon the availability of suitable alternatives to transplantation and the availability of donor organs. The success rate of transplantation also depends on these factors as well as the rejection reactions discussed earlier and the amount of tissue damage which the graft can tolerate and still function effectively. For example, a kidney graft can recover from a certain amount of damage following death of the donor before transplantation. It can also withstand some immunological damage caused by rejection reactions provided they are checked by immunosuppressive therapy. By contrast, the heart graft is liable to go into a fatal arrhythmia following only a moderate amount of damage.

Undoubtedly, the most successful transplantation programmes have been with kidney and cornea and success rates have improved with practice and statistical analysis of previous results in order to identify which factors are important in improving the level of graft acceptance and function (Fig.24.17). It appears that the acceptance of a graft depends on a balance of factors in the donor and the recipient (Figs.24.18 and 24.19).

organ	comment
kidney	alternative to dialysis in end stage renal failure, blood groups always matched, HLA matching advantageous
bone marrow	treatment of young patients with untreatable blood diseases, HLA matched siblings used to avoid GvH disease
skin	treatment for burns, temporary cover provided by allograft, permanent replacement by autograft
liver	for hepatoma and biliary atresia, not HLA matched, graft loss usually due to factors other than rejection
lung	not HLA matched, poor success rate but improving
heart	used in cardiac failure, insufficient donors to permit anything but ABO matching, graft losses due to rejection reactions
endocrine	include islets of Langerhans and parathyroid, tissue not HLA matched in spite of its immunogenicity, little used because of available hormone replacements

Fig. 24.16 Main areas of clinical tissue transplantation.

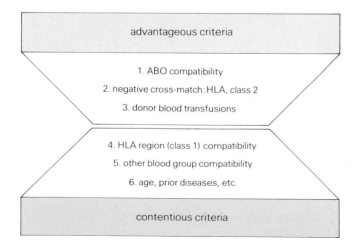

Fig. 24.17 Factors affecting kidney transplantation. There is no rigid consensus on the importance of all these criteria.

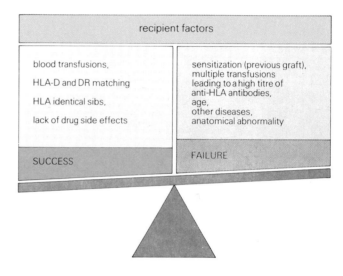

Fig. 24.18 Recipient factors affecting success in kidney transplantation. The success or failure of a kidney transplant depends on a balance of factors. Cross-matching the donor and recipient tends to produce success, especially if blood transfusions are performed prior to the operation – prior sensitization of the recipient to donor antigen is likely to end in rejection.

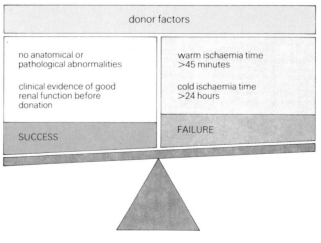

Fig. 24.19 Donor factors affecting success in kidney transplantation. Donor factors which affect graft success include the amount of time the donor organ is ischaemic, that is, lacking a proper blood supply. The length of time a graft can tolerate ischaemia depends on its temperature before transplantation, that is, 37°C (warm) or 4°C (cold).

24.7

IMMUNOSUPPRESSION

The success of any allogeneic transplantation is often due to the immunosuppressive measures adopted. These may be divided into two phases. Immediately after the graft has been implanted it is necessary to prevent sensitization of pre-existing mature T cells capable of recognizing the graft. After the graft has escaped the initial acute phase rejection reactions a cumulative unresponsiveness to the graft develops as the recipient is continually exposed to donor MHC. This stable state sometimes depends on the development of antigen-specific Ts cells. Unless the equilibrium is disturbed by other factors, such as infection, chronic rejection reactions may be avoided indefinitely. Immunosuppressive measures may be antigen specific or antigen non-specific.

Antigen Non-specific Immunosuppression

Antigen non-specific measures include the use of immunosuppressive drugs and other ways to specifically reduce T cell function. Many cytotoxic drugs are primarily active against dividing cells and therefore have some functional specificity for any cells activated to divide by donor antigens, but the use of these drugs is limited by the need not to damage other dividing tissues such as the gut epithelium. The drug cyclosporin A appears to have a greater specificity for lymphoid cells than others. It is an undecapeptide derived from the fungus *Trichoderma polysporum* and it is highly lipophilic. This drug acts at several levels of T cell activation but predominantly in the earliest phases of activation. Even so, it is not devoid of side-effects. Other measures directed at T cells include the use of anti-lymphocyte globulin at the time of transplantation and lymphoid irradiation prior to transplantation. A problem arising from all these measures is that the individual is more susceptible to infection and if infection occurs immunosuppression has to be suspended, at which time allogeneic reactions frequently develop.

Antigen-specific Immunosuppression

The ideal form of antigen-specific tolerance is that induced in the neonatal animal by infusion of donor cells (see 'Immunological Tolerance'). This is not, however, a practical proposition in human transplantation. Potentially more useful is the phenomenon of immunological enhancement. This occurs when graft survival can be prolonged by the seemingly paradoxical treatment with antibodies directed towards the graft alloantigens. This is referred to as passive enhancement (in an analogous way to passive immunization). It is possible to produce the same effect by an active pre-immunization with allogeneic cells. Various suggestions have been put forward as to the mechanism by which the enhancement occurs, including the removal of donor passenger cells or recipient Tн cells (Fig.24.20). Another suggestion is that the antibody shields the alloantigens on the graft from the responding host cells (Fig.24.21). In this sense the action of the antibody is similar to the action of anti-class 2 MHC antibodies in preventing T cell sensitization, and it is possible that transfusion does induce some anti-class 2 antibodies. None of these explanations seems wholly

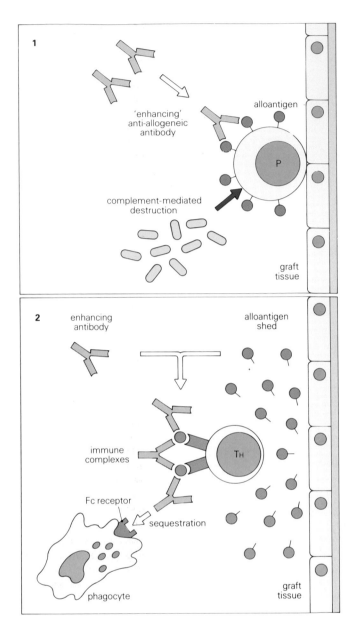

Fig. 24.20 Two hypotheses to explain the effect of enhancing antibody.
1. The antibody binds preferentially to passenger cells (P) in the graft which strongly express alloantigens. They are eliminated by complement-mediated lysis and so are unable to sensitize the recipient.
2. Antigens shed by the graft tissue bind to the enhancing antibody and the resulting complexes attach to recipient Tн cells capable of recognizing the alloantigens. These Tн cells are then removed by phagocytic cells via their Fc receptors.

satisfactory because the enhancing antibodies appear to have a long-term action in reducing reactions to the graft which extend beyond the short-term allogeneic reactions and in some instances there is a development of graft-specific Ts cells.

An interestingly similar phenomenon has been observed in human kidney grafting. In this case recipients immunosuppressed with steroids and azathioprine and previously sensitized by donor blood, either by pregnancy or by transfusion before operation, have improved

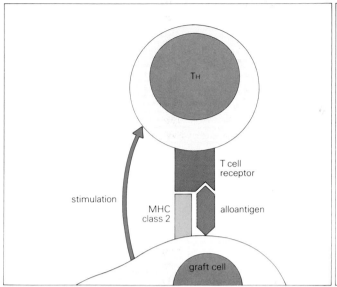
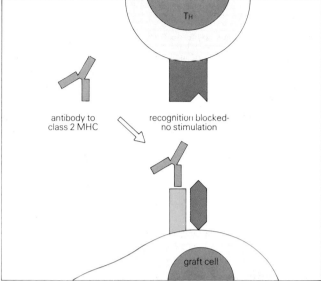

Fig. 24.21 Prevention of T cell stimulation using anti-class 2 antibodies. Normally T_H cells recognize a combination of MHC class 2 antigen and alloantigen, or recognize the foreign MHC or graft cells as an equivalent combination of stimuli (left). In this instance the graft cell is acting as an antigen-presenting cell. Antibodies to the class 2 MHC antigen (right) could block T cell recognition of the graft cell and thus prevent sensitization to it.

graft survival (Fig. 24.22). The mechanism for this observation is unknown but it may be related to those discussed above. The improvement noticed with blood transfusions to donors is less marked when donors and recipients are well-matched for MHC antigens, which again suggests that the manoeuvre is in some way removing antigen-presenting cells or donor specific T-helper cells. It is interesting to note that the preliminary indications are that if cyclosporin is used alone, or together with steroids then the pre-transplant blood transfusion does not affect graft survival. The main problem with blood transfusion is that a number of patients develop cytotoxic antibodies and these are a major bar to transplantation.

Another immunosuppressive technique, as described in 'Immunological Tolerance', is the induction of anti-idiotypic antibodies to the T cells which recognize the graft. These antibodies block the recognition of the MHC antigens on the graft but although there has been some considerable success in animals with this technique the induction of suitable anti-idiotypic antibodies during an extended period before the grafting presents difficult immunological and procedural problems in man. The various forms of immunosuppression are summarized in figure 24.23.

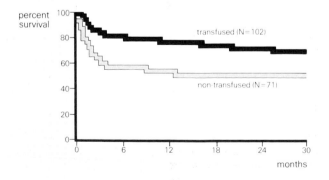

Fig. 24.22 The effect of blood transfusion on kidney transplantation. This graph plots the survival of kidney grafts in 102 transfused and 71 non-transfused patients.

antigen non-specific	antigen specific
1. cytotoxic drugs	6. neonatal tolerization
2. lymphoid irradiation	7. enhancing (anti-allogenic) antibodies
3. anti-lymphocyte globulin	8. anti-idiotype antibodies to receptors on T cells
4. cyclosporin A	9. blood transfusion in human kidney transplants
5. steroids/azathioprine (immunosuppressive)	

Fig. 24.23 Immunological suppression for transplantation. This table lists various immunosuppressive treatments. Items 6, 7 and 8 are of theoretical interest and have not found practical application in human organ transplantation.

FURTHER READING

Lachmann P. J. & Peters D. K. (1981) *Clinical Aspects of Immunology,* 4th edn. Blackwell Scientific Publications, Oxford.

Kahan D. (ed) (1984) *Cyclosporine A: Biological Activity and Clinical Applications.* Grune & Stratton Inc., New York.

Billingham R. E. & Silvers E. S. (1971) *The Immunobiology of Transplantation.* Prentice-Hall, New Jersey.

25 Immunological Tests

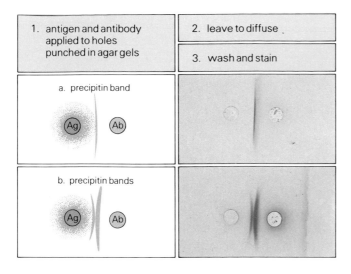

| 1. antigen and antibody applied to holes punched in agar gels | 2. leave to diffuse |
| | 3. wash and stain |

a. precipitin band

b. precipitin bands

Fig.25.1 Immuno-double diffusion I. Agar gels are poured onto slides and allowed to set (1-2% agar in buffer at pH 7–8.5). Wells are then punched in the gel and the test solutions of antigen (Ag) and antibody (Ab) are added. The solutions diffuse out and where antigen and antibody meet they bind to each other, crosslink and precipitate leaving a line of precipitation (a). If two antigens are present in the solution which can be recognized by the antibody two lines of precipitation form independently (b). The precipitin bands can be better visualized by washing the gel to remove soluble proteins and then staining the precipitin arcs with a protein stain such as Coomassie Blue (right).

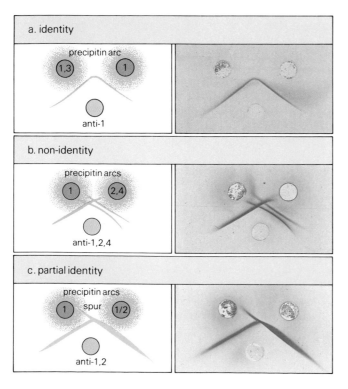

a. identity

precipitin arc

anti-1

b. non-identity

precipitin arcs

anti-1,2,4

c. partial identity

precipitin arcs

spur

anti-1,2

Immunologists employ a number of techniques common to other biological sciences. For example, the methods used to isolate and characterize antibody molecules are those of biochemistry and protein fractionation. Immunology has, however, developed a number of its own techniques, particularly those concerning the interaction of antigen with antibody and the isolation of different lymphocyte populations. A number of these techniques have been outlined in the previous chapters at appropriate places, others are used so generally in different experiments that they are described here. In addition, some of the techniques which are more commonly encountered in practical courses of immunology are also set out. Although these techniques were originally devised by immunologists they are finding increasing use in other biological sciences where it is now appreciated that the specificity of the antigen/antibody bond allows accurate identification and discrimination of any molecule to which an antibody can be raised.

ANTIGEN AND ANTIBODY

Precipitation Reaction in Gels

One of the first observations of antigen-antibody reactions was their ability to precipitate when combined in proportions at or near equivalence. By performing these reactions in agar gels it is possible to distinguish separate antigen-antibody reactions produced by different populations of antibody present in a serum – the immuno-double diffusion technique. The techniques have been extended to the examination of the relationship between different antigens (Figs.25.1 & 25.2).

Fig.25.2 Immuno-double diffusion II. The immuno-double diffusion technique may be used to determine the relationship between antigens (blue) and a particular test antibody (yellow). Three basic patterns appear. The numbers in the blue wells refer to the epitopes present on the test antigen. In reaction (a) the precipitin arcs formed between the antibody and the two test antigens fuse indicating that the antibody is precipitating identical epitopes in each preparation (epitope 1). This does not mean that the antigens are necessarily identical, they are only identical as far as the antibody can distinguish the difference. In reaction (b) the antibody preparation distinguishes the three different antigens which form independent precipitin arcs. In reaction (c) the antigens share epitope 1 but one antigen has an extra epitope (2). This is the same situation as in (a), but in this case the antibody can distinguish them, by virtue of being able to react against both epitopes. A line of identity forms with anti-epitope 1, with the addition of a 'spur' where the anti-epitope 2 has reacted with the second epitope, thus indicating partial identity between the antigen preparations.

Some antigen mixtures however, are too complex to be resolved by simple diffusion and precipitation and so the technique of immunoelectrophoresis was developed — antigens are first separated on the basis of their charge before being visualized by precipitation (Fig.25.3).

These gel techniques only identify antigens and antibodies qualitatively but by further modification, using the technique of single radial immunodiffusion they can be made quantitative (Fig.25.4). By applying a voltage across the gels to move the antigens and antibodies

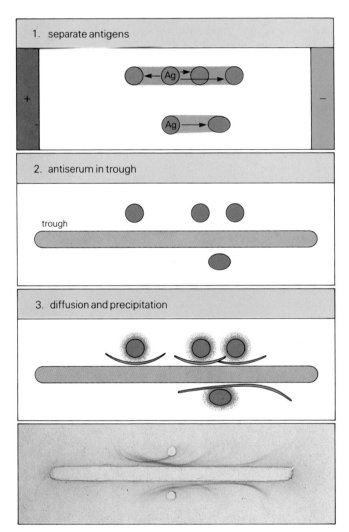

Fig.25.3 Immunoelectrophoresis. 1. Antigens are separated in an agar gel by placing an electric charge across it. The pH is chosen so that positively charged proteins move to the negative electrode and negatively charged proteins to the positive. 2. A trough is then cut between the wells, filled with the antibody and the plate left to diffuse. 3. The antigens and antibody form precipitin arcs. This method allows the comparison of complicated mixtures of antigens as found in serum.

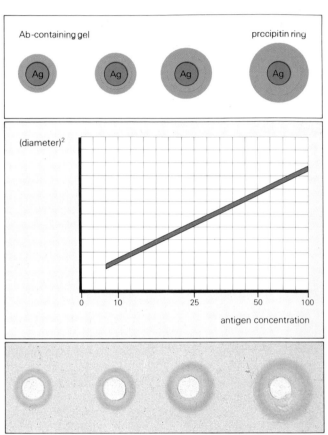

Fig.25.4 Single radial immunodiffusion. Antibody is added to the agar gel which is then poured onto slides and allowed to set. Wells are punched in the agar and standard volumes of test antigen of different concentration (Ag) are put in the wells. The plates are left for at least 24 hours, during which time the antigen diffuses out of the wells to form soluble complexes (in antigen excess) with the antibody. These continue to diffuse outwards, binding more antibody until an equivalence point is reached and the complexes precipitate in a ring. The area within the precipitin ring, measured as ring diameter squared, is proportional to the antigen concentration. Unknowns are derived by interpolation from the standard curve (graph). The whole process may be reversed to determine the concentrations of unknown antibody.

together immuno-double diffusion becomes countercurrent electrophoresis and single radial immunodiffusion becomes rocket electrophoresis (Fig.25.5). These techniques operate in the range 20 μg/ml to 2 mg/ml of antigen or antibody.

Haemagglutination and Complement Fixation

Antibody may be detected at lower concentrations by haemagglutination which relies on the ability of antibody to cross-link red blood cells by the antigen on their surface (Fig.25.6).

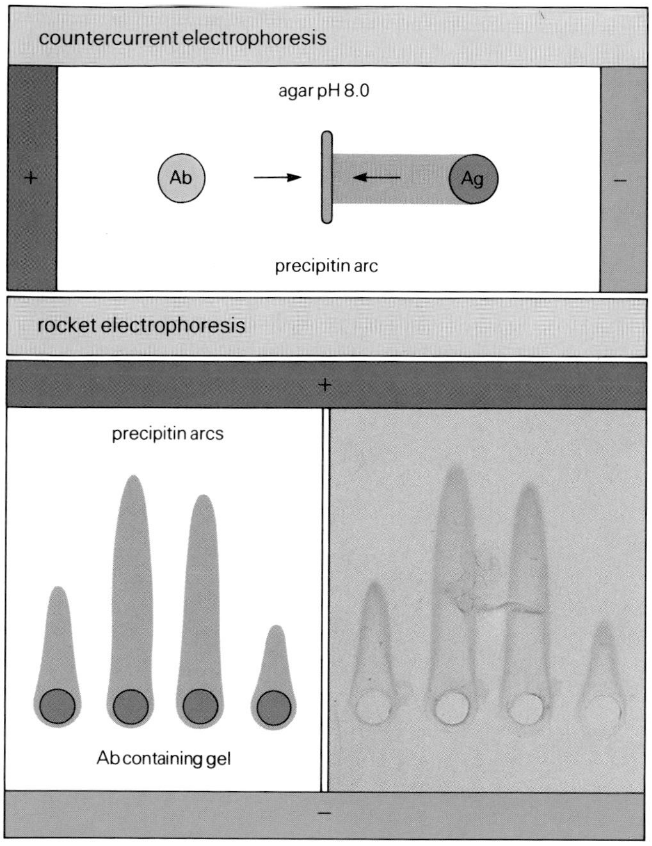

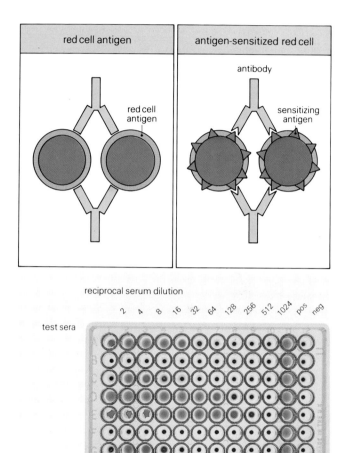

Fig.25.5 Countercurrent electrophoresis and rocket electrophoresis. Countercurrent electrophoresis is performed in agar gels where the pH is chosen so that the antibody is positively charged and the antigen is negatively charged. By applying a voltage across the gel the antigen and antibody move towards each other and precipitate. The principle is the same as immuno-double diffusion but the sensitivity is increased 10–20 fold. Antigens may be quantitated by electrophoresing them into an antibody-containing gel in the technique termed rocket electrophoresis. The pH of the gel is chosen so the antibodies remain immobile and the antigen negatively charged. Precipitin rockets form, where the height of the rocket is proportional to antigen concentration, and unknowns are determined by interpolation from standards. The appearance of stained rockets is shown on the right. Both these techniques rely on the antigen and antibody having different charges at the selected pH; this is true for most antigens since antibodies have a relatively high isoelectric point, pI (ie. they are neutrally charged at a more alkaline pH than most antigens). If the charges on the antigen and antibody are not sufficiently different the antibody or the antigen can be chemically modified to alter its pI. The rocket electrophoresis can be reversed to estimate antibody concentration if a suitable pH gel to immobilize the antigen (without damaging it or preventing antigen-antibody reaction) can be found.

Fig.25.6 Haemagglutination. The active haemagglutination test (left) detects antibodies to red blood cell antigens. The antibody is serially diluted (usually in doubling dilutions) in physiological saline and placed in the wells (1-10) of the haemagglutination plate. Positive controls (row 11) and negative controls (row 12) are included. A suspension of red cells (containing a protein to prevent the red cells agglutinating non-specifically) is added to each well to give a final concentration of about 1% cells. If sufficient antibody is present to agglutinate (cross-link) the cells they become cross-linked and sink as a mat to the bottom of the well (direct Coombs test). If insufficient antibody is present the cells roll down the sloping sides of the plate to form a red pellet at the bottom. Some antibodies do not agglutinate red cells very effectively and these may be detected in the indirect agglutination test (indirect Coombs test) by the addition of a second antibody which binds to the antibody on the red cell. By binding different antigens onto the red cell surface, either covalently or non-covalently the test can be extended to detect antibodies to antigens other than those present on red cells (right). Chromic chloride, tannic acid, glutaraldehyde and a number of other chemicals are used to cross-link the antigen to the cells.

It will be appreciated that the haemagglutination test is a direct development of the Coombs test described in 'Hypersensitivity – Type II'. Antigen-antibody reactions lead to immune complex formation which produces complement fixation via the classical pathway and this secondary reaction may be exploited in order to determine the amount of antigen or antibody present (Fig.25.7). These two techniques can detect antibody at levels of less than 1 µg/ml.

Direct and Indirect Immunofluorescence

Immunofluorescence is used extensively in the detection of autoantibodies and antibodies to tissue and cellular antigens (Fig.25.8). Although the techniques are considerably more cumbersome than the ones described above if a quantitative measure of antibody concentration is required, they do have a number of advantages. By using tissue sections (which contain a large number of antigens) it is possible to identify antibodies to several

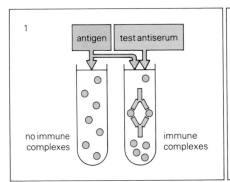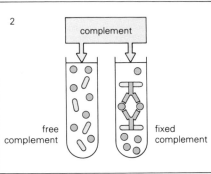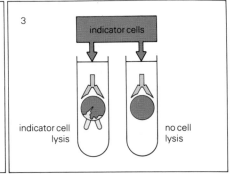

Fig.25.7 Complement fixation. The complement fixation test detects antibody. 1. A test antiserum is titred in doubling dilutions and a fixed amount of antigen is added to each well or tube. If antibody is present in the test serum, immune complexes will form. 2. Complement is then added to the mixture. If complexes are present they will fix complement and consume it. 3. In the final step indicator cells (red cells) together with a subagglutinating amount of antibody (EA, erythrocyte antibody) are added to the mixture. If there is any complement remaining these cells will be lysed; if it was consumed by immune complexes there will be insufficient to lyse the red cells. A quantity of complement is used which is

just enough to lyse the indicator cells if none is consumed by the complexes. The assay is often performed on plastic plates. By using constant amounts of antibody and titrations of antigen, the assay can be applied to testing for antigens. Appropriate controls are most important in this assay because some antibody preparations consume complement without the addition of antigen, for example, if the antibody preparation is the serum of a patient which already contains immune complexes. Some antigens can also have anti-complement activity. The controls therefore should include antibody alone and antigen alone to check that neither fix complement by themselves.

Fig.25.8 Direct and indirect immunofluorescence. A section is cut on a cryostat from a deep frozen tissue block. (This ensures that labile antigens are not damaged by fixatives.)
Direct. The test solution of fluoresceinated antibody is applied to the section in a drop, incubated and washed off. Any bound antibody is then revealed under the microscope; UV light is directed onto the section through the objective, thus the field is dark and areas with bound fluorescent antibody fluoresce green. The pattern of fluorescence is characteristic for each tissue antigen.
Indirect. Antibody applied to the section as a solution is visualized using fluoresceinated anti-Ig.
Indirect complement amplified. This is an elaboration of the indirect method for the detection of complement fixing antibody. In the second step fresh complement is added which becomes fixed around the site of antibody binding. Due to the amplification steps in the classical complement pathway one antibody molecule can cause many C3b molecules to bind to the section; these are then visualized with fluoresceinated anti-C3.

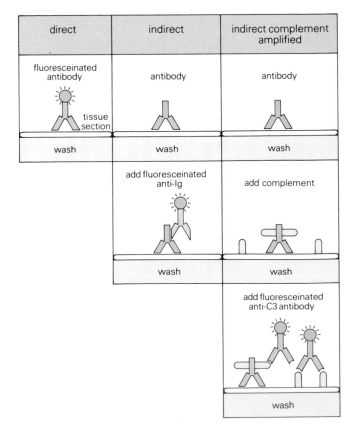

different antigens in a single test. The antigens are differentiated according to their different staining patterns. Furthermore, the immunofluorescence tests can be used to identify particular cells in suspension, that is, to identify antigens on live cells. When a live stained cell suspension is put through a fluorescent activated cell sorter (FACS) the machine measures the fluorescence intensity of each cell and then the cells are separated according to their particular fluorescent brightness. This technique permits the isolation of different cell populations with different surface antigens (stained with different fluorescent antibodies).

Radioimmunoassay and Enzyme-linked Immunoabsorbent Assay

These techniques are exquisitely sensitive for detecting antigens and antibodies, and they are extremely economical in the use of reagents (Figs.25.9 and 25.10).

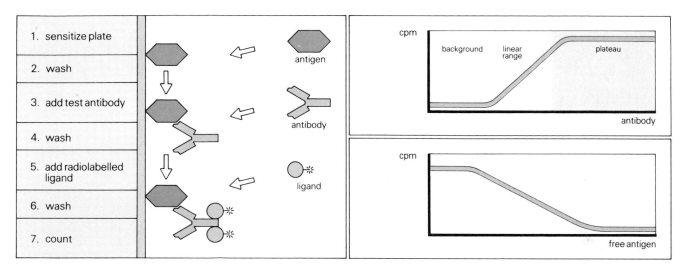

Fig.25.9 Radioimmunoassay (RIA). Antigen in saline is incubated on a plastic plate or tube (1). Small quantities become absorbed onto the plastic surface. Free antigen is washed away (2). (The plate may then be blocked with excess of an irrelevant protein to prevent any subsequent non-specific binding of proteins.) Test antibody is added, which binds to the antigen (3). Unbound proteins are washed away (4) and the antibody is detected by a radiolabelled ligand (5). The ligand may be a molecule such as staphylococcal protein A, which binds to the Fc region of IgG or more often it is another antibody specific for the test antibody. By using a ligand which binds to particular classes or subclasses of test antibody it is possible to distinguish isotypes. Unbound ligand is washed away and the radioactivity of the plate counted on a gamma counter. A typical titration curve is shown in the upper graph. With increasing amounts of test antibody the counts per minute (cpm) rise from a background level through a linear range to a plateau. Antibody titres can only be detected correctly within the linear range. Typically the plateau binding is 20–100 times background. The sensitivity of the technique is usually about 1–50 ng/ml specific antibody. Specificity of the assay may be checked by adding increasing concentrations of free test antigen to the test antibody at step 3; this binds to the antibody and blocks it from binding to the antigen on the plate. As shown in the lower graph, addition of increasing amounts of free antigen reduces the cpm.

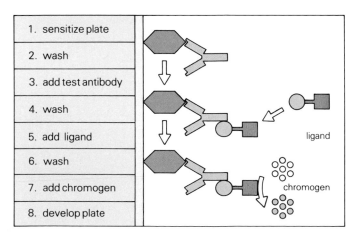

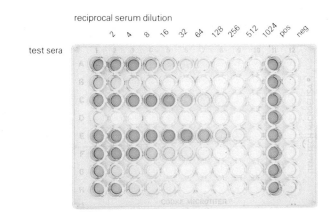

Fig.25.10 Enzyme linked immunoabsorbent assay (ELISA). The ELISA plate is prepared as a RIA plate up to step 4. At this point a different kind of ligand is used. The ligand is a molecule which can detect the antibody and is covalently coupled to an enzyme such as peroxidase. This binds the test antibody and after free ligand is washed away (6) the bound ligand is visualized by the addition of chromogen (7) – a colourless substrate which is acted on by the enzyme portion of the ligand to produce a coloured end-product. A developed plate is shown on the right. The amount of test antibody is measured by assessing the amount of coloured end-product by optical density scanning of the plate.

RIA and ELISA are probably the most widely used of all immunological assays for antibodies since large numbers of tests can be performed in a relatively short time. Modification of the basic system as illustrated by the RAST test allows identification of antibodies of a particular isotype (Fig.25.11). The radioimmunoassay can also be turned into a competition type of assay as illustrated by the RIST test and this may be used as a very sensitive assay for antigens (Fig.25.12). Indeed, this form of competition was the first type of radioimmunoassay. The serum concentration of a number of drugs and hormones are also measured by competition radioimmunoassay. (Note that in the RIST test the IgE being measured is acting as an antigen.)

Fig.25.11 The radioallergosorbent test (RAST). This test measures antigen-specific IgE in a radioimmunoassay where the ligand is a labelled anti-IgE antibody. The steps are identical to the standard radioimmunoassay except that the antigen (allergen) is covalently bound to a cellulose disc rather than non-covalently to a radioimmunoassay plate. By having much more antigen available on the disc this permits the high sensitivity necessary to bind the small quantities of IgE present in the test serum.

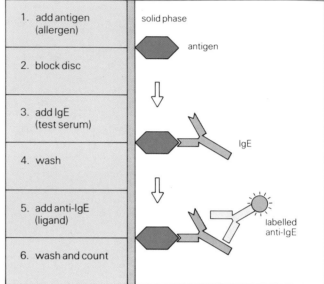

1. add antigen (allergen)
2. block disc
3. add IgE (test serum)
4. wash
5. add anti-IgE (ligand)
6. wash and count

solid phase
antigen
IgE
labelled anti-IgE

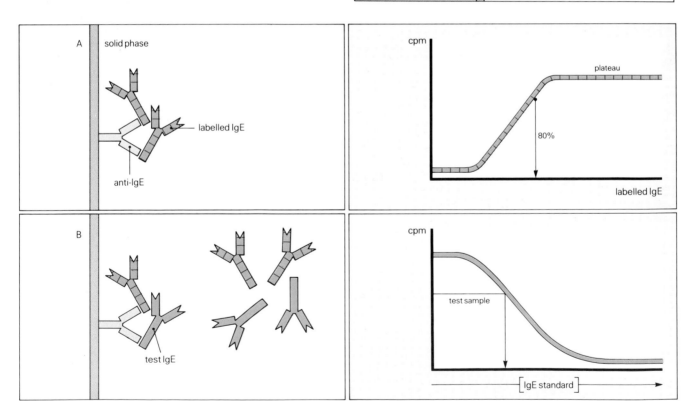

Fig.25.12 The radioimmunosorbent test (RIST). This is a competition radioimmunoassay for total serum IgE. The plate is sensitized with anti-IgE and increasing amounts of labelled IgE are added to the plate to determine the maximum amount of IgE that the plate can bind (A). A quantity of labelled IgE equivalent to approximately 80% of the plateau binding is chosen. In the test experiments (B) this amount of labelled IgE is mixed with the serum containing the IgE to be tested. The test IgE competes with the labelled IgE. Thus the more IgE that is present in the test serum the *less* the amount of labelled IgE that binds. This produces a standard curve of the type shown where dilutions of a serum containing a known IgE concentration are used. This type of test is widely used to measure hormone concentrations in serum.

Pure Antibodies

Affinity chromatography is the technique used where the isolation of pure antibody or pure antigen is the objective (Fig.25.13). Affinity chromatography is widely used in biochemistry but the use of antibody as the affinity binding reagent is a development of immunologists. Another more recent way of obtaining pure antibody of a defined specificity is in the production of monoclonal antibodies a technique which produces a cell which can manufacture a single antibody of defined specificity indefinitely, thus obviating the vagaries of antiserum production (Fig.25.14).

Although a monoclonal antibody is a well-defined reagent it does not have a greater specificity than a polyclonal antiserum which recognizes the antigen via a number of different epitopes.

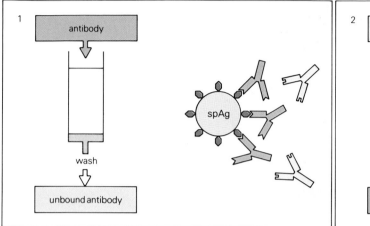

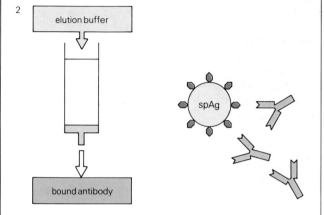

Fig.25.13 Affinity chromatography. Affinity chromatography may be applied to the isolation of a pure population of antibodies. A solid phase immunoabsorbent is prepared (spAg) which is an antigen covalently coupled to an inert support such as cross-linked dextran beads. The immunoabsorbent is placed in a column and the antibody mixture run in under physiological conditions. Antibody to the antigen remains bound to the column while unbound antibody is washed through (1). In the second step the column is eluted to obtain the bound antibody using elution buffer (eg. acetate pH 3.0, diethylamine pH 11.5, 3M guanidine, HCl) which dissociates the antigen-antibody bond (2). By placing antibody on the column the process can be reversed to obtain pure antigen. The technique can also be used for obtaining other types of molecule. For example, a lectin column will absorb all molecules with particular sugar residues and these can be eluted in buffer containing the free sugar, which competes with the bound protein for the attachment site on the lectin.

Fig.25.14 Monoclonal antibody production. Animals (usually mice or rats) are immunized with antigen. Once the animals are making a good antibody response the spleens are removed and a cell suspension prepared (lymph node cells may also be used). These cells are fused with a myeloma cell line by the addition of polyethylene glycol (PEG) which promotes membrane fusion. Only a small proportion of the cells fuse successfully. The fusion mixture is then set up in culture with medium containing 'HAT'. HAT is a mixture of Hypoxanthine Aminopterin and Thymidine. Aminopterin is a powerful toxin which blocks a metabolic pathway. This pathway can be bypassed if the cell is provided with the intermediate metabolites hypoxanthine and thymidine. Thus spleen cells can grow in HAT medium, but myeloma cells have a metabolic defect and so cannot use the bypass pathway, consequently they die in HAT medium. When the culture is set up in HAT medium it contains spleen cells, myeloma cells and fused cells. The spleen cells die in culture naturally after 1–2 weeks; the myeloma cells are killed by the HAT, but fused cells survive as they have the immortality of the myeloma and the metabolic bypass of the spleen cells. Some of them will also have the antibody producing capacity of the spleen cells. Any wells containing growing cells are tested for the production of the desired antibody (often by RIA or ELISA) and if positive the cultures are cloned, that is, plated out so that only one cell is in each well. This produces a clone of cells derived from a single progenitor, which is both immortal and produces (monoclonal) antibody.

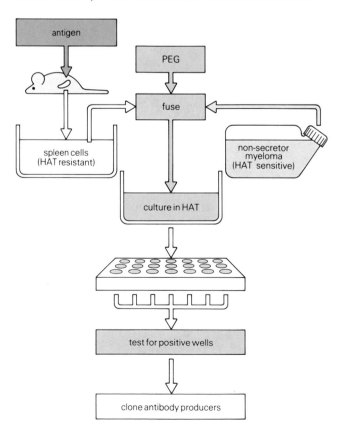

LYMPHOCYTE POPULATIONS

Antibody-forming cells are identified by the plaque-forming cell assay. This has been modified in a number of different ways to identify total antibody-producing cells and those producing specific IgG or IgM antibodies (Fig.25.15). Many of the experiments performed by immunologists use populations of lymphocytes either for *in vivo* or *in vitro* transfer experiments. Lymphocytes are isolated on gradients which separate them from other

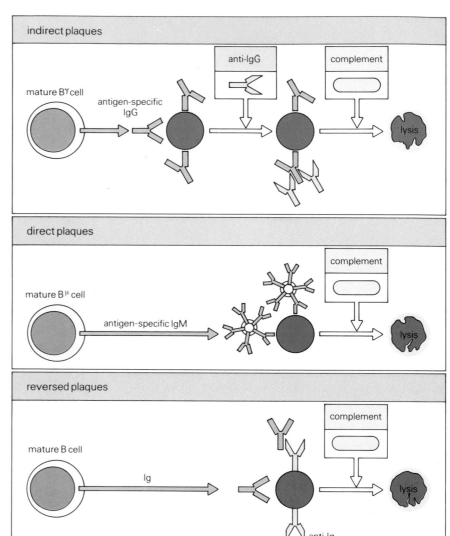

Fig.25.15 Plaque forming cell assays.
Plaque forming cell assays are used to detect antibody-forming cells The assay may be performed in three different ways.
Indirect Plaques. Cells producing antibody to a particular antigen release it, whence it diffuses and binds onto antigen on red cells. This may be red cell surface antigen, or the cells may be sensitized with another antigen as in the haemagglutination assay. To detect IgG antibodies bound to the red cells it is necessary to first add anti-IgG antibody and then complement. Complexes formed on the cell fix complement and produce a zone of erythrocyte lysis around the B cell.
Direct Plaques. Antigen-specific IgM antibodies are capable of causing complement-mediated lysis without the addition of an extra layer of anti-immunoglobulin. Thus the numbers of antigen-specific IgM and IgG plaque forming cells can be estimated separately.
Reversed Plaques. The reversed plaque method measures total immunoglobulin producing cells (not just antigen-specific cells). Released Ig binds onto red cells sensitized with anti-Ig. This complex can now fix complement and cause cell lysis. (Protein A, which binds IgG Fc regions, can substitute for the anti-Ig on the red cells in this assay).

Fig.25.16 Lymphocyte separation on Ficoll isopaque. Whole blood is defibrinated by shaking with glass beads and the resulting clot removed. The blood is then diluted in tissue culture medium and layered on top of a tube half full of Ficoll. Ficoll has a density greater than that of lymphocytes but less than that of red cells and granulocytes (eg. macrophages). After centrifugation the red cells and PMNs pass down through the Ficoll to form a pellet at the bottom of the tube while lymphocytes settle at the interface of the medium and Ficoll. The lymphocyte preparation can be further depleted of phagocytes by the addition of iron filings; these are taken up by the phagocytes which can then be drawn

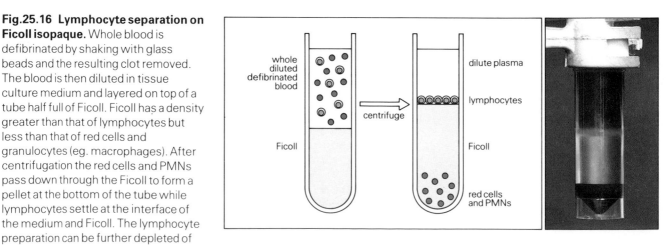

away with a strong magnet. Alternatively macrophages can be removed by leaving the cell suspension to settle on a plastic disk. Macrophages adhere to plastic, whereas the lymphocytes can be washed off.

cellular components of blood. This depends on the different density of lymphocytes compared with the other cell populations (Fig.25.16). Subpopulations of lymphocytes are usually obtained by rosetting or plating (Figs.25.17 & 25.18). Note that lymphocyte plating is a type of affinity chromatography but applied to lymphocytes.

Although this account of immunological techniques is by no means exhaustive they do form the basis of a great many experiments when used in combination, either together or sequentially. Furthermore, even complicated techniques found in research papers are frequently simple modifications of these basic systems.

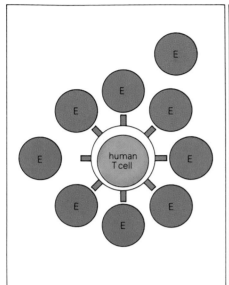

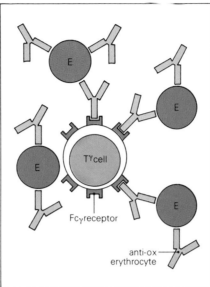

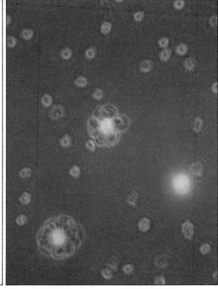

Fig.25.17 Lymphocyte populations — rosetting. Some cells have receptors for erythrocytes. For example human T cells have receptors for sheep erythrocytes (E), the function of which is unknown (left). They are not present on mouse T cells. When mixed together the T cells form rosettes with the erythrocytes; the T cells may now be separated from non-rosetting, B cells on Ficoll gradients. A modification of this technique to isolate cells with other receptors is shown here (middle). For example, some T cells have a receptor for the Fc of IgG (Fc^γ). These cells may be identified and isolated by rosetting with ox erythrocytes sensitized with a subagglutinating amount of anti-ox erythrocyte. A rosetted lymphocyte is shown on the right. Courtesy of Dr P. M. Lydyard.

Fig.25.18 Lymphocyte populations — plating. Cell populations can be separated on antibody-sensitized plates. Antibody binds non-covalently to the plastic plate (as for radioimmunoassay) and the cell mixture is applied to the plate. Antigen-positive cells (Ag^+) bind to the antibody and the antigen-negative cells (Ag^-) can be carefully washed off. By changing the culture conditions or by enzyme-digesting the cells on the plate it is sometimes possible to recover the cells bound to the plate. Often the cells that have bound to the plate are altered by their binding, for example, binding to the plate cross-links the antigen which can cause cell activation. Thus, the method is most satisfactory for removing a cell population. Examples of the application of this method include separating T_H and T_S cell populations using antibodies to Ly1 or Ly2, 3 and separating T cells from B cells using anti-Ig (which binds to the surface antibody of the B cell). By sensitizing the plate with antigen, antigen binding cells can be separated from non-binding cells.

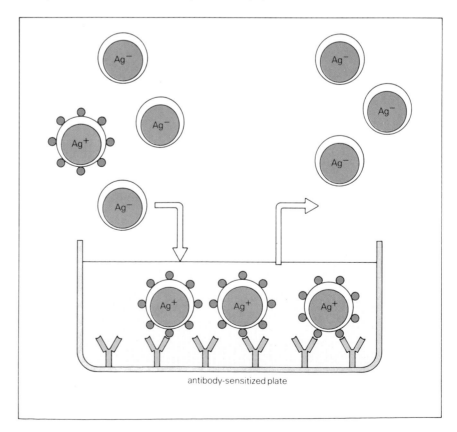

antibody-sensitized plate

FURTHER READING

Hudson L. & Hay F.C. (1980) *Practical Immunology* 2nd edn. Blackwell Scientific Publications, Oxford.

Johnstone A. & Thorpe R. (1982) *Immunochemistry in Practice.* Blackwell Scientific Publications, Oxford.

Nairn R.C. (ed.) (1980-1984) *Practical Methods in Clinical Immunology Series.* Churchill Livingstone, Edinburgh.

Weir D.M. (1985) *Handbook of Experimental Immunology* Vols I & II. 4th edn. Blackwell Scientific Publications, Oxford.

25.10

Glossary

ADCC (antibody-dependent cell-mediated cytotoxicity). A cytotoxic reaction in which Fc receptor-bearing killer cells recognize target cells via specific antibodies.

AFC (antibody-forming cells). Functionally equivalent to plasma cells.

APC (antigen-presenting cell). A variety of cell types which carry antigen in a form which can stimulate lymphocytes.

Adjuvant. A substance which non-specifically enhances the immune response to an antigen.

Affinity. Measure of the binding strength between an antigenic determinant (epitope) and an antibody combining site (paratope).

Affinity maturation. The increase in average antibody affinity frequently seen during a secondary immune response.

Allele. Intraspecies variance at a particular gene locus.

Allergy. Originally defined as altered reactivity on second contact with antigen, now usually refers to a Type 1 hypersensitivity reaction.

Allogeneic. Refers to intraspecies genetic variations.

Allotype. The protein product of an allele which may be detectable as an antigen by another member of the same species.

Anaphylatoxin. Complement peptides (C3a and C5a) which cause mast cell degranulation and smooth muscle contraction.

Anaphylaxis. An antigen specific immune reaction mediated primarily by IgE which results in vasodilation and constriction of smooth muscles, including those of the bronchus, and which may result in death of the animal.

Antibody. A molecule produced by animals in response to antigen which has the particular property of combining specifically with the antigen which induced their formation.

Antigen. A molecule which induces the formation of antibody.

Atopy. The clinical manifestation of Type I hypersensitivity reactions including eczema, asthma and rhinitis.

Autologous. Part of the same individual.

Autosomes. Chromosomes other than the X or Y sex chromosomes.

Avidity. The functional combining strength of an antibody with its antigen which is related to both the affinity of the reaction between the epitopes and paratopes and the valencies of the antibody and antigen.

β_1H. A cofactor of the complement system recently renamed Factor H.

β_2–microglobulin. A polypeptide which constitutes part of some membrane proteins including the Class 1 MHC molecules.

BCG (Bacille Calmette Guerin). An attenuated strain of *Mycobacterium tuberculosis* used as a vaccine, an adjuvant or a biological response modifier in different circumstances.

Bence Jones Protein. Free immunoglobulin light chain dimers found in the serum and urine of patients and animals with multiple myeloma.

Bursa of Fabricius. A lymphoepithelial organ found at the junction of the hind gut and cloaca in birds which is the site of B cell maturation.

C3b Inactivator. A factor of the complement system recently renamed Factor I.

Capping. A process by which cell surface molecules are caused to aggregate (usually using antibody) on the cell membrane.

Carrier. An immunogenic molecule, or part of a molecule, which is recognized by T cells in an antibody response.

Cell cycle. The process of cell division which is divisible into four phases: GI, S, G2 and M. DNA replicates during the S phase and the cell divides in the M (mitotic) phase.

Chemokinesis. Increased random migratory activity of cells.

Chemotaxis. Increased directional migration of cells particularly in response to concentration gradients of certain chemotactic factors.

Chimaerism. The situation in which cells from genetically different individuals coexist in one body.

Class 1/2/3 MHC molecules. Three major classes of molecule coded within the MHC. Class 1 molecules have one MHC encoded peptide associated with β_2– microglobulin. Class 2 molecules have two MHC encoded peptides which are non-covalently associated, and Class 3 molecules are complement components.

Clone. A family of cells or organisms having a genetically identical constitution.

CMI (cell-mediated immunity). A term used to refer to immune reactions which are mediated by cells rather than antibody or other humoral factors.

Cobra Venom Factor. A cobra complement component equivalent to mammalian C3b.

Cold agglutinins. Antibodies which agglutinate at temperatures below 37°C only.

ConA (concanavalin A). A mitogen for T cells.

Congenic. Animals which are genetically constructed to differ at one particular locus.

Conjugate. A reagent which is formed by covalently coupling two molecules together such as fluorescein coupled to an immunoglobulin molecule.

Cryoglobulin. An antibody or immune complex which forms a precipitate at 4°C.

Cyclophosphamide. A cytotoxic drug frequently used as an immunosuppressive.

Cyclosporin. An immunosuppressive drug which is particularly useful in suppression of graft rejection.

Cytophilic. Having a propensity to bind to cells.

Cytostatic. Having the ability to stop cell growth.

Cytotoxic. Having the ability to kill cells.

DTH (delayed type hypersensitivity). This term includes the delayed skin reactions associated with Type 4 hypersensitivity.

DNP. (dinitrophenol). A commonly used hapten.

Domain. A region of a peptide having a coherent tertiary structure. Both immunoglobulins and MHC Class 1 and Class 2 molecules have domains.

DsDNA. Double-stranded DNA.

Epstein-Barr virus (EBV). Causal agent of Burkitt's lymphoma and infectious mononucleosis. It has the ability to transform human B cells into stable cell lines.

Effector cells. A functional concept which in context means those lymphocytes or phagocytes which produce the end effect.

Endogenous. Originating within the organism.

Endothelium. Cells lining blood vessels and lymphatics.

Enhancement. Prolongation of graft survival by treatment with antibodies directed towards the graft alloantigens.

Epitope. A single antigenic determinant. Functionally it is the portion of an antigen which combines with the antibody paratope.

Exon. Gene segment encoding protein.

Fab. The part of an antibody molecule which contains the antigen combining site, consisting of a light chain and part of the heavy chain; it is produced by enzymatic digestion.

Fc. The portion of an antibody which is responsible for binding to antibody receptors on cells and the C1q component of complement.

Freund's adjuvant. An emulsion of aqueous antigen in oil: complete Freund's adjuvant also contains killed *Mycobacterium tuberculosis,* while incomplete Freund's adjuvant does not.

Genetic association. A term used to describe the condition where particular genotypes are associated with other phenomena, such as particular diseases.

Genetic restriction. The term used to describe the observation that lymphocytes and antigen-presenting cells cooperate most effectively when they share particular haplotypes.

Genome. The total genetic material contained within the cell.

Genotype. The genetic material inherited from parents; not all of it is necessarily expressed in the individual.

Germ line. The genetic material which is passed down through the gametes before it is modified by somatic recombination or mutation.

Giant cells. Large multinucleated cells sometimes seen in granulomatous reactions and thought to result from the fusion of macrophages.

H-2. The mouse Major Histocompatibility Complex.

Haplotype. A set of genetic determinants located on a single chromosome.

Hapten. A small molecule which can act as an epitope but which is incapable by itself of eliciting an antibody response.

Helper cells. A functional subclass of T cells which can help to generate cytotoxic T cells and cooperate with B cells in the production of an antibody response. Helper cells usually recognize antigen in association with class 2 MHC molecules.

Hereditary angioedema. A condition caused by congenital deficiency of C1 INH, and a pathological activation of the classical complement pathway.

Heterologous. Refers to interspecies antigenic differences.

HEV (high endothelial venule). An area of venule from which lymphocytes migrate into lymph nodes.

Hinge. The portion of an immunoglobulin heavy chain between the Fc and Fab regions. This allows flexibility within the molecule and allows the two combining sites to operate independently. The hinge region is usually encoded by a separate exon.

Histocompatibility. The ability to accept grafts between individuals.

HLA. The human major histocompatibility complex.

Homologous. The same species.

hnRNA (heteronuclear RNA). The fraction of nuclear RNA which contains primary transcripts of the DNA prior to processing to form messenger RNA.

Humoral. Pertaining to the extracellular fluids, including the serum and lymph.

Hybridoma. Cell lines created *in vitro* by fusing two different cell types, usually lymphocytes, one of which is a tumour cell.

Idiotope. A single antigenic determinant on an antibody V region.

Idiotype. The antigenic characteristic of the V region of an antibody.

Immune complex. The product of an antigen-antibody reaction which may also contain components of the complement system.

Immunoconglutinins. Autoantibodies which are formed against complement components.

Immunofluorescence. A technique used to identify particular antigens microscopically in tissues or on cells by the binding of a fluorescent antibody conjugate.

Interferons. A group of proteins which enhance antiviral immunity and are capable of modifying immune responses. There are several types of interferon. Interferon gamma (IFNγ), previously called immune interferon, is produced by lymphocytes.

Interleukins. The generic term for a group of peptides which signal between cells of the immune system.

Intron. Gene segment between exons not encoding protein.

Ir gene. A group of immune response (Ir) genes determine the level of an immune response to a particular antigen or foreign stimulus. A number of them are found in the major histocompatibility complex.

Isoelectric focusing. Separation of molecules on the basis of the charge. Each molecule will migrate to the point in a pH gradient where it has no net charge.

Isologous. Of identical genetic constitution.

Isotype. Refers to genetic variation within a family of proteins or peptides such that every member of the species will have each isotype of the family represented in its genome (eg. immunoglobulin classes).

K cell. A group of lymphocytes which are able to destroy their targets by antibody-dependent cell-mediated cytotoxicity. They have Fc receptors.

Karyotype. The chromosomal constitution of a cell which may vary between individuals of a single species, depending on the presence or absence of particular sex chromosomes or on the incidence of translocations between sections of different chromosomes.

Kupffer cells. Phagocytic cells which line the liver sinusoids.

LCM (lymphocytic choriomeningitis). A viral disease of mice.

Leukotrienes. A collection of metabolites of arachidonic acid which have powerful pharmacological effects.

Ligand. A linking (or binding) molecule.

Line. A collection of cells produced by continuously growing a particular cell culture *in vitro*. Such cell lines will usually contain a number of individual clones.

Linkage. The condition where two genes are both present in close proximity on a single chromosome and are usually inherited together.

Linkage disequilibrium. A condition where two genes are found together in a population at a greater frequency than that predicted simply by the product of their individual gene frequencies.

Locus. The position on a chromosome at which a particular gene is found.

LPR (lymphoproliferation gene). A gene found in MRL mice which is involved in the generation of autoimmune phenomenon.

LPS (lipopolysaccharide). A product of some Gram negative bacterial cell walls and which can act as a B cell mitogen.

Lymphokines. A generic term for molecules other than antibodies which are involved in signalling between cells of the immune system and are produced by lymphocytes (cf. interleukins).

Ly antigens. A group of cell surface markers found on murine T cells which permit the differentiation of T cell subpopulations.

MHC (the major histocompatibility complex). A genetic region found in all mammals whose products are primarily responsible for the rapid rejection of grafts between individuals, and which function in signalling between lymphocytes and cells expressing antigen.

MIF (migation inhibition factor). A group of peptides produced by lymphocytes which are capable of inhibiting macrophage migration.

Mitogen. Substances which cause cells, particularly lymphocytes, to undergo cell division.

Monoclonal. Derived from a single clone, for example, monoclonal antibodies which are produced by a single clone and are homogenous.

Myeloma. A lymphoma produced from cells of the B cell lineage.

NK (natural killer) cell. Natural killer cells are a group of lymphocytes which have the intrinsic ability to recognize and destroy some virally infected cells and some tumour cells.

Nef (Nephritic factor). An autoantibody to the alternative pathway C3 convertase which stabilizes the enzyme and potentiates the action of the alternative pathway amplifiction.

Neoplasm. A synonym for cancerous tissue.

NIP (4-hydroxy, 5-iodo, 3-nitrophenylacetyl). A commonly used hapten.

NP (4-hydroxy, 3-nitrophenylacetyl). A hapten which partially crossreacts with NIP.

Nude mouse. A genetically athymic mouse. It also carries a closely linked gene producing a defect in hair production.

NZB/W. A strain of mouse which is a model for systemic lupus erythematosus. The parental NZB strain also suffers from autoimmunity.

OKT. A group of monoconal antibodies used to identify T cell surface markers in humans.

Opsonization. A process by which phagocytosis is facilitated by the deposition of opsinins (eg. antibody and C3b) on the antigen.

PAF (platelet activating factor). A factor released by basophils which causes platelets to aggregate.

Paratope. The part of an antibody molecule which makes contact with the antigenic determinant (epitope).

Pathogen. An organism which causes disease.

PC (phosphorylcholine). A commonly used hapten which is also found on the surface of a number of microorganisms.

PCA (passive cutaneous anaphylaxis). The technique used to detect antigen-specific IgE, in which the test animal is injected intravenously with the antigen and dye, the skin having previously been sensitized with antibody.

PFA (plaque forming cell). An antibody producing cell detected *in vitro* by its ability to lyse antigen-sensitized erythrocytes in the presence of complement.

Prausnitz-Kustner reaction. A way of detecting antigen-specific IgE, in which antigen is injected into skin previously sensitized with IgE antibody.

PHA (phytohaemaglutinin). A mitogen for T cells.

Phagocytosis. The process by which cells engulf material and enclose it within a vacuole (phagosome) in the cytoplasm.

Phenotype. The expressed characteristics of an individual (cf. genotype).

Pinocytosis. The process by which liquids or very small particles are taken into the cell.

Plasma cell. An antibody producing B cell which has reached the end of its differentiation pathway.

Pokeweed mitogen. A mitogen for B cells.

Polyclonal. A term which describes the products of a number of different cell types (cf. monoclonal).

Prime. To give an initial sensitization to antigen.

Prostaglandins. Pharmacologically active derivatives of arachidonic acid. Different prostaglandins are capable of modulating cell mobility and immune responses.

Pseudoalleles. Tandem variants of a gene: they do not occupy a homologous position on the chromosome (eg. C4).

Pseudogenes. Genes which have homologous structures to other genes but which are incapable of being expressed (eg. $J_K 3$ in the mouse).

Pyogenic. Pertaining to a microorganism which causes pus production.

Reagin. Outdated term for IgE.

Receptor. A cell surface molecule which binds specifically to particular proteins or peptides in the fluid phase.

Recombination. A process by which genetic information is rearranged during meiosis. This process also occurs during the somatic rearrangements of DNA which occur in the formation of genes encoding antibody molecules.

Reticuloendothelial system. A diffuse system of phagocytic cells derived from the bone marrow stem cell which are associated with the connective tissue framework of the liver, spleen, lymph nodes and other serous cavities.

S (Svedberg unit). A measure of the sedimentation velocity of a molecule in a gravitational field, this being dependent on the size, density and shape of the molecule.

Segregation. The distribution of genes among gametes.

SLE (systemic lupus erythematosus). An autoimmune disease of humans usually involving anti-nuclear antibodies.

Somatic mutation/recombination. Various gene rearrangements which take place in the somatic cells (not the germ line cells). The rearrangements vary between individuals and between the cells within a particular individual, and the rearranged DNA segments are not passed on from generation to generation.

Splenomegaly. Increased spleen size, this is seen in a number of parasitic infections and is also used as an assay for graft versus host reactions.

Stoichiometry. Pertaining to the relationship and proportions in which substances react together.

Suppressor cell. A subpopulation of T cells which act to reduce the immune responses of other T cells or B cells. Suppression may be antigen-specific, idiotype specific, or non-specific in different circumstances.

Synergism. Cooperative interaction

Syngeneic. Strains of animals produced by repeated inbreeding so that each pair of autosomes within an individual is identical.

T15. An idiotype associated with anti-phosphorylcholine antibodies, named after the TEPC15 myeloma prototype sequence.

Tachyphylaxis. The process by which subsequent doses of a pharmacological reagent produce decreasing effects.

Tandem duplicates. Adjacent copies of related genes linked together on a chromosome.

THY. A cell surface antigen of mouse T cells which has allotypic variants.

Tolerance. A state of specific immunological unresponsiveness.

Transformation. Morphological changes in a lymphocyte associated with the onset of division. Also used to denote the change to the autonomously dividing state of a cancer cell.

Vasoactive amines. Products such as histamine and 5-hydroxytryptamine released by basophils, mast cells and platelets which act on the endothelium and smooth muscle of the local vasculature.

Xenogeneic. Referring to interspecies antigenic differences (cf. heterologous).

Index